MICROBIOLOGY
in
NURSING

MICROBIOLOGY *in* NURSING

R. Panjarathinam

PhD (Bact.); PhD (Medical); FZS (Cal.)

Department of Microbiology
B. J. Medical College, Ahmedabad, Gujarat, India
Formerly Visiting Professor of Microbiology
College of Nursing, Ahmedabad

New Central Book Agency (P) Ltd

LONDON
HYDERABAD ERNAKULAM BHUBANESWAR
DELHI KOLKATA PUNE

NCBA

REGD OFFICE

8/1 Chintamoni Das Lane, Kolkata 700 009, India
email: ncbapvtltd@eth.net

OVERSEAS

NCBA (UK) Ltd, 149 Park Avenue North, Northampton, NN3 2HY, UK

EXPORT

NCBA Exports Pvt. Ltd, 212 Shahpur Jat, New Delhi 110 049
email: ncbaexp@ncbapvtltd.com

BRANCHES

208B Peacock Lane, Shahpur Jat
New Delhi 110 049
email: ncbadel@ncbapvtltd.com

Shop Nos. 3 & 4, Vinayak Towers
681/B Budhwar Peth, Appa Balwant Chowk
Pune 411 002
email: ncbapune@ncbapvtltd.com

House No. 3-1-315, 1st Floor
Nimboliadda, Kachiguda, **Hyderabad** 500 027
email: ncbahydb@ncbapvtltd.com

GSS Shopping Complex, 1st Floor
Opposite College Post Office, Convent Road
Ernakulam 682 035
email: ncbaernk@ncbapvtltd.com

Shop No. 15, Bharati Towers, Ground Floor
Forest Park, **Bhubaneswar** 751 001
email: ncbabub@ncbapvtltd.com

MICROBIOLOGY IN NURSING

First Published: March 2004
Reprinted: July 2005, January 2011, January 2012

PUBLISHER AND TYPESETTER
New Central Book Agency (P) Ltd
8/1 Chintamoni Das Lane, Kolkata 700 009

PRINTER
New Central Book Agency (P) Ltd
Web-Offset Division, Dhulagarh, Sankrail, Howrah

COVER DESIGNER
Ankit, Kolkata

COVER PRINTER
Biswanath Studio, Kolkata

TECHNICAL EDITOR
Dr Mita Sen, MBBS

PROJECT SUPERVISOR
Prabir Ghosh

PROJECT TEAM
Sukumar Patra, Subas Maitra, and Prabhat Jas

ISBN: 81-7381-454-6

Price: ₹ 385.00

Dedicated to Divine Mother
Shri Aurobindo Ashram
Pondicherry

Preface

The paucity of a Text Book on Nursing **Microbiology in India** has prompted the author to bring out this comprehensive book to serve the nursing students of this country by covering the syllabi of Indian Universities as also the Nursing Council of India, New Delhi. The experience gained by the author as visiting Professor of Microbiology, College of Nursing, Ahmedabad, could help to solve the difficulties faced by the nursing students in the classroom through this book. Besides, this book could impart a clear, complete concept of this subject within a short time, when the nursing students are covering their vast nursing curriculum with ever increasing pressure due to the recent advances in nursing.

Much importance has been given to the application of the knowledge of Microbiology in nursing in hospital communicable disease unit, operation theatre, delivery room and in public health under Indian conditions.

Trained Professional Nurses in active service can also use this book for their reference purpose. In addition to various microbial infections, the chapters on immunisation, signs and symptoms of parasitic diseases, parasites of various organs, common parasites prevalent in India and a glossary of technical terms will be quite useful to the students as quick reference. This book has been generously illustrated to further aid the students in the learning of the subject. Any suggestion from my colleagues and students towards the improvement of the text will be highly appreciated.

6 March, 2004

R. PANJARATHINAM

Acknowledgement

I am thankful to Dr. R. C. Shah, M.B.B.S., M.Sc. (Medical) the Director of Medical Education and Research, Gujarat State, Ahmedabad, and Dr. V. V. Kollall, M.D. (Path. Bact.); D.C.P.; Professor and Head, Department of Microbiology, B. J. Medical College, Ahmedabad, for their kind permission and encouragement to write this text book.

I am indebted to Shri G. A. Gajjar, M.Sc. (Medical), College of Nursing, Ahmedabad, to my wife and children for their support and encouragement and to New Central Book Agency (P) Ltd., Publishers, Kolkata for their excellent endeavour to publish this book very elegantly.

Contents

SECTION IV

SECTION V

SECTION VI

SECTION VII

SECTION VIII

SECTION 1

CHAPTER 1

INTRODUCTION

Microbiology (Gr. **mikros**—small, **bios**—life, **logos**—science) is the science of minute organisms invisible to the naked eye, named microbes. It is the study of the laws of the life and development of microorganisms, and also of the change which they bring about in animal and plant organisms and in non-living matter.

According to the requirement of modern society, in the second half of the nineteenth century, microbiology was differentiated into general, agricultural, veterinary, medical and nursing microbiology.

Modern medical microbiology has become an extensive science and is divided into **bacteriology**—science of pathogenic bacteria (Gr. **bacteria**—rod); **virology**—science of infectious virus; **serology**—study of the reaction between antigen and antibody; **mycology**—study of fungi pathogenic to man; **protozoology**—study of pathogenic protozoa; **helminthology**—study of helminths (worms); **entomology**—study of insects (vectors) transmitting disease to man; **parasitology**—study of parasites (protozoa and helminths). In addition, medical microbiology also includes the study of the mechanisms of infection and immunity, the methods of specific therapy and prophylaxis of infectious diseases.

Nursing microbiology is the application of knowledge of medical microbiology at the bedside of patients during nursing care.

Nursing care in the hospital and community is of paramount importance to promote health. It is considered the backbone of public health. To attain perfection in this profession, nurses should acquire sound knowledge of nursing microbiology, as nursing is an interdependent profession influenced by the recent scientific and technological advances of nursing sciences.

HISTORICAL OUTLINE

In ancient times, at the beginning of civilisation, man used certain processes caused by the life activities of microorganisms, like fermentation of milk, wine, juice etc. Avicenna (980-1037 A.D.) thought all infectious diseases were caused by minute living creatures, invisible to the naked eye and transmitted through air and water.

The first person to see and describe the microbes was a Dutch scientist, A. Leenwenhoek 1632-1723. He himself made simple lenses which magnified 160-300 fold. In 1678, he published his letter on "**animalcula viva**",— live animalcules which he observed in water, faeces, infusions and teeth scrapings. Besides his discovery of microbes, he drew accurately the microbes. His discovery was the starting point of the study of the microbial population. After this wonderful investigation, more than 150 years had passed before the search of causative agents of infectious diseases was successfully completed.

The practical problems faced against the battle of epidemic diseases were solved by the knowledge of microbiology. In 1798, English physician, Edward Jenner (1749-1823) proved that vaccination of human beings with cowpox protected them from smallpox. Pasteur (1880-1890) developed vaccines against fowl cholera, anthrax, rabies. This discovery was very useful to combat these diseases in animals and human beings.

In the first half of the nineteenth century, the causative agents of the diseases were discovered. In 1839, D. Schoenlein established that the favus is caused by pathogenic fungus. In 1843, D. Gruby revealed the causative agent of trichophytosis (ring-worm). In 1849-1854, A. Pollender, C. Davaine, F. Bravell discovered the anthrax bacillus.

In the second half of the nineteenth century the methods of microscopy were developed with the help of better microscopes. During the study of microorganisms, much attention was paid to the biochemical processes, the ability of microbes to ferment organic substrates. Louis Pasteur (1822-1895), French scientist, chemist and microbiologist, proved that alcoholic fermentation and putrefaction were due to the activity of microbes. He investigated into the causative agents of fowl cholera, anthrax and rabies and prepared vaccines. Because of ubiquitous nature of microorganisms, Pasteur protected the nutrient media from the microbial contamination and proved that spontaneous generation of living microorganisms does not exist. His discoveries attracted many scientists towards him. Based on the microbial infection described by Pasteur, the English surgeon, Joseph Lister (1827-1912) introduced into surgery the principles of antiseptics (disinfection of wounds with chemical disinfectants).

The German physician, Robert Koch (1843-1910) made a detailed investigation of wound infections and developed a method of isolation of pathogenic bacteria in pure culture, attacked the problem of anthrax, developed the method of staining of bacteria and also described the method of cultivation on solid media. He established a school of microbiology and his pupils were K. Eberth, G. Gaffksy, K. Klebs, F. Loeffler, S. Kitasato and many others. In 1874 Hansen described the bacillus of leprosy. In 1880, Pasteur isolated the bacillus of fowl cholera and Eberth observed the bacillus of Typhoid fever. Adequate description of staphylococcus was made by Ogston (1881). Koch (1882) discovered tubercle bacillus. In 1885, Frankel isolated pneumococcus; Escherich, colon Bacillus. Nicolaier observed tetanus bacillus which was later cultivated by Kitasato in 1889. Welch and Nuttall described the anaerobic bacillus known as **Clostridium welchii**. In 1894, Kitasato and Yersin described independently the bacillus of plague which is now known as **Yersinia pestis**. In 1896, Van Ermengem described **Cl. botulinum** as causative agent of food poisoning. In 1897, Bang discovered the bacillus causing bovine abortion. Thus, by the end of nineteenth century, a great variety of microorganisms had been identified and found to be associated with human diseases. Joseph Lister, Professor of Surgery at Glasgow, devised a method of diluting a bacterial culture and preparing a series of subcultures with a small quantity of the original fluid which yielded a single bacterial cell, so Lister was the first bacteriologist, though he is basically a surgeon, to obtain a certainly pure culture of bacteria. Thus, the microbiological revolution inaugurated by Pasteur and extended by Koch spread far beyond the field of medicine. There were no appreciable advances in the knowledge of bacteriology of diseases during 1875 to 1900 as the techniques developed by Pasteur and Koch were only applied over a very wide field during this period.

The study of immunity (branch of bacteriology), derived from Pasteur's studies on chicken cholera, anthrax and rabies, has absorbed a large number of bacteriologists. From Metchnikoff's (1845—1916) investigations on the cellular reaction in infection as well as from the work of Buchner, Nuttall, Von Behring

(1890), Ehrlich (1854-1915), Bordet and others, more improved laboratory diagnostic methods of infectious diseases were devised and vaccines were obtained against enteric fever, cholera, plague and other diseases.

Discoveries of important causative agents of infectious diseases

Year	Discoverers	Microorganisms
1839	J. Schoenlein	Causative agent of favus
1843	D. Gruby	Causative agent of trichophytosis
1849-1854	A. Pollender *et al*	*Bacillus anthracis*
1859	D. Lambl	*Giardia lamblia*
1873-1874	A. Hansen	*Mycobacterium leprae*
1874-1885	T. Bilroth *et al*	Pathogenic streptococcus
1875-1903	F. Losh, F. Schaudinn	*Entamoeba histolytica*
1877-1916	L. Pasteur *et al*	Causative agent of gas gangrene
1878-1884	R. Koch, A. Ogston et al	Pathogenic staphylococcus
1879	A. Neisser	Gonococcus
1880	K. Eberth, G. Gaffky	*Salmonella typhi*
1880	A. Laveran	Malarial plasmodium
1882	R. Koch	*Mycobacterium tuberculosis*
1883	R. Koch	*Vibrio cholerae*
1883-1884	E. Klebs, F. Loeffler	*Corynebacterium diphtheriae*
1884	A. Nicolaier	Causative agent of tetanus
1885	T. Escherich	Colibacillus
1885	A. Frankel	Pneumococcus
1886-1914	D. Bruce	Brucella
1887	A. Weichselbaum	Meningococcus
1891-1898	K. Shiga *et al*	Bacteria of dysentery
1892-1906	G. Guarnieri *et al*	Small pox virus
1894	A. Yersin, S. Kitasato	*Pasteurella pestis*
1896	G. Ashard *et al*	*Salmonella paratyphi* A, B
1896	E. Van Ermengem	*Clostridium botulinum*
1898-1903	B. Babesh, A. Negri	Negri bodies in Rabies
1898-1903	W. Leishman	Leishmania
1901	W. Reed	Yellow fever virus
1905	F. Schaudinn, E. Hoffman	*Treponema pallidum*
1906	J. Bordet, O. Gengou	Bacillus of whooping cough
1908	C. Nicolle, L. Manceaux	Toxoplasma
1908-1910	K. Landsteiner, E. Popper	Poliomyelitis virus
1910-1916	G. Ricketts, C. Prowazek	Rickettsiae of typhus fever
1911-1917	Aragao, E. Paschen	Chicken pox virus
1914-1915	R. Inado, Y. Ido	Causative agent of leptospirosis
1915-1917	F. Twort, F. d'Herelle	Bacteriophage
1933	W. Smith *et al*	Influenza virus
1934	C. Johnson, E. Goodpasture	Virus of parotitis
1934-1938	M. Hyashi *et al*	Japanese encephalitis virus
1938	H. Plotz	Virus of measles
1942-1962	G. Findlay *et al*	Virus of epidemic hepatitis
1944	M. Eton *et al*	Causative agent of atypical pneumonia
1953	W. Row *et al*	Adenovirus
1957	S. Stewart, B. Eddy	Virus of polyoma
1983	Luc Montagnier *et al*	Lymphadenopathy Associated virus (LAV)
1984	Robert Gallo *et al*	Human T cell Lymphotropic virus III (HTLV-III). Human Immunodeficiency virus (HIV)

In the twentieth century, the field of specific prophylaxis of infectious diseases was developed. Ramon (1924-1925) prefected a method for the preparation of anatoxins (toxins rendered harmless by formalin, i.e. toxoid). Immunisation against diphtheria and tetanus was successfully carried out with the help of this toxoid (vaccine). Live, attenuated causative agent of tuberculosis was used for the preparation of vaccine against tuberculosis (Calmette and Guerin, 1919). Similarly, plague vaccine (Giard and Robic, 1931), tularaemia vaccine (Gaisky, 1939), and poliomyelitis vaccine (Sabin, 1954-1958) were prepared.

Modern medicine achieved a great success in the treatment of infectious disease, because of introduction of Salvarsan (Ehrlich), bacteriophage (d'Herelle), sulphonamide (Domagk *et al*), penicillin (Fleming *et al*), streptomycin (Waksman *et al*). The biochemical mechanisms of heredity and variations were revealed because of the genetics of bacteria and viruses. A new field of science — molecular biology — originated from genetics of bacteria and viruses.

The development of the study of infectious diseases, epidemiology, virology, immunology, surgery, hygiene etc. was due to the success of microbiology. It can be said firmly that medical science could have not progressed without the development of microbiology.

Historical relationship between Professional Nursing and Microbiology

About 150 years ago, during the war of Crimea (1854), when microbiology was at its early stage of development, professional nursing was practised by Florence Nightingale (1820-1910). In her time, the transmission of infection from man to man was not fully understood, though, she organised hospitals which minimised cross-infection. Lister's discovery of antiseptic surgery (1865) opened the door to the professional nurse to practice the whole field of operating room technique. Therefore, nursing profession should be indebted to Joseph Lister.

Since the discovery of preventive or prophylactic measures by the use of various vaccines (e.g., small pox vaccine, polio vaccine, measles vaccine, rabies vaccine, diphtheria and tetanus vaccines and antitoxins or immune sera), the education of the nurse in the principles of the preparation, use of vaccine and in the methods to administer them was necessitated.

More advanced microbiological training of the professional nurse for the collection of specimens and reporting laboratory specific findings immediately to the physician for early treatment is of great necessity for the microbiological laboratory diagnosis. Since nursing care is altered by the advent of chemotherapeutic agents and newer antibiotics, a golden opportunity is given to the professional nurse qualified in nursing microbiology.

The discoveries of the transmission of malaria, filaria and yellow fever (Ronald Ross, Reed *et al*, 1851-1902) by arthropods (vectors, insects) necessitated the professional nurse to study Entomology to prevent the transmission of disease from vector to man.

During nursing care in hospital and community every nurse should know as much as possible about nursing microbiology to assist in the recognition and prevention of the microbial diseases. Nurses should apply their knowledge of microbiology in their day-to-day nursing practice by their own judgements according to the different situations, instead of mechanically following the technical procedures. In due course of time, an intelligent student will realise that the fundamental information, acquired during the course of study of microbiology is very essential for professional nursing care.

SECTION 2

CHATPER 1A

BIOLOGICAL CLASSIFICATION OF MICROORGANISMS

Microorganisms may be defined as living creatures that are microscopic in size and relatively small, unicellular in structure. The diameter of the smallest body that can be resolved and seen clearly with the naked eye is about 100 μ (1 μ, or micron = 0.001 millimeter). All microorganisms are smaller than 100 μ. Therefore, a microscope is necessary for the observation. Light microscope can resolve down to 0.2 μ in diameter and thus includes all microbes except viruses which can be seen only under electron microscope whose limit of resolution is 0.0005 μ (i.e., 0.5 mμ = millimicron = 5 Angstrom Units). One Angstrom Unit = 1/10th of 1 mμ. When microorganisms grow on solid or semi-solid media, their progenies accumulate locally to form masses or *colonies* which are visible to the naked eye.

Microorganisms constitute a very antique group of living organisms which appeared on the Earth's surface almost 1.5 billion years ago. Some scientists believe that the microbes were the first living microorganisms of the Earth. It is now regarded that the organisms evolved along the following lines : Viruses containing Ribonucleic acid (RNA), Viruses containing Deoxyribonucleic acid (DNA), chlamydiae, rickettsiae, mycoplasma, bacteria, blue-green algae, lower and higher fungi, plants and animals.

In order to decide to which species the microorganism under investigation should belong, it is necessary, first of all, to study its main properties and then to identify it by these properties, and at last to determine its position in the classification of microbes according to a key.

In microbiology, the binomial system of nomenclature is accepted where each species has a generic and a specific name. The generic name is written with a capital letter and the specific name with a small letter. For example, *Staphylococcus aureus* (the golden pus coccus), *Bacillus anthracis* (the anthrax bacillus), *Corynebacterium diphtheriae* (the diphtheria bacillus), *Mycobacterium tuberculosis* (the tubercle bacillus).

International classification founded by an American bacteriologist, D. Bergey, is the most commonly used in microbiology. It is manual of determinative bacteriology. It includes descriptions of more than 1,500 species of microbes, though there are more than 3,000 known species of bacteria. All lower organisms of the plant kingdom, Protophyta, are subdivided into three classes :

Class I : *Schizophyceae* (blue-green algae);

Class II : *Schizomycetes* (microorganisms lacking chlorophyll);

Class III : *Microtatobiotes* (rickettsiae, viruses, filterable microbes).

Class I. *Schizophyceae*, consists of a large group of blue-green algae which are not pathogenic to man and animals.

Class II. *Schizomycetes* comprises 10 orders of 5 of which (II, III, VI, VII, VIII) are non-pathogenic to man and animals. Certain families and genera of the orders I, IV, V, IX, X contain species pathogenic to man and animals.

Class II. *Schizomycetes*

1. Order *Pseudomonadates* (motile cells, with polar flagellation and non-motile cells).

 7. Family *Spirillaceae*
 1. Genus *Vibrio*
 7. Genus *Spirillum*

2. Order *Chlamydobacteriales* (filamentous bacteria, motile and non-motile).

3. Order *Hyphomicrobiales* (bacteria multiplying mainly by budding).

4. Order *Eubacteriales* (true bacteria, rod-shaped, coccal-shaped, motile with flagella arranged peritrichously, and nonmotile).

 4. Family *Enterobacteriaceae*
 1. Genus *Escherichia*
 2. Genus *Aerobacter*
 3. Genus *Klebsiella*
 8. Genus *Proteus*
 9. Genus *Salmonella*
 10. Genus *Shigella*

 5. Family *Brucellaceae*
 1. Genus *Pasteurella*
 2. Genus *Francisella*
 3. Genus *Bordetella*
 4. Genus *Brucella*
 5. Genus *Haemophilus*
 6. Genus *Actinobacillus*

 6. Family *Bacteroidaceae*
 1. Genus *Bacteroides*
 2. Genus *Fusibacterium*

 7. Family *Micrococcaceae*
 1. Genus *Micrococcus*
 2. Genus *Staphylococcus*
 3. Genus *Kaffkya*
 4. Genus *Sarcina*
 5. Genus *Peptococcus*

 8. Family *Neisseriaceae*
 1. Genus *Neisseria*

 10. Family *Lactobacillaceae*
 1. Genus *Diplococcus*
 2. Genus *Streptococcus*
 5. Genus *Peptostreptococcus*

 12. Family *Corynebacteriaceae*
 1. Genus *Corynebacterium*
 2. Genus *Listeria*
 3. Genus *Erysipelothrix*

 13. Family *Bacillaceae*
 1. Genus *Bacillus*
 2. Genus *Clostridium*

5. Order *Actinomycetales* (actinomycetes, filamentous, branching cells).

 1. Family *Mycobacteriaceae*
 1. Genus *Mycobacterium*
 2. Family *Actinomycetaceae*
 1. Genus *Nocardia*
 2. Genus *Actinomyces*
 3. Family *Streptomycetaceae*

6. Order *Caryophanales* (large, non-motile, segmented cells, joined in filaments).

7. Order *Beggiatoales* (cells occur singly, in filaments sometimes spherical-shaped, sulphur globules and found in cells).

8. Order *Myxobacteriales* (slime bacteria, rod-shaped, non-rigid cells, motile, non-flagellate).

9. Order *Spirochaetales* (spirochaetes and treponemas, cytoplasm in the form of spirals with at

least one turn about a slender axial filament, non-rigid, non-motile).

1. Family *Spirochaetaceae*
2. Family *Treponemataceae*
    1. Genus *Borrelia*
    2. Genus *Treponema*
    3. Genus *Leptospira*

10. Order *Mycoplasmatales* (small, pleomorphic, filterable microorganisms, pathogenic species cause pleuropneumonia in cattle, agalactia in goats and sheep, atypical pneumonia in humans).

Class III. Microtatobiotes

1. Order *Rickettsiales*
    1. Family *Rickettsiaceae*
        1. Genus *Rickettsia*
        2. Genus *Coxiella*
    2. Family *Chlamydiaceae*
        1. Genus *Chlamydia*
        2. Genus *Miyagawanella*
    3. Family *Bartonellaceae*
        1. Genus *Bartonella*
    4. Family *Anaplasmataceae*
        1. Genus *Anaplasma*

2. Type viruses (Vira) are divided into two subtypes : Subtype Deoxyvira which includes viruses containing DNA and Subtype Ribovira which consists of viruses containing RNA.

The new classification of viruses was discussed at the Nineth International Congress of Microbiology. This classification is based on the type of nucleic acid (DNA or RNA), anatomy of viruses, type of symmetry (spiral, cuboid, binary), the number of capsomeres in the viruses with a cuboid symmetry and on the presence of an external membrane.

All the viruses known (more than 3,000) are grouped into 5 classes, 8 orders, 21 families. The families are composed of genera which in their turn are made up of species designated in Latin, according to the binomial principle (e.g. family — *Herpesviridae*; genus — *Herpesvirus*; species — *Herpessimplex*).

Viruses containing ribonucleic acid (RNA)

Mixoviruses: Viruses of influenza, parainfluenza, epidemic parotitis, measles, rabies.

Picornaviruses: Virus of epidemic poliomyelitis, Coxackie and Enteric Cytopathogenic Human Orphan (ECHO) virus, rhinoviruses, foot and mouth disease virus and infectious hepatitis.

Arboviruses: Viruses of tick-borne encephalitis, Japanese encephalitis, St. Louis encephalitis, haemorrhagic fever, yellow fever, Dengue fever, sandfly fever.

Viruses containing deoxyribonucleic acid (DNA)

Poxviruses : Viruses of smallpox.

Herpes virus : Viruses of human herpes, chicken pox, herpes zoster.

Adenoviruses.

Viruses of tumours (oncogenic viruses).

This classification does not include fungi and unicellular *Protozoa* which belong to independent phyla and are studied separately from bacteria, actinomycetes, rickettsiae and viruses.

MORPHOLOGICAL CLASSIFICATION OF MICROORGANISMS

The main groups of bacteria are classified by their morphology and Gram-staining reactions into :

I. **Lower Bacteria** — Simple, generally unicellular structures, never in the form of a mycelium or spherical filaments :

1. Cocci — spherical cells.
2. Bacilli — straight rod shaped cells.
3. Vibrio — curved rod-shaped (comma-shaped) cells.
4. Spirochaetes — thin, spirally twisted, flexuous filaments.
5. Spirilla — spirally twisted, non-flexuous rods (Table 1.1).

II. **Higher Bacteria** — Filamentous organisms sheathed or branching to form a mycelium e.g., *Actinomycetes* — simple branching filaments forming a mycelium; may form conidia; non-motile.

Size of Bacteria — The unit measurement of bacteria is the micron (μ) which is equal to 1/1000th of a millimeter. The size of bacteria varies from 0.1 μ for *Mycoplasma laidlawii*, the smallest bacteria, to 2-3 by 15-20 μ for *Spirillum volutans* and even up to 1 mm for the giant sulphur bacteria. *The majority of the pathogenic bacteria have dimensions from 0.2 to 10* μ. (Cocci — 1 μ in diameter; bacilli — 3 μ in length, 0.3 μ thick; spirochaetes — 4-16 μ in length and 0.1-0.6 μ thick).

Cocci (Lat. **Coccus** - spherical) : According to the mode of cell grouping and the reaction to Gram-stain, cocci are distinguished into :

1. *Diplococcus* (Gr. *diplos* - double) — Cells mainly adherent in pairs and slightly elongated in axis of pair; Gram-positive (e.g., *D. pneumoniae*).

2. *Streptococcus* (Gr. *Streptos* - Chain) — Cells mainly adherent in chains, due to successive cell divisions occurring in the same axis; Gram-positive (e.g., *Streptococcus pyogenes*).

3. *Staphylococcus* (Gr. *Staphyle* — cluster; bunch of grapes) — Cells mainly adherent in irregular clusters due to successive division occurring irregularly in different planes; Gram-positive (e.g., *Staphylococcus aureus*).

The genus *Micrococcus* is similar to *Staphylococcus*, but it is motile, weakly Gram-positive and differs in size.

4. *Gaffkya* — Cells mainly adherent in plates of four (tetrads) due to division occurring successively in two planes at right angles; Gram-positive (e.g., *Gaffkya tetragena* — Producer of four).

5. *Sarcina* (Lat. *Sarcio* — to tie) divide in three planes at right angles to one another and resemble packets of 8, 16 or more cells. They are not virulent and are frequently found in the air.

6. *Neisseria* — Cells mainly adherent in pairs and slightly elongated at right angles to axis of pair; Gram-negative (e.g., *Neisseria meningitidis*).

Bacilli : On the basis of Gram and Ziehl-Neelsen staining reaction and spore formation, they are divided into :

1. *Acid fast bacilli* (AFB) — The genus *Mycobacterium* includes *Mycobacterium tuberculosis* (tubercle bacillus).

2. *Gram-positive Spore forming bacilli* — The genera *Bacillus* (aerobic) and *Clostridium* (anaerobic) are primarily Gram-positive. The size, shape and position of spores may assist recognition of the species, e.g., the tetanus bacillus is characterised by its bulging, spherical, terminal spore (drum-stick form).

3. *Gram-positive non sporing bacilli* — These include several genera of which *Corynebacterium* is distinguished by its curving or club shape.

4. *Gram negative bacilli* — Include numerous genera belonging to the families *Pseudomonadaceae, Achromobacteriaceae, Enterobacteriaceae, Brucellaceae* and *Bacteroidaceae*. Pseudomonas is distinguished by its polar flagellation, whereas motile members of other families are peritrichously flagellate.

Vibrios and Spirilla : Vibrios are recognised as short, non-flexuous, curved rods (e.g., *Vibrio cholerae*) and spirilla (Lat. *Spira* - Twist as non-flexuous spiral filaments e.g., *Spirillum minus*). They are Gram-negative and mostly motile having polar flagella and showing a very active, "darting" motility.

Spirochaetes : The spirochaetes are slender, flexuous, spiral filaments and are Gram-negative. They can be distinguished from spirilla because they are capable of active flexion of the cell body and are motile without flagella. The pathogenic spirochaetes are classified into three genera :

1. *Borrelia* — are larger and more refractile than the other pathogenic spirochaetes and are more easily stained by ordinary methods. Their coils are large and open with a wave length of 2-3 μ. At least 8-12

fibrils of 0.02 μ thick are found twisted around the whole length of the protoplast under electron microscope (*Borrelia recurrentis*).

2. *Treponema*— are thin filaments with shorter wave length (e.g., 1.0 - 1.5 μ) coils typically similar to regular "corkscrew" form. They are feebly refractile and difficult to stain except by silver impregnation method. Under electron microscope, 2-3 fibrils are seen wound round the protoplast of the cell wall (e.g., *Treponema pallidum*).

3. *Leptospira* — have very fine and close coils of wave length of 0.5 μ, which are clearly seen under electron microscope, winding round a single axial filament. Under dark ground microscope, one or both the extremities of the spirochaetes are seen "hooked or recurved, so that they may take the shape of walking stick, an S or C" (e.g., *Leptospira icterohaemorrhagiae*).

Actinomycetes : Actinomycetales (mycelial bacteria) include three main genera :

1. *Actinomyces*— have tendency to fragment into coccal and bacillary forms, do not form conidia; are anaerobic and Gram-positive, non-acid fast (e.g., *Actinomyces israeli*).

2. *Nocardia*— are similar to *Actinomyces*, but aerobic and mostly acid-fast (e.g., *Nocardia farcinica*).

3. *Streptomyces*— their vegetative mycelium does not fragment into short forms; form aerial hyphae, conidia are formed in chains (e.g., *Streptomyces griseus*).

Table 1A.1 : According to morphology and staining reaction, lower bacteria can be divided into :

LOWER BACTERIA

- Cocci
  - Gram-positive
    - *Staphylococcus aureus*, *Staph. albus*, *Staph. citreus*
    - *Streptococcus pyogenes*, *Strep. viridans*
    - *Diplococcus pneumoniae*, *Gaffkya tetragena*, *Sarcina lutea*
  - Gram-negative
    - *Neisseria meningitidis*
    - *Neisseria gonorrhoeae*
- (A) Non-sporulating Bacilli
  - Gram-positive
    - *Corynebacterium diphtheriae*
    - *Listeria monocytogenes*
    - *Mycobacterium tuberculosis* (Acid fast bacilli)
  - Gram-negative
    - *Bordetella pertussis*
    - *Salmonella typhi*
    - *Salmonella paratyphi A, B*
    - *Shigella dysenteriae*
    - *Escherichia coli*
    - *Proteus vulgaris*
    - *Klebsiella pneumoniae*
    - *Pseudomonas pyocyanea*
    - *Vibrio cholerae*
    - *Yersinia pestis*
    - *Brucella abortus*
    - *Bacteroides fragilis*
- (B) Spore forming Bacilli
  - Aerobic
    - *Bacillus anthracis*
  - Anaerobic
    - *Clostridium welchii*
    - *Clostridium tetani*
    - *Clostridium botulinum*
- Spirochaetes, Vibrios, Spirilla (Gram-negative)
  - *Treponema pallidum*
  - *Borrelia recurrentis*
  - *Leptospira icterohaemorrhagiae*

CHAPTER 2

MORPHOLOGY : ANATOMY OF BACTERIAL CELL

Cell is a unit of organised living material or protoplasm. It consists of:

(a) the *protoplast*, surrounded by a thin semi-permeable which is known as *cytoplasmic membrane* or *plasma membrane*.

(b) *Cell wall* which is outermost and rigid.

The protoplast is distinguished into : the *cytoplasm*, the *nucleus*. The nucleus is an inner body filled with the thread-like chromosomes in the genes which are the hereditary determinants of character.

Microorganism is simple unicellular microscopic structure. On a solid medium, its progenies accumulate at the site of inoculation as *colonies* which are macroscopic. The microorganisms are differentiated into : primitive (prokaryotic) cells and more advanced cells (eukaryotic) cells.

Prokaryotic cells are — bacteria and related organisms (rickettsiae, chlamydiae and mycoplasmas). Eukaryotic cells are fungi, protozoa, helminths, plants and animals.

The characteristic features of prokaryotic cells :

1. Prokaryotic cell has a homogeneous, simple, nucleus without nuclear membrane separating it from the cytoplasm; the nucleus does not contain nucleotides, spindle and non-identical chromosomes.

2. It does not possess the internal membrane separating the respiratory and photosynthetic enzyme systems in specific organelles. Thus, the respiratory enzyme is located in the mesosome (convoluted structure) of the cytoplasmic membrane of the bacteria.

3. It has a rigid cell wall containing a specific mucopeptide which is strengthening element. The mucopeptide is the target of antibacterial action of antibiotics and lysozymes. It is absent in eukaryotic cell.

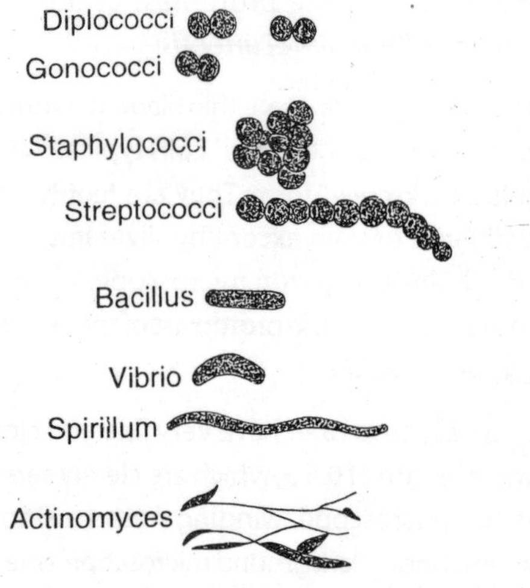

Fig. 2.1a : Classification of bacteria

Bacteria can be defined briefly as small microorganism with a prokaryotic form of cellular organisation. They are usually unicellular, however they may grow attached to one another in clusters, chains, filaments (hyphae) or a mycelium (*Actinomycetales*; higher bacteria). They usually measure from 0.4 to 1.5 µm and smaller than fungi and protozoa. They have rigid cell walls which are responsible for the maintenance of their characteristic shape; the shape may be spherical (coccus); rod shaped (bacillus); comma-shaped (vibrio); spiral (spirillum and spirochaetes) or filamentous (Fig. 2.1a)

The whole body of living material (protoplast or protoplasm) is surrounded by a very thin elastic and semi-permeable cytoplasmic membrane. A rigid, supporting, porous and relatively permeable *cell wall* covers very closely this membrane. The development of a transverse cytoplasmic membrane and a transverse cell wall or *cross wall* from the periphery to inwards is known as *cell division*.

The cytoplasm is made of watery sap packed with many granules known as *ribosomes* which are centres for protein synthesis and few convoluted membranes bodies known as mesosome which is site for respiratory enzyme. The *nuclear body* or *chromatin* is referred to the nuclear material; the bacterial nucleus cannot be seen under light microscope, though the word *nucleus* is now accepted.

The cytoplasm contains also *inclusion granules* of storage products such as metachromatic granules or volutin (polyphosphate), lipid (poly-β-hydroxy butyrate), glycogen or starch. A capsule, which is outside the cell wall, is a protective gelatinous covering layer; if it is too thin (less than 0.2 μm it is called as *microcapsule.* A loose slime is the soluble large molecular material disposed by the bacterium into the environment. There are two filamentous appendages protruding outwards from the bacterial cell wall : (a) *flagella* — which are organs of locomotion and (b) *fimbriae* (*Syn. pili*) — which are organs of adhesion. The cell wall, capsules or microcapsules, flagella and fimbriae have the special roles in the process of infection (Fig. 2.1d)

Bacterial nucleus (DNA)

Deoxyribonucleic acid (DNA) is double stranded long molecule occurring in the form of a closed circle of circular thread of about 1,000 μm long, coiled and tightly packed up in a bundle resembling a skein of woollen thread. it is considered by the geneticist as chromosomes containing genetic informations of bacterial cell. As the chromosome is not bound to the protein, it is stained like eukaryotic chromosome. The nucleus cannot be differentiated from the cytoplasm under light microscope and there is no nuclear membrane separating the nucleus from the cytoplasm and there is no nucleus.

Bacterial cytoplasm

The bacterial cytoplasm is a viscous watery substance. It contains organic and inorganic solutes and small granules known as *ribosomes.* There is no endoplasmic reticulum or membrane bearing microsomes, no mitochondria. It shows no amoeboid movement.

Ribosomes. Bacterial ribosomes can be seen under the electron microscope. They are strung together on strands of RNA to form *polysomes* and at this site that the code of mRNA is translated into peptide sequences. The antibacterial agent, like streptomycin, may interfere with bacterial metabolism at the ribosomal level without upsetting human ribosomal function.

Inclusion granules. In the cytoplasm of many bacteria, there are round granules which are not permanent or essential structures. They seem to be concerned with the cell metabolism, because they are in plenty when the energy-yielding nutrients are in abundance and disappear under energy source starvation. They are volutin (polyphosphate), lipid, glycogen, starch or sulphur.

Volutin and lipid granules, 0.1 - 1.0 μm in diameter are found in parasitic and saprophytic bacteria and very useful to identify certain bacteria; e.g., diphtheria bacillus, (pathogenic) can be differentiated mainly by its volutin from diphtheroids (non-pathogenic) which are common in the throat.

Volutin granules (Syn. metachromatic granules) have an affinity for basic dyes (e.g., methylene blue) and stained red violet with contrasting blue stained cytoplasm of the bacteria. It seems that polymerised inorganic phosphate is responsible for the metachromatic staining and volutin granules are rich source of energy and phosphate for cell metabolism, slightly acid-fast and appear highly opaque under electron microscope.

Lipid granules are spherical, varying in size, and consist mainly of polymerised β-hydroxy butyric acid and act as a carbon and energy storage product and have an affinity for fat soluble dyes like Sudan black, so they are stained black in contrast to the bacterial cytoplasm which is counterstained pink with basic fuchsin.

Polysaccharide granules. They may be glycogen or starch. If it is glycogen, it is stained red-brown; if it is starch it is stained blue by iodine. In *E. coli,* the cytoplasmic polysaccharide is glycogen and appears as minute granules under electron microscope.

Mesosomes. They are convoluted membranous bodies developed by complex invagination of cytoplasmic membrane into the cytoplasm which can be seen only under electron microscope. It is suggested that they are responsible for the compartmenting of DNA at cell division or at sporulation and for the excretion of material from the cytoplasm to the exterior.

Cytoplasmic membrane. It is 5-10 nm thick and is made of lipoprotein. It can be seen under electron microscope. It surrounds externally the cytoplasm and has little mechanical strength. The cell wall supports the cytoplasmic membrane. Cholesterol is absent in bacterial cytoplasmic membrane, but is normally present in animal cell cytoplasmic membrane. It acts as osmotic barrier which is permeable to many small molecular solutes like lipid soluble ones. It affects selective transport of specific nutrient solutes into the cell and that of the waste products out of the cytoplasm. Besides the enzymes (permeases) which carry out the active uptake of nutrients, the cytoplasmic membrane contains other enzymes — respiratory enzymes and pigments (cytochrome system), certain enzymes of tricarboxylic acid cycle and polymerising enzymes that manufacture cell wall and extra mural structure.

Cell Wall. It is 10-25 nm thick, strong, rigid, porous and permeable to small solute molecules of 1 nm in diameter. It maintains the characteristic shape of the bacterium and supports the weak cytoplasmic

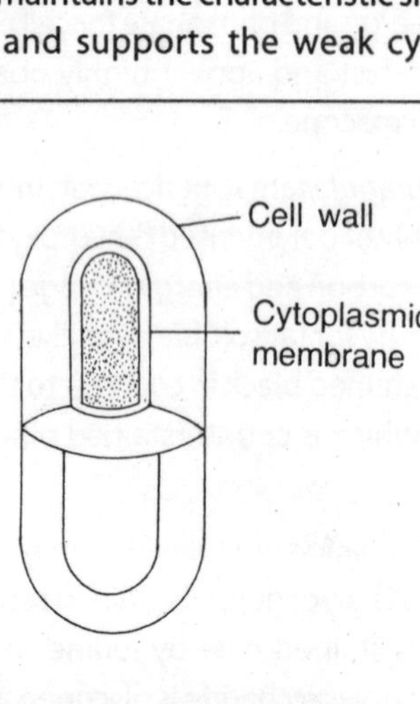

Fig. 2.1b : Cross section of bacteria

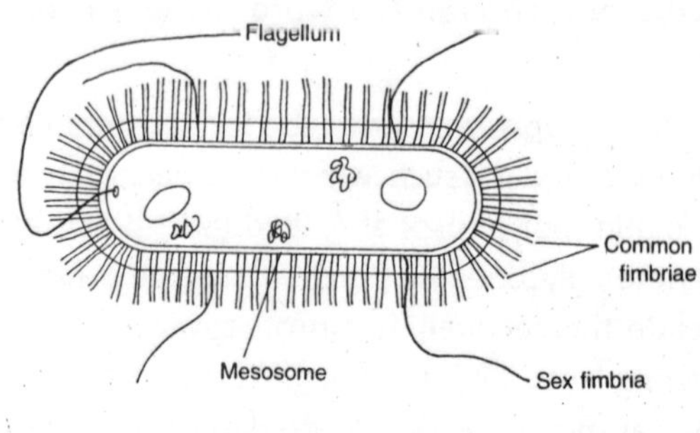

Fig. 2.1c : Structure of bacteria

membrane. Cell wall of bacteria may be compared to the outer cover and the cytoplasmic membrane to the inner tube of the pneumatic tyre of a motor car (Fig. 2.1b,c).

If the cell wall is weakened or ruptured, the protoplasm may swell from osmotic imbibation of water and the weak cytoplasmic membrane will burst. The bacterium will disintegrate and will be dissolved — the process is known as *lysis.* If the cell wall ruptures partially, the protoplasm will protrude out of the cell wall — the phenomenon is known as *plasmoptysis.* Bacterial cell wall substances can be hydrolysed by their own enzymes, known as *autolysis.*

Abnormal Forms. (Spheroplasts, free protoplasts, pleomorphic involution forms and L-forms or L-phage organisms) can be produced by weakening, removal or defective formation of the cell wall.

Pleomorphism. A considerable variation in size and shape which differs from the normal (e.g., swollen, spherical and sphere shaped forms, filaments with localised swellings, elongated filaments) *Streptobacillus moniliformis. Yersinia pestis* show this pleomorphism in old culture on artificial media with substance (penicillin, sodium chloride high concentration and organic acids at low pH).

Involution Forms. or degenerate forms are seen generally in abnormal cells; some are not viable, others will grow and revert to normal forms when they are grown in a suitable environment. This abnormal form may be due to defective cell wall synthesis. The growing cytoplasm expands the weakened wall to produce a swollen cell similar to a spheroplast that later bursts and lyses.

Free protoplasts and spheroplasts. If all cell wall material of bacteria is removed, the spheres are *free protoplasts.* If these spheres are enclosed by an intact but weakened residual cell wall, they are called *spheroplasts. Bacillus megaterium* can liberate protoplasts by dissolution of cell wall with egg white lysozyme. *Escherichia coli* can produce spheroplasts, when they are grown in presence of a substance (penicillin, bacitracin, oxymycin or glycine).

Protoplasts enlarge but do not multiply in an osmotically protected nutrient medium. Spheroplasts may multiply by fission in a nutrient medium with penicillin.

L-Forms of bacteria (*L-phage organisms*). These are abnormal forms derived from bacteria of abnormal morphology (cocci, bacilli, vibrio) due to variation in the laboratory. They lack rigid cell wall, they are viable, grow and multiply on suitable culture media. They are soft protoplasmic bodies, spherical or disk-like. They vary in size (0.1 µm - 20 µm). The smallest ones can pass through the bacteria stopping filters. Some L-forms are devoid of a cell wall. Colonies of L-phage organisms on agar media are small and have a characteristic 'fried egg' appearance. Though they are similar to mycoplasma organism, L-forms should be regarded as laboratory artefacts, degenerate growths, that do not occur or survive in natural habitats, the reason of which is not yet clear.

Capsules and microcapsules

Outside and immediately in contact with the cell wall, there is a discrete covering layer of relatively firm gelatinous material which can be seen under light microscope in the wet preparation and can be called as *capsules*. When this capsule is narrower, it can be demonstrated indirectly by serological reaction (capsular swelling reaction) or directly by electron microscope, it is known as *microcapsule*. The capsule is made of complex polysaccharide in most species. In some species it consists of polypeptide or protein.

Capsules cannot be demonstrated by ordinary method (e.g., Gram stain and Leishman stain). The most reliable method is by negative staining in wet films with India Ink. The carbon particles of the Ink make a dark background in the film and cannot penetrate into the capsule which appears as a clear halo around the bacterium.

Function of Capsule. It protects the cell wall against attack by various antibacterial agents (e.g., bacteriophages, colicines, complement, lysozyme) and against ingestion by the phagocytes. In *Bacillus anthracis*, the capsule is a polymer of D-glutamic acid. It protects the bacteria against phagocytosis and the action of a bactericidal basic polypeptide of animal tissues. When capsulate pneumococci are treated with type specific antiserum, the sharpness of outline of the capsule is greatly enhanced, which is known as the "capsular swelling reaction".

Loose slime or free slime is an amorphous viscid, colloidal material, that is secreted extracellularly by some non-capsulate bacterium and also, outside their capsules by many capsulate bacteria. In capsulated bacteria, the slime is chemically and antigenically similar to capsular substance, when slime forming bacteria are grown on a solid medium, they form watery "mucoid" colonies.

Flagella. Motile bacteria possess long thin filamentous appendages known as *flagella*, which act as organs of locomotion. The flagellum originates in the bacterial protoplasm and is extruded through cell

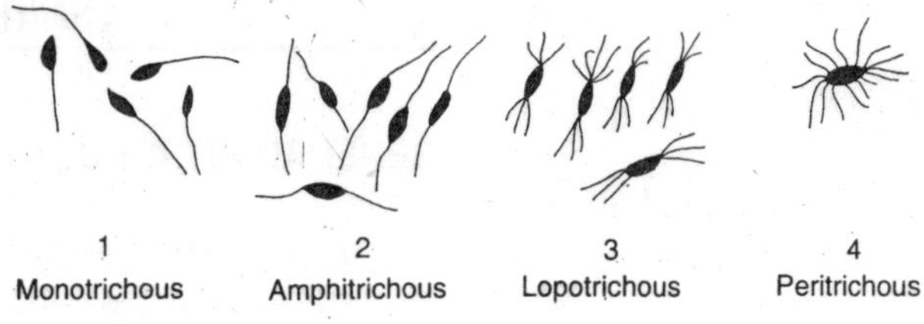

Fig. 2.1d : Distribution of flagella

wall. It is made of a protein *flagellin* chemically similar to myosin which is the contractile protein of muscle. It can be easily demonstrated by electron microscope or by Leifson stain. The flagella may be peritrichous or lateral when they originate from the sides of the cell; *polar* when they originate from one or both ends (Fig. 2.1d).

Motility of bacteria can be shown by hanging drop method or spreading growth on semi-solid agar medium.

Fimbriae. Certain Gram-negative bacteria (saprophytic intestinal commensal and pathogenic species) in the family enterobacteriacae possess filamentous appendages which are different from the flagella. These are called fimbriae or pili and occur in some non-motile bacteria; they are more numerous than flagella. Fimbriae act as organs of adhesion.

Bacterial spores. Some species, Bacillus and Clostridium develop a highly resistant resting phase or *endospore,* whereby the organism can survive in a dormant state, through a long period of starvation and other adverse environmental condition.

Each vegetative cell forms only one spore. This phenomenon is known as *sporulation.* Each spore gives rise to a single vegetative cell known as germination.

The appearance of the mature spore varies according to the species, being spherical, ovoid, elongated occupying a terminal, subterminal or central position.

In aerobic spore-forming bacilli, *Bacillus anthracis,* the spores are within the cell, not bulging, spherical or oval central. In anaerobic spore-forming bacilli, Clostridia, the spores are bulging, spherical, terminal, oval subterminal (Fig. 2.2).

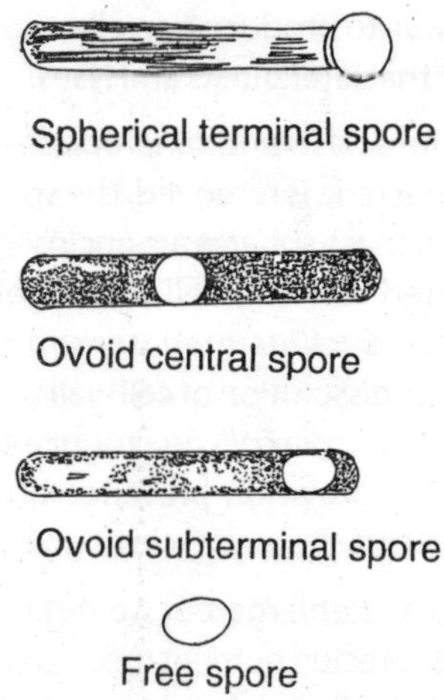

Fig. 2.2 : Spore position (Gram's stain)

Application to Nursing

In the daily practice of professional nursing, knowledge of morphology, structure and physiology of bacteria, is of very great importance — to associate the name of bacterium with the fact that this particular bacterium is resistant to heat as it forms spores; hence it has to be exposed to a higher temperature of hot air oven or autoclave; and is also responsible for a particular clinically diagnosed disease. The knowledgeable and professional nurse can understand the scientific names of microorganisms and the associated diseases appearing in the professional literatures.

An experienced professional nurse should be able to recognise and understand the scientific names of microorganisms in the microbiological laboratory reports with the specific disease, so that she can bring it *immediately* to the attention of the physician, if the organism isolated in the laboratory is responsible for the severe infectious disease. The prompt transmission of the laboratory report to the physician may be quite useful to the physician to switch over to specific treatment and to save from further damage to the patient's health.

CHAPTER 3

GENERAL INTRODUCTION TO VIROLOGY

History: Many common contagious diseases of animals and man were clinically known since ancient time for which no bacterial aetiology has been assigned. From pre-Christian times; Small pox was considered as a deadly infection and Hippocrates (460 -377 B.C.) described swollen neck in mumps, about 2,400 years ago. In 1884, Pasteur believed that Rabies of dogs is caused by a "microorganism infinitesimally small", as he could not detect bacteria in the infective material of rabid dogs. In 1892, Iwanowsky showed that the mosaic disease of tobacco plants was caused by a minute agent which was so small, ultramicroscopic and could pass through the pores of bacteria stopping filters. In 1898, Loeffler and Frosch have shown that foot and mouth disease of cattle was caused by a filterable infectious agent. In 1901, Walter Reed *et al* proved that yellow fever was caused by a mosquito-borne virus.

Viruses were originally described as ultramicroscopic and filter passing. Later, it was shown that the viruses cause serious diseases in animals such as foot and mouth diseases and rinderpest in cattle, distemper and rabies in dogs and fowl pest in poultry. Rous, in 1911, demonstrated that certain sarcomata of fowls could be transmitted with cell free filtrates of the tumours. Since that time, it was established that virus can cause tumour in animal and they are called "*Oncogenic viruses*". Fibromas, papillomas, and related tumours in rabbit and other mammals; mammary carcinomata, leukemias and parotid tumours (polyoma virus) in mice and leucosis in poultry were caused by *Oncogenic viruses*.

Insects are vectors of viruses which attack man, animals and plants. Nematodes, parasitic to pigs, spread swine influenza virus as in case of plant nematodes.

Twort in 1915 and d'Herelle in 1917 observed independently that viruses can infect and cause lysis of bacteria (clear zone of lysis — plaque), these viruses are called Bacteriophage — a name later abbreviated as "phage". This phenomenon of lysis was first noted in *Shigella shigae* — causative agent of bacillary dysentery. Because of this, knowledge of mechanism of phage infection and reproduction is much advanced than knowledge of the corresponding mechanism of animal viruses.

Definition of virus

Viruses (*Vira* — poison) were earlier defined as an ultramicroscopic agent which can be seen only under electron microscope, can pass through the bacteria stopping filters, reproduce by replication, can grow only in living cells, resist the action of antibiotics and contain Ribonucleic acid (RNA) or Deoxyribonucleic acid (DNA) covered by a protein coat.

Luria, in 1967, produced a composite definition incorporating all the accepted essential features of viruses :

"Viruses are entities whose genome is an element of nucleic acid, either DNA or RNA, which reproduces inside living cells and uses the synthetic machinery to direct the synthesis of specialised particles, the virions, which contain the viral genome and transfer it to other cells."

The recent definition is : A virus is one of a group of minute infectious agents characterised by a lack of independent metabolism and by the ability to replicate only within living host cells. They range from 15 - 300 nm in size and are morphologically heterogeneous (DORLAND'S MEDICAL DICTIONARY).

Following are two cardinal features of viruses :

1. They possess the genetic material which, when it is within the host cell, behaves as a part of the cell.

2. They also exist in an intracellular form, which is the product of the host cell under the control of the virus itself. The extracellular form — the *virion* — serves as a vehicle to carry the viral genome to other cells.

Viruses can reproduce only when they are within their host cells and are of necessity intracellular parasites. They have no ribosomes, no enzymes to generate high energy bonds, no mitochondria. They lack a rigid cell wall. Thus, there is no muramic acid in their outer coatings, hence, they are unaffected by antimicrobial agents. Indeed, viruses have no real cell structures and it is difficult to regard them as microorganisms. True microorganisms multiply by binary fission.

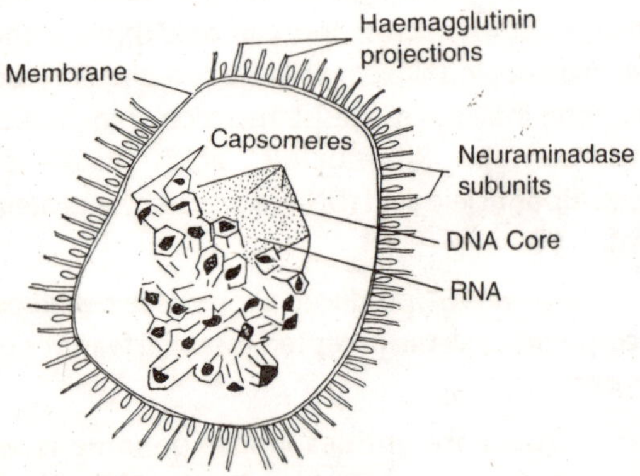

Fig. 3.1 : Structure of virus

Structure. A complete infective virus particle is called as virion and the genome is in core and consists of *either* deoxyribonucleic acid (DNA) or of ribonucleic acid (RNA) but not both. The outer shell of protein covering the nucleic acid is known as *capsid.* The protein and nucleic acids are closely integrated to form a nucleoprotein of distinct symmetry, when a virion enters the host cell, its protein capsid is stripped off and its nucleic acid is liberated within the host cell. At this stage, it ceases to exist as a particle although its nucleic acid is still present and intact. Component parts are still detectable. This stage in viral multiplication is known as the eclipse phase. All true viruses have an eclipse phase in their reproductive cycle (Fig. 3.1).

Classification of viruses

Animal viruses may be arranged into groups. The names of these groups end in the suffix-Virus e.g., adenovirus, herpesvirus and poxvirus. Members of these groups share similar features and constitute families ending with the suffix — idae, i.e., the family *Herpesviridae* would have as its type genus Herpesvirus which is a group that contains the *Herpes simplex*, varicella-zooster.

Following are the important distinguishing features of animal viruses : (1) type of nucleic acid; (2) chemical composition; (3) susceptible to chemical and physical agents; (4) size and measurement; (5) design and construction of virus; (6) antigenic characters.

Deoxyriboviruses, at present, are placed in five groups (Poxvirus, Herpesvirus, Adenovirus, Papavovirus, Parvovirus) and Riboviruses in nine groups (Orthomyxovirus, Paramyxovirus, Rhabdovirus, Togavirus, Arenavirus, Reovirus, Picornavirus, Leukovirus, Coronavirus).

There are many viruses that do not fit neatly into these groups. They are known as Arboviruses, because they are transmitted by the bite of arthropods.

Types of nucleic acid

DNA or RNA carries in their nucleic acids the genome and infectivity of viruses.

Most deoxyriboviruses have linear double stranded DNA; whereas, in the parvoviruses, the molecule is single stranded RNA.

When the protective capsids of the viruses are removed, some fragile viral nucleic acids retain their infectivity for some time, they can be seen and measured under electron microscope. Most of them are linear but some are circular.

Chemical composition

Proteins are the main components of all viruses. The most important function of these proteins is to provide the shield for the underlying delicate nucleic acid molecules. The surface proteins of the virion have special affinities for specific receptor sites on the host cell and provide a means of attachment of the particle to a position where it can enter the host cell and initiate the process of infection.

Viral antigens, which are protein in nature, stimulate the host immune response during infection. They are responsible for the distinctive serological characteristics of the viruses.

The capsomeres of most pathogenic viruses contain several different polypeptides. These polypeptides make up the surface configuration. They constitute the hemagglutinin prickles of ortho and paramyxoviruses and form a part of the mushroom-shaped projections of neuraminadase subunits.

Viral enzymes : There are many enzymes coded in the nucleic acids.

Lipids : When some mature viruses are liberated from nuclear and cytoplasmic membrane, they acquire a surface layer of lipoprotein derived in part from the host cell. The lipids may cement the proteins in the envelopes of the viruses. These viruses are inactivated by lipid solvents (ether, chloroform, bile salt).

Carbohydrates : Some viruses contain minimal amounts of carbohydrates.

Effects of Physical and Chemical Agents

Heat and Cold : The viruses causing the diseases in man and animals are readily inactivated by moderate heat (56° to 60°C for 30 minutes) except serum hepatitis and poliomyelitis viruses. Viruses are resistant to extremes of cold; freezing at –35°C or –70°C is a satisfactory common method for their preservation in the laboratory. The majority of viruses can be well preserved by freeze drying method.

pH variation. Viruses remain viable within a range of pH 5 to 9, but they are destroyed by extreme acidity or alkalinity.

Glycerol. Many viruses remain viable for many months or years in a 50 per cent solution of glycerol. Poliomyelitis, rabies and herpes simplex viruses can be kept for long period in glycerol at 4°C. Rinderpest virus and certain bacteria do not tolerate glycerol.

Virucidal agents : The most efficient disinfectants for use against viruses are oxidising agents (hydrogen peroxide, potassium permanganate and organic iodine derivatives). Formaldehyde (a reducing agent) is slower in action but is valuable in defined concentration in the preparation of inactivated poliomyelitis vaccines. Glutaraldehyde has an important role in the disinfection of apparatus used in renal dialysis units. Phenol and certain cresol disinfectants (i.e., lysol) are active against only a few viruses and are not to be recommended for material contaminated with the poliomyelitis or small pox viruses. Antiviral agents acting on Human Immunodeficiency virus (HIV) are : U-90.152 (drug); Zidovudine; Didanosine and Zalcitabine are currently licensed, Acyclovir acts on Herpes simplex and Varicella Zoster virus.

Ether. Viruses containing lipids in their envelopes are sensitive to ether. Naked viruses (polio, echo, coxsachie, adeno, papova and parvoviruses and some pox viruses) are resistant to ether, whereas herpes, orthomyxo and paramyxo, rhabdo, corona and leuko viruses are inactivated by ether.

Vital dyes. Acridine dyes, neutral red and toluidine blue permeate the nucleic acid and render virions vulnerable to ultraviolet rays. *Herpes simplex* and vaccinia viruses are more severely damaged than polioviruses. Double stranded DNA viruses stained with acridine dyes fluoresce with a yellow colour when seen under electron microscope, while single stranded DNA viruses fluoresce red.

Antibiotics and chemotherapeutic agents have no effect on viruses, but the agents of psittacosis lymphogranuloma group are susceptible to these drugs.

The unit measurement of whole virus particle is the nanometer (nm) or millimicron (mμ) or one-thousandth part of a micron (μ) or micrometer (μm)or 0.000001 nm or it is 10^{-9} meter; whereas the component parts or the internal structure (capsomere) of the virus is expressed as Angstrom (A°) which is one-tenth of a millimicron (0.0000001 mm). The Angstrom is the unit used to measure the wave length of light in microscope.

Virions vary in diameter from 300 to 18 nm. The largest ones are nearly half the size of small bacteria and can just be seen under an optical microscope. Most viruses can be seen only under electron microscope. Largest virus is vaccinia virus (330 × 100 nm), smallest one is picornavirus and parvovirus (40-20nm).

It is customary to include in a suspension of purified viruses some latex particles of known size (e.g., 88 nm) in electron microscope, so in electron micrographs, the size and shape can be determined accurately : Vaccina virus is brick shaped; influenza virus is round or filamentous; bacteriophage is sperm-like with head and tail.

Formerly, the size of viruses was measured by their capacity to pass through the filters or by their rate of sedimentation in a suspended fluid.

Design and construction of virus

A virion (the old term which is still in use) in its simplest form is a single molecule of nucleic acid enclosed within a protein capsid. It was known as "elementary body". The shape taken by the capsid is that of rigid spherical cage or of a tube; mainly the capsid protects the nucleic acid.

Viral capsids are made up of large number of "morphological units" or "capsomeres" that are attached to each other by their bonds.

Cubical capsids. Viruses with cubical symmetry take the form of an icosahedron. An icosahedron has 20 facets, each an equilateral triangle and 12 vertices or corners.

Antigenic classification of animal viruses depends upon the antigenic patterns.

Virus hemagglutinin. Many different viruses agglutinate red blood cells when virions and erythrocytes are in a suspension, they collide and adhere to each other; the cells become speckled with attached virions and they are bound to each other by viral bridges.

Inclusion bodies. During the course of multiplication, the viruses are associated with the appearance of large distinctive structures known as "inclusion bodies". They may be situated either in the cytoplasm (intra-cytoplasmic inclusion bodies) or in the nucleus (intra-nuclear inclusion bodies) or as in the case of measles, in both. The inclusion bodies are usually acidophilic and appear as pink masses in smears stained with Giemsa stain or Mann's eosin methylene blue stain; basophilic inclusion bodies are characteristic of psittacosis-lymphogranuloma group. They vary in size from 1-30 μ in diameter.

The presence of large intra-cytoplasmic acidophilic inclusion bodies in the nerve cells of hippocampus of the brain is the presumptive diagnosis of Rabies.

Acidophilic intranuclear inclusion bodies are of two types : Cowdry Type A is granular in appearance and of variable size (herpes simplex, zoster varicella, yellow fever); Type B is more round and multiple (Poliomyelitis, adenovirus).

Virus tropism. Viruses are classified according to their particular tissue predilection as dermotropic, neurotropic, pneumotropic, enterotropic and viscerotropic.

Viral pathogenicity. When the virus multiplies in the cell, it may spread from cell to cell producing a small focal lesion (Wart or molluscum contagiosum). When the viruses are deposited on the mucous membrane of respiratory tract, they infect, multiply inside the mucosa and spread over a large area producing common cold; when trachea and bronchi are infected, influenza ensues.

Transmission of virus infection. Inclusion conjunctivitis is transmitted by the direct contact between persons during intercourse from one concert to another. Later it reaches the eyes of the newborn as it passes through the infected birth canal. Polioviruses and other enteroviruses may be transmitted after the ingestion of food or drink.

Interferon. Among animal viruses, interference of one virus with the reproduction of another may be mediated by a protein called "*interferon*" which is produced by the cell after infection with the first virus.

Interferon is a protein with a molecular weight of 30,000 daltons. Because of its size, the interferon

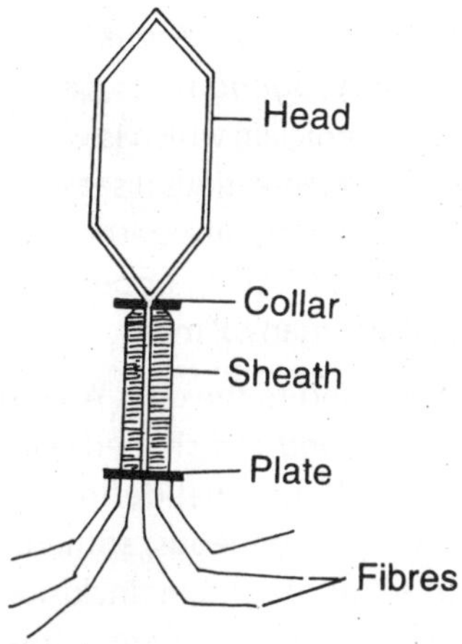

Fig. 3.2 : Bacteriophage

is released from cells and can diffuse in the body throughout the extracellular fluids.

Cultivation of Virus. Viruses can be grown in (1) The animal; (2) Chick embryo; (3) Tissue culture (*Refer* Chapter 62 on Laboratory techniques).

Bacteriophage. The structure of bacteriophage is complex and sophisticated than that of virus. The basic design is sperm shaped with a polyhedral head and a cylindrical tail.

The head of T_2 phage of *E. coli* is bipyramidal hexagonal prism and consists of an outer shell of about 1,000 subunits of a protein with a molecular weight of 80,000 and an inner central mass of DNA. The tail is about 100 mμ long and 25 mμ wide and is composed of contractile sheath surrounding a central hollow core. At the distal extremity of the tail, there is a hexagonal plate to which six fibers are attached. The sheath of the tail contracts less than half of the original length. The central core extrudes through the bacterial wall to enable the transference of DNA to the host cell (Fig. 3.2). The epidemiology of the disease can be studied by bacteriophage typing. The choleraphage typing method has obvious epidemiological uses in tracing the epidemic spread of cholera (Fig. 3.2).

Arthropod Borne Virus (ARBOR) Viruses

The term *arbor virus* is used to denote a large number of viruses transmitted by arthropod. These viruses are taken in by the arthropods, while sucking blood of man or animal. These viruses — multiplying within the body of the arthropods without causing damage to the tissues of the arthropod — produce the disease in man.

Slow and oncogenic viruses. They have in common the long continued association with the host. In general, the associated diseases occur sporadically and they exceptionally assume epidemic features (slow virus infections scrapie, Kuru, Animal virus tumours).

Application to nursing. Professional nurses - working particularly in communicable disease ward and public health should have a sound knowledge of virology and bacteriophage which is used to study the epidemiology of communicable diseases.

CHAPTER 4

GENERAL INTRODUCTION TO MYCOLOGY

Fungi (Lat. *fungus* — mushroom) are eukaryotes with a distinct nucleus and rigid chitinous cell wall and were formerly regarded as plants without *chlorophyll* and are now grouped with protozoa, slime moulds and most algae as Higher Prostita. Mycoses are infections caused by true fungi.

Eumycetes contains more than 80,000 species and can be classified morphologically into :

1. Phycomycetes are fungi with an unicellular, non-septate mycelium (500 species). The spores (endospores) are enclosed in special sporangia. Reproduction is sexual and asexual.

Atypical representative of Mucor (bread mould) is *Mucor mucedo*. Pathogenic species of this Mucor (mould) may cause infection of lungs, middle ear and general severe infectious process in man. The mould (filamentous) or mycelial fungi grow as long filaments (hyphae) and reproduce by formation of spores. The major part of the mycelium, the *vegetative mycelium*, grows and penetrates into the substrate absorbing nutrients for growth; other hyphae form *aerial mycelium* and protrude from the vegetative mycelium into the air. They form various kinds of spores and disseminate them in the air.

2. *Ascomycetes* or sac fungi (35,000 species) have a multicellular mycelium. They reproduce sexually by means of ascospores (spores which develop in spherical spore cases, *asci* — ascus (Gr. *askos* — sac) and asexually by conidia (exospores which have the function of asexual reproduction in many fungi).

The genus *Aspergillus* belongs to the class *Ascomycetes*. These fungi have divided septate mycelium and an unicellular conidiophore which terminates in a *fan-like row* of short sterigmata from which the spores are pinched off in chains — conidia (Gr. *Konis* — dust). The fruiting part of the aspergillus resembles a jet of water from a watering can and hence the name "Sprinkler" mould. *Aspergillus niger* is a representative of Aspergilla and is widespread in nature, certain species may cause aspergillosis of the lungs, ear and eye of man and may infect the whole body.

The genus *Penicillium* (Fig. 4.1) belongs to the class *Ascomycetes*. The mycelium and conidophore are multicellular. The fruiting body is in the shape of a brush. The conidiophore branches towards its upper part and terminates into *sterigmata* from which even-rowed chains of conidia are pinched off. This genus of fungi is widespread in nature (fodder, milk products, moist objects, old leather, ink, jam). The type species is *Penicillium glaucum*.

Certain species (*Penicillium notatum, Penicillium chrysogenum etc.*) are used for the production of penicillin which is widely used in the treatment of many infectious diseases. Some species of this genus of fungi are pathogenic and cause infection of the skin, nails, upper respiratory tract, lungs and other organs of man.

Yeasts belong to the class Ascomycetes. They are large, oval, round, rod-shaped cells. They have a double cell wall and welldefined nucleus. The cytoplasm is homogeneous, sometimes of a fine granular structure. It contains inclusions (glycogen, volutin, lipid) and also filamentous bodies — chondriosomes which are responsible for synthetic process of the cell. Yeasts multiply by budding, fission, sporulation and some of them reproduces asexually. Daughter cells produced by budding from the parent cell transform into independent individuals. The yeasts can also reproduce by sporulation. When there is lack of nutrition, 2, 4, 8 or 16 endospores are formed inside the cells of some species of yeast. Yeast cell forming the ascospores is called the *ascus* (sac), while sporulating yeasts are known as *Ascomycetes*, since the yeasts ferment various carbohydrates, they are widely used in brewing beer, in wine making and in baking bread. *Saccharomyces cerevisiae, S. ellipsoides* are typical representatives of the yeasts.

Among the asporogenic yeasts (family *saccharomycetaceae*), there are species pathogenic to man; they are called *Candida* which cause grave

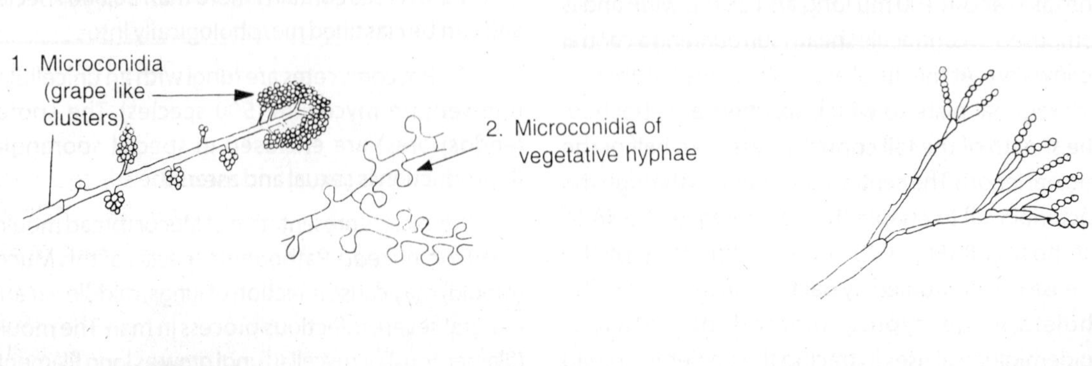

Fig. 4.1 : Penicillium

diseases known as candidiasis. They occur as a result of the growth inhibition of the normal microflora by antibiotics used for treating a number of infectious diseases and inflammatory processes.

3. *Basidiomycetes*. Fungi with a multicellular mycelium. These organisms predominantly reproduce asexually by basidiospores (basidia reproductive organs in which a certain number of spores develop, usually 4).

Certain species are free parasites. Two hundred species of mushrooms are used as food. Twentyfive species of mushrooms are poisonous.

Smut fungi invade grains crops causing disease known as smut. Rust fungi affect sunflowers and other plants producing orange-coloured spots on infected plants.

4. *Imperfect fungi (Fungi imperfecti)* are a rather large group of fungi consisting of a multicellular mycelium without either asco or basidio-sporangiophore, but only with conidia. Reproduction is asexual; but the sexual reproduction is unknown. To this class belong the orders *Hyphomycetales, Melanconiales and Sphaeropsidales.*

Among the *hyphomycetes*, which may be of great interest to the physicians are : *Fusarium graninearum* causing intoxication in human (drunken bread) and *Fusarium sporotrichicidales* causing intoxication in man and domestic animals who had eaten the grain crops which had remained in the fields during the winter.

Pathogenic species of imperfect fungi are causative agents of dermatomycoses (*superficial mycoses*) : favus (*Acharion schoenleini*); trichophytosis (*Trichophyton violaceum*), Microsporosis (*microsporum lanosum*) epidermophytosis (*Epidermophyton inguinale*).

PATHOGENIC FUNGI

Aspergilli. The pathogenic species are : *Aspergillus fumigatus, A. roseus, A. flavus, A. nigricans.* More than forty species have been recovered from patient suffering from various clinical forms of Aspergillosis. In human beings, they are responsible for lesions in the lungs, bronchi, cornea, ear canal and other organs and tissues. The disease is prevalent among millers.

Penicilli. There are more than thirty species of *Penicillium* pathogenic to man. They cause penicilliosis affecting the skin, nails, ears, upper respiratory tract and lungs (pseudotuberculosis). Pathogenic species are : *P. minutum, P. linguae, P. glaucum* and *P. album* (Fig. 4.1).

Mucor fungi. More than fifteen species of *Mucor fungi* cause mucor mycosis characterised by lung lesions similar to tuberculosis in their clinical manifestations, keratitis, otomycosis, vulvovaginitis, gamma of the skin.

Laboratory diagnosis of aspergillosis, penicilliosis and mucormycosis is made by microscopic examination of the pus, its inoculation into common nutrient media or Sabouraud's medium and subsequent cultivation at 25 - 28°C. The treatment is by nystatin.

IMPERFECT FUNGI

Many imperfect fungi have septate hyphae and asexual conidia resembling those of *Ascomycetes*, but sexual or "perfect" state has not yet been described for these fungi — hence they are called *Fungi imperfecti*. A majority of the pathogenic moulds, yeasts, yeast like fungi (candida) and dimorphic fungi (Histoplasma, Paracoccidioides) belong to this group —*Fungi imperfecti.*

Sporotrichum has a septate mycelium. Lateral branches extend from the hyphae bearing single conidia or clusters of conidia at their sides or ends. The *Sporotrichum* grows on common nutrient media (pH 6.5) producing the best growth on Sabouraud's medium at 25 to 28°C. Growth is slow. The colonies are leathery, fluffy, smooth or folded and quite frequently pigmented.

This causative agent enters the subcutaneous tissue and the lymph nodes through abrasions of the skin as a result gumma similar to that in syphilis and tuberculosis are produced in the pharynx, larynx, muscles and synovial membrane. It may also cause abscess of the bones, joints and internal organs. Antibiotics and sulphonamides have no effect.

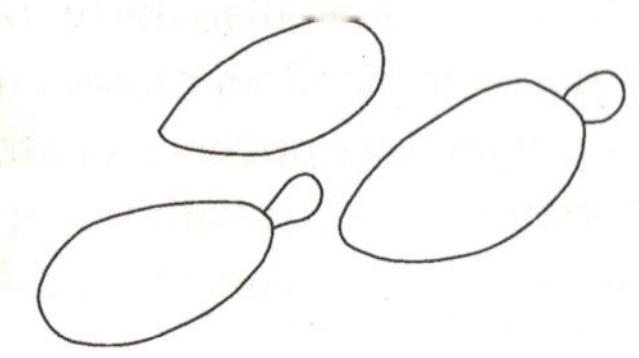

Fig. 4.2 : Candida albicans

Candida (Fig.4.2). They are unicellular organisms which reproduce by budding. Neither conidia nor ascospores are produced. They possess *no true mycelium*; the pseudomycelium is devoid of a membrane and septa and develops by successive or terminal budding.

Candida albicans and *C. tropicalis* are most important in human pathology. About 20 species of the genus candida are human pathogens and are present on the skin and mucous membrane of the mouth, gastrointestinal tract and urinogenital organs of man. They occur on fruit, vegetables and other foodstuffs, in bath sewage, washing from catering establishments and on dishes.

The infection is acquired when body is weakened and in the presence of unfavourable conditions (increased moisture, skin maceration, long term occupational contact with sugar containing fruit and vegetables, inadequately disinfected baths). Debiliated children, bath-house attendants, confectioners are susceptible to candidiasis.

Candidiasis associated with the long term use of antibiotics (penicillin, chlortetracycline etc.) have become of great importance. They cause profound disturbances of symbiotic relationship among normal microflora resulting into a condition of dysbacteriosis which enhances intensive multiplication, spread of the co-members into the buccal, intestinal and vaginal mucosa and their transformation from the saprophyte state into conditionally pathogenic and pathogenic forms. As a result, local and general lesions develop.

The yeast-like fungi affect the skin between the fingers and toes in the inguinal and axillary folds, the nails and nail folds, the mucous membranes of the lips and mouth corners, the tongue, fauces, esophagus, and, sometimes, the vagina with the development of white films. Infection of the mucosa is known as "Thrush".

The gastrointestinal, respiratory, urogenital and nervous system, liver, biliary tract, pancreas, bones, kidney are also involved in candidiasis. The most common candida infection is vaginitis or *vaginal thrush* which is characterised, in pregnant women, by a whitish discharge with a pH below 5.2 and, microscopically, some pus cells and many yeasts, including pseudomycelium, can be seen. In infection due to trichomonas and bacteria, the discharge is more purulent and less acid.

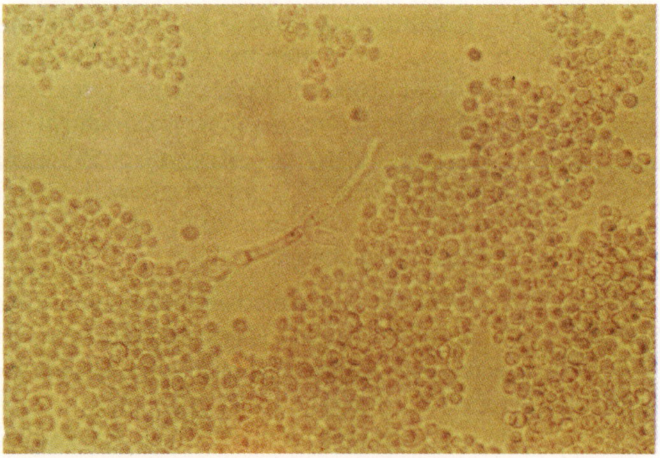

Fig. 4.2a : Candida albicans with germ tube x 400

Oral thrush occurs in debilitated or bottle fed infants. Creamy white patches are found covering red, raw areas of mucous membrane and tongue. It also occurs in adults in angular cheilitis, in sore mouth caused by ill-fitting dentures and, in all, too frequently, after prolonged courses of oral anitbacterial therapy.

Infections of the skin are common in diabetes and skin lesions are characterised by erythema, exudation and desquamation and occur most commonly in the axilla and groin, on the vulva and glans penis. It also affects the interdigital clefts, the skin folds round the nails and sometimes nail itself.

Infections of the intestine occur in infants, the aged and those on long courses of oral antibiotics. Symptoms are pruritus ani or diarrhea. The organism survives well in exudate collected on swabs and may even multiply if there is delay in transmission to the laboratory. It may be demonstrated microscopically in wet preparation or Gram-stained smears and grows readily on blood agar or Sabouraud's medium at 25 to 28°C (room temperature). The incorporation of antibiotics in medium may inhibit the growth of other bacteria.

Characteristic of *C. albicans* is the production of curved, elongated germ tubes within three hours when it is transferred from peptone water to mammalian serum at 37°C (Fig. 4.2a, 3).

On Sabouraud's medium, after two days, *C. albicans* produces high convex, off-white colonies of 1.5 mm in diameter (Fig. 4.3a). It ferments carbohydrates; but it *fails to split urea*; which is used in differentiating it from other yeasts.

Before undertaking the treatment, it is always advisable to correct the underlying disturbances (diabetes or poor hygiene). The usual treatment is to give the polyene, nystatin locally. Nystatin is very poorly absorbed from the gut so that the systemic infection must be treated with amphotericin B. Another polyene, trichomycin, is often used in vaginitis as it is effective against trichomonas and candida.

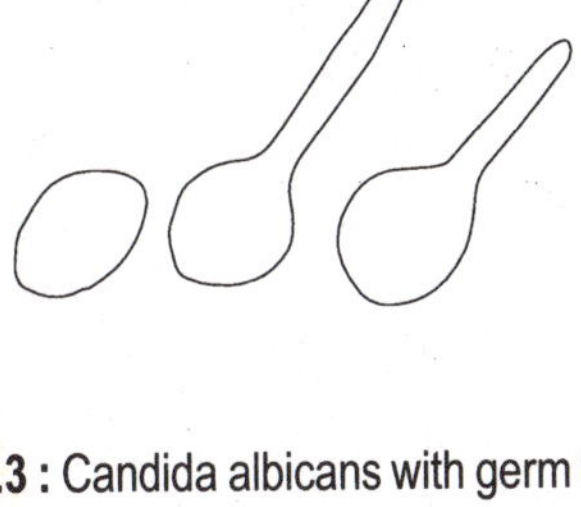

Fig. 4.3 : Candida albicans with germ tube

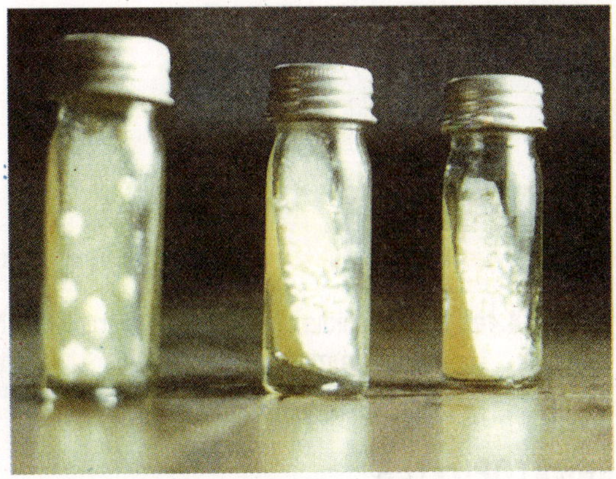

Fig. 4.3a : Growth of C. albicans on sabouraud's agar

Blastomyces dermatitidis and *Cryptococcus neoformans* cause Blastomycosis

Blastomyces dermatitidis is a large budding cell which is microscopic. Its mycelium is segmented, branching and with conidia protruding laterally. On blood agar at 37°C, the fungus produces white, moist, waxy, soft, wrinkled colonies of the yeast only. On Sabouraud's medium at 25°C it produces fluffy white colonies which turn brown. The disease becomes chronic with skin lesions on the face, hands and buttocks. Internal organs are rarely affected.

Cryptococcus neoformans is round and oval yeast like cell, with one or two buds, which is frequently surrounded by a capsule. On Sabouraud's medium, it forms mucoid, white colonies which later become brown and creamy in colour. This fungus causes in man a deep-seated, systemic chronic blastomycosis commonly in agricultural workers and animal breeders. The lungs, intestine, skin, subcutaneous tissue, lymph nodes, brain, meninges and bones are involved, and the mortality is very high. Laboratory diagnosis is by microscopic examination. The use of ineffective broad spectrum antibiotics is banned. The physical condition of the body should be strengthened. Special antibiotics (nystatin, neomycin, candicidin) are prescribed for blastomycosis and candidiasis.

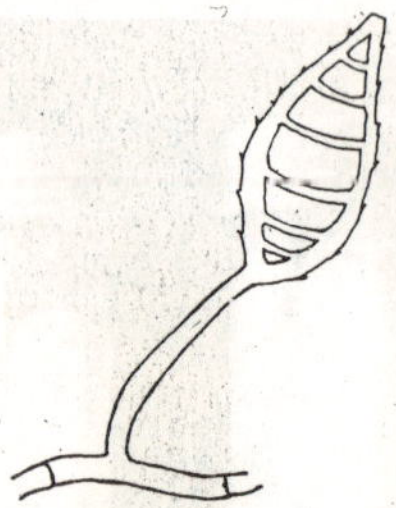

Fig. 4.4a : Macroconidia of microsporum

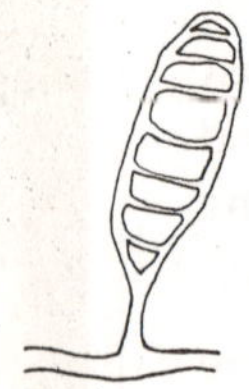

Fig. 4.4b : Macroconidia of trichophyton

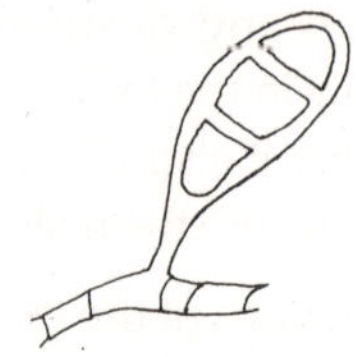

Fig. 4.4c : Macroconidia of epidermophyton

DERMATOPHYTES

Common (superficial) dermatophyte infections (ringworm or tinea) of skin, hair and nails are caused by the members of a group of thirty to forty related filamentous fungi that can digest keratin. These fungi are called "dermatophytes". This saprophytic members of the group, which normally live in the soil and from which the human and animal pathogens have probably been derived, play an important role in breaking down the keratinised tissue of dead animals. From 1843 till recently, only the asexual forms of the fungi were known and were placed under fungi imperfecti in three genera; *Epidermophyton, Microsporum* and *Trichophyton* distinguished by the morphology of their large asexual spores or "macroconidia" (Fig. 4.4a, b, c). In 1988, however, the sexual forms of perfect states of about half the Microsporum and Trichophyton species have been identified. They belong to two genera of the Ascomycetes. The species whose perfect states have been identified are mostly soil organisms but include some common pathogens. The following six species are responsible for ninety per cent of the dermatophyte infections of man. *Microsporum audouini; M. canis; Trichophyton rubrum; T. mentagrophytes; T. verrucosum* and *Epidermophyton floccosum.*

The dermatophytes causing infections in man live normally on the keratinised surfaces of man and domestic animals and do not invade non-keratinised tissues.

Their *morphology* consists of hyphae and arthrospores formed by segmentation of a hypha into a row of separate thick-walled cells. In artificial culture, two kinds of asexual spores, microconidia and macroconidia, are also formed. The microconidia are unicellular, small (2 to 5 μm), round or pear-shaped, borne laterally or terminally singly or in clusters. The macroconidia are multicellular and their shape, size and surface are used to differentiate the genera. In *Microsporum*, they are usually numerous *spindle-shaped*, with a rough surface and 5 to 15 segments and measure from 40 to 150 μm in length. In Epidermophyton, they are *pear-shaped* with a smooth surface and measure about 30-40 μm. Two or three often arise from the same hypha. In *Trichophyton*, they are usually scanty and often irregular in shape; characteristic ones are smooth, cylindrical, with 2 to 6 segments and 10 to 50 μm long.

At room temperature (25 to 28°C), Sabouraud's medium is suitable for isolation and is improved by adding cycloheximide which inhibits many common contaminants but does not affect dermatophytes.

Their spores are not killed by the mild wet heat of laundering so their destruction in clothings may require boiling or formaldehyde vapour. The benzoic and salicylic acids of Whitfield's ointment are fungicidal. Griseofulvin is fungistatic to all dermatophytes *in vitro* but not all infections respond to treatment with it. Ciclopirax Olamine (Batrafen) cream, miconazole nitrate (Zole) dusting powder are recent antifungal drugs. Sebefin has a broad spectrum fungicidal and fungistatic activity. Clobetasol propionate, gentamicin and miconazole nitrate cream (Lobate GM skin cream), Terbinafine HCl cream 1% (sebifin).

Diseases due to dermatophytes. The usual name given to these infections is ringworm or tinea and this name is qualified by the name of the site affected, e.g., tinea capitis or tinea pedis, but special names are also used in dermatology for particular manifestation, e.g., kerion, favus.

When the skin is infected, the fungus spreads radially in the dead keratinised layer in the form of branching hyphae with occasional arthrospores. The inflammatory reaction from living tissue below may be very mild and only little dry scaling or hyperkeratosis is seen. More commonly there is irritation, erythema, edema and some vesiculation especially at the spreading edge and this irregular pink periphery gives rise to the name "ringworm". The species that commonly attack the skin are Trichophyton sp. *E. floccosum* (groins and feet) and *M. canis.*

Infection of the nails renders them irregular, discoloured and friable. The fungus grows deep into the substance of the nail. The species usually responsible are *T. rubrum* and both human and animal strains of *T. mentagrophytes.*

When the scalp is infected the fungus grows in the horny layer of the epidermis and down into the hair follicles. The hyphae surround and invade the hair shaft and, once within it, they grow outwards. The hair continues to grow and the hyphae break up into long chains of arthrospores, in some species within the shaft (endothrix infections) but more commonly mainly on the outside (ectothrix infections). After two or three weeks' growth the weakened hair breaks off, leaving either a black dot at the follicle mouth as in endothrix infections.

Ectothrix infections are caused by *Microsporum* sp., and *T. mentagrophytes*, whereas endothrix infections are due *T. violaceum* and *.T. schoenleinii.* The last is the normal cause of favus.

Laboratory diagnosis of ringworm is based on direct microscopic demonstration of hyphae and arthrospores in the keratinised tissue and on colonial appearance and hyphal and conidial morphology in culture. Genera are distinguished according to the morphology of macroconidia and species by a combination of microscopic and colonial features.

The specimens of the nails should be collected after cleansing with 70 per cent ethyl alcohol. From skin lesions, scales of 2 to 3 mm in diameter should be scrapped outwards with a blunt scalpel from the active periphery of the lesion and the vesicles should be sniffed off.

Good material from nails can be obtained by scraping from the nail with a scalpel. The dusty stumps of ectothrix infections and the black dots of some endothrix infections can be recognised by the naked eye, the hairs when located can be plucked with fine forceps. Specimens should be folded up in black paper.

In the laboratory, the specimens are "cleared" with 20 per cent KOH and examined. The hyphae appear greenish, branching, running across the outlines of the colourless cells of skin or nail. In hairs, arthrospores are easy to see than the hyphae and their position within or outside the hair shaft may allow a presumptive diagnosis of the species.

Culture is carried out on Sabouraud's medium with added cycloheximide at 28°C (room temperature). Colonies of dermatophytes may be visible in two to three days. Cultures are usually reported as negative until after three weeks.

Oral griseofulvin is the treatment of choice for hair infection and those due to *T. rubrum.* It may be less effective for infections of the skin and nails, particularly those of the feet and those due to human strains of *T. mentagrophytes* for which Whitfield's ointment should be tried first.

INFECTIONS OF DEEPER TISSUES

These infections are mainly in warm climates in people whose bare skin is exposed to soil, dust or recurrent trauma. *Mycetoma* is the commonest and most widespread syndrome which is caused by filamentous fungi or higher bacteria under aerobic actinomycetes. *Chromoblastomycosis* and *subcutaneous phycomycosis* are two other syndromes caused by more than one fungus.

These infections are chronic, localised and acquired by the traumatic inoculation of opportunistic organisms normally present in the soil or on thorns.

Madura foot is characterised by a swelling often with sinuses discharging pus which may contain granules of varying size (0.5 to 2 mm) and colour (black, red, buff). The main actinomycetes responsible for this condition are : *Nocardia brasiliensis, N. asteroides, Streptomyces madurae.* They destroy soft tissue, bone, tendon and nerve.

Grains (colonies of the organisms) in the pus may be collected into the surgical gauze. Their size and colour suggest the species responsible.

After crushing the granules, wet preparations and gram-stained smears should be made. The size of the hyphae is more than 2 μm in width in fungus whereas in case of actinomycetes it is less than 1 μm.

Sabouraud's medium (without cycloheximide) at 26°C can be used to cultivate the fungi and Lowenstein Jensen medium at 37°C for actinomycetes. Some are sensitive to antibiotics *in vitro* but none is sensitive *in vivo.* Nocardia sp. may be semi acid fast and are sensitive to many antibacterial antibiotics, sulphones and sulphonamide-trimethoprim mixtures both *in vivo* and *in vitro.* The only effective treatment for fungal mycetoma is the surgery; nocardial and streptomyces infection respond to long course of dapsone and cotrimoxazole.

(a) Chromomycosis is a chronic warty dermatitis caused by traumatic inoculation of one of five closely related pigmented fungi : *Phialophora pedrosoi, P. compactum, P. verrucosa, P. dermatidis* and *Cladosporium carrionii.* Microscopically, the hyphae are brown and several types of spores are produced. Treatment is not satisfactory.

(b) Subcutaneous Phycomycosis can be caused by Absidia sp. and Rhizopus sp. by infecting and penetrating the mucous membrane of the nose, sinuses and stomach when patients are *in extremis.*

Dimorphic fungi. The majority of fungi are filamentous, some exist as yeasts and others change from one form to other depending upon the conditions of growth. The last are called dimorphic fungi and include a number of pathogens; *Sporothrix schenckii, Blastomyces dermatitidis, Paracoccidioides brasiliensis, Histoplasma capsulatum.* Another pathogen, *Coccidioides immitis,* is dimorphic in different way. The infections they cause are not communicable from man to man and acquired by inhalation. The process is slow with cellular granulomatous reaction.

Infection with *S. schenckii,* usually follows injury to the hands with the contaminated splinters or thorns but may be acquired from infected animals. A local "chancre" forms and small subcutaneous abscess develop along the line of inflamed drainage lymphatics.

Paracoccidioides brasiliensis causes "South American blastomycosis" which is chronic, progressive, pyogenic, granulomatous disease with a predilection for lymphatic tissue. It main lesions are common in mucous membranes, lymph nodes, skin, spleen and intestine. It is fatal if not treated. It is acquired by inhalation. Treatment is not yet very satisfactory.

Histoplasma capsulatum is a dimorphic fungus found in many parts of the world in soil enriched with the droppings of certain birds and mammals. When its spores are inhaled by a mammalian host they develop into yeasts which set up an intra-cellular infection of the histiocytes. The clinical manifestations in man vary from an asymptomatic pulmonary infection to fatal generalised disease. There are many parallels with tuberculosis. The usual outcome is a small calcified peripheral focus in lung.

Coccidioides immitis is a dimorphic fungus. Its infection is acquired by inhalation and is normally asymptomatic. It has many parallels with tuberculosis and histoplasmosis. The treatment is by amphotericin B. *Rhinosporidium seeberi* causes the development of polyps in the submucosa of the nose, mouth, conjunctiva, in the skin. Natural infections occur in man, horses, mules and cows in most parts of the world, commonly in India and Sri Lanka (Ceylon).

A portion of polyp may be crushed in water between slide and coverslip. Some large cysts and many small spores should be seen, if it is *Rhinosporidium seeberi.* Treatment is surgical.

CHAPTER 5

GENERAL INTRODUCTION TO MEDICAL PARASITOLOGY AND ZOOLOGICAL NOMENCLATURE

Medical Parasitology is that branch of Medical Science which deals with the parasites and their relationship with the host.

It consists of:

1. *Protozoology* — Study of Protozoa
2. *Helminthology* — Study of Helminths
3. *Entomology* — Study of insects or vectors.

Parasite is an organism which has adopted itself to live in or on the other organism on which it is mostly dependent for its nutrition or metabolism. Literally, `parasite' comes from the Greek word `parasitos', from `para' — beside, and `sitos' — com, bread, food. So 'parasite' means eating from the table of another or at other's cost.

Most of the parasites which attack man are of animal nature, i.e., they belong to one of the five main divisions of animal kingdom — the protozoa, the helminths and the arthropods.

Parasites can be classified on the basis of their relationship with the hosts:

1. An *ectoparasite* is one which lives on the surface of the body, e.g., the human louse, *Pediculus humanus.*

2. An *endoparasite* is one normally found inside the human body, e.g., the roundworm, *Ascaris lumbricoides*, lives in the human intestine.

3. *Commensal* is a parasite which lives in or on a host for its benefit but does not produce disease, e.g., *Entamoeba coli.*

4. *Pathogens* are parasites which are pathogenic to man, living at the expenses of the tissues, fluids and metabolites of their hosts, e.g., *Entamoeba histolytica.*

5. *Symbiosis* is a relationship when two organisms live in close association, so that each derives benefit from the presence of other.

Infection, when a parasite establishes itself within a host.

Infestation, when a parasite lives superficially on the host.

A *host* is any animal that harbours a parasite.

A host may be:

(a) definite
(b) intermediate
(c) a reservoir.

A *definite* host is one that harbours the vegetative, the adult or the sexual stage of parasite. Man is definite host for *Taenia saginata.*

An *intermediate* host is an animal which harbours the cystic, larval, immature or asexual stage of the parasites. Cattle is intermediate host of *T. saginata.*

A *reservoir* host is an animal which takes the place of man in the life cycle of a parasite, e.g., Antelope is the reservoir host of African Trypanosomiasis.

Following are several states of parasitism:

(i) *Facultative parasites* — are those parasites which have free living and parasitic forms, e.g., *Strongyloides stercoralis.*

(ii) *Obligatory parasites* — are those which are incapable of free living and completing their life cycle in the absence of their hosts. Example : *Toxoplasma gondii.*

(iii) *Erratic* or *ectopic parasite* — found in organs or tissues of the body which it does not normally invade, e.g., *Ascaris lumbricoides* are occasionally found in the bile duct or liver which they do not normally parasitise.

Classification of parasites can be explained as follows :

	Termination	Example
Phylum	—	Platyhelminthes
Class	—	Cestodes
Order	— idea	Cyclophyllidea
Superfamily	— oidea	Taenioidea
Family	— idae	Taeniidae
Genus	—	Taenia
Species	—	*Taenia saginata*

A. Mechanisms of Disease Production by Animal Parasites

The parasites may damage the host tissues :

1. By mechanical injury,
2. By detrimental effect of toxic substances.

These two effects may, sometimes, take place together as in *Plasmodium falciparum.* When this malaria parasite grows in the human red blood cells, it can mechanically destroy the architecture of red blood cells. At the same time, it liberates toxic substances which cause the rigors and clinical symptoms of malaria. Similarly, *Entamoeba histolytica* damages the human intestine by mechanical injury and by production of a histolytic enzyme and, ultimately, causes amoebic dysentery.

Mechanical injury may be

(a) by means of pressure as the parasite grows larger (Hydatid cyst).

(b) by obstruction of ducts —

— blood vessels (Strongyloides) causing infarction.

— Lymph vessels (filaria) causing elephantiasis.

— Intestine (*Ascaris lumbricoides*) producing intestinal obstruction, perforation and necrosis.

3. By competing with the host for food, e.g., *Diphyllobothrium latum,* fish tapeworm, deprives its host of vitamin B_{12}, this causing megaloblastic anemia. Similarly, the hookworm (*Ankylostoma duodenale*) infestation leads to iron-deficiency.

4. By bacterial infection — Bacteria may contaminate the wound or ulcer which is initially produced by parasite, *Dracunculus medinensis,* guinea-worm. Tetanus is the complication.

B. Host Reactions to the Parasites

These reactions may be tissue reactions or immunological response.

Tissue reactions occur when parasites invade certain tissues of the human body, there is excessive proliferation of the tissue, e.g., fibrosis (or cirrhosis) in the liver due to ova deposited by *Schistosoma mansoni* in the liver; hepatic fibrosis and hyperplasia of the biliary epithelium in liver flukes infection (*Clonorchis sinensis* and *Fasciola hepatica*).

Parasites of medical importance should be studied as per the scheme given below :

1. History of the discovery of the parasite,
2. Geographical distribution,
3. Habitat inside the human body,
4. Morphology,
5. Life cycle,
6. Modes of infection,
7. Pathogenicity and clinical features,
8. Laboratory diagnosis,
9. Treatment and prophylaxis.

PROTOZOOLOGY

Protozoa are single-celled or unicellular animals which are microscopic in size (*Proto,* primitive, *zoa,* animal).

Morphology: In general, there is a protoplasmic body or *cytoplasm* in which is embedded one or more nuclei.

The cytoplasm is usually divided into:

(a) an outer ectoplasm, and

(b) an inner endoplasm.

The ectoplasm performs the functions of locomotion, respiration, excretion, protection. The function of *endoplasm* is nutritive and reproductive.

Nucleus : It controls various functions and regulates reproduction. It consists of a nuclear membrane which encloses a network of fine delicate filaments. Usually, there is a mass in the centre of nucleus, the *Karyosome*, which may be minute. The nuclear membrane and fine filaments contain chromatin granules. The nucleus is useful to differentiate the genera and species.

Organelles of Locomotion : On the basis of the organ of locomotion, pathogenic protozoa can be classified into:

(a) *Rhizopoda* — which move with the help of pseudopodia (pseudo — false; podia, feet). These pseudopodia are also used by amoebae to engulf food (Entamoeba).

(b) *Mastigophora* — they have elongated thread-like filaments, flagellum (Trypanosoma).

(c) *Sporozoa* — which exhibit no movement, e.g., malarial parasite.

Ciliata — their movement is carried out by means of shorter processes — *Cilia*, e.g., *Balantidium coli.*

Protozoa have three stages in their life cycle:

1. Trophozoite — or motile stage which exhibits gliding movement and is capable of enclosing itself in a resistant wall to form a cyst (encystment).

2. Precystic stage — it has a blunt pseudopodium projecting from the periphery.

3. Cystic stage — it is a resistant stage. On reaching the anatomical site in the alimentary canal, the cyst gives rise to one or more trophozoites (excystation).

Metabolism. The protozoa may engulf food in a solid form or absorb it in a liquid state. Food material is digested in the endoplasm in "food vacuoles" into which digestive ferments and enzymes are secreted. Following digestion, food may be absorbed, or stored in the form of glycogen, volutin chromatoid bodies and other substances. The waste products left after digestion pass out into the medium in which the animal lives.

Nutrients metabolised by protozoa in vitro. Cultivation studies of protozoa showed that the malaria parasites and African trypanosomes metabolise large quantities of carbohydrates, e.g., glucose. The end product of metabolism in African trypanosomes is pyruvic acid; and lactase is known to accumulate in case of malarial parasites. Blood inhabiting protozoa require the following constituents of plasma for their growth and multiplication: amino acids, vitamins, inorganic salts and metabolic cofactors; whereas the intestinal protzoa differ from others in that they can only thrive in a bacterial flora.

Reproduction of protozoa may be asexual multiplication or sexual reproduction.

1. *Asexual multiplication*
   (i) by binary fission, that is, simple division into two, e.g., *E. histolytica* in the large intestine of man.
   (ii) by multiple fission or schizogony — In this process, more than two individuals are produced e.g., *Plasmodia* in the liver and red blood cells of the mammalian host.

2. *Sexual multiplication*
   (i) by conjugation — here a temporary union of two individuals takes place with the interchange of nuclear material, e.g., *Ciliata.*
   (ii) by syngamy or sporogony — that is, the process by which a male parasite unites with a female to produce a fertilised ovum or zygote which undergoes division into very numerous, thin rod-like structures known as sporozoites.

Members of the genus Trypanosoma of the class Mastigophora also reproduce asexually. In the African trypanosomes (*T.gambiense* and *T.rhodesiense*), the asexual reproduction takes place in the blood by repeated longitudinal fission. In the American trypanosome (*T. cruzi*), it occurs in the tissue cells where the protozoa round themselves up, dividing repeatedly to produce intracellular aggregations or 'nests' of young rounded parasites which elongate afterwards to the trypanosome form and re-enter the blood stream.

HELMINTHOLOGY

The word 'helminth' from Greek *helmins, — inthos* means 'worm'. All species of helminth belong to the subkingdom of the Metazoa and all are provided with tissues and organs derived from three embryonic body layers, the ectoderm, endoderm and mesoderm.

The helminths of medical importance are divided into two main divisions :

HELMINTHS
- Phylum PLATYHELMINTHES (Class Cestoidea and Trematoda)
- Phylum NEMATHELMINTHES (Class Nematoda)

Characteristics of Phylum Platyhelminthes

1. Flattened leaf-like or tape-like and segmented;
2. Mostly hermaphrodite;
3. Alimentary canal incomplete or entirely lacking;
4. Body cavity absent.

Characteristics of Phylum Nemathelminthes

1. Elongated, cylindrical, unsegmented bodies;
2. Sexes separate;
3. Alimentary canal complete;
4. Body cavity present.

General description of Cestodes (Tape-worms) :

1. They are long dorsoventrally flattened segmented, tape-like, so they are known as 'tape-worms';
2. They vary in size from a few millimeters to several meters;
3. They are found in the intestine of man and animals;
4. Adult worm has three regions (a) a head (Scolex), (b) a neck, (c) a body or trunk (Strobila) comprising of segments (proglottids);
5. They bear suckers (slit-like or cup-like) or hooks which are organs of attachment;
6. They are hermaphrodites (having organs of both sexes);
7. There is no body cavity and alimentary canal;
8. They have well developed organs of reproduction;
9. They have excretory and nervous systems.

Difference between Pseudophyllidean cestodes and Cyclophyllidean cestodes

(a) *Pseudophyllidean cestode has*
 (i) Two slit-like grooves (bothria);
 (ii) No branching uterus;
 (iii) Uterine pore;
 (iv) Common genital pore lying *ventrally in the middle line*;
 (v) Operculated egg hatching out ciliated larvae.

(b) *Cyclophyllidean cestode has*
 (i) four cup-like suckers;
 (ii) uterus with lateral branches;
 (iii) no uterine pore;
 (iv) a laterally situated common genital pore;
 (v) non-operculated eggs which do not hatch out ciliated larvae.

Pseudophyllidean tapeworms of man:

Superfamily Bothriocephaloidea.

Genus DIPHYLLOBOTHRIUM.

Species *Diphyllobothrium latum.*

Pseudophyllidean cestodes have

(a) Long chain of segments;

(b) Head bearing two slit-like grooves called *bothria*;

(c) *Ventrally* situated genital pores, not marginal (three genital orifices in each segment one male orifice and two female orifices);

(d) Scattered vitelline glands in the parenchyma;

(e) Uterus opening to the exterior through which eggs come out;

(f) Operculated eggs which can develop only in water and give rise to a single ciliated embryo (first stage larva - *coracidium*);

(g) Two more larval development stages - the second stage larva is called *Procercoid* and the third stage larve *Plerocercoid* in fish flesh.

ENTOMOLOGY

Entomology is that branch of biological science which deals with the study of insects (Greek *entoma* = insects).

Only insects (vectors) of medical importance are briefly described so as to enable the medical students, nurses and physicians to identify them in a very short time:

Phylum	ARTHROPODA
Order	DIPTERA — with one pair of membranous wings attached to the second thoracic segment; second pair of wings replaced by minute club-shaped balancing organs (halteres); mouth parts adapted for sucking; metamorphosis complete (egg → larva → pupa → adult).
Class	INSECTA
Species	*Anopheles calicifacies, Culex fatigans; Aedes polynesiensis* (mosquito);
Species	*Phlebotomus argentipes* (sandfly);
Species	*Culicoides austeni* (biting midgets);
Species	*Simulium damnosum* (black fly);
Species	*Musca domestica* (house fly);
Species	*Glossina palpalis* (tse tse fly).
Order	SIPHONAPTERA — Wingless, body strongly compressed laterally with an especially long pair of hind legs adapted for jumping; mouth parts adapted for sucking; metamorphosis complete (egg → larva → pupa → adult).
Species	*Xenopsylla cheopis* (rat flea).
Order	ANOPLURA (Sucking lice, literally insects which have an 'unarmed tail') wingless, body compressed dorso-ventrally; tarsi one clawed; mouth parts adapted for piercing and sucking; without metamorphosis (egg → nymph → adult).
Species	*Pediculus humanus* var. *capitis* (head louse);
	Pediculus humanus var. *corporis* (body louse);
	Phthirus pubis (pubic louse).
Order	ACARI (Ticks and mites) — Cephalothorax and abdomen united, not externally segmented, adults with four pairs of legs, — larvae with three pairs of legs.
Superfamily	IXODOIDEA (Ticks) — Hypostome large, with ventral recurved teeth, skin leathery, ventrally furrowed, adults with tracheae and

with one pair of stigmal plates near the bases of legs III or IV. Representative : *Ixodes, Dermacentor.*

Superfamily SARCOPTOIDEA — Palpi small, three jointed, eye lacking, tracheae lacking tarsi often end in sucker, ventral suckers at genital opening or near anal opening; body entire, surface provided with fine parallel lines or folds. Parasitic in all stages. Representative : *Sarcoptes scabiei.*

Subclass CRUSTACEA — they have two pairs of pre-oral antenniform appendages and three pairs of post-oral jaw-like appendages; chiefly aquatic, breathing through gills.

Order EUCOPEPODA (water flea) — Lacking compound eyes, females carry egg sacs. Representative : *Diaptomus, Cyclops.*

Eucopepods — These species are almost microscopically small, simple, aquatic with a pair of maxillae and five pairs of swimming legs. They lack compound eyes. They are elongated, convex on the dorsum, pyriform through the cephalic and thoracic regions, narrowed in the abdominal region and have two caudal furci. Medically, the genera *Diaptomus* and *cyclops* are important. *Diaptomus* are important intermediate hosts of *Diphyllobothrium latum.* Many species of cyclops are intermediate host of *Dracunculus medinensis.*

Order HETEROPTERA (true bugs) — Typically with two pairs of wings with basal part of front wings thickened, more or less leathery, but wingless in some families (i.e., bed bugs), body somewhat compressed dorsoventrally; tarsi two-clawed, mouth parts adapted for piercing and sucking; beak arises from front part of the head, metamorphosis gradual (egg → larva → pupa → adult).

Species *Triatoma infestans* (kissing bug, assassin bug).

ORDER DIPTERA IS DIVIDED INTO THREE SUBORDERS (NEMATOCERA, BRACHYCERA, CYCLORRHAPHA)

Order	DIPTERA
Suborder	NEMATOCERA
Class	INSECTA
Family	CULICIDAE (Mosquitoes)

STUDY OF MOSQUITO

Adult mosquito

1. Body consists of a head, 3 segmented thorax and ten segmented abdomen.

2. The head bears a pair of compound eye, a pair of fifteen jointed antenna, plumosed in male and pilosed in female, a pair of four jointed pulp and a biting and sucking type of proboscis.

3. Thorax is three-segmented, the mesothorax bearing a pair of wings and metathorax a pair of

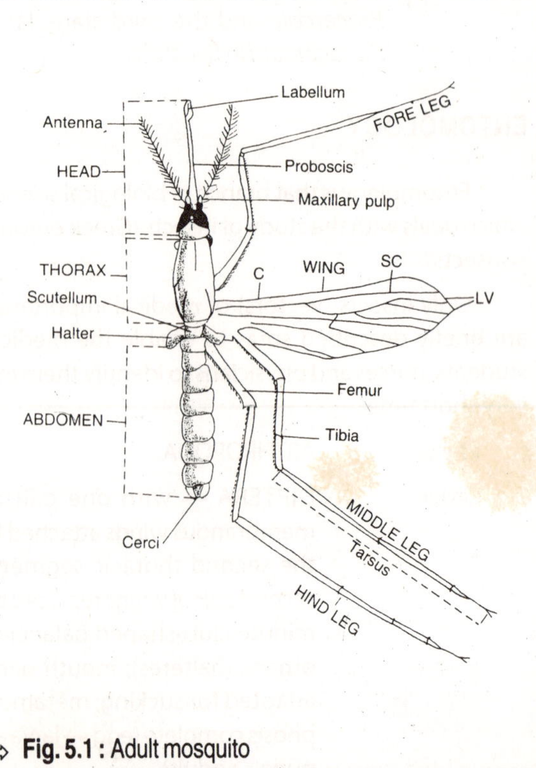

Fig. 5.1 : Adult mosquito

halteres — rudimentary hind-wings to maintain balance in flight. Each thoracic segment bear a pair of jointed legs.

4. The wings bear scales and the 2nd, 4th and 5th wing veins are forked (C, costal vein; Sc, sub-costal vein; Lv, longitudinal veins).

5. The abdomen is then segmented and the last two are transformed into sexual structure (Fig. 5.1).

Mouth Parts of Female Mosquito

1. Antennae which are scarcely hairy of pilosed, a pair of four jointed pulps, about one-third of the length of the proboscis.

2. The proboscis is elongated and consists of the following structures:

(a) an elongated labium ending in labellae
(b) a pair of maxilla distally serrated
(c) a pair of mandibules distally serrated
(d) labrum epipharynx
(e) hypopharynx.

The proboscis (mouth parts) of female mosquito is stout like needle, so that it can pierce through the skin — hence female mosquitoes are voracious blood suckers (Fig. 5.2).

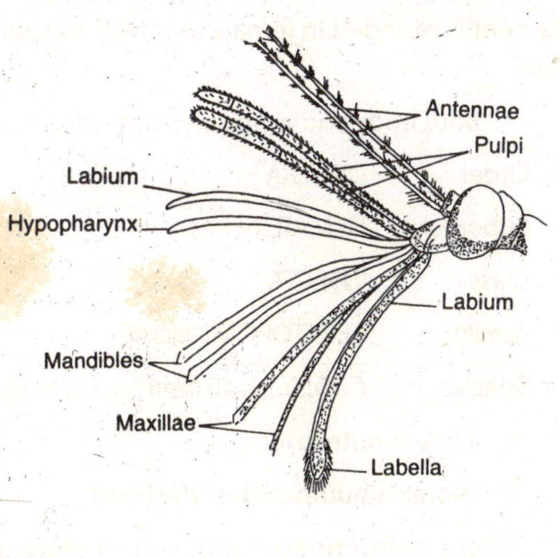

Fig. 5.2 : Mouth part of mosquito

Mouth parts of a male mosquito

1. Head bears a pair of compound eyes; a pair of fifteen jointed antennae which are thickly hairy or plumosed, a pair of four jointed pulps equal to proboscis and a sucking tube of proboscis.

2. Proboscis consists of the structures as in the female, but the maxillae and mandibles are greatly reduced — hence male mosquitoes are not voracious blood suckers.

Egg of mosquito

The raft is boat shaped and contains a large number of eggs — about 200. Each egg is ovoid, dark in colour, floats with narrow end upward and the broad end on the surface of water. To the broad end is attached a knob-like process. *Culex* egg; *Aedes* egg; *Anopheles* eggs (Fig. 5.3-5.7).

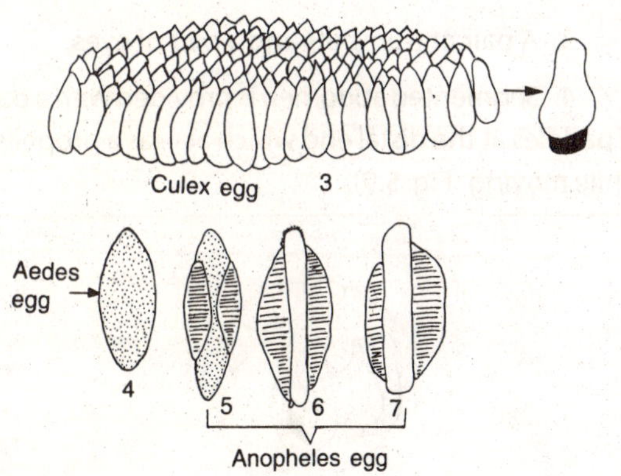

Fig. 5.3-5.7

Larva of mosquito

1. Round head with a pair of eyes and a pair of brushes near the mouth parts;

2. Wide unsegmented thorax;

3. A nine segmented abdomen ending in two pairs of gills;

4. Eighth segment bears a cylindrical syphon tube.

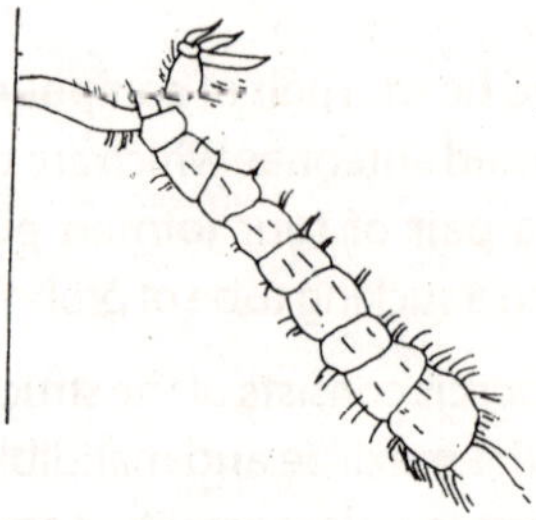

Fig. 5.8 : Larva

5. Larva rests either hanging or parallel to the surface of water with the syphon tube opening to the surface (Fig. 5.8).

Pupa of mosquito

1. Characteristic comma shaped.

2. No mouth parts, no feeding because the cephalothorax in ensheathed.

3. A pair of trumpets and a pair of eyes.

4. Segmented abdomen is provided with a pair of paddles at the distal end which acts as a propeller while moving (Fig. 5.9).

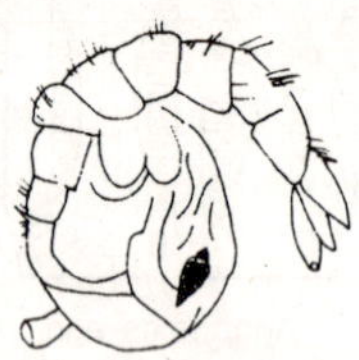

Fig. 5.9 : Pupa

Order	DIPTERA
Suborder	NEMATOCERA
Class	INSECTA
Family	PSYCHODIDAE
Species	*Phlebotomus argentipes* (sand fly)

1. Delicately built small insect.

2. Body consists of a head, three segmented thorax and ten segmented abdomen.

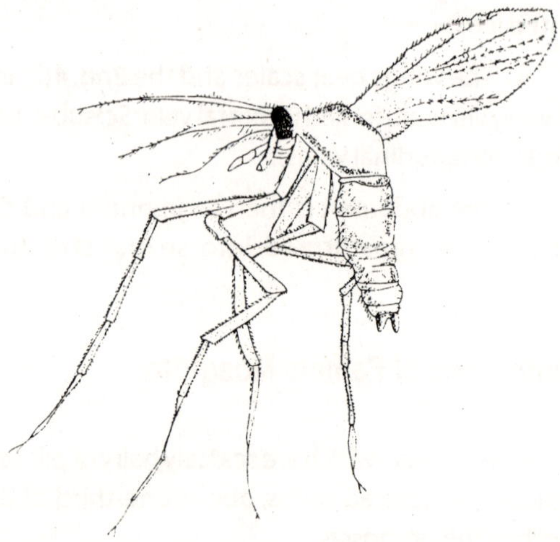

Fig. 5.10 :

3. Head bears a pair of sixteen jointed antennae, equally hairy in both sex, a pair of large compound eyes, a pair of five jointed pulp and a proboscis similar to mosquito.

4. Mesothorax bears a pair of wing, metathorax a pair of halteres and each thoracic segment bears long jointed legs (Fig. 5.10).

5. The wings are lanceolate and the second wing is forked twice.

6. The abdomen is ten segmented, the last segment is rounded in female and with claspers in male.

7. Both body and wings are covered with hair.

Order	DIPTERA
Suborder	NEMATOCERA
Class	INSECTA
Family	CERATOPOGONIDAE
Species	*Culicoides austeni* (biting midges)

1. It is a minute insect.

2. Thorax is humped over the head.

3. Long antennae plumosed in male and pylosed in female.

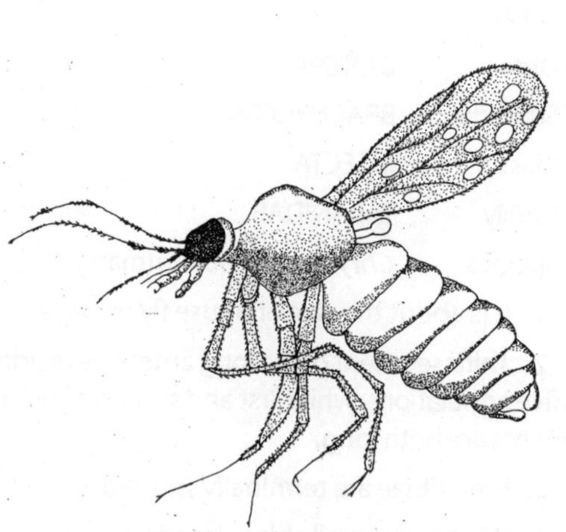

Fig. 5.11 :

4. Proboscis is short.
5. Wings are hairy and dappled (spotted).
6. Wing venation simple.
7. Anterior veins are short (Fig. 5.11).

Order	DIPTERA
Suborder	NEMATOCERA
Class	INSECTA
Family	SIMULIDAE
Species	*Simulium damnosum* (blackfly)

1. Minute, stout bodied with a humped back.
2. Stout, short legs.
3. Antennae are eleven, jointed, short and naked.
4. Conspicuous eyes.
5. Maxillary pulps are five, jointed.
6. Wings are unspotted.
7. They breed in running water.
8. Only females suck blood.
9. Mandibles function as a pair of scissors in snipping the skin. The maxillae tear open the wound. Thus the microfilariae of *onchocerca* are removed from the peripheral capillaries of host by labium-epipharynx and hypopharynx (Fig. 5.12).

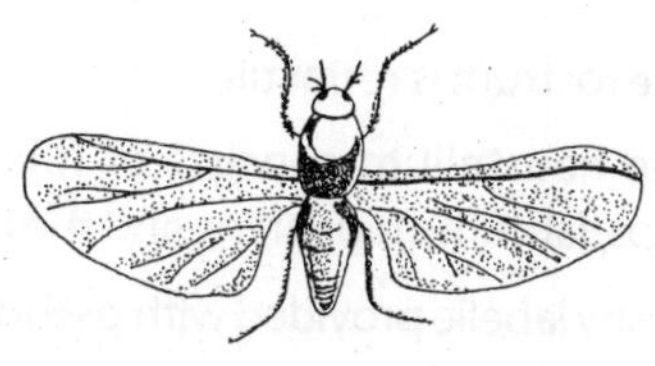

Fig. 5.12 :

Order	DIPTERA
Suborder	CYCLORRHAPHA
Class	INSECTA
Family	MUSCIDAE
Species	*Musca domestica* (common house fly)

1. Medium sized, slaty grey fly.
2 Body consists of head, three-segmented thorax and segmented abdomen.
3. Head bears a pair of compound eyes, a pair of short three-segmented antennae, with bilaterally plumosed arista, a pair of two jointed pulp and a sucking type of mouth part.
4. Thorax bears a few longitudinal stripes on the dorsum, three pairs of jointed legs and a pair of mesothoracic wings.
5. The wings are bare and the fourth wing vein curves anteriorly forming a closed apical cell.
6. Abdomen is segmented and tapering posteriorly (Fig. 5.13).

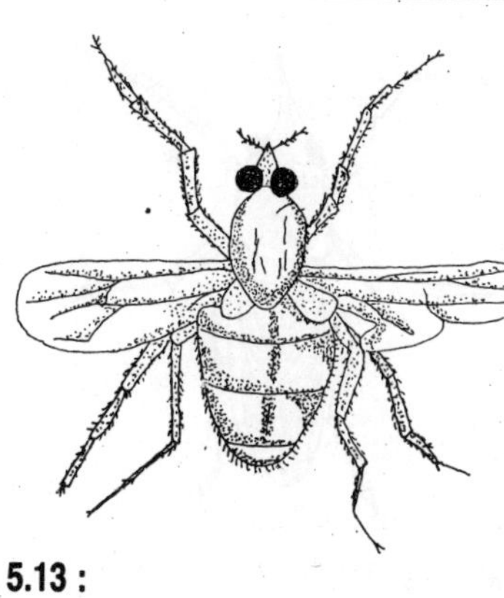

Fig. 5.13 :

Mouth parts of musca sp.

1. The rostrum Is retractile.

2. The haustellum consists of fulcrum, two jointed pulps, labrum epipharynx and the labium.

3. Fleshy labelle provided with pseudotracheal tubes.

Order	DIPTERA
Suborder	CYCLORRHAPHA
Class	INSECTA
Family	GLOSSINIDAE
Species	*Glossina palpalis* (tse tse fly)

1. It is honey brown.
2. It is of the size of a house fly.
3. The proboscis extends in front of head.
4. The wings have a characteristic venation and fold over one another straight back across the abdomen.
5. The antennae are larger and the bristles of arista are branched.
6. The maxillary palps are long, stout, extended organs with a flattened channel on their inner surface, in which proboscis lies.
7. The proboscis consists of a short, pyramidal rostrum and inconspicuous labella with rasps or teeth.
8. The labium enters the puncture wound made by the labellar teeth. Both males and females are voracious blood-feeders. The piercing organs are flexible like those of mosquitoes. They feed on capillary blood and that escape from the vessel (Fig. 5.14).

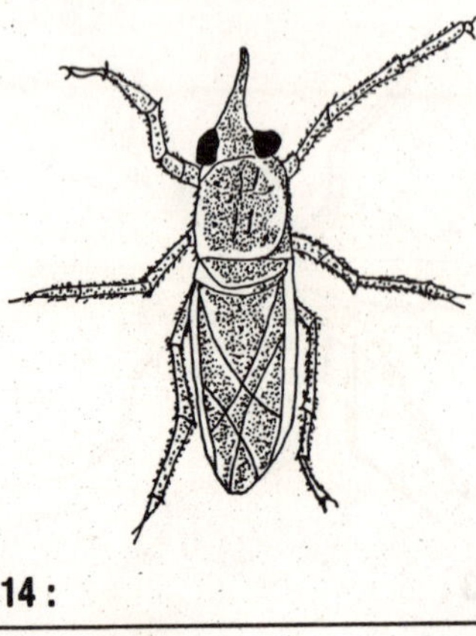

Fig. 5.14 :

Order	DIPTERA
Suborder	BRACHYCERA
Class	INSECTA
Family	TABANIDAE
Species	*Chrysops dimidiata* (mango fly)

1. It is about the size of house fly or larger.
2. Third segment of the long antennae divided into five annulations, while first and second antennal segments are both long.
3. Hind tibiae are terminally spurred.
4. Wings are usually black banded.
5. It has secondary eye-spots (Fig. 5.15).

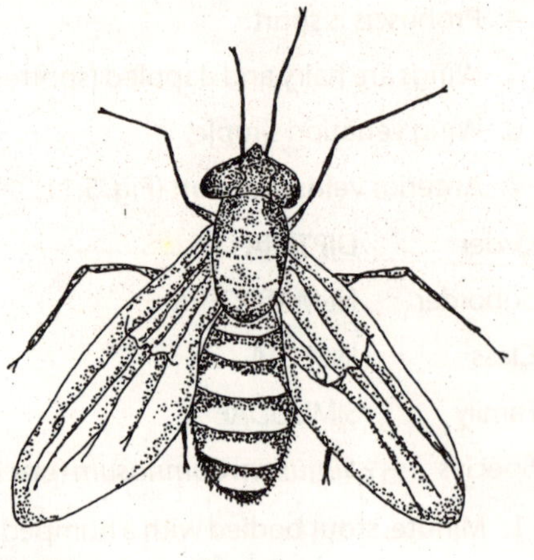

Fig. 5.15 :

Order	HETEROPTERA
Suborder	GYMNOCERATA
Class	INSECTA
Family	TRIATOMIDAE
Species	*Triatoma infestans* (assassin bug, kissing bug)

1. It is large in size.
2. Wings are well developed.
3. Ocelli present posterior to the eyes.
4. Head is more or less cone-shaped.
5. Abdomen is elongated, ovoidal and is not conspicuously flattened (Fig. 5.16).

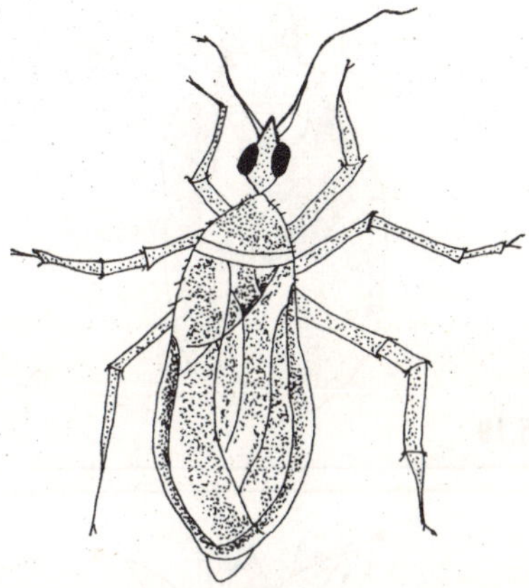

Fig. 5.16 :

Order	SIPHONAPTERA
Suborder	FRACTICIPTA and INTEGRECIPTA
Class	INSECTA
Family	PULICIDAE
Species	*Xenopsylla cheopis* (rat flea)

1. Body is laterally flattened and consists of head, three-segmented thorax and ten-segmented abdomen.

2. Head is roughly triangular and anteriorly rounded and bears two pairs of three jointed antennae in antennal groove, a pair of pigmented eyes(a).

3. Mouth parts are bitting and sucking types.

4. Genal comb at the ventral border of the head(d).

5. Thorax bears three pairs of jointed legs of which mesothorax pair is strongly developed.

6. Presence of sixteen pronatal comb at the posterior border of the prothorax(c).

7. On the 9th abdominal segment there is a saddle shaped structure known as 'pygidium'(d).

8. From the 7th abdominal segment, a pair of bristles overhangs the pygidium known as 'antipygidium'(c) (Fig. 5.17).

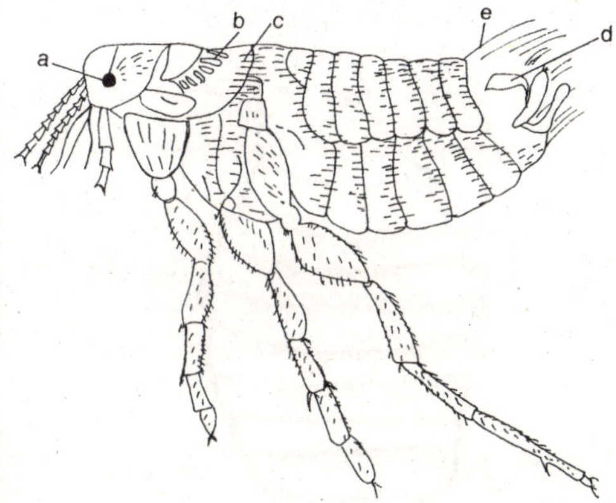

Fig. 5.17 :

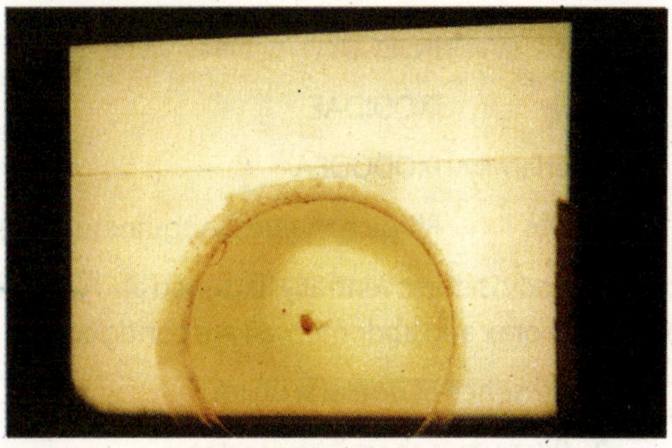

Fig. 5.17a : Xenopsylla cheopis (natural size)

Order	ANOPLURA
Suborder	GYMNOCERATA
Class	INSECTA
Species	*Pediculus humanus* (sucking louse)

1. Small insect with dorsoventrally flattened body.

2. Body consists of head, three-segmented thorax and ten-segmented abdomen.

3. Head is roughly conical, bears a five-jointed antennae, bitting and sucking types of mouth parts.

4. Thorax bears three pairs of jointed legs ending in claws(a).

5. Presence of mesothoracic spiracles.

6. Presence of large oval spiracle from second to seventh segment.

7. Abdomen is broad with festooned border.

8. Legs are provided with claws adapted for clinging to hairs or fibres (Fig. 5.18).

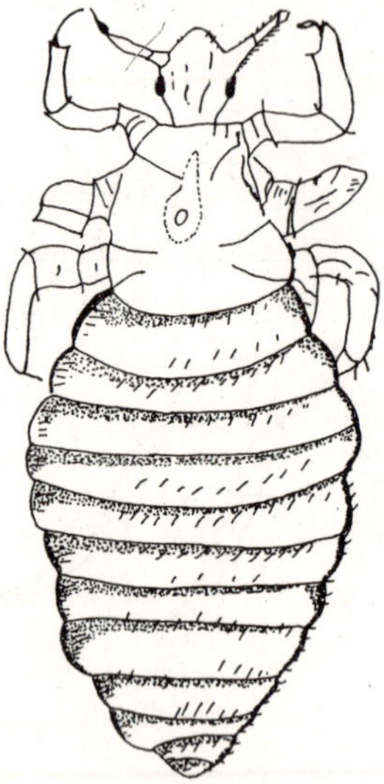

Fig. 5.18 :

Order	ACARI
Class	INSECTA
Family	IXODIDAE
Superfamily	IXODODEA
Species	Rhipicephalues sanguineus (tick)

1. Body is dorsoventrally flattened and consists of head, thorax and abdomen, all are contiguous.
2. Presence of dorsal scutum.
3. Rostrum is short (brevirostate).
4. Basis capitulum is hexagonal.
5. First coxae are deeply bifid.
6. Abdomen is festooned.
7. Eye is present.
8. Body is inornate.
9. Spiracle between third to fourth coxae (Fig. 5.19).

Order	ACARI
Calss	INSECTA
Superfamily	SARCOPTOIDEA
Family	SAROPTIDAE
Species	*Sarcoptes scabiei* (itch mite)

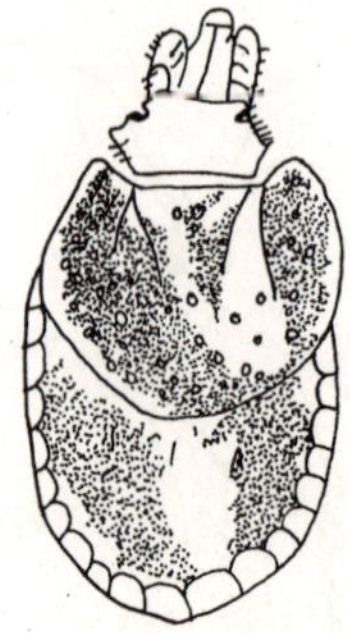

Fig. 5.19 :

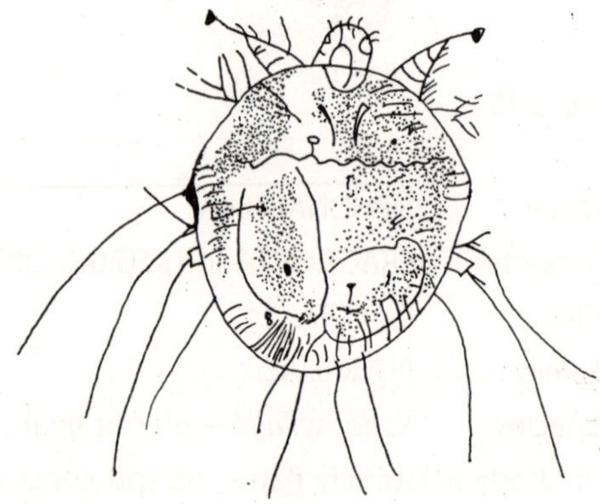

Fig. 5.20 :

1. Round or globular body.
2. Body is dirty white in colour with numerous scales and striations.
3. Anteriorly two pairs of legs coming out of the margin of the body.
4. The posterior legs remain within the body (Fig. 5.20).
5. Tarsi end in suckers.

Species *Demodex folliculorum* (mange mite)

1. Spindle-shaped body.
2. Body anteriorly round and posteriorly tapering.
3. Head, thorax and abdomen clearly differentiated.
4. Abdomen is elongated, posteriorly tapering with numerous transverse striations (Fig. 5.21).

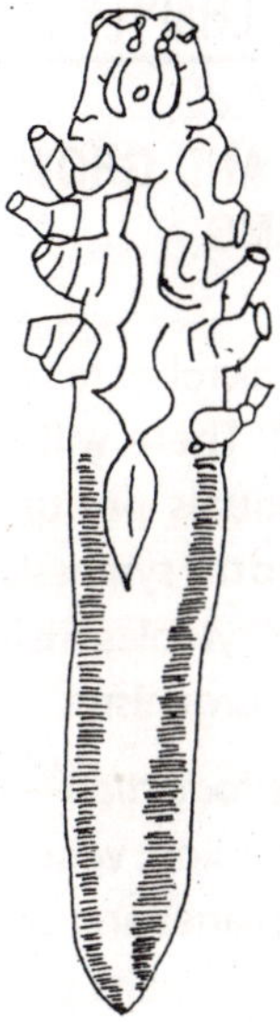

Fig. 5.21 :

VECTORS AND DISEASES TRANSMITTED		
Genus	**Common name**	**Diseases**
Anopheles (female)	Mosquito	Malaria
Anopheles, Culex, Aedes (female)	Mosquito	Filariasis
Glossina	Tse Tse fly	African sleeping sic'ness
Phlebotomus	Sand fly	Leishmaniasis (kala-azar, Oriental sore)
Culicoides	Biting midges	Loiasis, Non-periodic filariasis in Africa
Simulium (female)	Black fly	Onchocerciasis
Chrysops (female)	Mango or deer fly	Loiasis
Cyclops	Water flea	Diphyllobothriasis Dracunculosis
Musca	House fly	Amoebiasis
Xenopsylla	Rat flea	Hymenolepiasis
Triatoma	Kissing or Assassin bug	American sleeping sickness
Pediculus	Louse	Typhus fever
Ixodex	Tick	Typhus fever
Sarcoptes	Mite	Scabies

MOLLUSCS OF MEDICAL IMPORTANCE
Phylum MOLLUSCA (SNAIL)

Fleshy invertebrates lacking segmentation; with reduced body cavity, usually with an exo-skeleton which frequently takes the form of a shell.

Class GASTROPODA (SNAILS)

With asymmetrical organisation, a well-developed head having contractile tentacles and a shell spirally coiled, at least in the larval stage.

Many species are essential intermediate hosts of important trematodes of man.

Family MELANIIDAE. Fresh water species with broad snout, pedunculated eyes at outer base of tentacles (*Paragonimus westermani, Metagonimus yokogewaii*) (Fig. 5.22).

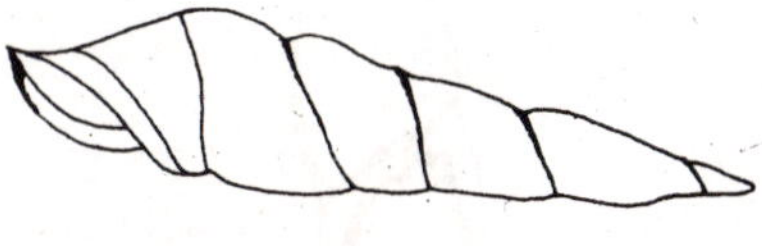

Fig. 5.22 : Melania libertina

Family CERITHIIDAE. Marine water species with broad, short contractile rostrum, widely separated tentacles, eyes or short peduncles (*Heterophyes heterophyes*).

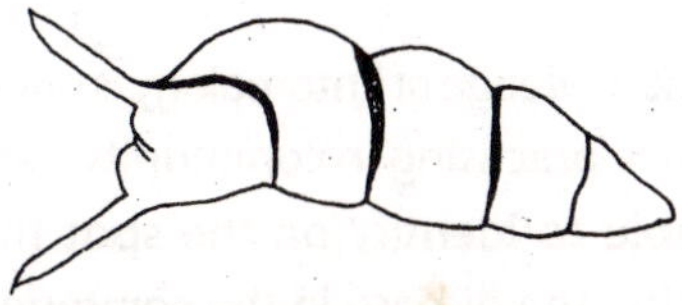

Fig. 5.23 : Lymnaea truncalata

Family LYMNAEIDAE. With oval or elongated shell. Many species of Lymnaea (Fig. 5.23) are intermediate hosts of flukes (*Fasciola hepatica*).

Subfamily SEGMENTININAE. Small discoidal shiny shells with or without internal partition. Segmentina sp, (*Fasciolopsis buski*) (Fig. 5.24).

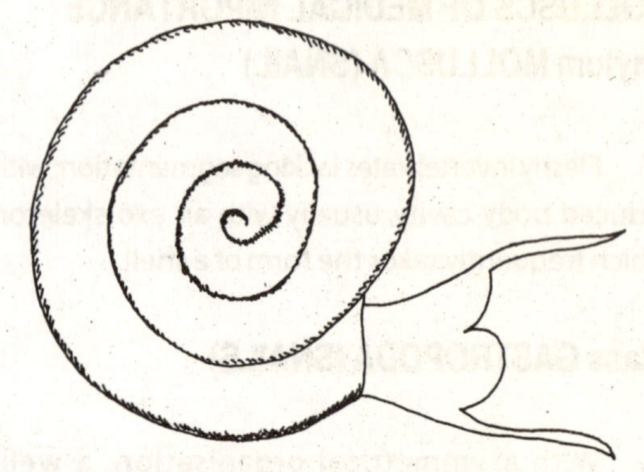

Fig. 5.24 : Segmentina

Family ANCYLIDAE. Foot oval, large; tentacles short blunt, cylindrical; with eyes at inner base; shell usually cap like. *Ferrissia tenuis (Schistosoma hematobium,* in endemic area, India) (Fig. 5.25).

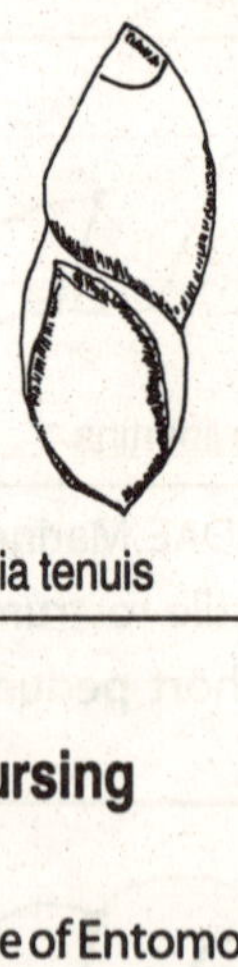

Fig. 5.25 : Ferrisia tenuis

Application to Nursing

The knowledge of Entomology is quite essential to the nurse practising in community health as she will be able to identify on the spot the vectors transmitting the disease in the community and to report immediately to the higher authorities for further necessary steps to check the transmission of the disease in the community by the destruction of the vectors. She will be able to explain in explicit language to the community about the identification of the vectors and the methods of the control during transmission of the disease.

CHAPTER 6

REPRODUCTION AND GROWTH OF MICROORGANISMS

The ability of microbes to self-multiply is known as "Reproduction". There will be increase in the number of individuals per unit volume during reproduction. Due to the synthesis of cellular material, the mass of bacterial cytoplasm is increased indicating the growth of microorganisms.

Method of Reproduction— Bacteria reproduce by simple binary division; vegetative reproduction occurs in different planes and produces many kinds of cells (clusters, chains, pairs, packets etc.). They also reproduce by budding, by conjugation, fusion of the chromatin matter of two related species of bacteria. Actinomycetes and many fungi reproduce by sporulation. One mother bacterial cell divides by the binary division in two equal daughter cells, representing a constant separation of daughter cells from the mother cell. After a certain number of generation, the mother cells age and die. This explanation does not support the concept of 'bacterial immortality'.

The rate of cell division varies among bacteria and depends on

(a) the species of bacteria,
(b) the age of the culture,
(c) the nutrient medium,
(d) temperature,
(e) carbon dioxide concentration, and
(f) other factors.

The length of the generation of *Escherichia coli, Cl. welchii, Streptococcus faecalis* is 15 minutes, while for cells of an animal tissue culture it is 24 hours. Thus bacteria reproduce almost 100 times faster than a tissue culture. The increase in the number of cells can be expressed in the following way :

1 – 2 – 4 – 8 – 16 – 32 – N number of cells.

0 – 1 – 2 – 3 – 4 – 5 – n number of generations.

The total amount of bacteria (N) after n generation will be equal to 2^n per cell of seeded material. If we take the original amount of bacteria inoculated into the nutrient medium as a single individual and the time for one division as 30 minutes then theoretically the total amount of bacteria produced for 24 hours would be equal to $N = 2^{48}$.

Reproduction of bacteria conforms to certain laws : The rate of reproduction; the size of the bacterial population expressed as logarithm of the numbers of live cells per milliliter of the medium.

There are eight principal phases of reproduction :

1. An *initial stationary phase* indicates the time from the moment of seeding the bacteria on the nutrient medium. Reproduction does not occur at this phase. The length of the initial stationary phase after seeding is 1 - 2 hours.

2. The *lag phase of reproduction.* Bacterial reproduction is not intensive during this phase, but the growth rate is accelerated. This phase lasts almost two hours.

3. *Phase of logarithmic growth.* In this phase there is a maximal division rate and decrease in cell size. The length of this period ranges from 5 to 6 hours.

4. *Phase of negative growth acceleration.* The rate of bacterial reproduction ceases to be maximal and the number of dividing cells diminishes. This phase lasts almost two hours.

5. *Maximal stationary phase* during which the number of newly produced bacteria is almost equal to the number of dead organisms. This phase continues for two hours.

6. *Accelerated death rate.* Here the equilibrium between the stationary phase and the bacterial death rate is interrupted. This continues for 3 hours.

7. *Logarithmic death rate* during which the cells die at a constant rate. This continues about 5 hours.

8. *Decelerated death rate phase.* In this phase cells which remain alive enter a dormant state.

The lengths of these periods are variable. The colibacilli divide every 15 - 17 minutes; salmonellae of enteric fever - every 23 minutes; pathogenic streptococci every 30 minutes; diphtheria bacilli — every 34 minutes and tubercle bacilli — every 18 hours.

CHAPTER 7

INFLUENCE OF ENVIRONMENTAL FACTORS ON THE GROWTH OF MICROORGANISMS

Chemical, physical, environmental and biological factors influencing the growth of microorganisms are : Nutrition, moisture, temperature, presence or absence of oxygen, osmotic pressure, pH etc.

A. *Chemical factors.* (1) Nutrition; (2) Oxygen; (3) pH; (4) Surface active substances; (5) Phenols; creosols and derivatives; (6) Dyes; (7) Salts of heavy metals; (8) Oxidising agents; (9) Formaldehyde; (10) Antiseptics.

B. *Physical factors.* (1) Moisture; (2) Temperature; (3) Dessication; (4) Light; (5) High pressure; (6) Osmotic pressure.

C. *Biological factors.* (1) Symbiosis; (2) Metabiosis; (3) Satellism; (4) Synergism; (5) Antagonism.

A. Chemical Factors

1. *Nutrition of microorganisms.*

(a) Metabolism means the digestion and utilisation of food to (i) synthesize the proteins, fats, carbohydrates and other substances of which living cells are made up and to (ii) furnish the energy necessary for living and reproduction. The protoplasm (cell substance) of all living cells is, therefore, identical. All living cells utilise and metabolise all foods by means of enzymic mechanisms. There are slight differences among different species of bacteria.

Food of microorganisms

Since Carbon (C), Hydrogen (H), Oxygen (O), Nitrogen (N), Phosphorus (P) and Sulphur (S) with smaller amounts of Magnesium (Mg), Iron (Fe), Copper (Cu), Sodium (Na), Potassium (K) and other elements are the main components of protoplasm and other structures of all living cells; the nutrients of all cells must contain all these elements. In addition, the growth factors, such as nicotinic acid (niacin), thiamine, riboflavine are utilised by bacteria in much the same manner as those cells of human body do. The composition and metabolism of human cells are similar to those of many microorganisms.

Organic compounds. Proteins, carbohydrates, fats.

Inorganic compounds. Sodium chloride, water, carbon dioxide, sulphur, iron, hydrogen.

Carbon source for growth. Like plants some non-parasitic bacteria are able to utilise carbon-dioxide (CO_2) as the main source of carbon and are called *autotrophs* (Gr. *autos* — self, *trophe* — nutrition) or *lithotrophs.* Energy is obtained in these organisms by the oxidation of inorganic compounds (Chemosynthetic autotrophs) or from the sunlight (Photosynthetic autotrophs). The majority of bacteria require organic nutrients, such as carbohydrates, amino acids, peptides or lipids to serve as the source of carbon and energy. These organisms are called *heterotrophs* (Gr. *heteros* — another, *trophe* — nutrition) or *organotrophs* and they obtain their energy by breakdown of the organic carbon source. They differ in the utilisation of organic compound. Thus some species of the genus *Pseudomonas* can utilise any one over a hundred organic compounds (sugars, acids, alcohols, etc.) as the sole source of carbon and energy. On the other hand, many bacteria are much more specific in their requirements.

Nitrogen source for growth. Bacteria differ widely in their ability to synthesize the main nitrogenous structural units - amino acids and nucleotides. Some are able to grow on ammonium salts as the sole source of nitrogen, while others require a variety of amino acids and nucleotides preformed in the medium.

2. *Influence of oxygen and redox potential*: Majority of bacteria are able to grow either *aerobically,* i.e., in presence of air and free oxygen or *anaerobically,* in the absence of oxygen and they are called as *facultative anaerobes* (e.g., *Salmonella typhi, Staphylococcus aureus,* and *Streptococcus pyogenes*). Certain other bacteria will grow only in the presence of air or free oxygen and are described as *obligate aerobes* (e.g., Tubercle bacilli, *Bacillus cereus,* common saprophytes of the soil). Still others will grow only in absence of free oxygen and are usually killed in its presence, they are known as *strict anaerobes* (e.g., *Clostridium tetani*). In the latter case, the ultimate determining factor is the state of oxidation of the environment, this being described in terms of oxidation-reduction or "redox" potential. A sufficiently low redox potential for the growth of strict anaerobes is usually provided by placing the culture media in an atmosphere of hydrogen with the complete exclusion of oxygen (e.g., McIntosh and Fieldes anaerobic jar). It has been suggested that in the presence of oxygen, a strict anaerobe is liable to produce toxic peroxides which it cannot destroy owing to lack of catalase, an enzyme present in most aerobes and facultative anaerobes. Finally, there is a group of organisms which grow best in the presence of a trace of free oxygen and often prefer an increased concentration of carbon dioxide (CO_2), these are called *microaerophilic.*

3. *Influence of hydrogen ion concentration*: *Hydrogen ion concentration.* Hydrogen atoms, when dissolved in water, immediately assume a positive electrical charge, they are called hydrogen ions and the acidity of any solution is due to them. Acids, such as hydrochloric or acetic acid, possess the property of acidity because they give off hydrogen ions (i.e., they ionize) in aqueous solutions. If a solution contains a large number of these ions, it is very acidic and it is said to have a high hydrogen ion concentration. If it is only slightly acidic or alkaline, it is said to have a low hydrogen ion concentration.

pH Hydrogen ion concentration is usually expressed by numbers used in the symbol of pH, which stands for hydrogen ion concentration. pH is an essential factor in bacterial metabolism and growth. The majority of commensal and pathogenic bacteria grow best at a neutral or very slightly alkaline reaction (pH 7.2 to 7.6). Some bacteria flourish in the presence of considerable degree of acidity and are termed acidophilic, e.g., *Lactobacillus.* Others are very sensitive to acid, but tolerant to alkali, e.g., *Vibrio cholerae.*

Most of the bacteria are rapidly killed by strong acid or alkali solutions, e.g., 5 per cent hydrochloric acid or sodium hydroxide but the mycobacteria (e.g., tubercle bacilli) are resistant to them.

According to their effect on bacteria, bactericidal chemical substances can be divided into surface active substances, phenols and their derivatives, salts of heavy metals, oxidising agents and the formaldehyde group.

4. *Surface active substances* change the electrical charges. Bacterial cells lose their negative charge and acquire positive charge which impairs the normal function of the cytoplasmic membrane.

Bactericidal substances with surface active action include fatty acids and soaps which harm only the cell wall and do not penetrate into the cell.

5. *Phenol, creosol and related derivatives* first of all injure the cell wall and then cell proteins. Some substances of this group inhibit the function of coenzyme (diphosphopiridine nucleotide) which participates in the dehydrogenation of glucose and lactic acid.

6. *Dyes* are able to inhibit the growth of bacteria. The basis of this action is the marked affinity for the phosphoric acid groups of nucleoproteins. Dyes with bactericidal properties include brilliant green, acriflavine etc.

7. *Salts of heavy metals* (lead, copper, zinc, silver, and mercury) cause coagulation of the cell proteins. Silver, gold, copper, zinc, tin, lead etc. have an oligodynamic action (bactericidal activity). Thus, for example, silver-plated objects, silverware in contact with water may render the metal bactericidal to many species of bacteria. The mechanism is that the positively charged metallic ions are adsorbed on to the negatively charged bacterial surface and alter the permeability of the cytoplasmic membrane. Thereby, the nutrition and reproduction are, possibly, disturbed. Under the influence of the salts of heavy metals, viruses may become irreversibly inactivated as they are very sensitive to these salts.

8. *Oxidising agents.* Chlorine is commonly used in decontaminating water, because chlorine acts on dehydrogenase, hydrolase, amylase, proteinase of bacteria; chloride of lime and chloroform are used as disinfectants. In medicine; iodine is used successfully as antimicrobial substance in the form of tincture iodine which oxidises proteins of bacterial cytoplasm and causes their denaturation. Potassium permanganate, hydrogen peroxide are other oxidising agents.

Many species of viruses are resistant to heat, chloroform, ethyl and methyl alcohol and volatile oils. All viruses are resistant to 50 per cent glycerine, except Rinderpest virus, sodium hydroxide, chloride of lime and chlorine can destroy viruses as they are oxidising agents.

9. *Formalin* (40 per cent formaldehyde) has bactericidal effect, because it possibly unites with the

amino groups of proteins and brings out denaturation of proteins. Formaldehyde destroys both the vegetative forms and the spores of bacteria. It is also used to decontaminate diphtheria and tetanus toxins and at the same time it detoxifies the toxins transforming them into *anatoxins* (toxoids). Phage and tobacco mosaic virus inactivated by formalin can sometimes renew their infectivity.

10. Antiseptic is of great importance in medical practice. The science of antiseptics played a great role in the development of surgery, brought a decrease in the number of post-operative complications like gas gangrene.

B. Physical Factors

1. *Moisture.* Since the bacterial cell consists of water, moisture is essential for its growth. Drying in air is injurious to many microorganisms; it may prevent the growth of microorganisms and may not kill them. One method adopted by microbiologists to keep certain microorganisms alive for long periods (20 years or more) is to dry them and store them in a refrigerated vacuum. Even delicate, non-sporing organisms may survive drying for many years if they are desiccated at a high vacuum (0.01 mm. Hg. or less) in sealed glass ampoule which is stored at room temperature in the dark. This is the basis of lypholisation or freeze drying process of preserving bacterial cultures or vaccines and viral vaccines in the laboratory or also during long-distance transport. Quick freezing of bacterial and viral suspension at a very low temperature provokes conditions at which crystals do not form and subsequent disruption of the microorganisms does not occur.

Certain fragile microorganisms, *Neisseria gonorrhoeae* (gonococci) causing gonorrhoea, *Treponema pallidum* causing syphilis, *Entamoeba* histolytica causing amoebic dysentery, die almost at once when subjected to drying, while *tubercle bacilli, Staphylococcus aureus* and small pox virus may survive for several months in sputum, pus, crust, respectively.

2. *Temperature.* Low temperatures halt putrefying and fermentative processes. The process of metabolism is inhibited, as a result bacteria die and the cells are destroyed under the influence of the formation of ice crystals during freezing. *Vibrio cholerae* loses its viability at a temperature of – 32°C. Some species of bacteria, remain viable at a temperature of liquid air –190°C and of liquid hydrogen (–253°C). *Diphtheria bacilli* are able to withstand freezing for 3 months and enteric fever bacteria (*Salmonella typhi*) are able to live long in ice. Bacillus spores withstand a temperature of –253°C for 3 days. Many microorganisms remain viable at low temperature and viruses are especially resistant to low temperatures. Thus, for example, Japanese encephalitis virus in 10% brain suspension does not lose its pathogenicity at –70°C for a year; the causative agents of Influenza and Trachoma at –70°C for 6 months and Coxsachie virus at –40°C for 1.5 years.

Only certain species of pathogenic bacteria are very sensitive to low temperature (e.g., meningococci, gonococci). During short periods of cooling, these species die quite rapidly. This is taken into account in laboratory diagnosis and the specimens for the presence of meningococci or gonococci should be sent to the laboratory protected from cold. Some microorganisms can grow best at a low temperature (4° to 10°C) and are said to be psychrophilic, whereas those bacteria growing best at higher temperature (from 20°C to 37°C) are called mesophils.

Most of the pathogenic non-sporing bacteria are killed at 58°C to 60°C for 30-60 minutes. Bacillus spores can withstand boiling (100°C) from a few minutes to 3 hours, but under the effect of dry heat at 160°C-170°C only 60 - 90 minutes. Heating at 121°C (15 lbs per square inch in gauge pressure) kills the bacteria and their spores within 20 - 30 minutes.

Some microorganisms will grow only at high temperatures ranging from 45°C to 75°C and are called thermophilic, e.g., *Bacillus stearothermophilus.*

The bactericidal action of high temperature is due to the inhibition of the catalase, oxidase, dehydrogenase activity, protein denaturation and an interruption of the osmotic pressure. High temperature causes rapid destruction of viruses, but some of the viruses (viruses of serum hepatitis, poliomyelitis) are resistant to environmental factors. They remain viable long in water, in the feces of patients or carriers and are resistant to heat at 60°C and to small concentration of chlorine in water.

3. *Dessication.* Dessication is accompanied by dehydration of the cytoplasm and denaturation of bacterial proteins. Gonococci, meningococci, treponema, leptospira and phages are sensitive to dessication. *Vibrio cholerae* persist for 2 days on exposure to dessication; dysentery bacteria for 7; plague bacilli for 8, diphtheria bacilli for 30; bacilli for enteric fever for 70; staphylococci and tubercle bacilli for 90 days. The dry sputum of tubercular patients remains infectious for 10 months.

Dessication in a vacuum at a low temperature does not kill bacteria, rickettsiae, viruses. This method of preserving cultures is employed in the manufacture of stable long storage of live vaccines against tuberculosis, plague, brucellosis, small pox, influenza.

4. *Light.* Direct sunlight has the greatest bactericidal action. Different kinds of light have bactericidal or sterilizing effects. They are ultraviolet rays (electromagnetic rays with a wave length of 200-300 mμ); X-rays (electromagnetic rays with a wave length of 0.005 - 1 mμ); gamma rays (short wave X-rays); beta particles or cathode rays (high speed electrons); alpha particles (high speed helium nuclei) and neutrons. Rays of short waves have a high bactericidal effect and are used for the disinfection of wards, infectious material, for the conservation of products, the preparation of vaccine, treating operation and maternity wards. Viruses are very quickly inactivated under the influence of ultraviolet rays with a wave length of 200-300 mμ. These waves are absorbed by the nucleic acid of viruses. Longer waves are weaker and do not render viruses harmless. Viruses in comparison to bacteria are less resistant to X-rays and gamma rays. Beta-rays are more markedly viricidal.

5. *High pressure and mechanical injury to microbes.* Bacteria withstand easily atmospheric pressure. Some bacteria, yeasts and moulds withstand a pressure of 3,000 atmospheric pressure. The movement of liquid media has a harmful effect on microbes. The movement of water in rivers and streams, undulations in stagnant water are important factors in self-purification of reservoirs from microbes. *Ultrasonic oscillation* (waves with a frequency of about 20,000 hertz per second) has a bactericidal activity and it is used for the preparation of vaccines and disinfection of various objects.

6. *Osmotic pressure.* Like other living cells, bacteria have a semipermeable cytoplasmic membrane which is subjected to osmotic pressure. Bacteria are very tolerant of changes in the osmotic pressure of their environment and can grow in media with widely varying contents of salts, sugar and other such solutes because of the thickness and mechanical strength of their walls. For most species, the upper limit of sodium chloride concentration permitting growth lies between 5 and 15 per cent, though holophilic (or osmophilic) species occur which can grow at higher concentration up to saturation. Sudden exposure of bacteria to solution of high concentration (e.g., 2 - 25 per cent sodium chloride) may cause plasmolysis (i.e., temporary shrinkage of the protoplast and its retraction from cell wall due to osmotic withdrawal of water, this occurs much more rapidly in Gram-negative than in Gram-positive bacteria). Sudden transfer from a concentrated to a weak solution, or to distilled water, may cause plasmolysis i.e., swelling and bursting of cell through excessive imbibition of water.

C. Biological Factors

1. *Symbiosis* is an intimate mutually beneficial relation of organisms of different species. They develop together better than separately. Sometimes, the adaptation of two organisms becomes so close that they lose their ability to exist separately (symbiosis of the fungus and blue green algae).

2. *Metabiosis* is one type of relationship in which an organism continues the process caused by another organism, liberating it from all its life activities and thus creating conditions for its own further development (nitrifying bacteria).

3. *Satellism*, a symbiont known as the favourable microbe, accelerates the growth of the other (some yeasts producing amino acids, vitamins etc. enhance the growth of microbes which are very specific regarding their nutrient requirements).

4. In *Synergism*, there is an increase in the physiological function of microbial association (Borrelia and fusobacterium).

5. In *antagonism* there is struggle for oxygen, nutrients and a habitat (antibiotics).

Application to Nursing

The nurse will use the methods of the control of the microorganisms by the knowledge of the relation of microorganisms to their environmental factors.

For example, high temperatures affect the living cell structures causing death; pathogenic bacteria are capable to produce infection or toxin according to the presence or absence of oxygen. The inhibition or destruction of microorganisms depends upon the removal of food, water and oxygen. In nursing practice, the microbial growth can be controlled by altering the temperature and subjecting the microorganisms to disinfectants.

In nursing situations (operating rooms, nurseries, communicable disease units, isolation wards, intensive care units) microorganisms can be destroyed by physical environmental factors (X-rays, gamma rays etc.). Introduction of antiseptics in surgical practice prevented the access of microbes into the wounds. Aseptics are attained by disinfection of the air and equipments of the operating room, by sterilisation of surgical instruments and materials and by disinfecting the hands of surgeon and the skin of the operating field.

Modern methods of aseptics have been well perfected, by which almost all operations are accompanied by primary healing of wounds without suppuration and the post-operative septicemia has been completely eliminated.

The nurse would be able to adopt the suitable method to control the growth of microorganisms according to their relationship with the environment. The growth of microorganisms can be slowed down or completely stopped by altering the environmental growth factors. The high temperature can affect the structure of the living bacterial cells, so that they may be completely destroyed. Anaerobic bacteria can grow very well in absence of oxygen and elaborate the toxin which is responsible for the pathogenic effect. In the presence of oxygen, the same bacteria cannot produce such toxin and, hence, they are not pathogenic. It may not be always possible to inhibit or destroy microorganisms by simple removal of food, oxygen, water. In nursing practice, the microbial growth can be controlled primarily by subjecting the microorganisms to the sterilisation and disinfection. Ultraviolet rays can be sometimes used to kill the microorganisms in nursing situations (operation rooms, nurseries, communicable diseases).

CHAPTER 8

ISOLATION OF BACTERIA IN PURE CULTURE

To determine accurately the specific causative agent of the disease by its diagnostic characters, the microbiologist must isolate a single bacterium, in pure form, from other bacteria with which it is mixed, as an alchemist purifies the metal from other metals or impurities. In clinical specimens (sputum, stool, urine etc.), the mixed microorganisms are common, may mask and confuse the diagnostic results. To avoid this confusion, a pure culture is needed. The extraneous organisms may change the pH, may damage or kill the desired microorganisms. A pure culture is the one which contains only one kind of microorganisms whereas a *mixed culture* contains two or more kinds of microorganisms. Pure culture may be compared to a bed of roses obtained in pure culture of roses.

The methods, used to isolate the bacteria in pure culture, consist of separating a single living bacterial cell and allowing it to multiply on a suitable culture medium, usually in a solid medium, to form a pure colony. Bacteria multiply very rapidly, so that a single bacterial cell deposited on a solid medium gives rise to a mass which is called a colony.

1. *Streaking or Plating* (inoculation of culture media). If the material containing bacteria is streaked several times on the surface of a solid medium with a platinum loop, without recharging, fewer and fewer bacterial cells will remain on the loop as successive streaks are made and finally it may deposit a single bacterial cell on the surface. This procedure will thus give separate colonies of the organisms present in the material.

2. *Dilution and Plating.* When the bacterial content of the material is expected to be high (e.g., feces), it is diluted with sterile nutrient broth or saline before plating.

3. *Use of selective medium.* Media which promote the growth of one type of organisms and inhibit or retard the growth of others are known as "Selective Media". Inhibiting substances like brilliant green, gentian violet, bile salts, potassium tellurite and penicillin are widely used in the preparation of such media.

4. *Differential Sterilisation by chemicals.* An example of this method is cultivation of *Tubercle bacilli* from sputum (which contains numerous other organisms) after preliminary treatment with dilute mineral acid or alkali. In Petroff's method, the specimen of sputum is mixed with three or four times its volume of 4 per cent sodium hydroxide solution, incubated for one half an hour at 37°C and centrifuged. The deposit is neutralised, in the presence of an indicator, by dilute hydrochloric acid and then seeded on a suitable medium. This treatment kills all other organisms except tubercle bacilli which are resistant to the action of dilute mineral acids, alkalis and other chemicals. "Antiformin" (Sodium hydroxide) can also be used instead of a dilute alkali.

5. *Differential sterilisation by heat.* This method is employed where the organisms to be obtained in pure culture are more resistant to heat than others present in the material, e.g., separation of spore bearing bacilli (which are more resistant to heat) from the non-spore bearers. The material is heated at 60°C for 30 minutes, cooled and then inoculated in a suitable medium. Only the spore-bearers which have survived, will grow.

6. *Inoculation of a susceptible animal.* This method is employed to isolate pathogenic microorganisms which are not easily grown on culture media or which are readily overgrown by the contaminating organisms. As example, we may quote isolation of tubercle bacilli from pus, peritoneal and pleural fluids by inoculating a guinea-pig and isolation of pneumococci by inoculating a mouse. In the latter case, the contaminating organisms are rapidly killed in the animal body whereas the pathogenic organisms multiply and can be recovered in pure culture from the tissues.

CHAPTER 9

SYSTEMATIC STUDY OF BACTERIA (Identification of Bacteria)

The identification of the bacteria isolated from a specimen may be carried out by the following studies:

1. *Morphology and staining* serve as preliminary criteria. The gram-stained smear shows the gram-

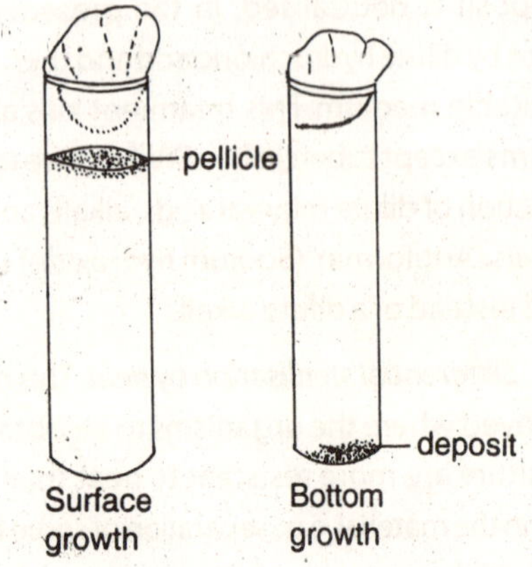

Fig. 9.1 : Bacterial growth in liquid medium

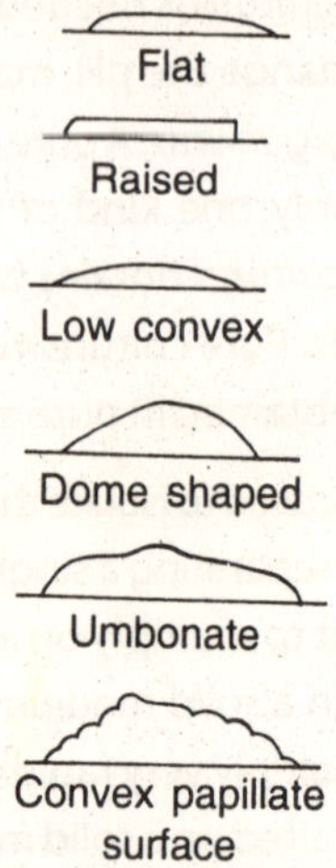

Fig. 9.2 : Colony appearance on solid medium

reaction, size, shape, groupings of the bacteria and intracellular position of the endospore. Special staining reaction can reveal the presence of capsule. Hanging drop wet preparation can be used to study the motility of bacteria. An unstained wet film is examined under dark ground illumination microscope to observe the exact morphology of delicate spirochaete. A smear is stained by Ziehl-Neelsen method to demonstrate the acid fast staining reaction.

2. *Cultural characteristics*. The growth requirement and the appearance of colonies on media to the naked eye are further criteria to assist the identification of bacteria. A culture is a growth of bacterium on artificial nutrient medium or culture medium prepared in the laboratory. Attempts are made to grow (to cultivate or culture) the bacteria on media of different compositions (glucose, inorganic salts mixture, meat extract or meat infusion with blood incubated under a variety of conditions (different temperatures, pH) in the presence of atmospheric oxygen (aerobically) or in it's absence (anaerobically). The ability or inability to grow on medium containing a selective inhibitor (e.g., bile salt, optochin, tellurite, bacitracin, malachite green, low pH, high pH) may also be useful to identify the bacteria.

The growth of bacteria in liquid culture medium (e.g., nutrient broth) may show:

(1) a uniform turbidity; (2) little deposit at the bottom; (3) surface growth(pellicle formation) (Fig. 9.1).

The appearance of the discrete masses of growth or *colonies* that can be grown from isolated bacteria on the surface of the solid medium (nutrient agar) can be used to study the size of the colonies (diameter in mm), their outline (whether circular, entire, indented or wavy or rhizoid), their elevation (low convex, high convex, flat, plateau - like, umbonate, or nodular), their transparency (clear and transparent) or opaque, whether they are colourless (white or pigmented) or whether they produce any change in the medium (e.g., haemolysis in the blood agar medium) (Fig. 9.2).

3. *Biochemical reactions*, e.g., fermentation of various sugars (carbohydrates). Morphology and cultural characters may not be able to distinguish some species of bacteria; but these same species may exhibit distinct differences in their biochemical reactions, e.g., typhoid and paratyphoid bacilli (glucose and mannitol are fermented without gas production by typhoid bacilli, whereas paratyphoid bacilli produce

acid and gas). Certain serotypes of the salmonella group may resemble one another in fermentation properties.

The growth of the bacteria in liquid medium will ferment particular sugars (glucose, lactose, mannitol) with the production of acid, which is detected by the change of colour of Andrede's indicator dye incorporated in the medium, the gas production is detected by the collection of air bubble in a small inverted tube (Durham's tube) immersed in the medium. Other tests are used to find out the ability of a bacterium to produce particular end products, e.g., Indole, hydrogen sulphide, nitrite and certain enzymes (oxidase, catalase, urease, gelatinase, collagenase, lecithinase, lipase) in culture media.

4. *Antigenic characters.* Species or types of bacteria can be easily, distinctly identified by "specific antibody reactions" observed in serological tests performed on a glass slide. This specific antibody (antiserum) is obtained from the animal (rabbit) immunised against a particular type of microorganism which agglutinates with the same antiserum. An unknown bacterium may thus be identified by demonstrating its reaction with one out of a number of standard known antisera. Similarly, the serum of a person suffering from a bacterial infection may contain specific antibody. The nature of the infection may thus be diagnosed by demonstrating that the patient's serum agglutinates one out of a number of known antigens of laboratory cultures, e.g., Widal test in Typhoid fever.

5. *Typing of bacteria : Bacteriophage sensitivity.* A single bacterial pathogenic species may include different types of strains which are distinguishable in minor characters. Recognition of the type of a strain isolated from a patient may be of great importance in epidemiological studies related to the source and the spread of the infection in the community. The typing of strains may be done by special biochemical or serological tests. Another important method of typing is by testing the susceptibility of the culture to lysis by each of a set of type specific, lytic bacteriophages.

6. *Animal pathogenicity.* Final identification of a toxigenic strain of tetanus bacillus may be done by injecting the toxin liberated by tetanus bacillus into the base of the tail of two mice, one of them has already been protected by prior injection of specific antiserum to tetanus toxin (a soluble poisonous protein secreted by the tetanus bacilli). The unprotected mouse shows the symptoms of tetanus, whereas the protected one without any tetanus symptoms identifies the culture as an organism producing tetanus toxin, as the injected antiserum neutralised toxin liberated by tetanus bacilli. Similarly, diphtheria bacillus is also identified by inflammation and necrosis of the skin of guinea pig brought about by diphtheria exotoxin.

7. *Antibiotic sensitivity.* The organism is tested for its ability to grow on artificial nutrient media containing different antibiotics and chemotherapeutic agents in different concentrations. In *disk diffusion test*, the culture to be examined is inoculated confluently over the surface of an agar plate and six to ten paper disks containing different antibiotics are placed in different areas of the plate. Antibiotic diffuses outwards from each disk into surrounding agar. On incubation, the bacteria grow on areas of the plate except those around the antibiotic disks to which they are sensitive. The width of each growth-free "zone of inhibition" is a measure of the degree of the sensitivity of the drug.

Information about the sensitivity patterns of strains (*antibiograms*) isolated from the patient is required as a guide to the *drug of choice for therapy* and may also be used as an epidemiological marker in tracing hospital cross-infection.

Application in Nursing

In daily nursing practice in the hospital, the knowledge of the identification of bacteria is very much essential to interpret "culture and sensitivity" test of the organism isolated in the microbiological diagnostic laboratory from the specimens (urine, stool, pus, sputum, blood, cerebrospinal fluid — CSF etc.) collected from the patients. The nurse will be able to understand clearly — with her sound knowledge of nursing microbiology acquired during her training — the causative agent of the disease, the information about the antibiotics to which the isolate (causative agent) is sensitive and to assist the physician by reporting immediately so that he can choose the drug for therapy for speedy recovery of the patient and he can also use the antibiogram as the epidemiological marker in tracing out the hospital cross-infection.

Nurse practising in community health should have knowledge of the serological typing, bacteriophage typing and antibiotic sensitivity test under the method of identification of the microorganisms, to recognise the type of strain isolated in certain localities of the communities and to conduct the epidemiological studies relating to the source and spread of the infection in the community.

CHAPTER 10

MICROBIAL PATHOGENICITY : SOURCES AND SPREAD OF INFECTION IN COMMUNITY

Pathogenicity is the ability of the microbes to initiate the infection. It requires three attributes :

1. *Transmissibility* or *communicability* from one host or reservoir to a fresh host;

2. *Infectivity* or the ability to breach the new host's defences;

3. *Virulence*, a variable factor that may enhance or reduce the capacity of the pathogen to cause overt infection.

Pathogens (Pathogenic microorganisms) cause diseases and they may be (a) opportunistic, or (b) true pathogens.

Opportunistic Pathogens. Many commensal or non-pathogenic microorganisms may be transmissible from person to person or derived from the environment and are present, in large numbers, on the skin, in the upper respiratory tract, in the intestine and lower urinogenital tract hence they are normal microflora of the body and sometimes they may act against invading pathogenic microorganisms and are unable to invade the tissues as they cannot overcome the healthy body defences. Sometimes, when the body defence mechanism is lowered and when these commensals leave their natural habitat and reach other parts of the body, e.g., coliform bacilli (*Escherichia coli*) are mostly harmless commensals in the intestine, but they may cause infection in the urinary tract; similarly *Clostridium welchii*, an intestinal commensal, can cause gangrene in locally damaged tissues; *Streptococcus viridans* is the commensal of the mouth; after tooth extraction they may invade the blood stream and settle on previously damaged heart valves as opportunistic pathogens.

True Pathogens. They are those microorganisms which are able to overcome the normal body defence mechanism and initiate the infection.

Several properties are essential for pathogenicity of microorganisms :

(a) *Transmissibility.* The ability of a pathogen to grow profusely in the body and to be shed in large numbers in body fluids or secretions which are capable of dissemination and reach new host after surviving in the adverse conditions, e.g., desiccation in the dry dust.

(b) *Infectivity.* Pathogenic microbes are able to initiate the infection by penetrating the healthy body's first line of defence, that is, skin, mucous membranes to which they readily gain access. To infect a person, only a few of the pathogens can cross the protective barriers in the respiratory and alimentary tracts. The pathogen may initiate a localised lesion at the site of infection, e.g., staphylococcal boil on the skin or streptococcal pharyngitis in the throat.

The capacity of the microbes to initiate the infection is mostly related to the dosage of the pathogen, its phase of growth and its virulence factors. In salmonella family, the infecting dose of *Salmonella typhi* is very small; whereas large number of *S. typhimurium* (food poisoning salmonellae) must be ingested to produce acute vomiting and diarrhoea. Microorganisms which are in the logarithmic stage of growth are more likely to overcome host resistance than those in the latent phase : *Streptococcus pyogenes* is more infective when transferred directly from a person with a sore throat than when it is inhaled after drying in dust particles, because *Strepto pyogenes* has the capsular M protein (antiphagocytic component) during the active phase of sore throat infection.

(c) *Virulence.* The virulence of a pathogen is the ability to kill susceptible animals(mouse, guinea pig etc.). The tubercle bacillus isolated from Indian patients with tuberculosis are often less virulent to the guinea pigs than strains isolated in Britain. The assessment of virulence for animal is not necessarily applicable to virulence of man. *Shigella dysenteriae* causes much more severe infection than *Sh.sonnei.* Similarly, the *gravis* strain of *Corynebacterium diphtheriae* causes more deaths than the *mitis* strain. Type 1 poliovirus is more likely to initiate epidemics of paralytic poliomyelitis than is type 2.

Pathogenesis

Pathogenic bacteria produce diseases by virtue of one or both of the main attributes : Toxigenecity and invasiveness.

Toxigenecity

Toxins may be (a) exotoxins or (b) endotoxins.

(a) *Exotoxins.* German and French workers were first to prove that the products of the diphtheria bacilli, diffused from the local infection or injected as bacteria-free filtrates of cultured diphtheria bacilli, could produce widespread systemic damage in guinea pigs. The toxin produced by diphtheria bacilli in the throat is carried by the blood stream (toxaemia) throughout the body. When the bacteria grow actively in broth culture, they secrete apparently the poison which is called as "exotoxin". Other bacteria which secrete highly potent toxins are tetanus bacilli and *Clostridium botulinum.* So 1.0 mg. of tetanus and botulinal toxin can kill more than one million guinea pigs and it is estimated that 3 kg of botulinal toxin can kill the world population.

Exotoxins are mainly produced by gram-positive bacilli (except Shigella bacillus neurotoxin and cholera enterotoxin) and have special affinity for specific tissues; for example, tetanus, botulinal and diphtheria toxins all affect different parts of the nervous system : tetanus toxin affects control mechanisms that govern motor cells in the anterior columns of the spinal cord; botulinal toxin paralyses cranial nerves by blocking the transmission of effector messages from their endings; and diphtheria toxin has affinity for peripheral nerve ending as well as for specialised tissues like heart muscle.

Exotoxins behave like enzymes : alpha toxin of *Cl. welchii* is a phospholipase (lecithinase C) which acts on phospholipids of cell membrane; diphtheria toxins depress the formation and / or release of acetylcholine in different parts of the nervous system.

(b) *Endotoxins*. They are complex phospholipid polysaccharide - protein macromolecules. Most of the endotoxins are lipopolysaccharides and additional endotoxin released by few gram-negative pathogenic bacteria (*Yersinia pestis* and *Bordetella pertussis*) is protein in nature and is present in the bacterial cytoplasm. They are released only after natural autolysis or artificial disruption of bacterial cells and therefore they are called *endotoxins*. Typical endotoxins are particularly associated with gram-negative bacteria (salmonella, shigella, escherichia, neisseria) and are distinguishable from exotoxins by the following properties :

1. They are present in the outer layer of the bacterial cell wall;

2. They are heat stable;

3. They are much less toxic and specific in their cytotoxic effects than exotoxins;

4. They cannot be converted into toxoids;

5 Homologous antibodies cannot render them non-toxic, if combined.

The complex phospholipid-polysaccharide-protein molecule can be separated by phenol extraction into :

(a) lipopolysaccharide moiety,

(b) protein fraction,

(c) phospholipid fraction.

The lipopolysaccharide moiety can be split further into different sugars including those that determine the antigenic specificity of the endotoxin and lipid which is mainly responsible for the toxicity.

Pyrogenic effect (fever) is the toxic effect produced by the smallest amount of endotoxin. If 0.002 μ g endotoxin per kg body weight is injected intravenously into rabbit or man, it causes within 15 minutes an elevation of body temperature which lasts for several hours.

Invasiveness. It is the other main attribute of pathogenic bacteria. It is its capacity to invade and multiply in the healthy tissues, e.g., pneumococcus produces the disease depending entirely upon the quality of invasiveness just as botulinus bacillus depends entirely on its toxigenicity. Thus, the diphtheria bacillus must be initially invasive in order to establish itself in the tissues of the oropharynx, where it manufactures its toxin; the *gravis* strain of diphtheria bacillus has the greater capacity to invade and multiply in the tissues with a consequent greater production of toxin than *mitis* strain. *Strepto. pyogenes* is mainly an invasive pathogen. It also produces an erythrogenic toxin which is responsible for the rash of the scarlet fever. The invasiveness of *Staph. aureus, Strepto. pyogenes* and *Cl. welchii* is due to their production of cytolytic and leucocidal toxins which enable them to breach tissue barriers and protect themselves against phagocytosis.

Pathogenic bacteria which are predominantly invasive are :

1. The *first category* — The pathogenic gram positive cocci initially attract phagocytes by chemotactic mechanisms, resist phagocytosis; but ultimately they may be engulfed and destroyed by phagocytes.

2. The *second category* — Tubercle bacilli, typhoid, brucella bacilli, though they are readily phagocytosed are more resistant to destruction when within phagocytes and become intracellular parasites which are disseminated by phagocytes throughout the body. There is fight between phagocytes and antiphagocytic bacteria; when specific antibody acting as opsonins come to the aid of the phagocytes in destroying the antiphagocytic bacteria, then these bacteria are destroyed by phagocytes and there is a dramatic fall in temperature — the crisis — as observed in pneumococcal pneumonia. In infection with intracellular parasites there is clinical illness that persists for some weeks with low fever.

Capsules and Pathogenicity. The bacterial capsule plays an important role in conferring the virulence on bacteria by enabling them to resist phagocytosis and bactericidal substances in body fluids, therefore the capsulation is important for the virulence of pneumococci, streptococci of Group A and Group C, the anthrax bacillus, the plague bacillus, *Kbesiella pneumoniae* and *Haemophilus influenzae.*

It has been observed that the non-capsulate bacteria are rapidly phagocytosed and, within a few hours, are mostly destroyed, whereas the capsulate bacteria remain free and soon multiply to large numbers. The mechanism of the antiphagocytic property of capsulate bacteria is not known, but it may be that the lipid containing cell membrane of the phagocyte's pseudopodia is inhibited from making contact with the hydrated capsule gel because of the surface charge. However, heavily capsulate harmless saprophytic bacteria and some non-virulent strains of bacillus anthracis and plague bacilli are fairly susceptible to phagocytosis.

Aggressins — Other non-toxic protective or aggressive factors that may contribute to the ability of capsulate and non-capsulate pathogens to invade and multiply in the host tissues are :

1. *Hyaluronidase* or spreading factor, is an enzyme that dissolves the hyaluronic acid or cement like substances that binds cells together and so allows pathogens (*Strepto. pyogenes, Staph. aureus*) to permeate through the tissues.

2. *Coagulase prothrombin* — like enzyme produced by all pathogenic staphylococci may help to protect the pathogen from phagocytosis into two ways :

(a) by forming fibrin barriers around staphylococci and staphylococcal lesions, and

(b) by inactivating the bactericidal substance present in the normal blood serum.

3. *Streptokinase* secreted by *Strepto. pyogenes* may promote the spreading of streptococcal lesions.

4. *Collagenase*, produced by *Cl. welchii*, may play some part in the pathogenesis of gas gangrene.

5. *Neuraminidase* produced by some bacteria and viruses acts on mucoproteins of cell surface and may facilitate attacks on the cell.

Organotropism. The affinity of many pathogenic microbes for specific tissues or organs is known as organotropism. Pneumococcus and meningococcus both have the natural habitat in the nasopharynx, but the virulent pneumococcus has a predilection for lung tissues and the meningococcus for the meninges of the brain, whereas gonococcus mainly affects the mucosa of urethra. *Brucella abortus* localises in the uterus of cows because of the presence of erythritol, a growth factor for *Br. abortus*, in the bovine placenta. However, *Coxiella burnetti* and chlamydiae localise in the uterus but they do not use erythritol.

Comparative Characteristics of Toxins

Exotoxins	Endotoxins
1. Composed of proteins, have the properties of enzymes, some have been obtained in crystalline state.	1. Composed of phospholipid, polysaccharide—protein complexes.
2. Easily diffuse from the cell into the surrounding medium.	2. Firmly bound within the bacterial cell.
3. Highly toxic, characterised by the selective affection of certain organs and tissues.	3. Less toxic, selective action poorly expressed.
4. Thermolabile.	4. Thermostable.
5. During parenteral injection, they produce highly active antibodies (antitoxins).	5. During parenteral injection, they produce precipitins, lysins, opsonins, agglutinins and complement fixing antibodies.
6. Under influence of 0.3 - 0.4 per cent formalin and a temperature of 38 - 40°C change to anatoxin (Toxoid).	6. Under the influence of formalin and temperature are partially rendered harmless.

CHAPTER 11

HOST FACTORS CONTRIBUTING TO INFECTION

Various host factors, affecting an individual or a community, contributing to the occurrence of the infection are :

1. Very young children and very old individuals are susceptible to infection, because of inadequate body defence mechanism.

2. Malnutrition favours the incidence and severity of infection in poor community.

3. Metabolic diseases like diabetes and hormonal upsets due to corticosteroid therapy predispose to the infection.

4. Haematological disorders like leukemia, neoplasm and renal diseases may reduce host resistance to infection.

5. Factors such as age, obesity, size of wound, wound drainage, duration of operation and length of stay before or after operation may affect the *nosocomial* infection (hospital acquired infection) caused by staphylococci and gram-negative bacilli.

6. Acquired immunodeficiency syndrome (AIDS) Patients are highly susceptible to various infections.

7. Community factors affecting host resistance are the complex components of poverty (over-crowding, inadequate food, clothing and housing, hypothermia and poor personal hygiene).

8. Drug addiction and alcoholism may predispose to infection.

SOURCES OF INFECTION FOR MAN

The term *infection* (Lat.*infectio* — to infect) signifies the sum of biological processes which take place in the human or animal body upon the penetration of pathogenic microorganisms in the host's body by injuring body tissues and producing a reaction on the part of the host. *Source of infection* is defined as the normal growth habitat of the microbes, e.g., a site in the body of the human or animal host. Objects contaminated with live or temporarily inactive microbes may be called *vehicles* or *reservoirs* of infection, not sources of infection.

Man acquires infection

A. From outside sources, which is known as *exogenous* infection, e.g., from human patients with clinical infections, healthy human carriers of the pathogenic microorganisms.

B. Within the patient's own body, the infection is said to be *endogenous*.

Exogenous infections

1. *Patients*. Some microbial infections are acquired from sick patients with active infections (pulmonary tuberculosis, leprosy, whooping cough, syphilis, gonorrhoea, measles, small pox, mumps and influenza).

2. *Healthy carriers*. Healthy persons, though they carry many species of pathogenic microbes, sometimes show a subclinical infection and are commonly capable of disseminating these pathogenic microbes to other persons who will manifest the signs and symptoms of illness; they are then termed as *carriers*; thus they are potential source of infection. Some infectious diseases are contracted from carriers much more frequently than from patients, e.g., streptococcal, staphylococcal, pneumococcal and meningococcal infections, diphtheria, typhoid fever, bacillary dysentery and poliomyelitis.

3. *Convalescent carriers* are persons in whom a limited, localised infection continues for a period of weeks or months after clinical recovery from a manifest infection.

4. *Contact carriers* are those persons who acquire the pathogen from a patient.

5 *Paradoxical carriers* are those who acquire the infection asymptomatically from another carrier. If the carriage persists for more than an arbitrary period of time, e.g., one year in the case of typhoid infection, the person is called chronic carrier.

Endogenous infections

Endogenous infections may occur in carriers of potentially pathogenic organisms, when these previously harmless bacteria invade. Other surfaces or tissues in the carrier, e.g., *Escherchia coli* derived from the bowel, where it is harmless, may cause acute suppurative infection in the urinary tract; *Staph. aureus* from the nostrils may cause boil in the skin or infection in a wound; and pneumococci from the nasopharynx may cause bronchitis and bronchopneumonia. The source of endogenous infection is thus the site in a patient's body (e.g., colon, skin or nasopharynx) where the organism grows harmlessly as a commensal.

Staphylococcal sepsis of the skin and wounds, which is mainly endogenous, may under certain circumstances become transmissible, as in hospital, where conditions may favour *cross-infection* between patients. Thus, the *cross-infected* patients suffer from exogenous infection. However, patients with endogenous infections caused by organism of low virulence are not likely to infect other persons, e.g., patients with bronchopneumonia due to pneumococci of less virulence are not a danger to relatives, nurses or other patients and there is no need to isolate them from other patients in hospital.

Modes of Spread of Infections

A variety of mechanisms can spread respiratory and alimentary infections from host to host, while a single mechanism, for which the parasite is specially adapted, can spread venereal and arthropod-borne blood infections :

1. *Respiratory infection.* The causative microbes are disseminated into the environment in masses of infected secretion, e.g., secretion transferred from the nose or mouth on floors, handkerchiefs, cups, spoons or secretions expelled in spitting or blowing the nose; they are also discharged to a less extent in the droplet spray produced by sneezing, coughing and speaking, but in normal breathing, they are very rarely disseminated. The secretion contaminates handkerchiefs, clothing, bedding, floors, furnitures and household articles (fomites) which may act as vehicles or reservoirs of infection. It dries in dust, most kinds of respiratory microbes may remain alive for several days, even for several months, if protected from direct sunlight, e.g., tubercle bacilli, diphtheria bacilli, streptococci, staphylococci and small pox virus.

(a) Infection may be passed to the recipient by contact, either (i) *direct contact,* i.e., touching of bodies as in handshaking, kissing and contact of cloth, or (ii) *indirect contact,* e.g., contaminated eating utensils, door handles, towels; the recepient may transfer the microbes from contaminated fingers to his sore or mouth.

(b) Infection may be *dust-borne* by inhalation of air-borne infected dust particles. The infected numerous dust particles are disseminated into the air from the skin and clothing during normal body movements; from dried contaminated handkerchiefs during its use, from bed sheets while bed making, from floor during sweeping and walking, and from furniture while dusting. The larger infected dust particles may settle within a few minutes on the floor and other exposed surface, e.g., skin, clothing, wounds and surgical supplies; whereas the smaller dust particles remain air-borne for up to 1 to 2 hours and may be inhaled into the recipient's nose, throat, bronchi, lung alveoli. Within the room of its origin, air-borne infection is very common and dangerous; but its spreading to other rooms in the same building is rare.

(c) The third least important means of respiratory infections is droplet spray, except in the case of the pathogens that are rapidly killed by drying, e.g., meningococcus, whooping cough bacillus, measles and common cold viruses. Sneezing, coughing, speaking and other forceful expiratory activities expel a spray of droplets derived from the saliva of the anterior mouth which is infected with small numbers of pathogenic microbes from the nose, throat, lungs. Numerous droplets are expelled, but only a few are infected. The large droplets (over 0.1 mm. in diameter) fly forwards and downwards from the mouth to the distance of a few feet (about 1 meter), they reach the floor or body surfaces (eye, face, mouth and clothing) or the persons standing in front of the other person producing the spray, within a few seconds. These particles cannot be inhaled. Measles, chicken pox and dog distemper are common viral infections spread by the larger droplets. The *small droplets* (below 0.1 mm. in diameter) evaporate immediately to become minute solid residues or *"droplet nuclei"* (mainly 1 to 10 μm in diameter) which remain air-borne and may be inhaled into the nose, throat, lung. Few of the droplet nuclei are infected with pathogenic microbes. Measles, chicken-pox, and dog distemper are common viral infections spread by the droplet nuclei.

2. *Mucous membrane, skin wound, discharges and burn infections.*

Gonococcal ophthalmia caused by gonococci and inclusion blenorrhoea caused by sub-group-A of chlamydia may be acquired from the infected genital tract of the mother, when the mucous membrane of eyes of new born infants gets infected as the infant passes down the infected birth canal.

Leptospira excreted in the urine of the infected animals enter the human body through the skin, similarly larvae of schistosoma and ankylostoma penetrate the skin.

The superficial infections may be acquired by (a) contact with infected hands, clothing or other articles, (b) by exposure to the deposition of contaminated droplet spray, pathogenic streptococci and staphylococci derived from respiratory tract are important causes of wound and burn infections; if pathogenic staphylococci are disseminated from pus discharge, they may cause infection of broken skin and burn wound.

3. *Venereal infections.* The diseases transmitted exclusively by sexual intercourse are called venereal diseases, since the causative agents, e.g., *Treponema pallidum* and *Neisseria gonorrhoeae* are highly susceptible to lethal effects of drying, they are to be transmitted only by sexual contact. Gonococcus which causes vulvovaginitis in young girls may be acquired, under unhygienic conditions, from the common use of towels and bathing facilities. This is non-venereal spread of infection in young girls. Sub-group A of chlamydia (*Lymphogranuloma Venereum* - LGV) infection is transmitted by sexual contact. Acquired immunodeficiency syndrome (AIDS) caused by Human immunodeficiency virus (HIV) can be transmitted through sex — commonly by homosexuality.

4. *Alimentary tract infections.* Persons with intestinal infection may disseminate the pathogenic microbes in excreta. These microbes are transmitted in various ways, the so-called *faecal-oral routes,* leading to their ingestion by the recipient, e.g., *Salmonella typhi.*

Most of the intestinal pathogens are not much resistant to drying, they may die within a few hours, they may survive on cloth, or in dust for several days. They are more likely to be spread by moist vehicles (*water* or *food*) in which they may survive for several weeks.

(a) *Water-borne infections :* May occur when faeces contaminate a water supply, e.g., river or well, which is used without purification for drinking purpose. In typhoid and cholera, water is the common vehicle of infection and the infecting dose may be small. Water is supplied to the citizen by the municipality after purification. Purification, which renders the water non-infective, is carried out on a large scale by storage, filtration and chlorination. Small amounts of water required for drinking purpose may be treated by boiling or by the addition of hypochlorite tablets.

(b) *Hand infections :* The hands of the nurses can get infected while attending the patients and touching the bed pans. Similarly the hands of the carrier can be contaminated with bacteria contained in the faeces. Such persons may contaminate the foodstuffs, eating utensils, wash basins, towels, door handles and other fomites (inanimate objects). A recipient may eat contaminated food or put in his mouth the contaminated utensils or may pick up the microbes on his fingers and then transfer them into his mouth.

(c) *Food-borne infections* may occur through :

(i) a carrier handling the food (food as a vector of disease);

(ii) preparation of the food in utensils contaminated by handling or washing in contaminated water;

(iii) files alighting on the food after feeding on infected faeces. Enterotoxins may be produced on the food contaminated by bacteria during their growth in favourable conditions, e.g., *Staph. aureus* and *Clostridium botulinum.* These preformed enterotoxins are prerequisites for bacterial food poisoning, whereas food-borne infections may result from the ingestion of only a few pathogenic microorganisms, e.g., *Sh. dysenteriae* which liberate enterotoxin.

5. *Urine.* Typhoid bacilli are excreted in the urine and feces, similarly leptospirae are excreted by animals through the urine and enter the mucous membrane and skin.

6. *Arthropod-borne infections.* In systemic infection, the causative microbes are present in large number in blood, so they may be transmitted to other individuals by blood sucking arthropods such as mosquito (malaria, filaria, yellow fever); flea (plague); louse (epidemic typhus fever); mite (scrub typhus) and tse tse fly (trypanosomiasis).

7. *Laboratory infections.* Laboratory workers may occasionally become infected from artificial cultures or infected diagnostic or necropsy materials collected from patients or experimental animals. Brucella, rickettsia and *Pasteurella tularensis* especially cause laboratory infections; while other organisms (tubercle bacilli, anthrax bacilli, pathogenic leptospires, borreliae, freshly isolated typhoid, dysentery bacilli, psittacosis organisms and serum hepatitis virus) should be handled very carefully. The pipetting of infected liquids by mouth leading to their accidental ingestion is certainly a danger of laboratory infections. Accidental self-inoculation with a syringe may take place or the conjunctiva may be sprayed when the needle becomes loosened from a syringe during an injection.

Many laboratory procedures (the expulsion of liquid from a pipette or the use of the mechanical blenders, the centrifugation of tubes bearing traces of liquid on their rim) or drop separated from an inoculation loop may cause laboratory infections, when working particularly with pathogens which may cause air-borne infection such as tubercle bacilli, thus it is necessary that all these procedures should be carried out within a especially ventilated protective cabinet or inoculation hood.

8. *Congenital transmission.* Serum hepatitis virus can be transmitted from the infected pregnant mother through the placenta to the fetus. Similarly, human immunodeficiency virus (HIV) can be transmitted through placenta to the newborn.

Congenital malaria is comparatively rare. The intrauterine transmission of malaria is well established. The congenital malaria is very common in non-immune infected mothers. It is also believed the passage of the parasite to the fetus occurs only when the placental barrier has been injured.

Congenital toxoplasmosis results from the congenital infection in infants and young children. It usually appears as a form of encephalitis, accompanied by chorioretinitis, hydrocephalus or microcephaly, mental retardation and convulsions. The infection passes from the mother through the placenta late in pregnancy when neutralisation of antibodies cannot take place. The child is usually born jaundiced with purpuric or maculopapular rash, enlarged liver and spleen.

Congenital trypanosomiasis in man is possible but is rare; a case was reported in a child born of an infected mother, in Germany, who died less than three months after birth, because of proven trypanosomiasis. Later, two more proven congenital infections in infants were reported.

Congenital filariasis. The microfilariae of *Wuchereria bancrofti* may pass from the infected pregnant mother to the new born through the placental filter.

BASIC PRINCIPLES OF DISEASE TRANSMISSION

Portals of entry and portals of exit are two basic principles of disease transmission :

1. *Portals of entry :*

Normally, microorganisms enter into the body through *certain routes* and cause the infection; but they cannot gain entrance through other abnormal portals of entry :

(a) Cuts or abrasions of the skin (e.g., bites of arthropods or animals); (b) mucosa of respiratory tract (nose, throat, lungs), eyes and mouth, gastrointestinal, genitourinary tracts are the most important common portals of entry.

Abnormal portals of entry. If harmless saprophytic microorganisms are introduced parenterally into the brain or into the peritoneal cavity by a hypodermic needle, they set up the rapid fatal infection.

Many organisms can cause the infection if they enter only through their *obligate* portals of entry.Thus, dysentery bacilli can produce severe bacillary dysentery, if they are consumed through water or food; if they are rubbed into the skin wound, they will not initiate any infection. Severe, even fatal infections (abscess, boil, carbuncle), can be produced if staphylococci are rubbed in the skin; if swallowed, they are ineffective. Some organisms can enter through any portal.

Path of organisms in the body. From the sites (portals of entry) of infection, organisms may pass into the blood stream and initiate a secondary (metastatic) infection in internal organs (i.e., in the meninges of the brain and spinal cord — meningitis).

When the *enteric pathogens* (typhoid bacilli, dysentery bacilli, *Vibrio cholerae*) are swallowed, they enter the stomach unaffected temporarily by gastric juice (especially in the presence of food), they set up ultimately gastro-intestinal infection.The *respiratory pathogens* locate in or on tonsils, throat (Streptococci, diphtheria bacilli, whooping cough bacilli) may cause the infection, if they pass down into the lungs, they may produce pneumonia (Pneumococci) and tuberculosis (tubercle bacilli). The organisms (*Treponema pallidum*, gonococci) find their portals of entry through genital mucosa.

2. *Portals of exit.* The pathway by which organisms leave the body of one patient to another patient or healthy individual to initiate the infection is known as Portals of exit.

VECTORS

Vectors may be animate or inanimate :

(a) *Inanimate Vectors* may be the food, discharges (faeces, saliva, pus), water, bandages, dressings, instruments, bedding, eating utensils and other inanimate objects (fomites) contaminated with infectious discharges.

(b) *Animate Vectors* are generally arthropods or mammals : female anopheles mosquito is the vector for malaria; vectors of rabies are dogs or other mammals. Other animate vectors are the *hands* (very common) of the patients, nurses, doctors and patient's relatives coming in contact with an infectious patient or his fomites. Since man cannot be disinfected with Dichloro Diphenyl Trichloroethane (DDT) or muzzled and put on a leash, he himself may be regarded as one of the most dangerous vector of the diseases (e.g., man is the only significant living vector of AIDS, poliomyelitis, measles and syphilis and he is the most frequent live vector of human tuberculosis).

Application to Nursing

An intelligent well-trained professional nurse should know how to deal with the pathogenic microorganisms leaving the patient's body to the environment. While attending the patient she should protect herself and the environment from these pathogens. The transmission of most infectious agents should be stopped by her at the portal of exit by immediate collection of and proper disposal of all bodily excretions, secretions, discharges, and tissues likely to contain the pathogens (faeces, urine, saliva, mucous, pus, tissue drainage, used bandage, etc.). In case of malaria, infected blood sucking female anopheles mosquito must be destroyed by Dichloro Diphenyl Trichloroethane (DDT) spray.

If the most probable portal of entry is intelligently understood by the nurse, she can adopt the appropriate methods of protection. For example, the respiratory portals of entry can be covered by masks; cuts or abrasions on the hand can be protected by bandage or surgical gloves. The alimentary canal is protected by appropriate selection and disinfection (as by pasteurisation of milk, chlorination of water and cooking) and sanitary preparation of food. The skin must be protected from the biting arthropods by clothing, and fly repellants. Tissues and blood can be protected from the infection by vaccination or by prophylactic use of antibiotics and chemotherapeutic agents.

SECTION 3

CHAPTER 12

CONTAINERS AND SWABS FOR COLLECTION OF SPECIMENS

Containers used for microbiological investigations should be sterile, leak-proof and strong. Each container should bear the name of the patient, from whom the specimen was collected and his case register number. The investigation requisition form should also accompany the specimen indicating the investigation required along with the probable clinical diagnosis and current chemotherapy. Details of previous immunisation should be furnished for serological investigation.

Glass tubes and universal containers. Specimens of exudate, pus, blood, cerebrospinal fluid, urine and faeces should be collected in strong, sterile, corked glass test tubes (4 × 3/8 inch). Before collection of samples, test tubes with loosely fitted cotton plug, or bark corks can be sterilised in hot air oven and then the corks should be pressed in.

Universal container. Screw capped bottle is a strong moulded glass bottle (3. 1/4 in height × 1. 1/8 in diameter) of one oz (28 ml) capacity with a flat base and wide mouth. It is sterilised with loose cap and then tightened. It cannot be sterilised in the hot air oven as the rubber washer will not withstand the temperature.

The screw capped universal container has many advantages over the glass test tubes. It is strong, the mouth of the container is sterile because of the screw cap; whereas in case of stoppered glass test tubes, the dust may collect at the rim of the test tube. The content of a container will not leak and will not be contaminated. It is quite stable at the base of the container and it is very convenient for collection of the sample at the bed side and it is very suitable for the collection of serous fluids, e.g., pleural or peritoneal fluids. The collection of the fluids that may be coagulable on standing can be done in the container to which 0.3 ml of a 20 per cent solution of sodium citrate is added prior to the autoclaving. This method of collecting fluid may be useful in performing cell count or centrifuging procedures.

Blood may be collected in a sterile universal screw capped container or test tube fitted with cotton plug for serological investigation. The streptokinase digested or minced blood clot may be cultured in a selective medium, e.g., for enteric organisms (Salmonella) or blood for culture may be collected and submitted to the bacteriological laboratory in a special blood culture bottle containing bile salt broth. Serum from clotted blood can be transmitted to the laboratory while preserved in sodium azide or merthiolate (1 : 10,000) in a sterile polysterine or polypropylene plastic container.

Faeces. May be collected in a small bottle of about 2 oz capacity or in a glass specimen tube or by a rectal swab. If the laboratory is situated at a far off place, the container may be transmitted with all precautions by post; the package should be labelled as "Pathological specimen". If there is a delay of some hours before laboratory cultivation can be performed, neutral glycerol saline should be added to the faeces. Rice water stool from cholera patient should be collected on a leaf or paper, but not in disinfected bed pan; because disinfectants can kill Vibrio cholerae. Specimen should be sent in transport medium, e.g., alkaline peptone water or Venkatraman-Ramakrishnan (VR) medium.

Urine— For the diagnosis of urinary tract infection, the urine, if required in small quantity, can be collected in a universal container; complete early morning specimens (large quantities of urine) can be collected in a 20 oz screw capped bottles.

Disposable Specimen Containers

Sterile screw capped waxed cartoons of 2 oz capacity (such as used for ice-cream) are suitable for the collection of sputum or faeces. These waxed cartoons cannot be sent through post because of postal regulations. Plastic polysterene or polypropylene containers of variable size are suitable for urine, faeces, pus, blood etc. Recently, disposable plastic specimen containers have become available from various manufacturers. All disposable containers should be destroyed in a furnace after use.

Swab— A swab consists of a piece of wooden (bamboo or broom) stick of about 6. 1/2 in long. Around one end of the stick a thin pledget of absorbent cotton wool is tightly wrapped for about 3/4 in. The stick is placed in a test tube (5 in × 1/2) and the top of the tube is plugged with a cotton-wool. This has the advantage that the stick can be broken off short when the swab has to be placed in transport medium in a screw-capped container. Besides collection of specimens, the swab can also be useful in the laboratory for seeding of medium for antibiotic disk sensitivity tests.

A variety of disposable swabs (Plain, serum coated, charcoal coated) in plastic tubes are available. They can be destroyed in a furnace after use or sterilised in autoclave before discarding.

Swabs are useful in collecting specimen from :

(i) *Throat*: in cases of suspected diphtheria, tonsillitis;

(ii) *Wound*: specimen from surgical conditions (fistula, sinus) or discharging ears can be collected by swabs;

(iii) *Postnasal or naso-pharyngeal space* : Specimens from suspected meningococcal carriers and whooping cough can be collected by using sterile postnasal swab which is made from a flexible copper wire or Nichrome (0.51 mm diameter), its terminal end (1/4 in) bent back through an angle of 45 degrees is tightly wrapped with a thin pledget of absorbent cotton wool. For the diagnosis of whooping cough, a prenasal swab is preferrable to the postnasal swab.

(iv) *Rectum*: Rectal swabs are very useful in bacillary dysentery in young children.

(v) *Cervix uteri*: A longer sterile stick or wire, 9 in, is preferrable for the specimens in gonorrhea and puepal infections.

In conditions where delicate pathogens are concerned, e.g., meningococcus, gonococcus or *Bordetella pertussis*, it is preferrable to place the swab in a sterile Bijou bottle containing transport medium, e.g., neutral glycerol saline.

For blood culture, medical flat bottle is used.

CHAPTER 13

METHODS OF COLLECTION OF SPECIMEN AND LABORATORY DIAGNOSTIC TECHNIQUES

A. Respiratory Tract Infection

1. **Upper Respiratory Tract Infection :** The upper respiratory tract is frequently the site of general and localised infection involving the mouth, pharynx, nose, nasopharynx, larynx, trachea.

The primary infection is often of viral origin and secondary bacterial infection is most often due to the potent pathogens resident in the upper respiratory tract, e.g., pneumococci, streptococci, *Haemophilus influenzae* and staphylococcus.

The most useful method is to take a swab direct from the surface, if exudate, membrane or pus is present, some of this should be sampled. Films may be prepared from the swabs after culture media have been inoculated, or smears may be prepared directly from the membrane, exudate or surface by means of swabs and stained by suitable stains.

Sore throat:This syndrome is mostly due to *Streptococcus pyogenes* and is characterised by acute inflammation of the tonsillar and faucial areas (acute tonsillitis, acute pharyngitis) with or without exudate, which may be loose or adherent. Acute adenitis, sinusitis, otitis media, rhinitis, laryngitis, tracheitis, peritonsillar abscess (quinsy) may accompany or follow the acute throat infection.

2. **Lower Respiratory Tract Infection :** In the lower respiratory tract (trachea, bronchi, bronchioles and lung tissue) there is often a primary infection by a virus (e.g., adenovirus, myxovirus, respiratory syncytial virus, herpesvirus, picornavirus) which is followed by a secondary infection by pathogenic meningococcus. From the upper respiratory tract and by spread through the blood and lymph channel or very rarely there is direct extension of infection from liver. In health, the mucous membrane of lower respiratory tract is sterile.

The direct examination of the lower respiratory tract infection is by bronchoscopy or by lung biopsy. This is not always possible in the routine diagnosis of the infection.

Sputum from patients with acute bronchitis, bronchiolitis and pneumonia should be examined bacteriologically. In most cases, the sputum may be the mixtures of exudate and the affected mucous membrane or lung tissue and saliva. In separate purulent material containing pathogens from saliva, it is necessary to spread the mixture in a petridish and then pick up directly the purulent material with a loop. Another method is the homogenisation of the sputum by adding saponin and incubating for half an hour or by shaking the sputum with glass beads or by digesting with pancreatin.

Direct film: Direct film is very useful in the diagnosis of pneumococcal and staphylococcal infection of the lung after Gram's stain and also of the pulmonary tuberculosis after Ziehl-Neelsen's method of staining for tubercle bacilli. The direct film may not give any indication about the number of viable organisms; besides, the saliva may contain commensal organisms.

Culture: Sputum is plated on blood agar for aerobic and anaerobic incubation and on heated blood agar under anaerobic condition with antibiotics disks. For differential diagnosis of pneumococci from *Streptococcus viridans*, an optochin disk is placed on the plate. Pneumococci are sensitive to optochin. Large number of causative organisms are isolated in specific infections with staphylococci, *Haemophilus influenzae* and pneumococci. In case of suspected tuberculosis, sputum can be homogenised and concentrated before culture on Lowenstein-Jensen medium and before guinea pig Inoculation.

B. Infection of the Intestine

Acute intestinal infection : Various causative microorganisms (bacterial, virus, protozoa) are responsible for acute intestinal infection. The most common pathogens are food poisoning, Salmonella enterotoxic strains of *Staphylococcus aureus*; less common are *Clostridium welchii, Clostridium botulinum*.The help of the diagnostic laboratory is essential for the diagnosis of the disease and the specimens should be sent for the bacteriological examination.

Specimen Collection

Faecal sample is much better than the rectal swab; but the rectal swabs may be of necessity to collect sample from the contacts of a patient. It is necessary to ensure that the swabs sample the content of the rectum and that they are not merely placed in the anal orifice. Faeces should be passed into a clean pot which does not contain any antiseptic and the specimens should be collected free from urine and be sent to the laboratory as soon as possible. If delay is anticipated, the specimen should be transported in glycerol-saline because it prevents the overgrowth of the intestinal commensals on any other enteric pathogens.

In case of cholera, the stool can be collected on a clean paper or leaf, never in a bedpan, because of the bactericidal effect of the antiseptic used in disinfecting the bedpan; *Vibrio cholerae* can be transported in alkaline peptone water or alkaline taurocholate tellurite liquid medium or sea water or its equivalent (Venkatraman-Ramakrishnan (VR) fluid) to the bacteriological laboratory for examination of motility "darting motility"—which is a very important aid for quick diagnosis of cholera.In amebic dysentery, the motile vegetative form of *Entamoeba histolytica* can be demonstrated within few minutes in the freshly passed faecal sample.

C. Infection of Urinary Tract

Bacteriological examination of the urine is of great necessity in the diagnosis of the urinary tract infection. Besides, the chemotherapy of the proven infection may be controlled by the *in vitro* antibiotic sensitivity tests.

Specimen Collection

Universal containers or disposable plastic pots with tight fitting lids may be used to collect the urine specimens. The wide mouthed containers of 12 oz capacity can be very useful to collect the mid-stream specimens from females.

A mid-stream specimen of urine (MSU) can also be collected from male patients. Formerly, for bacteriological examination, a catheter specimen of urine (CSU) was always collected from female patients to avoid contamination of the specimen with organisms from ano-genital region. This method is no longer advocated, since the catheterisation may introduce the infection. The patient should pass the urine with the labia separated and the middle of the stream is collected for the examination.

Once collected, the specimen must be transported to the laboratory *immediately* (without any delay) because the urine is the best culture medium for the rapid growth of many bacteria. If there may be a delay of 1-2 hours, the specimen can be stored in the refrigerator to check the multiplication of bacteria or it may be transported in a container of low temperature. Urine may also be preserved by adding boric acid to a final concentration of 1-8 per cent.

If the urinary tract is suspected for tuberculosis, the first urine passed in the day is the most suitable specimen (early morning urine). Three complete early morning urine samples should be sent to the laboratory where the microbiological, cultural and animal tests can be performed on the centrifuged deposit.

Bacterial viable counts can be carried out by :

(i) pour plate method;

(ii) inoculating the surface of the medium with known volumes of urine. Colony counts are made after incubation for 24-48 hours. There are two semi-quantitative methods of culture of urine :

  (a) the first in which a loop of standard diameter is used;

  (b) the second — the dip slide — in which a thin layer of agar — either as a coating on a slide or in a metal or plastic spoon — is dipped into a fresh specimen of urine.

In the loop method, the loop is charged with the uncentrifuged urine and plated on solid media. After overnight incubation, the plate culture is inspected for colonies and the results are evaluated by colony counting.

In the dip slide method, the slide or spoon coated with agar is dipped into a fresh specimen of urine, the excess of urine is drained off; the specimen or spoon can be sent in a suitable container to the laboratory.

Significant bacteriuria (counts greater than 10^5 organisms per ml) may sometimes be found in the absence of symptoms or pyuria, in patients who subsequently develop symptoms of urinary infection. There is good evidence of frequent association between a symptomatic bacteriuria and pyelonephritis.

D. Meningeal Infection

Patients suspected of having meningitis should always have a specimen of cerebro-spinal fluid (CSF) examined in the laboratory as soon as possible. The causal organism should be identified promptly. It is very important because the proper antimicrobial therapy cannot be prescribed until the exact bacteriological diagnosis is made.

Specimen Collection

Cerebrospinal fluid should be collected very carefully by lumbar puncture. It is safe to remove 5-10 ml of CSF as long as intracranial pressure is not increased.

One or two sterile screw capped containers can be used to collect the CSF. Test tubes with cotton plugs should not be used because, if they are shaken or fall over, the CSF may be absorbed by the plug. The specimen should be sent *immediately* to the diagnostic laboratory, because meningococci — being delicate — may die, leucocytes may disintegrate and the concentration of sugar in the CSF may be reduced. Specimen should not be kept in the refrigerator which kills *H. influenzae.*

Examination for Cells

There is a great increase in the number of leucocytes in the CSF which becomes turbid in acute bacterial meningitis. One mm^3 of CSF may contain up to several thousands cells and in early stages of the disease, almost all of them are polymorphs. But there are fewer cells in CSF (200-500 per mm^3) with predominant lymphocytes in tuberculous meningitis. In case of virus infections of the meninges, there are only 50-100 lymphocytes per mm^3 of CSF resulting in "aseptic" type of meningitis.

Biochemical Examination

Quantitative biochemical estimation of protein, sugar (glucose) and chloride content of the CSF should be conducted.

Examination for Microorganisms

(a) *Acute Purulent meningitis* : In this condition, the CSF is turbid. *Neisseria meningitidis*, pneumococci, *H. influenzae* are responsible for this type of meningitis as they may reach meninges via the blood stream, because of their simultaneous isolation by blood culture. The infections of middle ear, paranasal or frontal sinuses may spread directly to the meninges. Variety of organisms (*Staphylococcus aureus, Streptococcus pyogenes, Pseudomonas phyocyanea, Escherichia coli, Bacteroides,* anaerobic streptococci) may gain access to the meninges after careless lumbar puncture.

In the laboratory, films made from CSF centrifuged deposit are stained by Gram's stain and examined. The remaining deposits are cultured on blood and heated blood agar (chocolate agar) medium and incubated anaerobically, in 5-10 per cent CO_2 at 37°C. A primary antibiotic disk sensitivity test is done if large number of organisms is seen in the stained film.

(b) *Acute non-purulent bacterial meningitis :* *Mycobacterium tuberculosis* or *Leptospira icterohaemorrhagiae* may cause acute non-purulent bacterial meningitis and the CSF is not usually turbid. A veil clot appears in the CSF on standing, in the case of tuberculous meningitis and on microscopy by Ziehl-Neelsen's stain, acid fast bacilli can be demonstrated. CSF centrifuged deposit may be cultured on Lowenstein-Jensen medium and by guinea pig inoculation. Serological tests are useful to diagnose leptospiral meningitis.

(c) *Viral (aseptic) meningitis :* In this condition, the CSF is not turbid. Picorna virus, coxsackie virus, poliovirus (least) are responsible for this infection. Echovirus and coxsackie virus, though they are present in faeces, can be isolated directly from CSF. Hence, CSF and faeces should be sent to the laboratory. These materials can be stored up to 24 hours at 0° - 4°C or frozen at – 30°C or in 50 per cent glycerol saline.

CSF IN DIFFERENT TYPES OF MENINGITIS

Test	Normal	Acute bacterial meningitis	Tuberculous meningitis	Aseptic meningits
Appearance	Clean; colourless	Turbid	Clear or opalescent	Usually clear
Total protein	15-40 mg/ 100 ml.	Greatly increased	Moderately increased	Slightly increased
Sugar	50-70 mg/ 100 ml.	Greatly reduced	Reduced	Normal
Chloride	700-740 mg/ 100 ml.	Reduced	Reduced	Normal
Cell count	0-3 Lymphocytes per mm³	Greatly increased all lymphocytes	Increased mainly lymphocytes some polymorphs	Increased lymphocytes predominate
Culture on artificial medium	Sterile	Isolation of causative bacterium	Isolation of *Myco. tuberculosis*	Negative

E. Infection of Reproductive System

Coliform bacilli, streptococci, *Mycobacterium tuberculosis, Neisseria gonorrhoeae* are pathogens responsible for the infection of female genital tract.

Pueperal sepsis or septic abortions which are acute infections in the female after delivery are caused by *Streptococcus pyogenes, Clostridium welchii,* Bacteroides, Coliform bacilli.

Cervical swabs should be taken with the help of a speculum under direct vision, put in to Stuart's transport medium and sent to the diagnostic laboratory.

In acute vaginitis due to *Trichomonas vaginitis* and vaginal thrush due to *Candida albicans,* exudates can be readily obtained by swabbing and direct smears can be made on slides for microscopic examination or exudates may be collected by pipette or spoon for wet films.

Acute urethritis and prostatitis in male are due to *N.gonorrhoeae,* chlamydia or *Mycoplasma hominis.*

F. Wound Infection

Wound infection may be : (a) *endogenous,* or (b) *exogenous.*

Endogenous infections (*auto-infection*) are caused by organisms that were commensals elsewhere in the host body, e.g., organisms from large intestine may infect the abdominal surgical wounds after an operation that has involved the incision of the skin.

Exogenous infections are due to organisms from outside the host who has become infected.

Cross-infection is an example of exogenous infection where the causative organism is spread from person to person. Infection may occur after accidental or intentional trauma of the skin or other tissues : the latter type is known as "post-operative sepsis."

Specimen Collection

Swabs should be well soaked in pus or exudate from infected wounds. Syringe can be used to collect the pus or exudate specimens which can be transferred into a sterile test tube. Pieces of tissues removed at operation or curettings or other tissues can be sent immediately to the bacteriological laboratory and they should be homogenised in a tissue grinder before being used for bacteriological examination. Delay in the transit of specimens to the laboratory must be avoided, particularly in cases of swabs where the exudate may dry in the cotton-wool.

G. Infection of the Conjunctiva

Pseudomonas pyocyanea causes severe conjunctivitis due to the use of contaminated eye drops. Gonococcus (ophthalmia neonatorum), *Staphylococcus aureus* (sticky eye in new born babies), pneumococci, *Moraxella lacunata* and *H.influenzae*, certain viruses (herpes virus, adenovirus), TRIC agent (Trachoma, inclusion blenorrhea) produce conjunctivitis.

Swabs coated with exudates can be sent to the laboratory in Stuart's transport medium. Purulent exudate from inflamed conjunctiva can be considered as pus. Gonococcus can be shown by direct microscopy and can be grown on heated blood agar medium.

TRIC agents can be demonstrated in the scrapings taken from the conjunctiva, spread on slides, stained with Giemsa stain and examined for basophilic inclusion bodies or stained by a fluorescent conjugate antiserum and examined by fluorescent microscopy.

H. Pyrexia of Unknown or Uncertain Origin

Patients with a significant and persistent fever (greater than 100°F = 38°C) are classified as "Pyrexia of Unknown Origin" (PUO) since the cause cannot be readily diagnosed on clinical examination. PUO may be due to the infection which can be diagnosed by the presence of a specific pathogen in the blood or tissues. In addition to isolation (direct method) of causative agent, the serological tests (indirect methods) can also be performed to demonstrate the specific antibody. The possibility of an exotic infection may be included if the patient was abroad recently.

(i) *Examination of Blood*

(a) *Blood film*: The examination of blood films may rule out the presence of malarial parasites (Plasmodia) and reveal the white blood cell picture of the peripheral blood.

(b) *Blood culture* can be done on successive days or on several occasions each day or over a period of several hours as in the case of subacute bacterial endocarditis, because of the number of causative organisms which may be very small and of the inhibitory effects of antibiotics on the circulating pathogens and special media (Brucella or Albimi agar) are required for the isolation of Brucella and an atmosphere of 10 per cent carbon dioxide for isolation of *Brucella abortus*. *Salmonella typhi* can be isolated in a blood culture bottle containing the bile salt broth.

(c) *Animal inoculation*: Leptospira, Brucella, Rickettsiae can be isolated from the fresh blood on animal inoculation which is more successful than on artificial media.

(d) *Examination of Serum*: Part of the blood used for culture may be allowed to clot and the serum is used for serology. Serological studies should be done at an interval of 5 to 10 days during the acute stage of the disease and later during the convalescent stages to demonstrate rise or fall in the amount of antibody. Examination of paired specimens (5 to 10 ml each) should always be made for antibodies to the enteric group of *Salmonella* (Widal test) and *Brucella* species.

(ii) *Examination of Urine*: Routine examination should be carried out to exclude the infection of urinary tract. In chronic pyelonephritis, *Escherichia coli* may be present only on intermittent occasions. *Salmonella sp.* can be isolated occasionally from the urine. Repeated examinations may be necessary.

In genito-urinary tuberculosis, three entire morning specimens or a 24 hour specimen of urine should be collected; pyuria is usually present and *Myco. tuberculosis* can be seen after centrifugation and staining of the urine deposit; in leptospirosis, leptospires can be demonstrated by dark field examination of the fresh alkalised urine.

(iii) *Examination of Faeces*: In intestinal infection, Shigella, Salmonella, intestinal protozoa and the ova of helminths can be demonstrated in the faeces. In suspected virus infection it is advisable to watch the virus infection with the rise of the homologous antibody titre of the serum.

(iv) *Examination of Tissue* : Tissue, such as lymph node, may be cultured for *Myco. tuberculosis* after grinding it in a homogeniser or tissue blender. Tissue can be collected by biopsy.

(v) *Examination of other body fluids* can be done by microscopy or by culture. Aspirations of secretion of bile in suspected infections of the gall bladder, liver or biliary passage, CSF in meningitis and bone marrow in enteric fever are used to confirm the suspected infection.

(vi) *Skin tests* may be useful in the diagnosis of subacute or chronic infections. The inoculation of a small quantity of bacterial products, e.g., tuberculin, brucellin, the Frei antigen results in a localised delayed type hypersensitivity reaction.

Body fluids and discharges with infectious organisms and fomites likely to be contaminated :

Body fluids discharges with infectious organisms	**Articles fomites etc. likely to be contaminated by microorganisms**
Faeces and Urine Salmonella Shigella (only in faeces) *Vibrio cholerae* (faeces) Brucella, *Escherchia coli* Infectious hepatitis virus Leptospira (urine only) Poliomyelitis virus (faeces) Helminths, protozoa	Bed linen, clothing, **nurse's hands,** eating utensils, bedpans likely to be contaminated by faeces or urine.
Sputum, Nose and Throat Discharges any organism causing pneumonia *Corynebacterium diphtheriae* *Streptococcus pyogenes* *Bordetella pertussis* *Neisseria meningitidis* *Mycobacterium tuberculosis* Influenza virus Poliomyelitis virus Measles, chicken pox, Mumps virus Small pox virus.	Bed linen, clothing, handkerchiefs, towels, tooth brush, eating utensils, books, pencils, sputum bottles, thermometer, tongue depressors, throat swabs, medicine spoons, spray from coughing, sneezing; nurse's mask, gloves, apron; *nurse's hands.*
Pus or Exudate from Local Lesions Staphylococcus, Streptococcus *Neisseria gonorrhoeae* *Treponema pallidum* Body fluids, discharges with infectious organisms.	Bandages and dressings; clothing, bed linen, toilet seats; *nurse's hands* Articles, fomites likely to be contaminated by microorganisms.
Blood *Salmonella typhi* (first week) *Brucella melitensis* Plasmodium Leptospira *Neisseria meningitidis* (early stage) Arthropod borne bacterial, Viral diseases, rickettsial diseases (early stage) Hepatitis B virus.	Syringes, needles, gauze used to soak blood, sheet, clothing, or wash water contaminated with blood, obstetric instruments, dressings, vectors of the disease; *nurse's hands.*

CHAPTER 14

REMOVAL, INHIBITION AND DESTRUCTION OF MICROORGANISMS

History. When it was assumed that the communicable diseases were caused by microorganisms, the methods of sterilisation, disinfection and sanitation were adopted in daily practice. In early nineteenth century, the hospitals were dirty buildings accommodating the patients on mats spread on the floor, overcrowded together, dead and dying in the same beds. Surgeons wore black coat with linen thread wound around the button of his coat, which was used as suture material. His scalpel, kept attached to his breast pocket, was used periodically for the incision and was sharpened on the heel of his boot. The doctors washed their hands when they were soiled with pus and blood. The sleeve of the coat was rolled back to prevent from getting it spoiled. Such unhygienic conditions prevailed in those days in the hospital.

Then, during this 19th century came, Louis Pasteur (1863) who proved that the microbes caused the diseases. Robert Koch (1865) described many microbial diseases and isolated the causative microbes in pure culture. Later, Lister (1867) advocated in surgery the use of dilute carbolic acid as disinfectant. In obstetric and gynecology practice, the hand washing before delivery and operation was made compulsory. The practice of antisepsis and disinfection started from 1867.

About 200 years ago Napoleon Bonaparte ordered to serve better food for his armies. In order to obey his order, a French scientist, Nicholas Appert, developed a process which was called an "Appertizing" which involved steam, heat, and pressure — as in autoclaving. This principle is even now adopted in the modern method of sterilisation in every hospital. Later Pasteur advocated a method to check spoilage of beer by subjecting it to a temperature of 50° - 60°C for a few minutes and named it "Pasteurisation" which is used in our day-to-day practice, i.e., *Pasteurisation* of milk.

Koch sterilised the culture media by a method of intermittent heat at 100°C. Tyndall modified and perfected the method and called it as "Tyndallisation".

In 1880, Pasteur constructed a miniature early autoclave similar to the modern pressure cooker. In 1890, for the first time in the world, an autoclave was installed in Rochester City Hospital, New York.

It is well established that the microorganisms (both harmful and harmless) are ubiquitous in nature i.e., they exist everywhere. The pathogenic (harmful) bacteria should be killed or eliminated completely — particularly in surgery, surgical environment, hospital and public health. This procedure can be accomplished by the professional trained nurse by her skilful intelligent application of her nursing microbiology knowledge in the medical and nursing practice.

In bacteriological laboratory, mostly *pure cultures* grown on nutrient media are dealt with. Therefore, the disinfection and sterilisation methods advocated for pure cultures were followed in the diagnostic laboratory, whereas, in nursing practice, the situations are different unlike laboratory. So the ingenious professional nurse has to deal with *mixed cultures,* e.g., resistant forms and vegetative forms of microorganisms living in tissues, exudates, discharges, faeces mucus, pus, blood, Therefore, the intelligent well-trained nurse must exercise her own judgement after evaluating each situation to adopt the best methods to remove, disinfect, inhibit or destroy completely the pathogenic microorganisms.

The following are the best possible procedures :

1. Removal by
   (a) Passing the fluids through very fine filter which retains bacteria;
   (b) High speed centrifugation.
2. Inhibition by
   (a) Low temperature (dry ice);
   (b) Desiccation (drying process);
   (c) Combination of low temperature and desiccation;
   (d) High osmotic pressure (brine);
   (e) Microbiostatic chemicals and drugs

(i) dyes — eosin, methylene blue, crystal violet;

(ii) chemical agents — sulphonamide, antiseptics.

3. Destruction by

(a) Heat — dry (hot air oven); moist (autoclave);

(b) Chemical agents (disinfectants);

(c) Radiation (X-rays, ultraviolet);

(d) Mechanical agents (crushing).

INHIBITION OF MICROORGANISMS : ANTIMICROBIAL AGENTS

Antimicrobial agent is a chemical which inhibits the growth and causes the death of organisms.

The agents can be grouped accordingly :

1. If the substance merely causes a cessation of growth of microorganism — which is reversed when the chemical is removed — it is called *static* agent, if the substance kills the bacteria, it is called *cidal* agent. A static agent may become cidal if the concentration is increased. The disinfectants have a cidal action, while chemotherapeutic agents are often static at the concentration used.

2. Agents acting on bacteria are *bacteriostatic* or *bactericidal*, those acting on fungi are fungistatic or fungicidal.

3. In practice, chemotherapeutic agents can be distinguished :

(a) *Disinfectants* are chemicals used to kill potentially infective organisms normally present on inanimate objects, surface, water etc. They are potentially toxic to man, when they come in direct contact with man.

(b) *Antiseptics* (mild disinfectants) are relatively non-toxic and non-irritant, antimicrobial agents which may be used for the topical application on the body surface to kill or inhibit the pathogenic microorganisms.

(c) *Chemotherapeutic agents* are chemicals used to inhibit or kill bacteria already established in the body tissues and are used for the therapeutic purposes in the treatment of microbial infections.

Chemotherapeutic agents should act at a concentration that can be tolerated by the tissues of the host and, therefore, they must have a selective toxicity for the microorganisms compared with the host cells. The most widely used chemotherapeutic agents are the *antibiotics* which are naturally occurring antimicrobial agents produced by the microorganisms. The most common groups of antibiotic producers are actinomycetes and fungi.

Sulphonamides. The discovery of sulphonamides in 1935 by Domagk, a German chemist, began with the finding that the red dye, Prontosil, was capable of causing inhibiting infection with *Streptococcus pyogenes*, Prontosil itself had no effect on streptococci *in vitro*, but to be effective, it has to be broken down in the animal to sulphonamide. Sulphonamide itself is effective in non-toxic doses. By substituting different organic groups (represented by R groups in the formula below). For example, the addition of a pyridine group gave sulphapyridine, a thiazole gave sulphathiazole and so on. In this way, thousands of derivatives called sulphonamides were produced and many of them were found to be effective antimicrobial agents. Because of the development of newer antibiotics, relatively few sulphonamides have found a practical therapeutic use. It was observed that yeast and meat extract had the property of overcoming the inhibitory effect of sulphonamides on bacteria *in vitro*. The sulphonamide "antagonist" in the extracts was isolated and was shown to be para (p)-amino benzoic acid (PABA). It was also shown that PABA is an essential metabolite in any organism and was converted by them to dihydrofolic acid then to tetrahydrofolic acid, which acts as a co-factor in reaction leading to the synthesis of nucleic acids and proteins required for cell growth.

It was found that the sulphonamides inhibit the first stage of the synthesis of dihydrofolic acid from para-amino benzoic acid. The drug, trimethoprim, which was later discovered and introduced into the medicine at much later date, inhibits the conversion of dihydro-folic acid into tetrahydrofolic acid (Fig. 14.1).

Summary

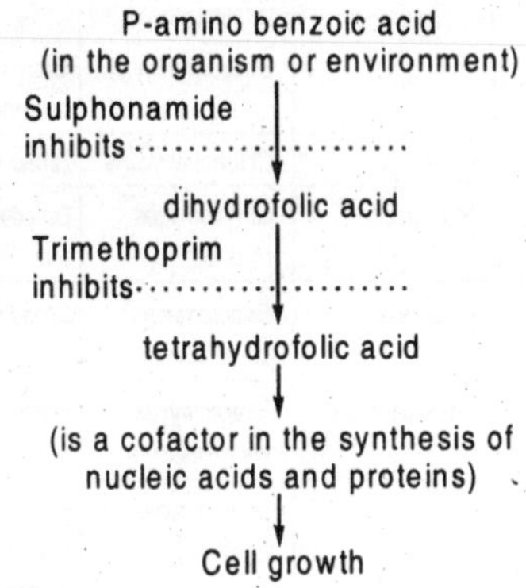

Fig. 14.1

Since p-amino benzoic acid and sulphonamides have similar chemical structures (Fig. 14.2), there is *competition* between sulphonamide and PABA for the active site on the surface of the enzyme initiating the conversion of PABA to dihydrofolic acid. To inhibit the conversion of one molecule of PABA into folic acid, a large number of sulphonamides molecules are required in the *competitive* inhibition (Fig. 14.2).

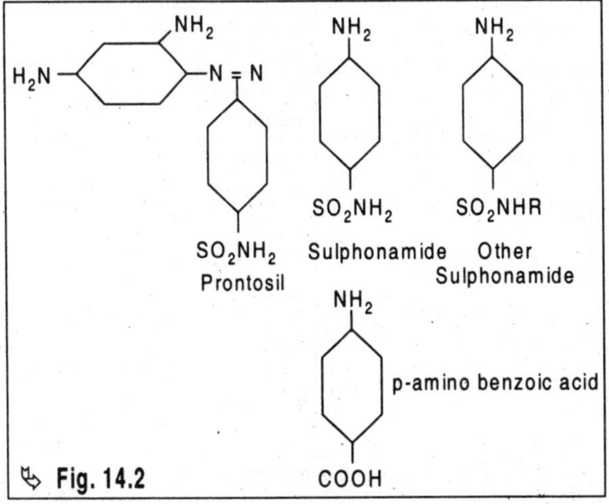

Fig. 14.2

Antibiotics inhibiting cell wall synthesis

Mucopeptide of the bacterial cell walls is responsible for their mechanical strength. If the synthesis of mucopeptide is inhibited, while synthesis of other cell components continue, then the cell can be expected to be lysed rapidly in normal osmotic environment. Penicillin inhibits the conversion of a complex nucleotide (uridine diphosphate UDP-N-acetyl muramic acid pentapeptide) into mucopeptide (Fig. 14.3)

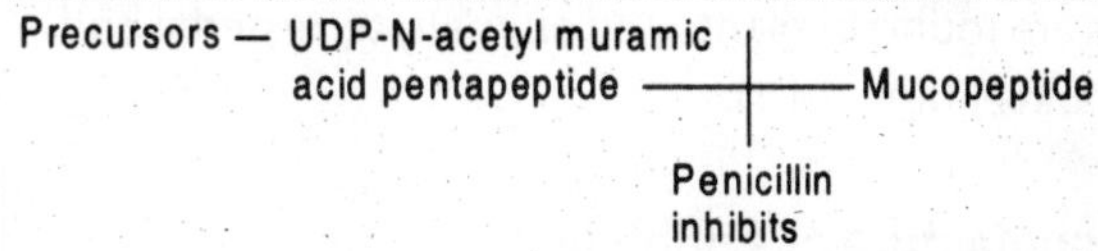

Fig. 14.3

Penicillin was discovered by Alexander Fleming in 1922.

Antibiotics affecting protein synthesis

A number of antibiotics (Streptomycin, Kanamycin, Tetracyclines, Erythromycin and Puromycin) are known to inhibit protein synthesis. Streptomycin, discovered by Waksman, was the first antibiotic to be introduced clinically after penicillin.

Antibiotics affecting nucleic acid synthesis

Few antibiotics combine with and alter the functioning of nucleic acids though they are generally toxic for therapeutic use. Ribonucleic acid (RNA) synthesis is prevented by Actinomycin, because it forms a complex with double stranded Deoxyribonucleic acid (DNA), but not with single stranded DNA; however, at higher concentrations, DNA synthesis is inhibited. On the other hand, mitomycin links complimentary strands of DNA resulting into blockage in DNA synthesis.

Antibiotics acting on the cytoplasmic membrane

Polymyxin acts on the cytoplasmic membrane as a cationic detergent binding to the membrane, as a result the semipermeable properties are lost and essential low molecular weight intermediates and coenzymes pass into the environment causing the death of bacteria. Polymyxin should be used with caution as it binds also with the membrane of the host cells.

Source of Antibiotics

Unlike synthetic sulphonamides, most of the antibiotics are produced in the culture media during the growth of certain microorganisms (Streptomyces, Bacillus, Penicillium, Aspergillus). New antibiotics are found in plants and animals, terresterial and marine (Table 14.1).

Manufacture of Antibiotics

The desired antibiotic producing organism is cultivated in large tank of suitable liquid medium for a predetermined length of time. The culture is then centrifuged and filtered to remove the microorganisms. The filtered fluid, containing the antibiotic is then subjected to purification and concentration process. These at length yield crystals of the pure antibiotics which are then tested for purity, sterility, then packed and distributed.

Classes of Antibiotics

Antibiotics may be grouped as follows:

Group I. (Penicillin, Streptomycin, Bacitracin, Polymyxin B) can be used together, they are often synergistic; never antagonistic. For example, when penicillin and streptomycin combined they are valuable in endocarditis. The combination is more effective than the sum of both.

Group II. (Tetracyclines, Chloramphenicol, Erythromycin, Carbomycin, Neomycin, Oleandromycin, Novobiocin) is neither antagonistic nor synergistic. Th's sometimes works well in combination with antibiotics of first group. This second group is generally of the "broad-spectrum" type. There are many other broad-spectrum antibiotics. The usual response to antibiotic therapy and antibiotic resistance or drug fastness are two important properties of organisms.

Table 14.1 : Antibiotics in common use

Antibiotics Common name	Trade name	Source	Characteristics
Penicillin		*Penicillium nutatum*	Gram positive bacteria Treponema Neisseria
Paromomycin	Humat	*Streptomyces rimosus*	*Entamoeba histolytica*
Streptomycin		*Streptomyces griseus*	*Myco.tuberculosis*
Dihydrostreptomycin		*Streptomyces* Sp.	Gram negative bacteria
Tetracyclines	Achromycin	Chlortetracycline	Broad-spectrum
Oxytetracycline	Terramycin	*Streptomyces rimosus*	Broad-spectrum
Chlortetracycline	Aureomycin	*Streptomyces aureofaciens*	Broad-spectrum
Chloramphenicol	Chloromycetin	*Streptomyces venezuelae*	Broad-spectrum
Erythromycin	Althrocin	*Streptomyces erythreus*	Broad spectrum (not Enterobacteriaceae)
Carbomycin	Magnamycin	*Streptomyces halstedii*	Broad spectrum (not Enterobacteriaceae)
Oleandromycin	Matromycin	*Streptomyces* Sp.	Broad spectrum
Neomycin B	Flavomycin	*Streptomyces fradiae*	Mycobacteria
Viomycin	Viocin	*Streptomyces funiceus*	Gram positive bacteria, Treponema.
Amphotericin B	Fungizone	*Streptomyces nodosus*	*Candida* sp.
Kanamycin	Kantrex	*Streptomyces kanamyceticus*	Broad spectrum
Nystatin	Mycostatin	*Streptomyces noursei*	Pathogenic fungi
Cycloheximide	Actidione	*Streptomyces griseus*	Saprophytic fungi
Griseofulvin	Grifulvin	*Streptomyces griseus*	Pathogenic fungi
Bacitracin		*Bacillus subtilis*	Gram positive bacteria, *Treponema, Neisseriae*
Polymyxin B		*Bacillus polymyxa*	Gram positive bacteria
Pyocynin*		Miscellaneous	*Pseudomonas aeruginosa*

*One of the first known antibiotic substances. Not used medicinially.

Use of Antibiotics

Some of the antibiotics can be used only by oral route; some in ointment only; others are suitable for intravenous or subcutaneous injection. Some are effective chiefly against Gram-positive organisms and some against Gram-negative organisms. Others have a wide range of activity. They are known as *broad-spectrum antibiotics.*

Drug Resistance or Drug-Fastness. Microorganisms often undergo genetic mutations. These mutations generally result in alterations in enzymic equipment in the mutant cells. If mutation occurs in few cells of a species of microorganisms (e.g., *Staphylococcus aureus*) altering the enzymatic equipment of these cells which are multiplying in a patient treated with penicillin. These mutated few cells will produce penicillinase or beta lactamase enzyme acting on beta lactam ring of penicillin become resistant to penicillin and grow in presence of penicillin. They are called as antibiotic resistant or drug fast. There resistant cells may grow and finally predominate in spite of the drug. The predomination is very dangerous to the patient and for every one around him who may acquire the organisms (e.g., sulphonamide-resistant gonococci). The sufficient quantity of the chemotherapeutic drug in the blood stream affecting even the most resistant species of the infecting organism before it can start growing, can be maintained by using adequate doses. This blood level maintenance can stop the development of such drug-resistant microorganisms.

Blood Levels Maintenance

The amounts of drug in the blood can be maintained by repeated doses at proper intervals of time. If delayed, the patient has to combat a *drug-fast* infection and may succumb to the infection. Therefore, the nurse responsible for giving repeated doses of such drugs should be very careful that the patient receives the drug *on time* so that his blood levels may not decrease to dangerous low levels.

Table 14.2 : Microorganisms Response for Antibiotics

Microorganisms	*Usual response for proper antibiotic treatment.*	*Frequency of appearance of resistance in strains in patients*
Pneumococcus Meningococcus Gonococci Beta streptococci Shigella Treponema	Rapid	Rare
Staphylococcus	Rapid	Very Frequent.
Alpha and gamma streptococci Coliform Proteus Pseudomonas Tubercle bacilli	Slow or incomplete	Frequent
Erucella *Salmonella typhi* Rickettsiae	Rapid relapses require repeated treatments.	Frequent Rare (once) Frequent (recently)

CHAPTER 15

STERILISATION AND DISINFECTION

Sterilisation and disinfection: These two terms are used to describe the killing or removal of microorganisms. The sterilisation is an *absolute term* which denotes the complete killing or removal of microorganisms of all kinds, while the disinfection is a relative term indicating a mere removal of burden of pathogenic microorganisms on the article.

Sterilisation is the process of freeing of an article from all living organisms, including viruses, bacteria and their spores, fungi and their spores, both pathogens and non pathogens. Sterility is an absolute state. An article can never be "relatively sterile".

Sterilisation of culture media, containers and instruments is essential in bacteriological work for the isolation and maintenance of pure culture. In nursing practice, surgery and medicines, the sterilisation of the instruments, drugs and other supplies is important for the prevention of the disease and it is also required for medical and surgical instruments and materials used in procedures that involve the penetration into the blood, tissues and other normally sterile parts of the body, e.g., surgical operation, intravenous transfusion, hypodermic injections and diagnostic aspirations.

Disinfection is a method of freeing an article or instrument from some or all living pathogens which may produce the infection during the use of the instruments contaminated with the pathogens. This term is relative since the effectiveness of disinfection depends upon the proportion of the pathogenic microorganisms, killed or removed. In circumstances where the sterility is not necessary or sterilising procedures are unwanted and impracticable, the disinfection should be adopted, e.g., bedpans, baths, wash basins, furniture, eating utensils, bed clothes, fomites, which may spread the infection in the hospitals, cannot be sterilised but they can be easily disinfected. Similarly, it is not practicable to apply sterilising procedures to the skin. The non-spore forming bacteria present in the skin mostly infect the surgical wound, hence it is of great necessity to disinfect the operative site as a valuable pre-operative precaution to kill the vegetative bacteria.

Sterilisation can be effected by the following methods:

I. Physical methods
   (a) Heat
      (i) Dry heat (inceration, red hot, flaming, hot air oven, infra red radiation);
      (ii) Moist heat (Pasteurisation, boiling water, steam steriliser, autoclave).
   (b) Radiation
      (i) Non-ionising radiation (Ultraviolet radiation);
      (ii) Ionising radiation (X-ray, gamma ray).
   (c) Filtration (Berkfeld, Chamberland, Seitz, sintered glass, cellulose membrane filters).

II. Chemical methods

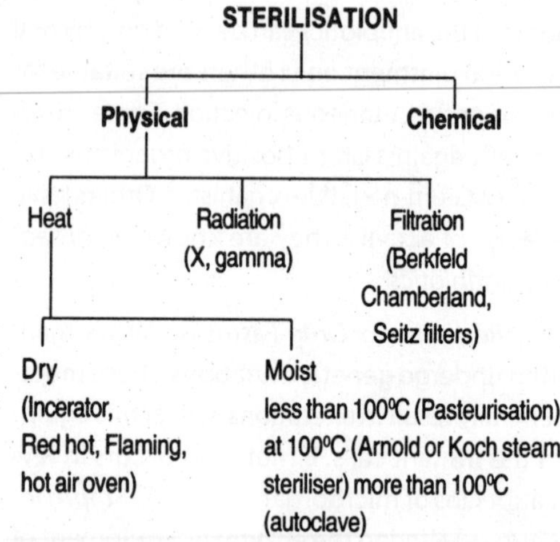

Basic Principles of Sterilisation by Heat

Moist heat is more effective than dry heat by sterilising at a lower temperature in a given time, or in a shorter time at a given temperature. Moist heat kills the microorganisms by *coagulating* and *denaturating* their *enzymes* and their *structural proteins*, a process in which the water participates. *Sterilisation, e.g., killing of the most resistant spores requires exposure to moist heat at 121°C for 10-30 minutes.* Dry heat is believed to kill the microorganisms by causing *destructive oxidation of essential cell constituents. Killing of the most resistant spores by dry heat requires a temperature of about 160°C for 60 minutes in hot air oven.*

Factors influencing Sterilisation by Heat

1. The temperature and the time of exposure;
2. The number of microorganisms and spores;
3. The species, strains and spore forming ability.

1. The temperature and the time of exposure for sterilisation are inversely related. At higher temperature, shorter time exposure is sufficient, e.g., the

heating must be hot enough. For surgical and bacteriological sterilisation, an exposure of the organisms to moist heat at 121°C for 10-20 minutes is sufficient for killing of all pathogenic spore forming organisms and all saprophytes except some strict thermophiles which grow best at more than 40°C. Sterilising time (holding period) is the time during which the microbes themselves should be held at the given temperature and *does not include* the heating up time. The amount of time allowed for heating up is known as *heat penetration time.*

2. The rapidity of the sterilisation is affected by *the number of microbes and their spores.* In practice, before applying heat for sterilisation, the cleaning of all the articles or instruments should be done to reduce the burden of contaminated bacteria for better and rapid sterilisation.

3. The susceptibility to heat is affected by the *species, strains and spore forming ability of the microorganisms.* The amount of heat required to kill a given strain or species of bacteria is related to the temperature and time of exposure and it is stated that the *thermal death point* when the lowest temperature is required to kill completely the bacteria within 10 minutes or the *thermal death time* when the shortest time is required to kill completely the microbes at a particular temperature. The most reliable method of measurement of the thermal death point and time is the *decimal reduction time* or *D value* which is the time (in minutes) required to achieve a tenfold reduction in the viability of a bacterial suspension at a given temperature under standard condition.

Effect of Moist Heat

A temperature of 50°C to 65°C may kill within 10 minutes the vegetative forms of most bacteria, yeasts and fungi and animal viruses. *Treponema pallidum* is fragile and killed at 43°C in 10 minutes *Coxiella burnetii* causing Q fever in man is heat resistant. *Bacillus stearothermophilus* is extremely resistant to heat. Poliomyelitis virus is killed at 60°C for 30 minutes and serum hepatitis virus is killed at 60°C for 10 hours. Bacteriophages are killed at the temperature of 65-80°C for 15-30 minutes. The most resistant forms of spores of actinomycetes, yeasts and fungi are killed at 80-90°C in 30 minutes. The spores of *Clostridium tetani, Cl. welchii* are killed at 100°C for 10 minutes, whereas *Cl. botulinum* in 8 hours.

Effect of Dry Heat

Dry heat at 160°C for 60 minutes will kill vegetative bacteria and spores which are susceptible to moist heat at 60°C in 30 minutes and heat resistant spores.

High content of organic substances protect spores and vegetative forms against the lethal action of heat. The heat resistance of spores is diminished with increased acidity and alkalinity. The effect of alkali is used in the disinfection of metal instruments by boiling at 100°C in water containing 2 per cent sodium carbonate; but this method is not reliable as autoclaving.

Sterilisation by Moist Heat

Microorganisms can be killed by moist heat if they come in contact with water or steam; otherwise if they are protected from wetting, as by grease or in a relatively impervious container exposed at the same temperature; the moist heat will have the weaker effect than the dry heat.

Method of Sterilisation by Moist Heat

In sterilisation, moist heat can be used:

(a) at temperature below 100°C;

(b) at a temperature of 100°C (either in boiling water or in free steam); or

(c) at a temperature above 100°C (in saturated steam under increased pressure) which ensures the complete sterilisation and killing of the most *highly resistant* spores.

Basic Principles of Moist Heat Sterilisation

Because of its greatest lethal effect on microorganisms, quicker heating up effect on the exposed articles and its penetrating power through porous materials (paper, cloth wrapper, bundles of surgical instruments, wool stoppers, cotton), saturated steam is a more efficient sterilising agent than the hot air.

When the cooler surface of the article comes in contact with the steam, the steam condenses into a small volume of water and liberates its large latent heat to that cooler surface of the article (e.g., 1,600 ml of steam at 100°C condense, at atmospheric pressure, into 1 ml of water at 100°C liberating 518 calories of heat). The contraction in volume causes immediate suction of more steam to the same site and this process continues till the temperature of the article is raised to the temperature of the steam. The condensed water provides moist conditions for killing of the exposed microbes. Since the penetration by the steam is hindered by the air, the air should not be trapped inside the autoclave; only pure steam is used. The loss of water by evaporation by heating is prevented by the saturated steam. Hence, culture media (both solid and liquid) can be sterilised by the steam under pressure. In the autoclave or steamer, the cotton wool stoppers can be drenched, this drenching can be avoided by covering the stopper with kraft paper. If a wire basket containing test tubes is used, it can be covered with a sheet of paper folded down the edges of the basket.

Moist Heat at a Temperature Below 100°C

The process which kills all non-spore forming pathogens (*Mycobacterium tuberculosis, Brucella abortus, Salmonella*) in milk by subjecting the milk to a temperature of 63°C for 30 minutes (the holder method) or 73°C for 20 seconds (the flash method) is known as "*Pasteurisation of milk.*"

Serum or body fluids containing coagulable protein can be sterilised by heating for 1 hour at 56°C on several successive days in water bath. Care must be taken not to allow the temperature to rise above 59°C, which may cause inspissation. Vaccines can be prepared in a vaccine bath at a temperature of 60°C for 1 hour.

Moist Heat at a Temperature of 100°C

Boiling at 100°C. Boiling at 100°C for 5-10 minutes does not ensure the complete sterility, but it is enough to kill all non-sporing organisms and few spore-forming bacilli (e.g., strains of *Cl. tetani* may survive boiling for 1-3 hours). Sometimes, in microbiology and medicine, this boiling method is used, when the absolute sterility is unwanted for pipettes, measuring cylinders, rubber stoppers, instruments (scalpels, forceps, scissors, metal or glass syringe) which do not withstand higher temperature. If water supply is hard, the instruments after removal from boiling water may become covered with a film of calcium salts; to avoid this effect, distilled water should be used. Addition of 2 per cent sodium bicarbonate may promote the sterilisation.

Long handed-forceps, kept immersed in 3 per cent lysol to a level approaching the finger grip, can be used to remove the articles and instruments from boiling water. If the instrument was taken into the hand, while it is wet, its working end (e.g., scalpel blade or syringe needle) may get contaminated with skin bacterium flowing from the fingers in the film of water.

However, boiling water can generally be used for contaminated dishes, bedding and bedpans, because these articles do require neither sterility nor the destruction of spores. Only disinfection is necessary for these articles. At altitudes over 5,000 feet, the boiling time should be increased by 50 per cent, because the water boils at this altitude at a temperature of 95°C or below.

Boiling (at 100°C) for 10 minutes kills the vegetative and actively multiplying cells of pathogenic bacteria, rickettsiae, all viruses except hepatitis and poliomyelitis viruses, if these microorganisms are not protected by the blood, food, faeces, mucus etc. It also kills or damages the cysts of protozoa, ova of helminths, ascospores of pathogenic yeasts, conidia of molds. Since the spores of *Clostridium tetani*, *Cl.welchii* and *Bacillus anthracis* and hepatitis virus are resistant to boiling even for 10 minutes, so boiling at 100°C for 10 minutes is not effective. Spores present in soil, faeces, dust, on instruments, bandages contaminated with blood, dust may be a risk of infection. Whereas anthrax spores occur only in areas where the infected animals died of anthrax.

Boiling at 100°C for 10 minutes is a sure means of disinfection (not sterility), if the spores and viruses are not present, of instruments and glasswares, if they are not soiled with blood, faeces, food etc. The margin of safety can be increased by boiling for 30 minutes.

Summary

1. Vegetative forms of all bacteria and fungi pathogenic to man; rickettsiae pathogenic to man; helminths and their ova; many viruses (except hepatitis virus); bacterial toxin (except staphylococcal enterotoxin) are killed or inactivated by boiling at 100°C for 10 minutes.

2. Bacterial spores; Hepatitis virus; ascospores of fungi; conidia of some fungi pathogenic to man; staphylococcal enterotoxin are not killed or inactivated by boiling at 100°C for 10 minutes.

Steaming at 100°C is commonly used in the microbiological laboratory to sterilise the culture media (both nutrient broth and nutrient agar). It is not as effective as autoclaving. *Koch* or *Arnold steam steriliser* or "Steamer" is a vertical metal cylinder with a removable lid having a small outlet for the steam escape and at its bottom it contains water which is heated up. Above the water level, a tray bears the articles to be sterilised. Frequent opening of the steamer should be minimised, because the air permitted inside the steamer ultimately interferes with the sterilisation.

Sterilisation can be carried out as follows:

(a) By a single exposure at 100°C for 90 minutes.

(b) By intermittent exposure at 100°C for 20-45 minutes on each three successive days.

(a) Single exposure at 100°C for 90 minutes is not suitable as the spores of thermophilic and some mesophilic bacteria can survive this exposure.

(b) Intermittent exposure at 100°C for 20-45 minutes on each three successive days is also known as "Tyndallisation". In this method one exposure will destroy all the vegetative organisms between the heatings, the spores in favourable nutrient medium become vegetative forms which are killed during the subsequent heating. This method is suitable for the medium containing sugars which may be decomposed at higher temperature and for gelating medium which, after prolonged heating, may not solidify on cooling.

Moist heat at temperature above 100°C

Sterilisation in the autoclave

Principle employed in the autoclave — water boils when its steam pressure equals to atmospheric pressure, or it can be interpreted as the water boils at 100°C at normal atmospheric pressure (i.e., 760 mm Hg; 14 lb per square inch pressure). So when the water is boiled within a closed vessel at increased pressure, the temperature at which the water boils and that of its steam will rise above 100°C. The most effective method of sterilisation of culture media (in the bacteriological laboratory) and surgical materials or supplies (in the hospital) is Autoclaving.

The steam should perforate all parts of the articles to be sterilised in the autoclave and should be *hot*, saturated (i.e., point of condensing to liquid water) and dry (i.e., free from particles of liquid water).

This dry saturated steam affects the sterilisation because of its high temperature (latent heat). The ideal minimum holding time Is 15-30 minutes at 121°C (15 lb per square inch gauze pressure).

Air discharge. To expose all articles in the autoclave to the pure steam during sterilisation, it is necessary to remove all the air from the autoclave, because (a) the mixture of steam and air results in a lower temperature at a particular pressure, (b) the penetration of steam in the interstices of porous materials (e.g., surgical dressings), syringes, etc., may be interferred by the air, and (c) the air, being denser than the steam from a cooler layer at the bottom of the autoclave, which prevents the sufficient heating of the articles at the lower level.

There are two types of autoclaves :

(a) The simple non-jacketed laboratory autoclave;
(b) Steam-jacketed autoclave with automatic air and condensate discharge.

(a) The simple non-jacketed laboratory autoclave (Fig. 15.1) is also called as "pressure cooker type". It is made up of a vertical or horizontal gun metal or stainless steel cylinder of about 18 inches in diameter and 30 inches in length with a supporting stand. The lid (door) is tightened by screw clamps and is rendered air tight by means of an asbestos washer. The water level inside the cylinder should be up to 3. 1/2 inches for a vertical cylinder of 19 inches internal length. The autoclave is heated by a gas burner or electric heater from below the cylinder. The articles to be sterilised are placed on a perforated tray situated above the water level. The lid of the autoclave is provided with a discharge tap for the air and steam, a pressure gauze and a safety valve which is adjusted to blow off automatically at any desired pressure.

Operating of the simple autoclave. Inside the autoclave, the water should be up to required level, i.e., below the perforated tray. The materials to be sterilised are placed on the tray and the heater should be turned on. The lid should be placed in position and fastened by screw clamps, the discharge tap should remain *open* and the safety valve is to be adjusted to the required pressure. In some autoclave, the pressure has been predetermined and adjusted by the manufacturers. When water boils inside the cylinder of the autoclave, the steam rises, mixes with the air in

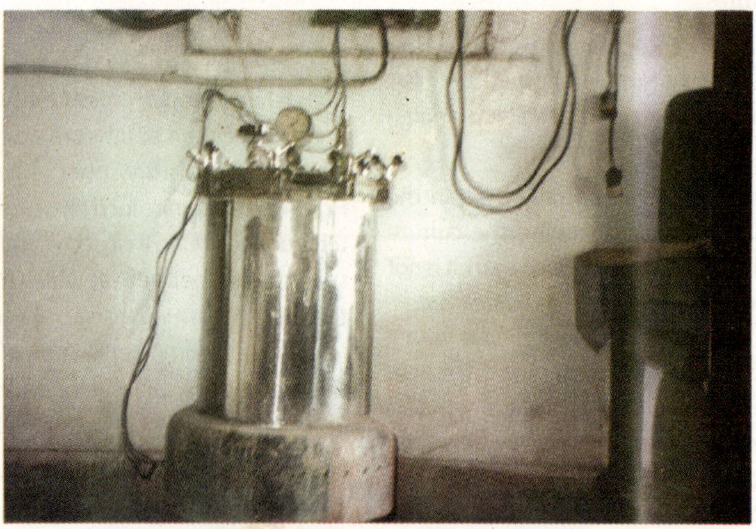

Fig. 15.1 : Autoclave (Laboratory type)

the chamber and expels out this air through the discharge tap. The operator should allow *the steam and air mixture to escape freely till all the air is completely removed from the autoclave*, which can be adjusted by connecting a rubber *tube from the* discharge tap into a container of cold water into which the steam condenses and the air rises as bubbles to the surface. This procedure can be followed by an inexperienced operator for his own satisfaction, when there is no trained nurse. If the air has completely escaped, the discharge tap should be closed. The steam pressure rises till it reaches the desired level, e.g., 15 lb per square inch for 121°C, when the safety valve opens automatically and allows the excess steam to escape. From this point, the *holding time* begins and continues for 15 minutes. The heater should be turned off, the discharge tap should be opened gradually and the autoclave should be allowed to *cool* till the inside pressure equals to the atmospheric pressure (0 lb per square inch) which may take about 1 hour; when the chamber pressure is still high, if the discharge tap is opened, there is possibility of danger of explosion of autoclave lid, culture media will boil and spill from the container. An excess amount of water will be evaporated and lost from the media if the discharge tap is not opened until the pressure has fallen much below the atmospheric pressure. It is necessary to have surgical linen and dressings wrapped in paper or cloth for quick drying of the materials after sterilisation. These wrapped articles are moistened by the condensation of the steam; when damp, even several layers of paper and cloth wrappings could not check the entry of contaminating bacteria into the sterilised articles. Therefore, *the sterilised articles* should not be kept in contact with unsterilised objects until their wrappings are dry.

(b) *Steam-jacketed autoclave* (Fig. 15.2) is mostly used in the hospital to sterilise the linen, surgical materials etc. It is a horizontal cylinder. At the front, there is a swing door which is tightened by screw clamps or by a "capstan head" with its radial bolts and it locks automatically while the chamber pressure is raised. This safety door, locked automatically by pressure, can prevent the possibility of a dangerous explosion, if the operator opens early the autoclave by mistake.

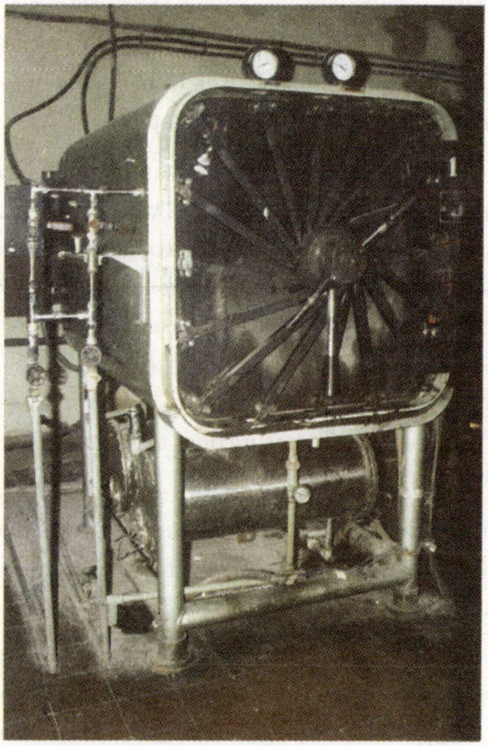

Fig. 15.2 : Autoclave (Hospital type)

The autoclave consists of (1) a steam supply from outside (e.g., an independent boiler), (2) a steam jacket which heats the sidewalls of the autoclave, (3) a channel discharging air from the bottom of the chamber, (4) a thermometer in the discharge channel, indicating the temperature above the lowest and coolest part of the chamber, (5) vacuum system to assist drying of the load, (6) an air intake with a self-sterilising filter for introducing warm sterile air in the chamber, (7) a cooling system to hasten the cooling of the liquids without violent boiling, (8) an automatic control system for heating up, holding, cooling and drying.

Steam supply. The steam supplied to the autoclave should be dry, i.e., free from excess of water, and *saturated,* i.e., not superheated.

Wet steam. The steam released from the boiler at a long distance may become "wet" and inefficient sterilising agent because of (a) cooling and condensation, (b) soaking of porous materials which prevents further penetration, and (c) the particles of water possess no latent heat. Thus, the pressure of the main steam supply should be usually 55 lb per square inch. The reduction in pressure dries the steam.

Superheated steam is not satisfactory because it abstracts the water from the exposed materials, may cause the less lethal effect and is still more destructive as dry heat.

Operating of steam jacketed autoclave. A space between the double sidewalls of the chamber (Jacket) is filled throughout the day with the steam at 121°C introduced from the boiler. Water of condensation from the steam is drained off through the jacket discharge channel which is thermostatically controlled. The operator should ensure that there is no obstruction of this discharge channel.

Loading of the chamber. The articles to be sterilised should be arranged loosely so that the steam circulates freely and the air is displaced.

Heating up and air displacement period. The swing door should be closed hermetically. The steam from the jacket should enter through a baffle at the back of the chamber. The pressure and temperature should be maintained in the chamber as in the jacket. The cooler and denser air should be displaced by the steam under pressure. If more steam is introduced under pressure, it displaces the air downwards through the articles to be sterilised and the air is discharged out through the chamber discharge channel situated at the bottom of the chamber. At the same time, the water of condensation on the cool load and the door of the chamber should be drained off through the same channel. As soon as all free air is eliminated, the inflow of pure steam raises the trap's temperature to 121°C, it closes automatically and it prevents further escape. The steam replaces the air in about 5-10 minutes.

Holding period of sterilisation. Holding period will start when the thermometer in the discharge channel reaches the temperature of 121°C. The exact duration of the holding period depends upon the nature of the load. A "near to steam" trap is essential as it opens when the temperature falls by 1°C below that of the pure steam.

Cooling and drying period. The steam supply to the chamber is stopped at the end of the holding period. The steam inside the chamber starts to cool by loss of heat through the door and pressure falls slowly.

High Pre-vacuum Steriliser

High vacuum surgical steriliser is the only method of sterilisation that can overcome the effects of bad packing or overloading of the steriliser. Tightly packed load is heated rapidly and uniformly to the sterilising temperature for a shorter time, e.g., 135°C for 3 minutes. The damage to heat sensitive materials is avoided by greatly shortening the time. The steam, admitted to the chamber, heats the whole load to 135°C within 2-3 minutes. The holding period is maintained for 3 minutes, the temperature reaches 135°C. The load is then dried within a few minutes by exhaustion of the chamber to a high vacuum.

Automatic control system. Carries through the whole sterilisation process — heating up, holding, cooling and drying accurately to the fixed time, temperature and pressure. Once the autoclave is started, no further attention is needed till it is cooled. The error due to negligence can be rectified by the control system. The sterilising process can be reported by the monitoring system, if the fixed temperature falls below at any time.

Temperature record. Recording thermometer can help the operator to avoid the errors in timing the holding period.

The overall efficiency of the autoclave can be judged by the following two methods : Chemical indicators and Spore indicators.

(a) *Chemical indicators* which show a change of colour or shape after exposure to a sterilising temperature, may be placed under the load. For example, (i) a sulphur pellet kept in a small glass tube will show a change of shape by melting when exposed to 120°C for a few minutes. (ii) Brownel's control tubes contain a red solution which turns green when heated at 115°C for 25 minutes (Type 1); or 15 minutes (type 2) or at 160°C for 60 minutes. These tubes should be stored at less than 20°C to avoid the deterioration and premature change in colour. (iii) Bowie-Dick tape, applied to packs and articles in the autoclave, develops diagonal lines when exposed to the sterilising temperature for the correct time. (iv) *Sterilometer* is a cellulose tape having on it a chemical indicator which changes its colour when properly heated in the autoclave.

(b) *Spore indicators. Bacillus stearothermophilus* grows best at 55°C-60°C. But a preparation of its dried spores is killed at 121°C in 12 minutes when placed within the load in the autoclave. After autoclaving, it can be tested for its viability on the culture media.

Nurse using the autoclave should be sure that

(a) all the air is allowed to escape and is replaced by the steam;

(b) the pressure of the steam reaches at least 15 pounds to the square inch and remains there;

(c) the thermometer reaches at least 121°C for 20 minutes.

Sterilisation by Radiation

Nonionising Ultraviolet radiation. Ultraviolet rays of sunlight have the bactericidal effects which depend upon the wave length. It is bactericidal when it reaches a wave length of 330 mμ (3,300 A° or Angstrom units). Angstrom is unit of measurement of wave length. Thus, as the wave length decreases, the effectiveness of the ultraviolet light increases as sterilising agent. The shortest ultraviolet rays of sunlight reaching the surface of the earth have a wave length of more than 200 mμ; however, most commonly used mercury vapours can emit even more effective radiations of 240-280 mμ.

High intensity ultraviolet radiation is applied with great precautions to protect the skin, to the site of the operation to check the post operative sepsis. Rays from ultraviolet lamps can reduce the bacterial load in the atmospheric dust. Pathogenic microorganisms on the floor and furnitures in rooms can be destroyed by the daylight passing through the ordinary glass windows.

Ionising radiation. In practice, sterilisation by radiation is achieved by the use of high speed cathode rays (electrons), X-rays and short X-rays (gamma rays) from an apparatus (linear accelator) or gamma rays from an isotope source (cobalt 60). This method is very costly for hospital use; but it is used commercially only for the sterilisation of prepacked disposable plastic syringes, transfusion sets and catheters which cannot withstand the heat. It is known as *cold sterilisation.*

Sterilisation by Filtration

In this process, the fluids (bacterial fluid cultures) can be freed from bacteria by passing through special filters. This method of sterilisation by filtration is specially useful to prepare toxin from bacterial growth and to sterilise the liquids (sugars, serum, antibiotic solutions) which are liable to be damaged by heat. These sterilising filters should be considered as rendering a liquid, bacteria free, but not virus free and are satisfactory for laboratory purposes; but, in clinical practice, such fluid (e.g., glucose, serum) sterilised by Seitz filtration are not safe.

Type of Filters

For bacteriological work, the following types of filters are used :

1. Earthenware candles, e.g., Berkefeld, Chamberland filters;

2. Asbestos and asbestos paper disk, e.g., Seitz filter;

3. Sintered glass filters;

4. Cellulose membrane filters.

1. (a) *Berkefeld Filters.* They are made from a fossil diatomaceous earth found in deposits in Germany and other parts of the world and are of three grades of porosity, e.g., V (Veil) the coarsest, W (Wening) the finest, and Normal (N) intermediate. Berkefeld V is often used. A small organism (*Serratia marcescens*) should pass through this filter.

(b) *Chamberland Filters.* They are made of unglazed porcelain of various grades of porosity. The finer grades will pass only certain viruses of extreme minuteness (e.g., Foot and Mouth Disease virus). The most porous grade L_1, clarifying filter, allows many microorganisms to pass. The next three L_{1a}, L_2 and L_3 are comparable with the Berkefeld V, N, and W candles, respectively. These filters can also be used to obtain bacterial toxin.

2. *Seitz Filters.* Consist of asbestos disk through which the fluid is passed. The disk is inserted into a metal holder which is jointed tightly by screw clamps. The whole filter is wrapped in kraft paper and sterilised in the autoclave. The asbestos disk is discarded after each filtration and is replaced by another new disk for fresh filtration. The disks are available in three grades : clarifying (K), normal, and "special EK." The normal and "special EK" do not allow the ordinary test bacterium *Serratia marcescens* to pass through.

3. *Sintered glass filters.* They are made of finely ground glass attached to the filtering apparatus and sterilised as in case of Seitz filter. After use, they should be washed with running water in reverse direction and cleaned with warm sulphuric acid to which potassium nitrate is added.

4. *Cellulose membrane filters.* There are two types of cellulose membrane filters : The gradocol membrane (older type) consists of cellulose nitrate and the modern membrane filter is made of cellulose acetate. The size of many viruses can be determined by these cellulose membrane filter; these filters can retaia *Serratin marcescens.*

Advantages of cell membrane filters are :

(a) They are much less absorptive and the rate of filtration is much greater;

(b) Bacteria retained on the surface of this filter can be cultivated by placing this filter on culture media.

5. The development of high efficiency particulate air (HEPA) filters or fiberglass filters has made possible to deliver clean air to an enclosure (cubicle or room). This type of air filteration together with a system of LAMINAR AIR FLOW is now recommended as air disinfection and used very extensively to produce dust and bacteria free air in vaccine sterility testing laboratory and it is expensive.

CHAPTER 16

CHEMICAL AGENTS OF DISINFECTION

Chemical sterilising agents are widely used as disinfectants and antiseptics.

Disinfectants are :

(a) chemical agents which are capable of destroying pathogenic microorganisms, but not resistant spores;

(b) potent and toxic;

(c) suitable only for application to *inanimate* objects.

Antiseptics are :

(a) chemical agents which kill microorganisms or prevent their growth;

(b) non-toxic;

(c) suitable for superficial application, to *living* tissues.

1. *Volatile antiseptics,* e.g., Chloroform. In the sterilisation and preservation of serum for culture media, chloroform can be used in the proportion of 0.25 per cent and later be removed by heating at 56°C.

Alcohols (Isopropyl alcohol, ethyl alcohol) are bactericidal in 70-75 per cent concentration. Chlorhexidine or Iodine is superior to alcohol alone for skin disinfectant before venepuncture or hypodermic injection.

2. *Antiseptics of the Phenol Group.* Lysol (liquor cresolis saponatus) and cresol (black and white fluid) are powerful disinfectants; they are used for sterilising surgical instruments, discarded cultures and killing cultures accidently split on the floor or table. Lysol is generally used in a 3 per cent solution and Phenol in 0.5 per cent for preserving sera. Sudol is less toxic substitute for Lysol. Dettol is less toxic, irritant and also less active. Hexochlorophane is an even blander agent and is incorporated in various antiseptic preparations. It is effective against Gram-positive and Gram-negative bacteria. It is potentially toxic and should be used with care.

3. *Metallic salts or organic compounds of metals.* Mercuric chloride (1 : 1,000) is used as disinfectant. Merthiolate, a proprietary name for sodium ethylmercuric thiosalicylate, is used in a dilution of 1 : 10,000 for preservation of antisera or sera. A drop of *Silver nitrate* (1 per cent) solution is used for prophylaxis of gonococcal ophthalmia in newborn babies. It is replaced by chlorhexidine (modern antiseptic).

4. *Formaldehyde* is an irritant water soluble gas which is highly lethal to all kinds of microbes and *spores,* killing bacterial spores as readily as the vegetative forms.

It is cheap and non-injurious to cloth, fabrics, wool, leather, rubber, paints and metals. So it can be used to disinfect the rooms, furnitures and a wide variety of articles which are liable to be damaged by heat (e.g., woollen blankets and clothing), shoes, gum elastic catheters). It can be applied as an aqueous solution or in gaseous forms.

Disinfection with aqueous Formaldehyde solution. A 40 per cent (W/V) solution of formaldehyde in water containing 10 per cent methanol to inhibit polymerisation is known as "commercial formalin". Formaldehyde diluted in water (5-10 per cent) is a powerful and rapid disinfectant when applied directly to a contaminated surface. Bacterial cultures and suspensions are also killed by this disinfectant.

Cleaned metal instruments may be sterilised by overnight immersion in a borax-formaldehyde solution :

Sodium tetraborate 50 g

Formaldehyde, 4 per cent in water, 1,000 ml.

Glutaraldehyde is bacterial sporocidal, more effective and less toxic. It is used to sterilise cystoscopes, anesthetic equipments, plastic materials and thermometers.

Disinfection by Formaldehyde gas. The articles which can be damaged by wetting or cannot be wetted completely with formaldehyde solution can be disinfected by Formaldehyde gas provided that the conditions, suitable for the action of gas, are maintained.The atmosphere must have relatively high (80-90 per cent) humidity and the temperature should be 18°C. Since the penetration of the gas into the porous fabrics is slow,the materials should be arranged in such a way the gas can have access to all contaminated surfaces.

Spraying, heating formalin or heating solid paraformaldehyde can liberate the gas. When spraying cold formalin, its polymerisation can be prevented by adding an equal volume of industrial spirit to cold formalin. Formalin diluted with sufficient water can be boiled to produce an adequate atmospheric humidity.This is a best method,because of the tendency of the gas to polymerise to paraformaldehyde and a maximal vapour concentration attainable at 20°C is 2.0 mg per litre of air, which is a desirable concentration. Higher concentration obtained at high temperature may be explosive. After disinfection, the articles may contain paraformaldehyde emitting irritant vapour for a long period which may be neutralised by exposure to ammonia vapour.

Exposure for at least 3 hours to formaldehyde gas in an airtight metal or painted wooden cabinet is sufficient to disinfect small articles (instruments, shoes, hair brushes).The gas is introduced inside the cabinet by boiling formalin in an electric boiler to the extent of 50 ml 40 per cent of formaldehyde per 100 cu ft of air space.Similarly, blankets and the surfaces of mattresses are disinfected in a large cabinet where they are hung *unfolded* so that the fabric can absorb formaldehyde gas (e.g., 500 ml. of formalin can be used for 100 lbs fabrics).Finally, the vapour is vented to the open air. *Folded* blankets and clothings can also be disinfected only if some heat is applied. They are packed in the chamber of steam jacketed autoclave; then 100 ml. formalin per 100 cu ft is placed at the bottom of the autoclave and the chamber is heated at 100°C for 3 hour by passing free steam through the jacket. At last, the vapour is vented through the autoclave vacuum system.

5. *Ethylene oxide.* It is a colourless liquid boiling at 107°C. It is moderately toxic gas above to this temperature and forms an explosive mixture when more than 3 per cent is present in air. A non-explosive mixture (10 per cent ethylene oxide in CO_2 or in halogenated hydrocarbon) can be used for sterilisation. It destroys bacteria and viruses, and kills the spores almost as easily as vegetative forms.

This is a gaseous disinfectant killing microorganisms and spores. It can diffuse more rapidly into dry, porous materials and is of great importance to sterilise articles which are liable to be damaged by heat (e.g., plastic, rubber articles, blankets, pharmaceutical products, lung heart machine etc.).

CHARPTER 17

STERILISATION METHODS IN MEDICAL PRACTICE

A. Sterilisation of Bottled Fluids

Hydrated fluids used for therapeutic intravenous infusions can be sterilised at 121°C for 12 minutes as the contaminating bacteria are already moist and can be easily destroyed at this condition. Similarly sterile water used in the operation theatre can be sterilised in the autoclave.

B. Sterilisation of Empty Bottles and Impervious Bottles

Empty and dry bottles can be sterilised in the autoclave, if they are not tightly stoppered so that the steam can enter and displace the inside air.They are arranged on their sides in the autoclave to permit a horizontal pathway for the entry of steam and escape of air. If unstoppered, they can be sterilised quickly; if stoppered with cotton wool or loosened screw cap, the displacement of air is slow and the holding period is 121°C for 30 minutes. Since the displacement of air from the stoppered container is not certain, it is always better to sterilise the stoppered empty container in hot air oven. The rubber liner inside the screw cap cannot withstand the high temperature (160°C) of hot air oven. This problem can be overcome by using silicon rubber liner.

C. Sterilisation of Wrapped Dry Goods and Surgical Dressings

When dry porous goods (e.g., paper), apparatus wrapped in cloth and surgical linen and dressings are to be sterilised by autoclave, it is essential that (a) the steam should displace by gravity completely the air from the autoclave; (b) the sterilised articles should be dry before they are removed from the autoclave. In this method, the load should be carefully packed so that there will be adequate spaces for the circulation of the steam. Glass and metal containers are kept open or covered only loosely. Metal drums and caskets must be provided with ports which must not be obstructed by the contents packed against them and must always be fully open during sterilisation and the steam should flow freely from top to bottom. A wrapping of two layers of good muslin is recommended for surgical packs. A single layer of coarse brown (Kraft) paper is also satisfactory.

Surgical dressings and other cloth articles should be arranged in packs no bigger than 12 × 12 × 20 inches (30 × 30 × 50 cm) and placed on edge in the autoclave so that the layers of cloth are vertical. Rubber gloves are powdered and packed loosely in muslin cloth to allow access of the steam to all parts. It used to be customary to autoclave rubber gloves at 5 to 10 lbs pressure for a short time to avoid the deterioration, but this exposure does not guarantee sterility, so the gloves should be autoclaved at the same temperature as for other goods. Instruments and syringes must be free from oil and grease, jointed instruments open and syringes disassembled. The chamber of the autoclave should not be overloaded and the perforated tray should not be removed.

D. Sterilisation of Surgical Instruments

Boiling is effective when 2 per cent sodium bicarbonate or a germicide is added to the water. There is the risk of recontamination when the instruments are washed before use to remove these substances.

Heat can blunt the sharp instrument, this effect is mainly due to oxidation, but the pure steam cannot damage. Ethylene oxide and formaldehyde are the only established chemical sterilising agents and can be used to sterilise the instruments (scalpels). Pasteurisation at 75°C or treatment with chlorhexidine in 75 per cent ethanol is recommended to sterilise the instrument (Cystoscopes).

Sterilisation of Syringes. In hospital wards and in microbiological laboratories, the syringes are very important in day-to-day use; therefore much heed is to be paid to their use, care and sterilisation. Sterilisation by chemical agents are not satisfactory, but the sterilisation by heat is the best method.

All glass syringes have many advantages over the glass metal type of syringes; the glass metal syringe is more difficult to clean and is more likely to break on heating due to the differences of expansion of glass and metal; it cannot be sterilised when assembled and it is difficult to keep sterilised until ready for use. The solder uniting the glass and metal may melt in hot air oven and autoclave. Syringes with cement at the glass metal junction which withstand 200°C are available. The mounts of the stainless steel needle of good quality must fit accurately the nozzle of the syringe.

All glass syringes. All new syringes must be well washed in soap and water with test tube brush according to their sizes. After washing in clean, warm water the barrel and piston should be dried. The syringes should be assembled, wrapped, sterilised and ready for use. If this facility is not available, all glass syringes should be sterilised just before use by boiling in a fish kettle or saucepan. Distilled water is preferable if the tap water is hard. The syringes should always be dismantled, the barrel and piston are placed in cold water which is brought to boil and kept boiling for 5-10 minutes. When *cool* and *dry*, the barrel and piston should be assembled with sterile forceps or clean, dry fingers, touching only the outside of the barrel and the top of the piston. The sterile syringes should be used immediately. The needle should also be boiled at the same time and affixed to the nozzle by means of sterile forceps. It is always better to sterilise all glass syringes in the hot air oven after they are wrapped with kraft paper; or the syringe with fitted needle should be accommodated in a test tube with cotton wool plug and the whole thing should be wrapped in kraft paper and sterilised in hot air oven at 160°C for 1 hour. It is sterile indefinitely and is ready for use, and also sterilised in the test tubes plugged with cotton wool.

Syringes used for blood culture or aspiration etc. should be immediately washed in cold solution of 2 per cent lysol. If blood is clotted in the syringe, it is difficult to remove the piston. Hot water should not be used, as it will coagulate the protein and the piston will stick. The syringe is cleaned in soapy water with a brush, washed in clean, warm water, dried and sterilised in hot air oven. The needle is washed with warm water, the bore of the needle is cleaned with a stilette and the mount of the needle with a piece of cotton wool to remove the blood. The needle is washed with warm water, then with alcohol and dried. After washing, the syringe and the needle are returned to the test tube in which they were sterilised.

Glass metal (Record) syringe is washed out immediately after use, and the needles are cleaned and sharpened. The piston and barrel are wrapped separately in kraft paper and sterilised in the autoclave.

E. Sterilisation of Rooms

After a patient with infectious disease has been discharged, the room occupied by him has to be fumigated with gaseous disinfectants; the fumigation was commonly adopted. Sulphur dioxide, generated by burning sulphur, was a common agent, but it is effective if the relative humidity is sixty per cent or more.

If the environment is contaminated with organisms of serious infectious diseases (anthrax, tuberculosis, small pox, hepatitis), the terminal disinfection is carried out by fumigation with formaldehyde.

Disinfection of room by spraying formalin is a more effective method of disinfection of the furniture and interior of the room. The room should be well sealed by covering ventilators, fire places etc. with brown paper and adhesive tape. The fully protected operator sprays 10 per cent formaldehyde solution (1 volume of formalin and 3 volumes of water) over the surfaces of the walls, floor, furniture and finally saturates the atmosphere by spraying undiluted formalin to the extent of 1 liter for 1,000 cu ft (3.3 cu m) The room is closed by sealing the door and left for 24 hours. A tray of ammonia solution is then introduced and left to evaporate for several hours to neutralise the formaldehyde and the excess of ammonia is removed by ventilation.

Disinfection of Room by Formaldehyde vapour

The room is sealed as described above and heated to 18°C. Formalin is boiled within the room in an electric boiler having a safety plug and a time switch set to cut off the current prior to this; 500 ml. of 40 per cent formaldehyde plus 1,000 ml. water are boiled per 1,000 cu ft (3.3 cu m) of air space. The room is kept sealed for 2 hours and the operator wearing a respirator then introduces a cloth soaked in ammonium solution (250 ml per liter of formalin used) which neutralises the formaldehyde within 2 hours.

Disinfection of Bed clothes

The bedding of a patient or carrier may become heavily contaminated with pathogenic bacteria (*Staphylococcus aureus, Streptococcus pyogenes*) and, if disturbed, may liberate many organisms in the air. Cotton and linen sheets and cotton blankets and synthetic fibers may be sterilised by boiling during laundering. These cotton blankets can be recommended to replace the woollen blankets which shrink during boiling. Woollen blankets can be disinfected by chemical agents (formaldehyde vapour and ethylene oxide) or, alternately, by impregnating the blankets in the quaternary ammonium disinfectant or synthetic phenolic compounds.

Disinfection of the Skin

The skin bacterial flora may be

(a) resident and (b) transient flora. The resident flora are found in the glands and hair follicles of the skin and it is very difficult to remove them and are harmless commensal organisms (*Staph.albus*, corynebacteria, sometimes *Staph.aureus*). The transient flora are essentially pathogens acquired from the environment. In skin disinfection, the first step is to wash thoroughly and to scrub in warm water with soap or some other surface-tension reducing agent (cetrimide cetavlon). Repeated use of a detergent containing 2 to 3 per cent hexachlorophane can reduce the skin flora. After washing the skin, the skin may be washed with 70 per cent ethanol, which dries quickly with less bactericidal effect. The addition of 0.5 per cent chlorhexidine improves the action of alcohol.

In surgery, sterile rubber gloves, impervious to the organisms of the skin, are to be worn. There is a great danger if the gloves are perforated during use. Before wearing the gloves, it is quite essential and important to remove all skin bacteria as much as possible by washing the hands as described above. The number of bacteria deposited in the gloves can be reduced by the addition of neomycin and bacitracin. If the operator's hands are to be disinfected repeatedly, the non-irritant agents are always preferrable. Stronger disinfectants (tincture of iodine or 5 per cent phenol solution, a strong solution of chloroxylenol-Dettol) can be used as single application for preparing the skin of the patient for incision or puncture. Recently, 0.5 per cent chlorhexidine in 70 per cent ethyl alcohol is found to be as effective as 1 per cent iodine in alcohol and also to be free from sensitation and irritation.

CHAPTER 18

USES AND PREPARATIONS OF DISINFECTANT OR ANTISEPTIC LOTIONS

Phenol Group Antiseptics

Lysol (*liquor cresolis saponatus*) and cresol (black and white fluid) are general powerful disinfectants.

Lysol, in 3 per cent solution, is generally used for sterilising discarded cultures; Sudol is less toxic substitute for Lysol.

Phenol (0.5 per cent solution) is effective in preserving sera; Chloroxylenol (Dettol) is less active toxic and irritant. Hexachlorophane is incorporated in various antiseptics preparations and reduces the skin flora, if it is used repeatedly as detergent containing 2-3 per cent hexachlorophane.

Metallic Salts

Mercuric chloride (1 : 1,000) is an useful disinfectant; merthiolate (1 : 10,000) can preserve antisera; silver nitrate (1 per cent) is employed for prophylaxis of gonococcal ophthalmia. Chlorhexidine (Hibitane — modern antiseptic) replaces silver nitrate and is effective against both Gram-positive and Gram-negative bacteria.

Formalin (40 per cent solution of formaldehyde in water) is a powerful and rapid disinfectant to decontaminate the surface and disinfect the bacterial cultures.

Borax — formaldehyde solution (Sodium tetraborate - 5 g.; Formaldehyde, 4 per cent in water, 1,000 ml) can be useful to sterilise the cleaned metal instruments.

Tincture of iodine or 5 per cent phenol solution or stronger solution of chloroxylenol (Dettol) can be used as a single application for preparing the skin of the patient for incision or puncture.

Recently, the addition of 0.5 per cent chlorhexidine in 70 per cent ethyl alcohol improves the action of 70 per cent alcohol and is also as effective as 1 per cent iodine in alcohol and also to be free from irritation.

Cetrimide (Cetavlon). This solution has pronounced surface tension lowering properties and, on shaking, it produces a prolific foam. It is incompatible with soap and similar anionic detergent. It has both powerful detergent and bactericidal properties. It is more effective against Gram-positive bacteria and to a lesser degree against Gram-negative bacteria. Aqueous or alcoholic solution of Cetavlon do not kill spores. It is specially useful to remove tar, oil or grease.

For all practical purposes, it is highly active against bacteria in concentration as low as 0.1 per cent; one per cent solution can be used for its full detergent power. 0.1 per cent solution of Cetavlon in 10 per cent alcohol is sufficient to effect a satisfactory degree of sterility within 2 minutes. For a more rapid sterilisation, higher concentration should be used.

A one per cent aqueous solution of Cetavlon has been found to be efficient preparation in the preoperative "Scrub up" of the hands. If soap and water are first used, the hands can be finally rinsed with a 0.1 per cent solution of Cetavlon to give the necessity of persistent bactericidal film.

One per cent solution of Cetavlon can be used in preliminary cleaning dirty, contaminated wounds. Oils, grease can be removed.

One per cent solution of Cetavlon is very useful to clean dog bite wound, adjunct to routine antirabic vaccination. Basins, bowels, tables can be readily cleaned and disinfected by rinsing with one per cent aqueous solution. Surgical instruments can be effectively cleaned by rinsing with one per cent aqueous solution of Cetavlon in a closed container. To prevent rusting, sodium nitrate is thoroughly mixed in the proportion of 4 g per liter of solution. Solutions used for storing instruments should be changed at weekly intervals. The instruments should be rinsed and dried when removed from the solution after use.

Preparation of Cetavlon. Aqueous solution of Cetavlon is rapidly and simply prepared by adding the concentrate to water. When solutions are being prepared for the storage of sterilised instruments, it is preferable to use boiled or distilled water.

Cetavlon concentrate 20%. It contains 20% Cetavlon in aqueous solution distinctly coloured with a non-staining yellow dye A 1% solution of Cetavlon is prepared by mixing 35 ml of the concentrate with about 7 litres of water.

Cetavlon tincture. An alcoholic solution contains 0.5% Cetavlon coloured by adding a harmless red dye. When applied to the skin, it eliminates bacteria and stains the area so that the site of operation is clearly defined. The dye may be removed by washing and will not harm the dressings.

Cetavlex cream. Contains 0.5% Cetavlon in an emolient cream base, it can be used in treatment of wounds and burns during emergency.

Savlon concentrate combines the advantages of two outstanding antiseptics of proved value it contains the new antiseptic 'Hibitane' (Chlorhexidine gluconate, 1.5% W/V) together with "Cetavlon" (Cetrimide, 15% W/V). Cetrimide possess antiseptic and cleaning properties; it is the most powerful for its detergency. It is highly active against Gram-positive organisms and Gram-negative organisms such a *Pseudomonas pyocynea.* The combination of these two antiseptics provides a most powerful antibacterial solution with a wide-spectrum of activity and high speed of killing.

A 1 in 200 dilution in water is recommended for disinfection of wards and hospital equipments.

For preliminary treatment of wounds and burns, in rinsing of hands, a 1 in 100 dilution is used. For preoperative preparation of skin and scrub up of surgeon's hands a 1 in 30 dilution in water should be recommended.

CHAPTER 19

STERILISATION AND DISINFECTION IN NURSING

Sterilisation and Disinfection in Nursing

1	2	3	4	5
In medical and surgical wards, in a general hospital	Terminal disinfection	In the operation room or delivery rooms	In the communicable disease unit or hospital	Disinfection in public health nursing

↓ (1)

1. Hand washing
2. Thermometer technique
3. Syringe and needles
4. Surgical dressings
5. Transfer forceps
6. Catheterisation
7. Reverse precaution

↓ (4)

1. Bedside equipment
2. Dishes
3. Secretions and Excretion

The application of sterilisation and disinfection in the practice of Nursing :

A. In Medical and Surgical wards of a General Hospital

1. *Hand washing.* Careful hand washing is always very essential in the following circumstances :

(i) after taking care of each patient;
(ii) before compounding the medicines;
(iii) after dressing an infected wound;
(iv) before each surgical dressing;
(v) after handling bedpans and urinals;
(vi) before the patient is served with food;
(vii) before taking her own food.

The following procedures should be adapted in good hand washing to prevent the transfer of the microorganisms by means of hands; all areas of the hands should be adequately soaped with soap suds by mechanical frictions, should be frequently, resoaped and completely cleaned. Before assisting a surgical operation, the nurse should scrub thoroughly her hands without fail.

2. *Disinfection of Oral Thermometer.* The recommended procedure :

(a) the thermometer should be wiped clean with gauze or cotton moistened in a mixture of equal parts of tincture of green soap and 70 per cent ethyl alcohol;
(b) rinsed completely with clean water; and
(c) submerged deeply in a solution of 1 per cent iodine and 70 per cent ethyl alcohol for 10 minutes or only in 70 per cent ethyl alcohol which is less effective without iodine. Formaldehyde and phenolic disinfectants are not fully effective against tubercle bacilli so they cannot be used. After disinfection, the thermometer should be rinsed several times in the water, kept in a clean, dry container until further use.

Rectal Thermometer. Before use, the rectal thermometer should be lubricated in water-soluble lubricant. Petrolatum or other oily lubricants cannot be used as they prevent thorough cleaning and disinfection. *Well wiped* thermometer can also be sterilised with germicidal vapours, if available.

Syringes and Needles should be sterilised in the hot air oven or autoclaved since they are used mainly for hypodermic or intramuscular or intravenous injections or for withdrawal of venous blood. Boiling should not be advocated for this purpose as the spores and some viruses (Serum and infectious hepatitis virus) may resist the boiling for a longer duration.

While handling the syringes, care should be taken so that the plunger and the inside of the barrel are always sterile. With the help of sterile forceps, the shank of the needle should be carefully held and mounted on the nozzle of the syringe. The bevelled edge (point) and the shaft of the needle should be protected by dry, sterile cotton or gauze. A needle should be sterile or a test tube with needles in it should be sterilised and then the needle should be used. It is not advisable to handle with fingers the sterile gauze or cotton soaked in disinfectant which is to be placed over the sterile needle, because the skin microorganisms may trickle down from the contaminated fingers and contaminate the sterile needle. The loaded syringe which is properly mounted with protected needle should be carried to the patient with a bottle containing skin disinfectant (1 per cent iodine in 70 per cent alcohol).

Sterile disposable, plastic syringe with needle attached is available for ready use, which can save time and avoid the contamination and infection.

Sharp instruments, which cannot withstand the sterilising heat, can be mounted on racks in jars containing disinfecting solution (isopropyl alcohol, 65.26 per cent; methyl alcohol, 2.75 per cent; formaldehyde, 8 per cent; hexachlorophane, 0.5 per cent, water 23.49 per cent) which can destroy spores within 3-5 hours.

Surgical Dressings. Nurse should remove the surgical dressings with a sterile forceps, but never by her fingers and these dressings should be transferred onto a newspaper, properly wrapped and put in a covered trash can for subsequent incineration. The contaminated forceps should be discarded in a covered container and boiled, cleaned and sterilised in hot air oven or autoclave. An infected wound can be carefully covered with a new sterile dressing by touching only the outer layer of the dressing with finger or with sterile forceps. The nurse should never touch any incision or cut wound as there is possibility of transferring pathogenic microorganisms to the wound from her fingers.

Transfer Forceps. It is a sterile instrument which is always found on a surgical tray. If this transfer forceps is used properly, there is less chance of contamination. This instrument should always be sterilised in hot air oven or autoclave daily. The transfer forceps is used *only* to transfer sterile instruments or dressings from one sterile place to another sterile place. If this transfer forceps touches accidently any unsterile objects, it should be discarded and resterilised. This instrument should be kept always submerged deep in a chemical disinfectant solution contained in a jar, it should be removed or returned to the jar in such a way that it will not touch its rim or cover. In this case, the chemical disinfection is done only to keep the instrument *sterile*, but *not to sterilise the transfer forceps.*

Catheterisation (removal of urine from the urinary bladder). Before following this procedure, the nurse should wash thoroughly her hands and wear immediately the sterile gloves. The external meatus of the urethra should be thoroughly washed with sterile normal saline or mild antiseptic solution to remove simply the burden of the microorganisms present in the meatus which may be introduced into the urethra or urinary bladder during the process of catheterisation. The catheter already sterilised in the autoclave should be sufficiently lubricated with *sterile water* soluble lubricant and it should be inserted gently without trauma to the delicate tissues, since the damaged tissues are vulnerable to the infection.

Reverse precautions are the special precautions ordered by the doctor for the patient (premature baby, patient with recent cardiac surgery, patient with artificial kidney, severe and extensive burn patient, debilitated patient), when the body resistance is lowered and is very susceptible to any infection. For reverse precautions, the nurse should know that any one coming in contact with the patient should wash thoroughly the hands, wear gowns, masks and caps before entering the rooms. The visitor with slightest infection should *not* be *allowed* to come in contact with the patient; hence, there should be a restriction for the visitors to enter the room. In short, *everything entering the room should be cleaned or sterilized.* So, vacuum cleaner or mops or cloth soaked in moist disinfectant can be used to clean and to dust. Wet mops (clothes) will not allow the dissemination of the dust in the room.

Terminal disinfection. After discharge of a patient, particularly of communicable disease, the ward, unit or room occupied by the patient should be cleaned thoroughly; the linens or covers should be washed with soap and water, dried and ironed, the equipment should be boiled and cleaned; the mattress and pillows are autoclaved, the blankets are washed; careless terminal disinfection may lead to the transfer of antibiotic resistant *Staphylococcus aureus* in the hospital.

Dishes. The silverware plates used for eating food by the patients of communicable diseases should be boiled for 5-10 minutes, so to kill all pathogenic organisms and then washed with clean water. The waste food from the infectious disease hospitals should be disposed off after burning or disinfecting. In communicable disease hospitals, used paper plates, paper cups etc. are burned completely.

Secretions and Excretions. Tissue papers used by the patient to receive the respiratory secretions and as well as the wipes should be completely burned. Copious respiratory secretions from tuberculosis patient should be collected in a waterproof container which should be packed later with sawdust or fine newspaper strips to absorb moisture from the secretions. The container should be wrapped very carefully with newspaper and burned in the incinerator. If glass or metal container is used, it should be immersed in saponated 5 per cent solution of cresol or strong chlorine bleaching solution for one hour. The container is then washed and used again.

Urinary and intestinal excretions collected in urinal or bed pan from a communicable disease patient should be disinfected by 5 per cent chlorinated lime.

Bed and body linens used for the patients in an infectious disease hospital should be soaked in saponated cresol (2 per cent) or in laundry bleaching solution overnight or autoclaved or boiled. Dressing from infected skin lesions should be burned completely.

B. In the Operation room or Delivery room

All articles (instruments, linens used for drapes, gowns and gloves) should be autoclaved. Some delicate eye surgery instruments, which are liable to be damaged by heat sterilisation, are sterilised by chemical agents (ethylene oxide or beta propiolactone). The tube containing sutures can be broken in a sterile towel and the sutures are transferred to the sterile place with sterile forceps.

The nurse must clean and open all instruments so that all surfaces of the instruments are exposed to the (autoclave or hot air oven) sterilisation and she should keep ready all sterilised instruments before the surgical operation or delivery. At the same time she should also keep ready sterile drapes and dressing. In operation room, she should cover her hair with a cap so that the hair or dandruff will not fall off and will not contaminate the operation theatre. To prevent the spread of the infection to the patient, she should wear the gauze mask over the nose and mouth.

Preparation of the Patient

The skin of the operative area should be thoroughly washed:

1. The skin of the operative area should be thoroughly washed;

2. This area should be shaved to remove all hair;

3. Fatty skin secretions can be removed by the application of ether or acetone or skin disinfectant (1.5 to 3 per cent alcoholic iodine solution).

4. The cleaning of an operative area of the skin removes the microorganisms and also superficial organic material. The removal of organic material may facilitate the penetration of the disinfectant.

Before assisting the surgeon for the surgical operation, the nurse should scrub her hands and forearms at least three times with water and soap containing hexachlorophane, 3 per cent. This soap is commonly used in all hospitals. After soap and water scrub, all soap should be completely rinsed with clear running water. Then the hands should be immersed in mild disinfectant solution (70 per cent ethyl alcohol). The nurse should wear a sterile gown and rubber gloves, assist the surgeons during the operation, should be responsible for the sterility during operation, if any breach in the sterility technique, she should bring it immediately to the notice of the surgeon.

Sterilisation by boiling in the hospital ward. Boiling (at 100°C) for 10 minutes kills vegetative pathogenic bacteria, rickettsiae, all viruses (except serum and infectious hepatitis virus). This method is used to disinfect instruments or syringes under circumstances where killing of vegetative forms of bacteria are required for ordinary purposes.

C. In the Infectious Disease Hospital

In the infectious disease hospital, pathogenic organisms can be transferred from patient to patient; patient to nurse; patient to visitor and, hence, outside of the hospital.

Bedside equipment. During the entire infectious phase of the disease, the same bedpan and thermometer should be used. The bedpan and urinal should be boiled for 5-15 minutes after each use to kill all pathogenic microorganisms. The equipments used occasionally between patients should be disinfected or sterilised. Otoscopes, stethoscopes and other instruments used for examination of the patients should be sufficiently immersed in the disinfectant, which is more effective than wiping with ethyl alcohol. These instruments may also be thoroughly wiped with saponated cresol solution (1 per cent) followed by cleaning with clean water and drying. It is a useful method.

D. Disinfection in Public Health Nursing

The intelligent professional nurse should be able to adapt the principles of disinfection, destruction and removal of microorganisms according to the various circumstances prevailing in public health.

The public health nurse should always pay much attention to hand washing after visiting each patient, as she is going from house to house and patient to patient. She must wash her hands thoroughly so that she does not carry the infection from patient to patient.

Before leaving the headquarter, the nurse should keep ready all syringes and needles sterilised in the autoclave or hot air oven and carry with her all these sterile items or she can also carry sterile disposable plastic syringe. In an emergency, where facilities are not available, she can disinfect needles and syringes by boiling in a covered saucepan for 30 minutes for ordinary purposes.

A home oven can be used as hot air oven. Similarly, a pressure cooker can be substituted for the autoclave; the rinsing of the syringes and needles with a disinfectant solution before each injection is not advisable.

Thoroughly washed and wiped thermometer may be placed in a screw cap plastic tube cushioned with the cotton at the bottom and around the wall of the tube and filled with 70 per cent alcohol. In case of communicable disease, the public health nurse can set up an isolation room for the patient at home by keeping bedside equipment exclusively for his use. Dishes and linens used by him should be disinfected by boiling for 30 minutes. She should also educate in explicit language the members of the family about the isolation technique so that they may continue this technique later in the absence of the public health nurse.

CHAPTER 20

BLOOD IN RELATION TO MICROBIOLOGY AND INFECTION

It is well-established that the blood supplies food to the various cells and tissues of the human body and removes all waste products from them. It also destroys the invading bacteria and their toxin and disposes off with the help of living cells and certain substances contained in it. The blood also plays a great role in the production, transmission, prevention, diagnosis and cure of the disease.

Blood Composition

Plasma. The fluid portion of the fresh uncoagulated blood is known as plasma which makes up 55 per cent of whole blood. It is yellowish and transparent. It contains proteins, food for the body tissues and waste products from the tissues. It consists of 91 per cent water, 1 per cent minerals (salts of Na, K, Ca, Mg, P); 1 per cent various substances (uric acid, urea, amino acids, glucose, carbon dioxide, oxygen, lipids and hormones). It carries the red blood cells, white cells and platelets which constitute remaining 45 per cent. Plasma contains fibrinogen which is involved in the clotting of the blood, which occurs when the soluble fibrinogen is converted into insoluble fibrin. Other proteins (albumins and various globulins) maintain the water balance of the body. *Gamma globulin* is of the globulin fraction or component. Blood is a rich source of antibodies. These antibodies can be used for treatment and prophylaxis of certain diseases and play an important role in the antibody mediated or humoral immunity.

Red blood corpuscles. Human erythrocytes (Greek, *erythros*, red; *kytos*, cell) are non-nucleated, biconcave disks. They have a life span of 130 days and are constantly replaced. In adult male, they number about 5 millions per cubic millimetre and in women, it is about 4.5 million per cubic millimeter. Red blood cells are manufactured in the bone marrow and released into the plasma of the blood. Hemoglobin (respiratory pigment) forms a loose chemical bond with oxygen when exposed to air in the lung, carries oxygen to the tissues of the body and releases it to them. Hemoglobin is released into the surrounding when the red blood cells rupture. The process is known as haemolysis (Greek, *haima*, blood, *lysis*, to disrupt or dissolve). *In vivo* and *in vitro*, red blood cells can be lysed by certain bacterial toxins.

White blood corpuscles. They are also known as leucocytes (Gr. *leukos*, white). They are larger and less in number than the red blood cells. They are about 7,000 per cubic millimetre of the blood. They act as scavengers or policemen in the blood. They engulf any foreign particle (dead tissues or bacteria) entering the blood stream, they ingest these particles directly, they move with the help of *pseudopodia* and enter between the tissue cells of the body. If the bacteria enter into the leucocytes through their thin cell membrane, they may be killed and digested by digestive enzymes of the leucocytes. This process is known as *phagocytosis*. Leucocytes can move out of the blood vessels by their amoeboid movement between the cells lining the blood vessels. Leucocytes can be attracted by the chemotaxis to the area of the inflammation caused by foreign particles (bacteria).

In the infected spot or boil the white, creamy material consists of dead leucocytes (pus cells), dead bacteria, tissue debris, fluid from blood and tissues and is known as "Pus".

Platelets. They are irregular and disk shaped particles of varying sizes and smaller than erythrocytes. They are about 3,00,000 per cubic millimetre of blood and look like fragments of cells. Their origin is yet unclear and they are also responsible for coagulation of blood. Blood with low platelets may not clot quickly and may cause surgical hazard.

Plasma	Serum
1. Yellowish fluid portion of whole blood.	1. Straw coloured fluid remaining after clothing of blood.
2. It contains fibrinogen; in blood clotting, soluble fibrinogen is converted into insoluble fibrin, the jelly like substance of the clot.	2. It contains no fibrinogen;
3. It contains antibodies (antibacterial substances) and bacterial toxins.	3. It contains antibodies and bacterial toxins.
4. In microbiology (Serology) it is used to diagnose some diseases as it may contain antibodies against some infections.	4. It is used in the diagnosis of diseases as it contains antibodies against the diseases.
5. It plays a great role in humoral immunity.	5. It plays an important role in humoral immunity.

Blood Circulation

Left ventricle of the heart pushes the blood continuously through the arterial system to the remotest branches - microscopic arterioles, venules or capillary vessels. The wall of the capillary vessels are of one cell thickness. Nutrients and other substances (hormones, oxygen etc.) filter through these thin membranous walls diffuse into the fluid (lymph) which is constantly bathing the tissue cells. The nutrients are brought from the gastro-intestinal tract and liver by the blood. Waste metabolic products (acids, carbon dioxide etc.) diffuse from the tissue cells into the lymph; then from the lymph into the blood stream of capillary venules and venous system which is in continuity with arterioles. These waste products in the venous (impure) blood are carried to the right auricle of the heart and are pumped to the right ventricle through the lungs when the red blood cells and plasma take up oxygen from the air and give off carbon dioxide. This purified blood returns to the left auricle and then to the left ventricle which pushes again the purified blood to the tissues. In this way, the blood circulates in the body for the benefits of the body (nutrition, metabolism, growth; protection against diseases etc.).

Blood and Disease. When blood passes through the tissues infected with toxin producing pathogenic microorganisms (e.g., diphtheria, tetanus) carries with it toxin (toxemia) and if bacteria (Salmonella) enter the blood stream (bacteriemia). The toxin and bacteria are carried alongwith the blood and are distributed to various parts of the body where they set up the infections, e.g., brain abscess, osteomyelitis (inflammation of bone), otitis media (middle ear infection). Blood borne diseases (malaria, filariasis, yellow fever etc.) can be transmitted by arthropods (mosquitoes) from person to person. The blood carries drugs and antibiotics injected or swallowed to abate the infection.

Blood and Immunity. Cell and antibody mediated immunities against the infection are performed through the circulating blood, leucocytes in the circulating blood are responsible for cellular immunity, whereas the antibodies for the humoral immunity. Antibodies (Gamma globulins) are soluble protein molecules secreted into the blood by lymphoid cells which are stimulated by the foreign proteins (Refer to chapter on immunology).

Infection. The term infection is used to designate an entry and the presence of organisms, whereas the *disease* to designate the response of the host to the infection.

Host parasite relationship is a part of science *ecology*, where the organisms live together and help mutually. A host parasite relationship develops during the evolution of many species of living organisms to thrive with each other. *Symbiosis* or *mutualism* is a host parasite relationship; when the organisms are mutually antagonistic they are *antibiosis. Parasitism* or *predation*, when some organisms live at the expense of the others. The infectious disease is an example of *parasitism* relationship.

Commensalism is a also an example of host relationship where the organisms thrive side by side peacefully after some struggle for their existence.

During the process of infection, immunity and allergy, many host-parasite relationship and adaptation are established.

Infection is a condition where the microorganisms enter into the human body tissues, grow in or on them, may damage them and the host may react to this damage by manifesting the symptoms like fever, chills, nausea and headache. Infection may be fatal or serious. A pimple is a simple reaction to the infection of the skin; whereas Typhoid is serious if untreated by antibiotics.

Factors of Infection

(a) Dose of infecting microorganisms.

(b) Virulence of microorganisms :

- (i) aggressiveness and
- (ii) toxigenicity.

(a) *Dose of infecting microorganisms*. There is possibility of infection, if the number of microorganisms entering the body is very large; a million of organisms may set up the infection, if the tissue resistance is lowered by fatigue, disease or alcoholism; or after entry into the body, by overcoming the host defence mechanism; whereas a single bacterium (coccus or bacillus) may not be able to establish in the healthy body.

(b) *Virulence of organisms* is the ability of organisms to enter, establish, infect, damage the tissues and produce the disease. The virulence depends upon two factors : (i) aggressiveness, and (ii) toxigenicity.

(i) *Aggressiveness.* Skin inhabiting bacteria are not very aggressive as they are unable to penetrate the skin barrier of the body. If they get entry into the skin, they will become aggressive in the favourable environment for their growth. Heavily capsulated organisms (Pneumococci, anthrax bacilli, klebsiella) are highly aggressive and dangerous as they cannot be engulfed by leucocytes.

(ii) *Toxigenicity* is the ability of organisms to elaborate the toxin. Bacteria producing toxin may not be aggressive (i.e., invasive), but they damage the body tissues by their toxin. For example, toxigenic strains of diphtheria bacilli lodging on the tonsils or in the throat will produce the toxin which is absorbed in the blood (toxemia) carried to various parts of the body and ultimately can cause the death. Tetanus bacilli are also toxigenic as diphtheria bacilli.

Toxins. Toxigenic strains of organisms produce two types of toxins which are proteins in nature. Toxin may damage the tissues of the body after combining with nerves, heart muscle, liver.

1. *Endotoxins* (Greek, *endon*, inside). They are found in the cytoplasm enclosed by the cytoplasmic membrane. These intracellular toxins, known as *endotoxins*, are released after the death and lysis of bacterial cells (e.g., Gram-negative bacteria, gonococci, typhoid bacilli) produce endotoxin.

2. *Exotoxins* (Greek, *exo*, outside). Toxin producing bacteria liberate toxins, through their cytoplasmic membrane, which are known as *exotoxins*. *Corynebacterium diphtheriae*, *Clostridium tetani* produce exotoxins. Few bacteria produce both endotoxin and exotoxin.

Specificity of toxin. Toxins of organisms are specific in their action. Tetanus toxin has an affinity for nerve cells, causing spasm of jaw muscles, i.e., lockjaw. Diphtheria toxin has affinity for heart muscle, death in the severe infections is usually due to acute myocarditis and heart failure. This toxin may lead to such sequelae as post-diphtheric paralysis. In staphylococcal food poisoning, *enterotoxin* of *Staphylococcus aureus* produces vomiting and diarrhea. This *enterotoxin* is also known as preformed toxin, as this toxin is preformed in the food contaminated by *Staphylococcus aureus* and consumed later.

Application to Nursing

A nurse should know that plasma and serum contain antibodies (Gamma globulins) which play a major role by protecting from diseases. She should also be aware of the fact that the patient with low platelet count may be affected by surgical hazard, as his blood may not clot immediately. A knowledge of blood clotting mechanism is necessary, the soluble fibrinogen is changed into insoluble fibrin which causes clotting. Antibiotics and drugs injected or swallowed are carried by the blood to combat the infection. A sound knowledge of toxin is essential, as the toxins are responsible for many diseases.

SECTION 4

CHAPTER 21

IMMUNOLOGY

The study of immune responses of the human body is known as *Immunology.*

History

The inhabitants of East Africa have succeeded in vaccination against the bite of poisonous snakes from time immemorial, they could immunise artificially against tick borne relapsing fever and could protect their cattle from contagious pleuropneumonia by their old method of vaccination. In 2,000 - 3,000 B.C., children were vaccinated against small pox in South East Asia by the folk methods of direct contact of hands of the children. Only after 100 years after Jenner's work, Immunology was enriched with his own methods built on the scientific works of Louis Pasteur.

ANTIGEN

Such substances (egg white, serum, milk, snake venom, dead and living bacteria, bacterial exotoxins and endotoxins, plant or animal tissue) containing proteins may act as antigen when introduced into the deeper tissues of the body. Protein taken in the gastrointestinal tract as food may not act as antigen under normal conditions because they are rapidly destroyed by the gastric juice. To act as antigen, a protein must gain entrance to the blood and other tissues in a chemically unaltered state. Entrance is commonly by *injection* or *infection* (i.e., by routes other than the gastrointestinal tract) or by *parenterally.*

An antigen (Gr. *anti.* against, *genos* - genus) is a foreign protein (organic substances of colloidal structure) which when introduced parenterally (Gr. *para,* beyond or outside of; *enteron,* intestine), by route other than the gastrointestinal tract into the human body, it will provoke the lymphoid tissue of the human to produce antibodies which will react specifically with the same antigen and not with other substances.

Antigens have the following main properties.

(a) *Antigenicity* (the ability to cause the production of antibodies);

(b) Antigenic *specificity* (the ability to enter into an interaction with the corresponding antibodies).

The small portion of a molecule may be called as unit of antigen. This unit is known as antigenic determinant. This determinant is a contour which locks

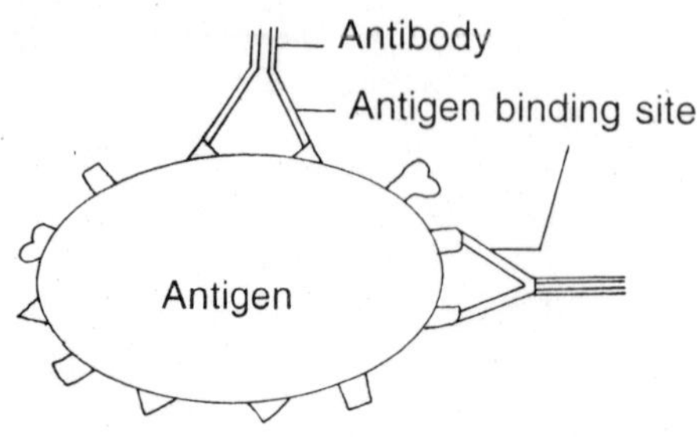

Fig.21.1: Antigenic determinant sites

one molecule of antibody. As antigenic determinants have a three-dimensional structures, the antibody molecule can approach or can get attached to any of the wide range of possible configurations in a single determinant (Fig. 21.1).

The specificity of the antigen is dependent upon antigenic determinant (epitope), i.e., chemical groupings of the antigen molecules. When the antigen comes in contact, the animal reacts. This is known as "acquired immune response". The acquired immune response may be of two forms : (a) the humoral or circulating antibody response; (b) cell mediated response. An antibody directed against an antigenic determinant of a particular antigen molecule will react only with this determinant or another very similar structure. Even minor chemical changes in the determinant will reduce the ability of the original antibody to react with the altered determinant. Antigens which are capable of stimulating an immune response is known as *Immunogens.*

Antigens may be *complete* or *partial.*

Complete antigens are substances which cause the production of antibodies and react with them *in vivo* and *in vitro* (e.g., foreign proteins, bacteria, toxins, rickettsiae, viruses).

Partial antigens are known as *haptens.* They do not produce antibodies but react with the antibodies produced by another substance. They are lipids, complex carbohydrates and other substances of low molecular weight. The addition of protein to haptens in small quantity will convert the hapten into complete antigen. In this case, the protein carries out the function of a conductor.

The antigenic function of bacteria, rickettsiae and viruses is characterised by species and type specificity. *Salmonella typhi* antigen induced immunity against Typhoid and it will not produce immunity against Paratyphoid fever. So this antigen is species and type specific. The type specificity is associated with the presence of special polysaccharide complexes in the bacterial cell.

In the laboratory, there is cross-reaction between antisera to certain bacterial antigens and antigens present in cells such as erythrocytes. These antigens are known as *heterophile antigens.* Antisera to such antigens will cross-react with cells of different species of animals and various microorganisms. Chemical groupings of *heterophile* antigens are not yet known. The best known of the heterophile antigens is the *Forssman* antigen which is present in the red cells of many species as well as in the bacteria such as pneumococci and salmonella. Another heterophile antigen is found in *Escherchia coli* and human red cells of Group B.

Semihaptens (iodine, bromine, quinine, antipyrin, colloidal iron, azoprotein) are not antigenic themselves, but in combination with the protein of the body, they acquire the properties of complete antigen.

All natural proteins are inherited with the properties of chemical, structural and functional specificity. Proteins of different species of animals, plants, bacteria, rickettsiae and viruses can be differentiated by immunological reactions.

Chemical Nature of Antigens

Antigens may be proteins, polysaccharides or lipids. Antigens of cell wall of bacteria (streptococci, staphylococci, corynebacteria) are rather less well defined and appear to be complex mucopeptides, sometimes associated with lipids. Capsulated microorganisms (pneumococci) have complex high molecular weight polysaccharides in their capsules.

General Properties of Antigens

1. Antigen should be foreign, egg albumin is an excellent antigen in the rabbit, but fails to produce an antibody response in fowl;

2. More foreign, it is more powerful antigen;

3. It should have a molecular weight of 5,000. Sometimes, some substances of low molecular weight (aspirin, penicillin, sulphonamides) can act as antigen when applied to the skin.

4. The ability of antibody to form a strong bond with an antigen depends on *intermolecular forces* which act strongly only when two molecules come in contact in a very precise manner. The better they fit the stronger the bond.

Isoantigens. Isoantigens are those substances which have antigenic properties and are contained in some individuals of a given species. They are found in erythrocytes of animals and men. At first it was established that there are two antigens (A and B) in the human erythrocytes and in the sera, there are two antibodies (anti-A and anti-B). Only heterogenic antigens and antibodies (agglutinins) are found in human blood. These combinations may be represented as below :

Antigens of erythrocytes (Blood Groups)	*Serum antibodies*
O	Anti-A Anti-B
A	Anti-B
B	Anti-A
AB	O

On the basis of antigenic structure, the erythrocytes of all people can be divided mainly into four groups. Consequently, variants of antigens of erythrocytes in the second (A) and fourth (AB) groups were isolated. The Group A consists of two sub-groups A_1 and A_2.

The AB groups containing A_1 B and A_2 B and the antigens M and N and M_2 and N_2 etc. have been revealed. At present 30 antigens are known. Besides, there is rhesus factor in the erythrocytes. All these groups are taken into account during blood transfusion.

Autoantigens are those substances (eye lens, spermatozoa, skin, kidney, lung) which do not, under normal condition, come in contact with the immune system of the body, then the antibodies are not produced against such cells and tissues. However, if these tissues are damaged, then the autoantigens may be released and may cause the production of antibodies which react with the corresponding autoantigens of the cells resulting in the development of glomerulonephritis, interstitial thyroiditis, orchitis, corneal opacity). The cooling, radiation, drugs (amidopyrine, sulphonamides), virus infection (virus pneumonia, infectious mononucleosis, bacterial proteins, toxins of streptococci, staphylococci, tubercle bacilli) and other factors may release autoantigens from the tissues.

ANTIBODIES (Immunoglobulins)

History

Von Behring and Kitasato in Berlin in 19th century recognised antibodies in the blood stream of an immunised animal against tetanus and diphtheria they observed clumping or agglutination of microorganisms and precipitation of soluble antigens by the serum of the immunised animal. They practised also the serotherapy method.

Serotherapy is the injection of antiserum, for the therapeutic use, from an immunised animal to nonimmune patient. They also carried out the fragmentation of immunoglobulins by pepsin digestion.

Antibodies are synthesised under the influence of antigens which penetrate into the body and disturb the normal blood composition. Antibodies are specific substances in the bodies of the vertebrates secreted in the tissue fluids from the lymphoid cells that have been stimulated by foreign substances (antigens) with which they react *specifically.*

Antibodies appear in the blood due to the infection or immunisation by live (attenuated) or dead bacteria, rickettsiae, viruses, toxins or toxoids etc. Antibodies which occur under the influence of active immunisation are named *immune antibodies* in contrast to normal antibodies which are found in the sera of men and animals which had not been infected or exposed to immunisation. Normal and immune antibodies can render harmless the causal agents of infectious diseases.

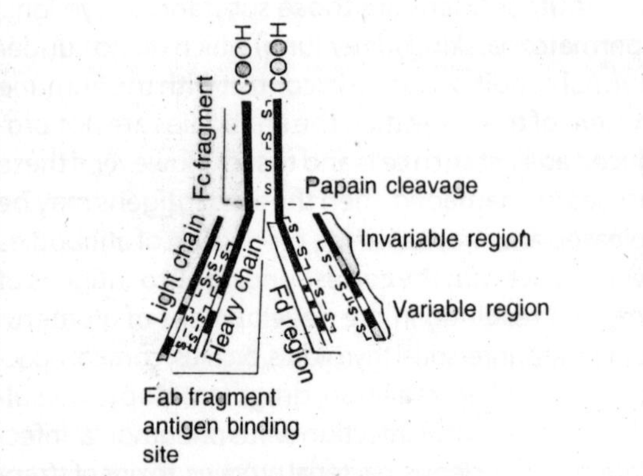

Fig.21.2: Structure of Immunoglobulin

Nature of Antibodies

1. Antibodies are globulins which have been altered under the influence of antigens;

2. Molecules of antibodies, like normal serum globulins are probably asymmetrical;

3. Antibodies are found in globulin fractions;

4. The transformation of normal globulin into immune globulin is due to alteration in the spatial configuration of active atomic groups of the protein molecules. A change in protein metabolism is responsible for this process. The mechanism of antibodies production is not yet clear, though many theories are put forth;

5. Antibodies do not differ greatly from normal globulins;

6. They have almost similar isoelectric points, viscosity molecular weight (from 100,000 to 1,000,000) and are sensitive to the temperature and to other denaturating agents.

7. Antibodies are thermolabile and denatured on heating at 70°C for one hour;

8. The pH of the medium and other factors affecting proteins can also affect the activity of antibodies;

9. Antibodies are not denatured by precipitation with ethyl alcohol at low temperature (from 0 to +4°C) but are denatured by alcohol at high temperature. Natural salts (magnesium sulphate, ammonium sulphate and sodium sulphate) can cause the precipitation of proteins, but do not denature antibodies. Ethyl alcohol at low temperature and natural salts can be used for fractionisation of immune sera to obtain them in a pure state.

There are five types of human immunoglobulins : IgG; IgM; IgA; IgD and IgE, on the basis of polypeptide chain structure consisting of heavy chains and light chains joined by disulphide bond.

Immunoglobulin G or IgG. Seventyfive per cent of total serum constitutes IgG. It is the major immunoglobulin component of serum and has a molecular weight of 150,000 in man. The molecule has two antigen combining sites which are called as Fab (antibody binding) portions of the molecule. Fab fragment has both light and heavy chains. Light chains are of two types. They are known as K or L (K, Kappa or L, Lambda) chains. The heavy chain or Y chain exists in four forms : IgG_1, IgG_2; IgG_3 and IgG_4. The molecule has also Fc fragment for complement fixation.

IgM, IgA, IgD and IgE

Like IgG globulin, each of these classes of immunoglobulins in man contain K and L light chains. The heavy chains are unique for each of the types of immunoglobulins. IgM contains μ chain, IgA alpha chain, IgD δ chain and IgE ε chain.

Table 21.1 : Human Immunoglobulins

Ig Class	*Serum concentration mg/100 ml.*	*Molecular weight*	*Light Chain*	*Heavy Chain*	*Properties*
IgG	900 - 1800	160,000	K & L	Y	Late antibody precipitation, complement fixation antibody.
IgM	67 - 145	960,000	K & L	μ	Early — Agglutination.
IgA	156 - 294	170,000	K & L	α	Surface protec-
IgD	0.3 - 40	184,000	K & L	δ	Not known.
IgE	10 - 130	188,000	K & L	ε	Reaginic antibody (hypersensitivity— Intradermal).

Structure and Function of Immunoglobulins

In the Fab portion, the heavy chain component (Fd portion) contains as much as 85 per cent of the antigen-binding ability. The light chain seems to act together with the heavy chain to form a stable antibody-combining site. The Fc portion of the IgG molecule is responsible for activation of complement system. On combination with antigen, the IgG molecule springs open at the hinge region exposing the Fc portion which can activate the complement. If IgG molecule has not combined with antigen, it will be unfolded. A single IgM molecule can get attached to a red cell by multiple combining sites (Fig. 21.2) and can bring about lysis; but for the same effect, 1,000 IgG molecules are required.

Agglutination is due to linkage of a particulate antigen (red blood cell or bacteria) by two Fab fragments of IgM. The IgM is of large size, so it is confined in the blood stream and plays an important role in the protection against blood invasion by microorganisms. IgM deficiency may result into septicemia. Diphtheria toxin, lysozyme or virus (poliovirus) can be neutralised by IgG antibodies and IgG antibodies can neutralise more effectively than IgM antibodies. Fc fragment of IgG molecule may assist the Fab fragments in neutralisation of virus infectivity and also helps in the selective transport of IgG. The characteristic feature of IgE class immunoglobulin is responsible for the hypersensitivity reaction in man which is due to the activity of Fc portion of IgE molecule. IgM antibody specific for particulate antigen (bacteria) makes the antigen more susceptible to the phagocytosis by coating the surface of particulate antigen, so it is called as opsonising antibody (Opsonin).

Selective Transport of IgG

In pregnant women, IgG globulins can pass through the placenta and reach the foetal circulation; this process is not due to the mere filtration but due to the selective transfer of IgG molecules which is brought about by a part of Fc fragment of IgG heavy chains. This property is a characteristic feature only of the y chain of IgG and is not found in the μ chain of IgM and α chain of IgA. This mechanism of selective transport is mainly observed in primates. Similarly, immunoglobulins are absorbed from the colostrum through the intestinal epithelium of the ruminants.

IgA globulins are selectively secreted into saliva, respiratory, intestinal mucous secretions and into the colostrum. This is another mechanism of selective transport. There are two types of IgA : serum IgA and dimer IgA.

Dimer form of IgA is manufactured locally and has an attached secretory transport piece which is not found in serum IgA. This transport piece is added to the IgA molecule during its passage into the mucous secretions from the lamina propria of the intestinal and respiratory tract. This secretory IgA would protect from the infection. The dimer form of IgA acquires the ability to fix the complement after attaching to Gram negative organisms.

The monomeric form of IgA can also pass from the lamina propria to the blood stream via lymphatics so that the infection of the intestine may lead to increased serum IgA levels. Local application of vaccine may stimulate dimer IgA.

Types of Antibodies

Opsonins. These antibodies render the microorganisms more susceptible to phagocytosis by altering the surfaces of the antigens.

Cytolysins. They help to dissolve the cells that stimulated their production.

Antitoxins are formed due to the stimulation of exotoxins which are protein in nature and soluble in water. These antibodies are inactivated or neutralised by the exotoxins.

Hemolysins. If a rabbit is injected several times with minute quantity of washed erythrocytes of another species of animal, e.g., sheep, the serum of the recipient rabbit acquires the property of destroying the erythrocytes of the sheep. This is due to the formation of cytolysins that sensitise the sheep red blood cells to complement and cause the lysis of the sheep erythrocytes. The hemoglobin escapes into the surrounding fluid. This process is called hemolysis. The haemolytic cytolysins are called *haemolysins.*

Precipitins. These antibodies combine with the molecules of soluble proteins and bring about a cloudiness in the fluid or visible flakes. This flocculent turbidity is known as precipitate as seen in Venereal Disease Research Laboratory (VDRL) test; they may form line of precipitation when they react with soluble antigens.

Agglutinins. They bring about the clumping of particulate antigens (bacteria, red blood cells) — hence agglutination. Many diagnostic tests are based on bacterial agglutinins. For example, Widal test is used to diagnose Typhoid fever.

Hemagglutinins are responsible for the agglutination of red blood cells or hemagglutination; cold hemagglutinins; viral hemagglutinins; and isohemagglutinins.

(a) *Cold hemagglutinins* are substances that appear in the blood of person with certain respiratory diseases, e.g., atypical pneumonia of unknown or viral origin and trypanosomiasis. The sera of the patient in dilution of 1 : 10,000 agglutinate their *own* erythrocytes (auto-agglutination) when cooled to 2°C; but not at 37°C. This agglutination at low temperature is known as cold hemagglutination.

(b) *Viral hemagglutinins.* Agglutination of red cells is brought about by several respiratory virus (Influenza virus) *not by antibody.* The virus itself attaches to the red cells of the chick at 5°C and agglutinate them. It can be separated (eluted) from them by mixing with saline solution followed by an incubation at 37°C. The viral hemagglutination tests are useful in the study of viruses and the diagnosis of viral diseases. In some infections, antibodies may prevent the viral agglutination of erythrocytes. They are called as hemagglutination-inhibition (HI) antibodies.

(c) *Isohemagglutinins.* These antibodies are formed in response to one or more antigens (A, B, Rh, M) found in human erythrocytes. They do not agglutinate one's own red blood cells, but cause agglutination, at body temperature (37°C), of red blood cells of another person. They play an important role in blood transfusion. If the serum of the recipient agglutinates the red blood cells of a donor or vice versa, then there is possibility of reaction or death of the recipient. It is not necessarily that the sera of all donors should agglutinate the erythrocytes of all the recipients and vice versa, because there are numerous classes or groups of blood with respect to isohemagglutinins, called *blood groups.*

Blood Groups. One major system of blood groupings consist of A, B, AB and O groups. It detects the presence or absence of the agglutinogens (antigens) in the erythrocytes of the persons to be identified and grouped. For example, any one person may have antigen A (Group A) or B (Group B) or both (Group AB) or neither (Group O). A person's own serum never contains agglutinins against his own Erythrocytes, but only against the absent agglutinogens.

A person's blood group is a physiological constant determined by the basic Mendelian laws of inheritance. It is possible to avoid the hemagglutination, by properly selecting donors and recipients of compatible group. Blood banks collect citrated blood donations already grouped and store in the refrigerator until needed.

Blood Grouping. A nurse should have the knowledge of grouping the blood. A drop of the patient's (recipient) blood should be added to a small amount of physiological saline (0.9 per cent sodium chloride) on a microscopic slide and then mixed with rabbit sera containing pure anti-A and anti-B antibodies. A readily visible agglutination will appear of the patient (recipient).

If the cells of the patient (recipient) are agglutinated by both anti A and anti B rabbit sera, then the cells of the patients are of group AB.

If the cells are agglutinated by neither sera, they are of Group O. If anti A serum agglutinates them and anti B serum does not, then the blood cells are of Group A; if anti B serum agglutinates them and anti-A serum does not, the cells are of Group B.

Certain irregularities in reaction can be eliminated and the blood groupings can be ascertained by testing the serum of the recipient against the red cells of the donor.

Table 21.2 : Isohemagglutination. International system of Blood Group

Sera from persons of Group.	Agglutinate the erythrocytes of patients of Group.			
	AB	B	A	O
AB	–	–	–	–
B (anti-A)	+	–	+	–
A (anti-B)	+	+	–	–
O (anti-A and anti-B)	+	+	+	–

+ = agglutination; – = no agglutination.

Hemagglutination in blood grouping. Anti B serum and anti A serum have been mixed on a glass slide with erythrocytes of Groups O, A, B and AB. Anti B serum agglutinates erythrocytes of persons of Group B and AB; anti A serum agglutinates erythrocytes of persons of Groups A and AB.

Universal Donor. A person of Group O is sometimes called as Universal donor because his red blood cells are not usually agglutinated by serum of recipients of any other groups; but he must receive only Group O blood because his serum agglutinates cells of all other groups in the A-B-O system.

Direct cross-matching between recipient and donor is necessary to have a "safe universal donor". There are several other antigen antibody systems in human bloods, e.g., Rh factor, M-N-S, P types which may cause serious transfusion reactions irrespective of A, B, O or AB groups.

Rh factor. When erythrocytes of Rhesus (Rh) monkeys are injected into rabbits, the serum of the rabbits contained anti-Rh agglutinins which agglutinate erythrocytes of 85 per cent or more human beings. The antigen in the human red cells which reacted with anti-Rh rabbit serum was designated as the Rh agglutinogen. The person having the Rh agglutinogen is called as Rh positive (+). If the Rh agglutination is absent in red blood cells of the remaining 15 per cent whose red blood cells do not react with the anti-Rh rabbit serum, they are called as Rh-negative. The Rh agglutinogen is complex and corresponds to several antibodies or blood factors - hr, hr', rh', hr', rh'. The most important is Rh factor.

Rh factor and transmission. If an Rh negative person receives a blood transfusion from a person who is Rh positive, the recipient develops in about two weeks antibodies that agglutinate the red cells of all Rh positive persons. Now, if a subsequent transfusion is given from an Rh positive donor and the Rh antibody titre (concentration) will rise to maximum, thereby all the red cells of the donor are agglutinated and ultimately haemolysis leading to severe transfusion reaction and death. Therefore, it is essential — before each blood transfusion — to evaluate the Rh factor and blood group.

Erythroblastosis foetalis (Hemolytic disease of the newborn). If Rh negative woman becomes pregnant by an Rh positive man, the child will most probably inherit Rh antigen in its blood cells. During pregnancy, if the child is Rh-positive (i.e., Rh factor), fetal red blood cells with Rh antigen often cross the foetal barrier, pass into the mother's blood circulation and the foetal Rh factor stimulates the maternal tissue to produce Rh antibodies. These Rh antibodies diffuse back into the foetal blood circulation. In any initial pregnancy, since the mother's Rh antibody titre is too low, there will be no detrimental effects in the foetus; when Rh antibody concentration increases with subsequent pregnancies, the red cells of the foetus are destroyed by Rh antibodies. Hence, the child with Rh factor (i.e., Rh positive) and Rh antibodies may be born dead (uncommon) or with hemolytic disease of the newborn (erythroblastosis foetalis) which is common. This type of condition may prevail if Rh negative mother has received a blood transfusion from Rh positive donor.

The periodic check up of the maternal blood for rising titre of Rh agglutinins is of great importance as a precautionary measure.

ANTIGEN-ANTIBODY REACTION

The interaction of the antigen and antibody is a chemical reaction and is specific. The molecules of the antigen and antibody bind with their terminal groups (Fig. 21.1) and form firm complexes. When molecules of antibody and antigen are brought together in solution, they interact with each other by the formation of a link between an *antigen binding* (ab) site on the immunoglobulin molecule (part of the Fab fragment) and the particular chemical groupings which make up the *antigenic determinant* of the antigen molecule. The molecules are held together by intermolecular forces which are effective only when the antibody combining site and the antigenic determinant group are able to make close contact.

The study of the reaction between the antigen and antibody is known as "Serology".

Serology is classified into :

1. Precipitation;
2. Agglutination;
3. Complement fixation;
4. Neutralisation;
5. Immobilisation;
6. Intradermal reaction.

1. *Precipitation*, in which the reaction takes place between antibody and antigen molecules which are *soluble* in nature; it is specific, sensitive and can detect even diluted antigen (1 : 1,000,000 - 110,000,000). VDRL, Kahn test for syphilis; gel diffusion test; counter immuno-electrophoresis.

2. *Agglutination*, in which there is reaction between antibody and *particulate* antigen (erythrocyte, bacteria) in the presence of electrolyte (0.85 per cent sodium chloride solution) in definite proportions. (Coombs' test, blood groupings; Widal test; Weil-Felix test; tube agglutination test for Brucellosis);

Coombs' test. The Coombs' test (antiglobulin test) is used, in particular, to detect incomplete agglutinins in rhesus negative mothers. To determine the fixation of agglutinins by the patient's erythrocytes, antiglobulin serum is added which, in saline solution, is capable of causing marked agglutination of erythrocytes sensitised by incomplete agglutinins. A molecule of antiglobulin binds two molecules of incomplete agglutinins fixed to two different erythrocytes, due to which the agglutination reaction takes place.

3. *Complement fixation reaction*, in which the antibody molecules, after reaction with antigen activate the serum complement which gets fixed with the antibody antigen complex — Wassermann test for syphilis.

4. *Neutralisation test* is used in virus identification; *Antitoxin-toxin neutralisation test* (in tetanus).

5. *Immobilisation* test for motile bacteria;

6. *Intradermal test* for the reaginic antibody characteristic of skin hypersensitivity.

IMMUNITY

The term *immunity* (Lat. *immunis* — freed from homage, save from something) means resistance of the body to the pathogenic microbes, their toxins or to other kinds of foreign substances. In other words, it can be defined as the body resistance power to infections immunity.

1. natural (innate),
2. acquired.

1. *Natural immunity* (*non-specific resistance*) is present from birth. The innate resistance mechanisms are non-specific in the sense that they are effective against a wide range of infective agents. The innate immunity is genetically controlled.

Determinants of Natural Immunity

(a) *Species and Strains.* Different species of animals are susceptible to different diseases, e.g., the guinea plg and man are not susceptible to diphtheria, whereas the rat is susceptible to diphtheria. Only man is susceptible to syphilis, gonorrhoea, typhoid. Rabies and Brucellosis affect both men and animals. American Indian and the Negro are genetically more susceptible to tuberculosis than Caucasians.

(b) *Individual Difference and Influence of Age.* Sickle cell anaemia (sickling) disease is genetically controlled. Sickle cell anaemia patients are resistant to malaria, as *Plasmodium falciparum* cannot parasitise red blood cells of sickle cell anaemia.

Because of the immaturity of the immunological mechanisms affecting the lymphoid system, children and young animals are highly susceptible to infections, older persons have diminished resistance as a result of the probable waning of the activity of immune response.

(c) *Hormonal Influences, Sex.* Patients of diabetes mellitus, hypothyroidism, adrenal dysfunction have decreased resistance to infection. The reasons are not yet well propounded. Sexes will not show the marked differences.

(d) *Nutritional Factors.* Inadequate diet may be associated with the increased susceptibility to various *bacterial diseases.* It has been experimentally proved that when a large number of animal species were undernourished, they become less susceptible than normal animals to a variety of viruses including vaccinia virus and certain neurotropic viruses, e.g., poliovirus. The same condition may be observed in case of malaria. When the nutrition level is lowered, there may be deficiency of paraaminobenzoic acid essential for the multiplication of malarial parasites.

Mechanism of Natural Immunity

(a) Mechanical barriers and surface secretion,
(b) Bactericidal substances of the tissues and body fluids:
  (i) Lysozyme,
  (ii) Basic polypeptides.
(c) Phagocytosis and inflammation:
  (i) Phagocytin,
(d) Temperature,
(e) Complement system.

(a) Mechanical Barriers and Surface Secretions

1. The intact skin and mucous membrane of the body give protection against non-pathogenic organisms and a high degree of protection against pathogens. Because of the horny layer of the skin consisting mainly of keratin, which is not digestible by most organisms and protects the living cells of the epidermis from the organisms and toxins, the skin is a most resistant barrier.

2. *Sebaceous secretions and Sweat of skin* contain bactericidal and fungicidal fatty acids and have a protective mechanism. The microorganisms are trapped by the sticky, mucous secretion covering the mucous membrane of the respiratory tract. They are swept down by the cilia or hair-like processes of the mucosa along with the mucous secretion towards the oropharynx and are swallowed. In stomach, most of the microorganisms are destroyed by the acid secretion.

Nasal secretion and saliva containing mucopolypeptide inactivate some viruses. The tear and mucous secretions of respiratory, alimentary and genito-urinary tract contain lysozyme which is active against some Gram-positive bacteria.

(b) Bactericidal Substances and Body Fluids

(i) *Lysozyme* is a basic protein present in leucocytes and body fluids except cerebrospinal fluid, sweat and urine. It splits the sugars of the cell wall of Gram-positive bacteria and causes lysis of bacteria. Egg white and human tear are rich source of lysozyme.

(ii) *Basic Polypeptide* is basic protein derived from the damaged tissue and blood cells. It has a bactericidal activity.

(c) Phagocytosis and Inflammation

When the microorganisms invade the blood stream or tissue fluids, they are engulfed rapidly by various circulating and tissue fixed phagocytic cells.

These cells are of two types :

(a) polymorphonuclear leucocytes or microphages of the blood;
(b) mononuclear leucocytes or macrophages, distributed throughout the body. The cells fixed in the tissues are the cells of the reticuloendothelial layer lining liver sinuses (Kupffer cells), red bone marrow, spleen and lymph node. Macrophages in the blood are known as monocytes, those in the connective tissue are known as histiocytes, those in spleen, lymph and thymus are known as the sinus lining macrophages (called as littoral cells).

Inflammation is a defensive response of living body tissues to any irritating or injurious agent. The inflammatory reaction is a complex process involving several physiological process which (1) *removes* the cause of the irritation and (2) repairs the damage, i.e., to heal the wound or lesion.

The inflammation may be due to :

(a) mechanical factors (trauma, cut),
(b) chemical agents (acids, excessive application of mustard, gases, bee stings),
(c) physical agents (excessive heat, cold, ultra violet rays),
(d) Living agents (microorganisms, worms).

Four cardinal sings of inflammation are :

1. *rubor* (redness, hyperemia);
2. *tumor* (swelling);
3. *calor* (heat);
4. *dolor* (pain) can be observed in a boil or in an inflammed area. The increased amount of blood in the dilated local blood vessels may cause the redness; the compression and injury of the sensory nerve branches in the tissue may result into pain. The dilatation and increased permeability of the blood vessels resulting in the collection of fluid under slight pressure in the spaces between the tissue cells is responsible for swelling (often called *edema* — inflammatory exudation of fluid).

Hyperemia is due to increased amount of blood in an inflammed area. *Thrombi* or clots are formed in the tiny vessels all around the point of injury due to the slowing down of blood flow in that particular area and prevent the entry of microorganisms into the general circulation.

Pus formation. When the blood flow slows down or stops, the leucocytes begin to migrate in between the cells of the vessel walls by amoeboid motion called *diapedesis.* The leucocytes become *pus cells.* In intense inflammation as in gonorrhoea, much pus is formed and discharged, but a mild inflammation may heal without pus formation.

Temperature changes. The inflamed area is usually hot compared to the temperature of the body surface which may be due to the warmth of the deep body blood brought rapidly to the body surface or warmth due to the chemical changes in the infected area.

Defensive of fibrin. The inflammatory area is filled and surrounded by a continuous network of fibrin fibres. At the periphery of the infected area, connective tissue cells (fibroblasts) begin to grow among these fibres. The acute inflammatory area is therefore soon surrounded by a wall of fibrin that tends to confine the inflammatory process and prevent the spread.

A closed sac formed by pyogenic membrane, is filled with pus, microorganisms and walled off forming abscess, pimple, boil, carbuncle. Several intercommunicable abscesses are called carbuncle.

Enzymes produced by various microorganisms digest the wall of the abscess nearest to the exterior finally making an opening through which the abscess drains. By this process, the boil heals.

Types of inflammation :

(a) *Acute inflammation* is of short duration (for few days).
(b) *Chronic inflammation* is of long duration (weeks, months, years).
(c) *Catarrhal inflammation* is of mild type seen in the throat, nose in cold or influenza.

(d) In *serous inflammation*, the serum like fluid is more and the fibrin is less. If pus formed is more, the process is described as *purulent* or *suppurative*. A fluid may be *sanguinopurulent* or *fibrinopurulent*.

Healing and scar formation. As soon as the infection or injury is brought under control by fibrin formation and other body defensive mechanism, tissue cells (fibroblasts) and blood vessels start to grow into the area of healing from periphery and form new healthy tissue. This early healing process is known as *Organisation*. The tissue thus formed is solid, tough connective tissue. This tissue constitutes *scar tissue* and this process is known as *cicatrisation*.

When there is inflammation, there is a response, there is initial polymorph infiltration; bacteria are digested and disintegrated within one hour or two, probably due to acid and digestive enzyme of phagocytes.

Phagocytin. Polymorphs contain acid soluble protein (phagocytin) which is bactericidal to Gram-negative bacteria.

Temperature

Mycobacterium marinum, which infect cold blooded animals, cannot infect man. Anthrax bacilli cannot infect fowls because of fowl's high temperature, 107°C. If the temperature of the fowl is lowered, it can infect fowls. High temperature (above 40°C) can kill Gonococci and Treponema.

Complement System

Complement is a heat labile serum component which has the ability to lyse red blood cells and destroy Gram-negative bacteria. It is an extremely complex group of serum proteins present in low concentration in normal serum. Components of complement are C_1, C_2, C_3, C_4, C_5, C_6, C_7, C_8, C_9. The complement is responsible for the biological activity of complement fixing antibodies.

Recently, a new pathway for complement activation has been described. C_1, C_4 and C_2 components are not involved. The activation starts at C_3 and proceeds to the later components :

$$C_3 - C_5, C_6, C_7 \rightarrow \begin{matrix} C_8 \\ C_9 \end{matrix} \left| \begin{matrix} \text{Cell} \\ \text{lysis} \end{matrix} \right.$$

Function

1. Complement action is of considerable importance because of its ability to get fixed with various types of cells such as Gram-negative bacteria or human red blood cells after they have been interacted with specific antibody; and

2. renders bacteria susceptible to lysozyme by digesting holes in the polysaccharide which protects inner lysozyme sensitive layer of mucopeptide in the cell wall;

3. complement also plays an important role in the attraction of polymorphonuclear phagocytes to the sites of antigen - antibody interaction. This chemotaxis appears to depend on the components of $C_{5, 6}$, C_6 C_7 interacting with C_1, C_4, D_2, C_3 complex.

ACQUIRED SPECIFIC IMMUNITY (Specific Resistance)

Microorganisms that overcome the innate non-specific resistance are faced, after an interval, by the host's second line of defense, i.e., specific immune response. Acquired immunity is *specific* in the sense that it protects against a particular pathogen or its toxic product.

The specific immune response takes two forms :

(a) *Humoral immunity* depends on the appearance of globulins or antibodies in the blood. These antibodies combine specifically with antigens that stimulated their production. Examples, antigen molecule or particles of bacteria may be clumped, their toxins may be neutralised and subsequently they are ingested and digested by phagocytes. Cells are lysed by the activation of complement.

(b) *Cell mediated immunity* depends upon the development of lymphoid cells which are specifically sensitised to the inducing agents and which react directly with the antigen to bring about cytotoxic effects. The function of lymphoid tissue is not yet well understood.

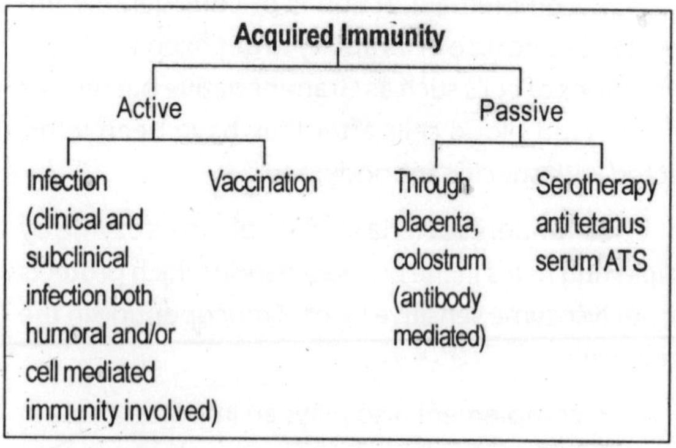

Actively acquired immunity is due to

1. *Infectious agents* which may be of two types :

(a) Some infections — diphtheria, whooping cough, small pox and mumps induce a long lasting immunity,

(b) Some infections like common cold and influenza confer immunity lasting for a short time.

2. *Vaccination* is an artificial process which stimulates the lymphoid tissue and is adapted to meet practical requirement. It is under human control. Several such artificial processes are used for artificial immunity. Vaccines are cheapest and most effective means of controlling deadly infectious diseases.

(A) Vaccine prepared from living attenuated organisms

Active specific immunity may be acquired artificially similar to subclinical infection, by means of injection of living attenuated (weakened) organisms in the human body which cannot cause a severe infection, e.g., Bacille Calmette Guerin (BCG) vaccine; small pox vaccine; Anti Rabies vaccine — *vacca*, (Latin for cow).

1. *BCG vaccination.* Calmette and Guerin, French scientists, developed a BCG vaccine consisting of live tubercle bacilli of low virulence for human being as an immunising agent against tuberculosis.

Cholera vaccination. A live oral cholera vaccine is recently used.

2. *Small pox vaccination* is carried out by inoculation of living cowpox virus into the human body which could give protection against small pox virus because of their antigenic relationship. The vaccine was available in freeze dried form, when small pox was in existence. Now small pox is completely eradicated.

3. *Anti-rabies vaccine.* Semple vaccine is prepared from the brain of sheep infected with the fixed rabies virus. Infected sheep brain suspension inactivated by 0.5 per cent phenol vaccine may cause paralysis in small proportion (1 : 4,000 to 1 : 10,000) of human beings, because of the presence of nerve cells in the vaccine (allergic type of encephalitis).

4. *Avinised Rabies vaccine.* To avoid the nervous symptoms, the vaccine is prepared from virus cultivated repeatedly in successive live embryonated avian eggs, inactivated by formalin, ultraviolet irradiation or phenol and finally the vaccine is dehydrated. This vaccine is reconstituted, used safely and effectively than sheep brain tissue vaccine.

Human Diploid Cell Strain (HDCS) *vaccine* is highly antigenic free from side effects and is costly. It is a recent vaccine against Rabies.

(B) Vaccine prepared from dead organisms

The active artificial immunity can be produced by another method, i.e., by injecting the actual organisms that cause the disease into the body. The body reacts and produces the antibodies. In this method, the organisms are *dead* or *killed* by heat or chemical disinfectant.

Many types of bacteria vaccines are used. Typhoid vaccine and Whooping cough (Pertussis) vaccine are very common. These vaccines are prepared by submitting the bacterial suspensions to a heat of 60°C for 1 hour to kill the living bacteria. It is customary to give three successive injections of the vaccines at intervals of one month and an annual booster dose.

1. *Mixed vaccines.* Vaccines containing *more than one* kind of organisms is known as mixed vaccines, e.g., Triple vaccine (Tetanus, Pertussis, Diphtheria, TPD) vaccine is not only effective, but it saves many extra pricks.

2. *Sensitised vaccines.* Organisms meant for the preparation of vaccine are sometimes treated before use with the serum of a person or animal immune to the bacteria. These bacteria combine with the antibody in the serum, so that *they are acted upon quickly by the blood, tissues or phagocytes of the person into whom they are infected* and ultimately immunity is produced rapidly and effectively. Such vaccines are called as *Sensitised vaccines.*

3. *Viral vaccines. Killed* viral vaccines are the vaccines against Influenza and Salk vaccine against Poliomyelitis. *Live* viral vaccine is Sabin Oral Poliomyelitis vaccine.

(C) Injection of modified bacterial exotoxin

1. *Toxoid.* Certain bacteria damage the body tissue by elaborating the toxins. When these toxins are detoxified by formaldehyde, they can be used as immunising agents against the diseases, e.g., Tetanus toxoid (TT) against tetanus; diphtheria toxoid against diphtheria.

Passively acquired immunity. Administration of immune serum from another species,. e.g., horse - diphtheria antiserum, tetanus antiserum (ATS) and gas gangrene antiserum were used therapeutically until the advent of antibiotics. Still now, it is used. Passive immunity due to maternal antibody may be transferred to foetus by the passage of maternal antibody across the placenta in some species — man and rabbit - where a particular part of immunoglobulin polypeptide chain has been found necessary for effecting the transfer. In other species, such as dogs and rats, antibodies are transmitted through the colostrum via the intestine and via placenta; the other animals, lamb and calf receive this form of immunity only by means of the colostrum. Pooled human immunoglobulin is also used as a source of antibody in a number of infections (measles, small pox and serum hepatitis) during the period of incubation to *modify* or prevent the infection.

THE IMMUNE RESPONSE

(A) Humoral Immune Response

After first contact of the tissue with the antigen, there is an interval of about two weeks before antibody can be found in the blood and, during this initial period, there is intense activity in the antibody forming tissues.

After primary antigenic stimulation, there is a rapid increase in cell proliferation and in the synthesis of protein in cells of the lymphoid organ.

The antibody which can be detected during the "primary immune response" does not reach its peak. Then, after a day or two, there is a remarkable rise in the level of antibody which reaches its peak. This "secondary immune response" can be boosted to even higher levels by a further injection of antigen (booster or recall dose) until no further increase occurs and it slowly falls. Once an animal has responded to a single dose of a live attenuated (e.g., small pox or polio vaccine) antigen the animal retains a "memory" of the antigen so that months or years later it responds with a rapid mobilisation of anti-forming cells. Vaccination with even nonliving agent such as tetanus or diphtheria toxoid, if given in two spaced doses provides, several years of useful protection against infection even though soon after vaccination the level of antibodies falls to a low level, the "memory" is retained. To obtain a maximum response, the interval between the primary and secondary injection should not be too short and an interval of less than ten days is likely to reduce the level of the secondary response. This allows time for a maximal increase in the number of antibody forming cells which can be stimulated by subsequent injection.

Determinants of Acquired Specific Immunity

1. *Form.* The natural ability of antigen to induce an immune response may be enhanced by altering or mixing it with another substance known as

adjuvant. The antigen can be absorbed on a mineral gel such as aluminium hydroxide or aluminium phosphate, e.g., Alum precipitated antigen. Such particulate form of antigen seems to be able to initiate antibody production much more effectively than the same antigen in non-particulate form. The effect is not yet fully understood, but it may be due to the direct effect of the particulate antigen on the lymphoid cell membrane leading to more effective transformation of the cell for antibody formation than that can be brought about by antigen in solution.

Another method has been developed to enhance antibody response, i.e., preparation of a water-in-oil emulsion. The emulsion forms a depot of antigen in the tissues from which small quantities of antigen are released continuously, sometimes for a year or more. Example, Influenza vaccine.

Route. If an antigen is given intravenously, most of the antibody is produced by spleen, and some in lung and bone marrow; if given subcutaneously or intradermally, the antigen travels via lymphatics to local lymph nodes where antibody is produced initially.

Dose. The antibody response is proportionate to the dose of antigen. If the antigen dose is increased, the immune response is small, so if a particular level of antigen is increased then there will be specific paralysis of the antibody forming tissues - Immunological tolerance.

(B) Cell Mediated Acquired Immune Response

Cell mediated immunity occurs particularly in infections by microorganisms that enter and grow within the tissue cells such as viruses, tubercle bacilli, brucella and some salmonella. It seems likely that the cell mediated immune response is involved in protection against infective agents, particularly those causing intracellular infection.

Cell mediated immunity is manifested by delayed hypersensitivity around the site of infection. The cell mediated response is initiated in different areas of spleen and lymph node (white pulp of spleen and paracortical areas of lymph). These areas are controlled by *thymus*— so these lymphocytes are called T-cells.

Very recently a number of yet uncharacterised non-antibody lymphocytic factors (non-specific antibodies) are described and are called as *lymphokines*. They are released by sensitised lymphocytes, T-cells, in contact with antigen.

Functions

Lymphokine has

1. The property of inhibition of the *in vitro* migration of macrophages on glass slide.
2. Macrophages can be grown in culture in capillary tube and will normally migrate out of the open end of the tube into the culture fluid.
3. A factor released by lymphocytes exposed to antigen will prevent this migration by causing the macrophages to stick together. This factor is likely to be released also *in vivo* and may be responsible for the accumulation for macrophages in cell mediated immune reaction.
4. Another factor released from sensitised lymphocytes after exposure to antigen causes stimulation and proliferation of normal unsensitised lymphocytes. This is known as mitogenic factor.
5. Another lymphokine has a chemotactic effect on macrophages attracting them to the site of the inflammatory response.
6. A cytotoxic effect due to a lymphokine (lymphotoxin) has been demonstrated to damage the different types of cell.
7. A factor which increases capillary permeability (skin reactive factor) can also be shown to be released by sensitised lymphocytes.
8. It is generally thought that the lymphokines are the main effector mechanism in the cell mediated response.

Tissue Involved in Immune Response

Lymph nodes, spleen and bone marrow are mostly engaged in the immune response, while lung and, to some extent, the liver, can take part in immune response. The specialised lymphoid organs (spleen and lymph nodes) take up foreign antigen and initiate the immune response. The lymph nodes and spleen are made up of three types of cells which are involved in the initiation of the immune reaction. The three types of cells are lymphocytes, plasma cells and phagocytic cells of reticuloendothelial system. The lymphoid tissues responsible for humoral antibody production are associated developmentally with the gut and consist of lymphocytes and plasma cells of the lymph nodes and spleen.

In the humoral immune response, immunoglobulins are secreted into the blood by the lymphoid cells, predominantly plasma cells situated in the spleen and lymph nodes.

In man, lymphoid tissue appears first in the thymus at about eight weeks' gestation. Peyer's patches are distinguishable by the fifth month and immunoglobulin secreting cells appear in the spleen and lymph nodes at about 20 weeks. From this period onwards both IgM and IgG globulins are synthesised by the foetus with IgM predominating. At birth the infant has a blood concentration of IgG comparable to, or sometimes higher than that of maternal serum having received IgG but not IgM via placenta from the mother. The rate of synthesis of IgM in the infant increase rapidly within the first few days of life and does not reach adult levels until about a year. Cell mediated immune reactions can be stimulated at birth but these reactions may not be as powerful as in the adult.

Cells Concerned in the Antibody Production

Cell cooperation between thymus dependent (T) lymphocytes and bone marrow derived (B) lymphocytes has been shown to occur. The (T) lymphocytes assist (B) lymphocytes in some as yet undefined way, possibly by concentrating antigen on their surface and presenting it to B cells or perhaps by releasing a *lymphocyte activation product* (lymphokine) to stimulate the B cells to respond to antigen.

In the spleen, the cells engaged in antibody production are found in the red pulp, whereas in lymph nodes, they are found in germinal centres of the cortex.

Individual immunoglobulin producing cells synthesise the whole molecule of immunoglobulin both heavy and light polypeptide chains. Individual cells make only one class of immunoglobulin and the light chains are restricted to one of the two types (K and L). T and B lymphocytes are morphologically similar.

Initially, B cells produce IgM antibody and then switch over to IgG production. Antibody secreting "Russell body" is found in plasma cell. B cells are responsible for immunoglobulin (Ig) synthesis and can either react to the direct contact with antigen or cooperate with T cells which are helper cells.

Protection and Immunity

A particular microorganism may become pathogenic if it is capable to overcome the immune response system of the human host:

1. **Human host can be protected from the bacterial infections by**
   (a) Antibody mediated immunity, or
   (b) Cell mediated immunity.
   (a) *Antibody Mediated Immunity in Bacterial Infections.* Because of the production of the exotoxin, some microorganisms (i.e., *Corynebacterium diphtheriae, Clostridium tetani, Cl.welchii, Cl.botulinum*) are pathogenic. Antibodies acquired by immunisation or previous infection or given passively as antiserum are able to neutralise the bacterial toxins. Bacterial toxins are enzymatic in nature; most probably, the antibody interacts with the active site of the enzyme and neutralises effectively the toxin.

When bacteria do not produce exotoxins, antibodies get attached to the surface of the bacteria. The most important effect of this attachment is to encourage phagocytosis by blood macrophages or polymorphs (*opsonisation*).

The mechanism is that the antibody alters the surface change of organisms and makes them more susceptible to phagocytosis. The phagocytes can also destroy the organisms by digesting by various enzymes produced in the intracellular lysosomes; but *Streptococcus pyogenes, typhoid* bacillus, *Mycobacterium tuberculosis* are able to resist the digestion by enzymes. If immunity exists due to previous infection or artificial immunisation, streptococcus is susceptible to intracellular digestion, whilst the smooth strains are able to resist the digestion.

In case of enteric infections (typhoid and paratyphoid due to salmonella) antibodies are secreted into the intestinal lumen and attack these organisms before they invade the intestinal mucosa. These antibodies are known as "copro antibodies" and they are of IgA type which is selectively produced in mucous membrane of respiratory and intestinal tract.

Other effects of antibody attachment to the surface of the organism are :

(i) The lysis of Gram-negative bacteria brought about by the activation of complement system. The effect of the complement is to digest the cell wall of lipopolysaccharide so that the structural mucopeptide is exposed to the attack by lysozyme.

(ii) Attachment of bacteria to red blood cells in presence of antibody and complement. This phenomenon which is known as "*Immune adherence*," may encourage the phagocytosis.

(iii) Antibody precipitated on the surface of certain parasitic nematodes can block the excretory orifices of the nematodes.

(b) *Cell mediated Immunity in Bacterial Infections.* Macrophages from animal immune to tubercle bacilli are more actively phagocytic than those taken from a normal animal. Similarly, macrophages from brucella infected animals showed enhanced cellular immunity. The same was observed in *Listeria monocytogenes.*

2. **Immunity in viral infections**

(a) *Antibody Mediated Immunity.* In virus infection, the antibody is mostly efficacious, if the virus passes through the blood stream to reach its target organ. For example, poliovirus initially crosses the intestinal route, invades the blood stream and passes on rare occasions to the spinal cord and brain where it proliferates. Antibody present in the blood stream can neutralise the virus before it reaches its target cells in the nervous system.

A number of virus behave in the same way (e.g., virus of measles, small pox, mumps, rubella and chicken pox). In case of Influenza and common cold, the viruses do not pass through the blood stream as their target organ is the respiratory mucous membrane. In this type of infection, a high level of antibody will be less effective against these viruses in comparison with its effect on blood borne viruses. Most of the antibody should pass through the mucous membrane into the respiratory secretion to act on such respiratory viruses. There is very little IgG and often no IgM in the content of mucous secretion, as this mucous membrane is not, most probably, very permeable to there classes of antibody. But IgA is the predominant immunoglobulin in the mucous secretion. IgA is manufactured by the plasma cells in the lamina propria of the mucous membrane and secreted in the nasal secretion. IgA has neutralising activity against common cold viruses. Intranasal administration of live attenuated Influenza virus can stimulate local production of IgA antibody in the mucous membrane of the nose.

The high degree of immunity was provided by live attenuated oral poliovirus may be due to locally produced antibody in the gut by neutralising the virus even before it reaches the blood stream. After oral vaccination, IgA against poliovirus has been demonstrated in the faeces, in duodenal fluid and in saliva, whereas no antibody was demonstrated after injection of inactivated poliovirus vaccine.

(b) *Cell Mediated Immunity*: The children with congenital hypogammaglobulinaemia can recover from virus infection without producing any demonstrable virus neutralising antibody, because of cell mediated immunity. The patients with Swiss type agammaglobulinaemia and an additional cell mediated deficiency are very much susceptible to virus infection and ultimately they may die.

3. **Immunity to protozoa and helminths**

The life cycle of parasite is complicated and the immune response can be effective, if the life cycle is interrupted at a stage when the parasite is accessible to immune process. The antibody may, most probably, have the access to the parasite if the permeability of the red blood cell membrane is altered so that the immunoglobulin can enter and attack the parasite. In protozoal infection, immunoglobulin production is increased and all classes of immunoglobulins are involved.

Life cycle of helminths is also complex as in protozoa. Protective immuno responses may act only at an early stage in the life cycle.

IgE (reaginic) antibody with pulmonary eosinophilia will appear in the parasitic infections and the immediate hypersensitivity reactions of anaphylactic type (Type 1) is involved in the pathogenesis of helminth infections.

ALLERGY (HYPERSENSITIVITY)

Von Pirquet coined the term allergy (Gr. *allos,* altered, changed; *ergon,* action) to describe the altered reactivity of an animal after exposure to a foreign antigen. The allergy included both immunity and hypersensitivity. It is now, restricted to refer only to *hypersensitivity.*

There are two forms of hypersensitivity reactions:

1. Immediate allergy, and
2. Delayed allergy.

1. The *immediate form* appears rapidly after exposure of a sensitised person to further dose of antigen and usually depends upon the liberation of *histamine* — pharmacologically active mediator substance which is formed under the influence of antigen antibody combination.

2. The *delayed form* appears more slowly (usually after 24 hours) and depends upon the immunologically activated lymphoid cells.

Various classifications of hypersensitivity reactions have been proposed, but the most widely accepted one is that of Coombs and Gell. The classification of Coombs and Gell recognises four types of hypersensitivity reactions, three of which come under the heading of immediate reaction.

Type I : *Anaphylactic* reactions;

Type II : *Cytotoxic* or cytolytic reactions;

Type III : *Toxic-complex* syndrome;

Type IV : *Cell-mediated* delayed hypersensitivity form of reaction.

Very recently, Type V, *mixed* type, *mixed antibody and cell mediated* reaction has been recognised.

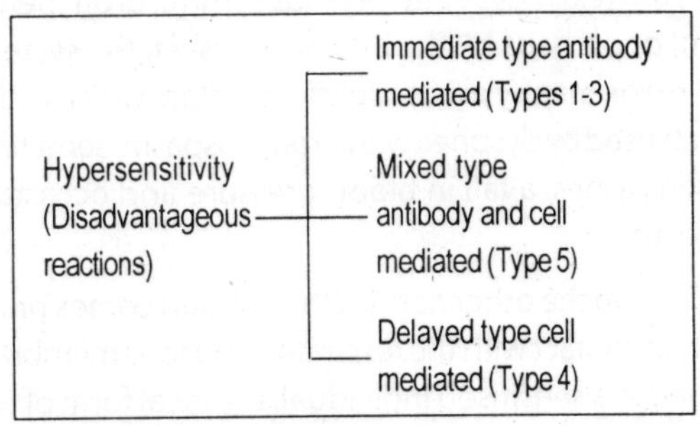

1. *Anaphylactic reactions* (Anaphylaxis) Type-I. If a guinea pig is injected with a small dose of a foreign antigen (egg albumin), no adverse effects are observed. When a second injection of egg albumin is given intravenously after an interval of ten days, a condition known as "anaphylactic shock" develops — the guinea pig becomes restless, starts to chew and rubs the nose with its own front paws, its respiration is laboured; the animal becomes cyanosed, may develop convulsions and, ultimately, die.

The initial injection of antigen is termed - "sensitising dose" and the second dose is known as "shocking dose". During the interval between the two injections, the animal has formed antibody which gets attached on the surface of cells; later, there will be interaction of shocking dose of antigen with the newly formed antibody on the surface of cells ultimately leading to "anaphylaxis".

In anaphylactic reaction, four pharmacologically active substances have been implicated — the most important is histamine. The release of histamine can be demonstrated *in vitro* by exposing antibody sensitised pieces of tissue to the contact of antigen. (Sensitisation may be induced by prior injection of antigen into the animal supplying the tissue which makes antibody as described above or tissue may be sensitised passively by the addition of antibody produced in other animal). The typical contractions induced in isolated strips of uterus and intestine are called *Schultz — Dale* reactions after the discoverers.

In man, there are two types of reactions, *systemic* and *local*, which are related to the mode of entry of the shocking dose of antigen into the body. If the antigen is injected parenterally as in the case of serum (e.g., *horse* anti-tetanus serum), drug (penicillin) or perhaps by the bite of an insect, the systemic form of anaphylaxis is likely to develop, which is characterised by dyspnea with bronchospasm, sometimes skin rashes, a fall in blood pressure and occasional death.

On the other hand, if the antigen comes primarily in contact with the respiratory mucous membrane, then in a sensitised individual, the local form of anaphylaxis may develop, i.e., hay fever, asthma. When the appropriate antigen (e.g., nuts, fish, strawberries) come in contact with the intestinal mucous membrane of a sensitised individual a mixed form of reactions may develop with the intestinal symptoms, urticaria, skin rashes and sometimes symptoms of asthma.

Antibodies in Anaphylactic Reactions

In man, reaginic antibody is responsible for the sensitisation of the tissues for anaphylactic reactions. This antibody has an affinity for tissues and can readily be detected in the serum of a sensitised individual by injecting a small quantity of this serum into the skin of a normal recipient, which is followed by introduction of the appropriate antigen into the same site of injection, after an interval of 24-48 hours. A *wheal and flare* erythematous reaction develops within about 20 minutes at the site of injection, just like a response to an injection of histamine. This reaction is known as *Prausnitz-Kustner* (PK) test according to its originators.

2. *Cytotoxic or cytolytic reactions, Type II.* The antibody directed against a cell which is associated with an antigen brings about cytotoxic or cytolytic effect which involves participitation of complement :

(a) In *incompatible blood transfusion*, the cytolytic effect of antibody on foreign red blood cells was observed.

(b) *Haemolytic disease* of new born has a similar mechanism.

(c) *Sedarmid purpura* is a cytotoxic reaction which is due to the union of the drug sedarmid with platelets, as a result an antibody response against the platelet absorbed drug brings about destruction of the platelets and thus cause purpura. Therefore, the drug sedarmid is withdrawn from the market.

A variety of infectious diseases due to salmonella and Mycobacteria are associated with haemolytic anaemia. Studies of salmonella infections revealed that the haemolysis is apparently due to an autoimmune reaction against a lipopolysaccharide endotoxin which becomes coated on the erythrocytes. A detailed study has been conducted in *Salmonella gallinarum* infections in chickens.

3. *Toxic complex syndrome*, Type III. This reaction is due to the combination of antigen with circulating antibody leading to formation of microprecipitates in and around small blood vessels with consequent inflammation and subsequent mechanical blockage of the vessels causing interference with the blood supply to surrounding tissues. There are two types of reactions :

(a) Systemic form — Serum sickness;

(b) Local form — Arthus phenomenon.

(a) *Serum sickness* develops in individuals given injection of foreign serum and it is described soon after the parenteral administration of horse antitetanus serum (ATS). Symptoms are asthma or laryngeal edema. The organs affected are kidney, heart and joints. Nowadays the most likely causes of serum sickness are drugs (penicillin) which form drug-protein complexes in the host.

(b) *Arthus phenomenon.* Like serum sickness, Arthus phenomenon is brought about by the formation of antibody-antigen complexes, but in this case, the phenomenon is local at the site of injection. Arthus reaction occurs in the walls of small blood vessels in the presence of large quantities of IgG antibody, which forms microprecipitates with antigen. This reaction may occur in diabetic patients who have received many injections of insulin and have developed high levels of IgG antibody to antigenic constituents in the insulin preparation. Similar reaction is also noted in case of anti-Rabies vaccination.

4. *Delayed hypersensitivity,* Type IV or *Cell Mediated* hypersensitivity. This type of reaction occurs after 24-48 hours after injection of antigen. The classical example of this type of reaction is *tuberculin* response which occurs, when an individual previously or currently infected with tubercle bacilli is given an intradermal injection of 0.1 ml. of a 1 : 1,000 dilution of a protein extract of tubercle bacilli (purified protein derivative, PPD), 24-48 hours later an indurated inflammatory reaction of variable size can be seen in the skin. The injection site is infiltrated with large number of mononuclear cells — lymphocytes. The mechanism is not yet well understood.

Macrophages in delayed hypersensitivity reaction sites may contribute lysosomal enzymes from their intracellular granules and thus cause further inflammatory changes.

When macrophages come in contact with antigen, the sensitised lymphocytes release a number of non-antibody factors (i.e., lymphokines) which are :

(a) a factor inhibiting macrophages migration;

(b) a chemotactic factor; and

(c) a cytotoxic factor. The role of these substances in delayed hypersensitivity is not clear.

Delayed hypersensitivity reactions are observed in brucella, salmonella, mycobacterium, pathogenic fungi and a wide range of virus (herpes simplex, measles, small pox, vaccinia) infections. It can develop after sensitisation to a variety of metal (nickel and chromium) and dyes (hair dyes).

Skin sensitisation to penicillin is common after topical application of the antibiotic ointment or cream — clinical signs are redness, swelling, vesicles scaling and exudation of fluid.

Types of Allergy

Whether immediate or delayed allergy, the basic explanation of allergic manifestation is that a reaction between antigen and its specific antibody has occurred in the body. If this reaction occurs in the blood, it will not cause allergic response and is the normal defensive process. If antigen-antibody combination occurs in or *on the tissue cells,* there is *allergy.* There are two types of allergy :

1. *Immediate allergy* is due to *precipitin* reaction occurring *in* or *on* certain *tissue cells.* It is characterised by the painful itching wheals known as "hives". This type of allergy may occur after eating certain foods or after injections of therapeutic serum; other manifestations are : intense gastroenteritis appearing within few minutes after consuming certain foods to which the victim is allergic and asthma after contact with pollen or with certain animals.

Shock tissue. The signs, symptoms and appearance of immediate allergic reactions depend upon the tissue cells which suffer precipitin reaction. The tissues that suffer are known as "shock tissues".

If the tissues are smooth muscle fibres, the muscle contracts. If the muscle fibres of gastrointestinal tract contract, diarrhoea and cramps may result; if the gravid uterine muscle contracts, there is abortion; asthma may occur, if the bronchioles contract. Besides smooth muscle contraction, edema and inflammation of mucosa are manifested in the allergy. 0.5 to 1 ml. of 1 : 1,000 epinephrine quickly reduces the swellings.

Anaphylaxis is one of the most dramatic manifestations of the immediate type of allergy.

2. In *delayed allergy,* the tissue response appears after 24 hours.

The tuberculin reaction is a best example of delayed allergy.

Histamine in allergy. In immediate allergy, an initial substance called *histamine* is released by tissue cells. The histamine causes many of the symptoms seen in hay fever, bee stings, serum reactions, antibiotic reactions and common colds. These discomforts can be relieved by *antihistaminics* which cause contractions of blood vessels.

Some Common Allergies

Pollen allergy. The pollen (sperm cells) of many plants — grasses, roses, ragweed — may cause allergy in some persons. When the proteins of the pollen come in contact with nasal and respiratory mucous membrane of the individuals, they are absorbed locally and set up a hypersensitivity condition of these tissues. When the individual inhales later more of the pollen proteins, the nose and throat become irritated, swollen and edematous. Because of the severity of the reactions against pollen, there develop a symptom of severe "cold" which is commonly known as "hay fever" or nose fever. These conditions may be relieved by antihistaminics and nasal decongestants.

Food allergy. A person may become sensitised to certain foods (strawberries or cod fish). Due to a slight gastrointestinal irritation, lesion or disturbance, some of the food is absorbed *undigested* through the stomach or intestinal wall into the blood, the result is the same as if the protein has been injected. The next time or perhaps every time, the same person eats strawberries or cod fish, he will react very violently. There will be allergic manifestation in the form of rash or blotches on the skin which itch persistently. These conditions are known as "hives". Some other victims may exhibit nausea, vomiting, gastrointestinal irritation and general symptoms. Antihistaminics are useful in these conditions.

Infection allergy. Due to microbial proteins entering into the blood stream, certain cells of the body may become sensitised to these microbial proteins resulting into the delayed allergy. A person suffering from tuberculosis may become allergic to tuberculosis. The relapses in rheumatic fever are due to repeated allergic responses (with damage to heart muscles) to reinfection with certain streptococci to which the patient is already allergic.

Allergy may also develop in viral, fungal, worm infections, such allergy is called as *Infection allergy.* Most of the damaging effect of infectious diseases is due to infection allergy.

Serum reactions. There are two forms of serum reactions : one is acute and serious form resembling anaphylaxis characterised by collapse, dyspnea, occurring after a few minutes after the injection of therapeutic serum (e.g., diphtheria antitoxin); the other one is milder, delayed form known as serum sickness. Both forms depend upon the precipitin in the patient. Either type of serum reaction is due to animal (horse) protein in the therapeutic serum, *not to the specific antitoxin.* Symptoms are chill, nausea, extensive painful itching hives or serum rash. Pain in the joints may occur later. If the patient is serious, there may be fatal end.

Delayed serum reactions. Serum sickness may appear after ten to fifteen days after a therapeutic use of horse serum. It is assumed that, during this period, the precipitin to horse serum protein may accumulate in the tissues. After reaching a certain concentration, the precipitins react with the proteins (even in residual portion) of the therapeutic *horse* serum which still remain in the body. If the therapeutic horse serum is to be given parenterally; a preliminary skin test for hypersensitiveness to horse serum may be performed as described below. If the test is positive, the patient should be *desensitised* by giving a number of a very small (0.1 to 1 ml.) doses of the serum at intervals of an hour or so before the main injection. The possible shock to the patient is lessened. This process is called as "desensitisation".

Persons with previous injections of serum usually require desensitisation. Sometimes, even in the persons who have not had the previous injections of serum, the serum sickness may also occur.

Atopy. Some individuals inherit not allergy itself, but a certain increased tendency to form *reagins* and thereby to develop allergic reactions (i.e., asthma, hay fever) and perhaps certain forms of arthritis and rheumatic heart disease. These persons are called atopic (and are called unfortunate).

Drug idiosyncrasies. Certain plant perfumes, cosmetics, drugs, rubber goods, dyes etc. may also cause immediate allergy like responses (hives, dermatitis, asthma) which may be basically different from true allergy and which may not be previously dependent on specific antibodies at all. These allergy like reactions restricted to only to certain individuals are known as drug *idiosyncrasies.* The mechanism is not yet well understood.

Binding Power of Tissues

Because of natural infections or artificial injection of certain antigens (bacterial cells and exotoxins), cutaneous and mucosal tissues often acquire the property of combining with and holding fast to these specific antigens entering the body. This is a defense mechanism and is probably one manifestation of allergy. These tissues are said to be *sensitised* to the antigens. Once sensitised, the tissues tend to hold on and bind to these specific antigens, infections or toxins to prevent their further spread from the site of localisation whenever, they gain entry into the body. The tissues may be damaged locally, but generalised infections or intoxication is prevented. The binding power of the tissues is the basis for the beneficial effect of several methods of artificial immunisation as per example, Bacillus Calmette Guerin (BCG) vaccine. This is also of great importance in resistance to brucellosis, syphilis and other chronic diseases.

Skin Tests for Hypersensitiveness

When a very small dose of sensitising dose is injected or scratched into the skin of a person or animal hypersensitive to that particular antigen, a wheal (a large, red, swollen area) will develop after an interval of time. This allergic reaction persists for an hour or more. Hypersensitiveness to horse serum is tested in this way by injecting a very small quantity of the serum to be used therapeutically.

Similarly, for testing food or pollen allergy, alcoholic or aqueous extracts of various foods or pollens, likely to be involved, are introduced into (not under) the skin either by scarification or injection and the results are noted.

Application to Nursing

The intelligent professional nurse, who acquired a sound knowledge about allergy during her training, will be able to understand and handle the untoward reactions encountered when certain sensitised individuals come into contact with that particular antigenic (allergic) substances — sera, antibiotics, some drugs, vaccines, some foods. A severe allergic reaction may ensue following the injection of an antigenic substance. This reaction can be prevented and the patient's life can be saved by the perceptive nurse. For example, since the patient is under constant observation of the nurse on duty, the patient may narrate that he is allergic to eggs (foreign protein); if the physician, unaware of this allergic reaction, prescribes a viral vaccine prepared from chick embryo, the nurse should inform immediately the physician about the allergy of the patient to the egg, so that a severe, possible fatal allergic reaction can be averted. If the patient who had a previous injection of horse serum receives again a dose of antitoxic serum prepared in horse, may have a severe and even fatal reaction to the serum, which, although given to provide the patient with immediate protection against a specific disease, becomes a very highly fatal dose to the patient, since the patient is allergic to horse serum.

It is quite essential to understand that the patient reaction to the antitoxic serum is not due to antibodies present in it; but due to *animal* (horse) *proteins* in the serum. Thus, the proteins may react to any horse serum irrespective of presence of antibodies. The well informed and trained nurse should keep in readiness epinephrine and antihistaminics to avoid such a fatal allergy which may occur due to the parenteral administration of horse serum for passive immunity and she should always be careful about immediate and delayed allergy to an allergenic substance and advise the patient to avoid in future the injections of this particular allergic substance.

AUTOIMMUNITY

Immune response of an animal does not, under normal circumstances, react against its own body constituents. It is a fundamental characteristic. However, there is a mechanism that makes the cells of the immune system to recognise what is "foreign" and what is "self".

Ehrlich and Morgenroth (1900) after immunising a goat with red blood cells of other goats found that the animal readily made antibody against the red blood cells of other goats, but this antibody failed to react with the animal's own red blood cells. Thus it was understood that the immunological response to self antigen was prevented.

Coombs *et al* (1946) developed a technique to detect the presence of antibody globulin on red blood cells by adding an antiglobulin serum which, after reacting with the globulin coating the cells, linked the cells together and agglutinated them. This technique is known as "Coombs" or "antiglobulin" test and could detect a variety of human and animal diseases in which antibody capable of reacting with a number of different antigens of the individual own tissue.

Haemolytic anaemia in man, in which red blood cells are coated with antibody globulin, was first discovered with Coombs' test. *Systemic lupus erythematosis* (SLE) in which antinuclear factor (ANF), — an antibody to nucleus of the cell, is involved. This autoantibody serum factor is present in the blood of patients suffering from connective tissue disease. This (SLE) disease was the second discovery by adopting Coombs' technique. *Interstitial thyroiditis*, (known as Hashimoto's disease) in which an antibody to thyroglobulin is involved, was the third discovery.

The control mechanism for autoimmunity tolerance could be overcome by two ways :

1. The first category is the evasion circumvention of a normal functioning mechanism, and

2. The second one is the failure of the mechanism itself.

In the first category, evasion may occur in two ways :

(a) a particular body antigen is not normally accessible to the cells of the immune system as the antigen is *hidden* within a cell or tissue; in the second category, a tissue antigen is *altered* in some way by a chemical, a drug, or an infective agent. The sperm antigen and lens antigen of the eye are *sequestered* (hidden) antigens; whereas antigen in the human colon is *altered* antigen.

1. In the human colon, there is an antigen which can be extracted. This antigen is similar to a polysaccharide antigen present in *Escherchia coli* O_{14}. So, it is believed that the inflammatory conditions of the colon known as "ulcerative colitis" in which anti-colon antibodies are involved and produced as a result of the immune response initiated by the cross-reacting bacterial antigen.

2. Group A streptococci causing rheumatic fever have an antigen common with that of human heart. Antibody to the antigen of streptococci may cross-react with the antigen of human heart causing heart lesions.

3. Streptococci carry surface antigen similar to that found in human glomeruli and so streptococcal infection is associated with the development of acute glomerulonephritis.

4. The association of *Mycoplasma pneumoniae* with primary atypical pneumonia may cause the development of IgM agglutinins which, in the cold, react with the patient's own red cells and may produce haemolytic anaemia.

Studies on the effect of herpes or rabies viruses on tissue culture cells suggested that the viruses are able to bring about alterations of cell membrane. The association of virus with lymphocyte membrane may possibly interfere with normal lymphocyte reaction to antigen.

Pathogenesis of Autoimmune Diseases

Three types of hypersensitivity reactions are involved in autoimmune diseases:

(i) *Cytotoxic reaction.* Autoimmune haemolytic anaemia is an example of the cytotoxic reaction in which two types of antibodies are involved.

1. *IgM antibodies* which agglutinate the patient's own red cells in the cold.
2. *IgG type antibodies,* which do not cause direct agglutination of the red cells, can be detected by Coombs' test with antiglobulin serum.

In mycoplasma infections, the IgM cold agglutinins react with a common red cell antigen known as the I antigen.

(ii) *Toxic complex type reaction.* Complex of antibody and tissue antigens, particularly nuclear antigens are the cause of glomerulonephritis and systemic lupus erythematosis (SLE) where a wide variety of anti-tissue antibodies is found.

(iii) *Cell mediated reaction.* In both man and animal the development of a number of autoimmune states is paralleled by the existence of cell mediated reaction of the delayed hypersensitivity type demonstrated by skin test with tissue antigens.

There is an association between the reactions of cell mediated immunity and humoral antibody in induced autoimmune orchitis in guinea pigs.

Other disease associated with autoimmune states is rheumatoid arthritis in which IgM antibody called rheumatoid factor is present in the patient serum. This factor can be detected *in vitro* by its ability to agglutinate red blood cells or latex particles coated with IgG globulin.

CHAPTER 22

IMMUNISATION
(Prevention is better than cure)

Almost 200 years after Edward Jenner's discovery of small pox vaccination, mankind benefits from this process more than ever before. Several new vaccines were evolved and are now made available to eradicate many diseases, e.g., Jenner's own first small pox vaccine has finally banished. In our time (1977), small pox disappearance from the earth.

The basic principle of vaccination remains quite the same as in Edward Jenner's day; Jenner noticed that milk maids who suffered from cow pox, a relatively harmless but contagious disease in cattle, did not contract the small pox. So, Jenner took some cow pox germs from Sarah Nelmes, a young milk maid, who had fresh cow pox lesions on her fingers and inoculated an eight year old boy (James Phipps) with it. Later, he inoculated the boy again with the small pox germs and proved that the disease could not develop in the boy as the immune system of the boy started to act against small pox germs.

Louis Pasteur, almost hundred years later (1870-80), discovered that a deadly germ could also offer protection against the disease it caused, if the germ is altered or killed and then injected. This provides a basis for developing at least 20 good vaccines. But recent advances in molecular biology and genetic engineering have led to a new era in vaccinology.

The first genetically engineered vaccine approved in 1986, was designed to prevent hepatitis B which affects an estimated 200 million people around the world. This vaccine was produced by using simple yeast cells into which was inserted the gene for the production of the disease causing virus's outer coating. The outer coat itself is not infectious but, on recognising the outer coat, an immune response can trigger a protective reaction against the whole virus.

Though there was already a vaccine against hepatitis B virus, made by altering live viruses extracted from the blood plasma of patients infected with the disease, it is suspected that all vaccines derived from blood products may carry the Acquired immunodeficiency syndrome (AIDS) virus or Human immunodeficiency virus (HIV). There will be no such risk in the new genetically engineered vaccine.

Recently, when a vaccine of bacterial meningitis was found to be only partially effective for babies under two, it was reengineered and an improved vaccine was produced.

Yet all these new findings and techniques have not made vaccine production easier in some cases, e.g., the common cold has no vaccine, because more than a hundred known viruses cause common cold. So, it is not possible to have a vaccine for each virus. And the influenza virus can change its form in every season. Therefore, any vaccine can become useless in a year.

Even worst is the HIV virus which changes its form at least twice as fast as influenza virus. Besides AIDS itself is a disease of immune system. However, a vaccine was produced which prevented AIDS in monkey using inactivated monkey AIDS virus. This vaccine cannot protect human beings against AIDS, as this monkey AIDS virus shares only 40 per cent of the genetic make up with the human AIDS virus. Most experts believe that a human AIDS vaccine may take at least another five to ten years. Antiviral therapy against AIDS is under experimentation.

In Bombay (India), since 1950, work was carried out for a leprosy vaccine. In 1965, the researchers could grow in the laboratory artificial medium a bacterium seems similar to a close cousin of *Mycobacterium leprae*. They studied every characteristic of these new bacteria, treated them with radiation, experimented on animals injected into the first human subject in 1979. The first human subject had a single white patch on the skin. In a short time, the single white patch disappeared. Today, some 30,000 persons have been injected with this vaccine as a part of field trials in Maharashtra (India). None of these persons living in close contact with leprosy patients had any sign of leprosy infection. Yet this vaccine must wait more trials before it is sold.

During an epidemic of infectious diseases, a great significance is given to specific immunoprophylaxis and immune therapy. Prophylaxis (Greek, *pro*, before, *phylassein* to guard or protect), is generally thought of being used in advance to prevent disease or infection. *Vaccine* (Lat. *vacca*-cow) received its name from the anti-small pox preparation from the virus of cow pox. Vaccines are preparations consisting of attenuated or dead causative agents or products of their life activity, while the method of inoculation is known as *vaccination* or *immunisation*.

Vaccines are introduced parenterally or orally or intranasally within a definite period of time (from several days to several weeks). Vaccines give active immunity. Vaccines should be highly immunogenic (capable of causing sound and long immunity) and should not be toxigenic.

Modern vaccines which are under routine use :

1. Vaccines from live causative agents with a decreased (attenuated) virulence;
2. Vaccines from dead cultures of pathogenic microorganisms (bacteria, rickettsiae, viruses);
3. Vaccines from the products of chemical cleavage of some bacteria (chemical vaccines);
4. Antitoxin (detoxified toxin by formalin at a temperature of 38° to 40°C);
5. *Associated* vaccines (diphtheria, pertussis, whooping cough and tetanus — DPT) vaccine.

Serotherapy. Sera are employed for treatment and prophylaxis of tetanus, gas gangrene, botulism. The length of protective action of sera by serotherapy (passive immunity) is from eight to twenty days. *Gamma globulins* obtained by the method of fractionation of serum protein by means of alcoholic solution of at temperature lower than 0°C, are used for prophylactic purposes against measles, poliomyelitis, whooping cough, serum hepatitis, small pox and are completely harmless as they do not contain hepatitis B virus and causative agents of other diseases.

Immunisation is an answer to the life saving protection against childhood diseases.

Five gentle pricks for life saving protection against childhood diseases. An infant has to be immunised five times before he completes first year of life.

1. Soon after birth	One BCG injection against tuberculosis.
2. At the age of 1½ months	One DPT injection against Diphtheria, Pertussis, Tetanus and first dose of polio drops.
3. At the age of 2½ months	Second dose as above.
4. At the age of 3½ months	Third dose as above.
5. At the age of 9 months	One injection against measles.

THREE IN ONE (3 in 1)

For protection against three killer diseases (diphtheria, pertussis — whooping cough and tetanus), three vaccines are given together in a single injection called DPT. Dose of polio drops are also given alongwith DPT to avoid repeated visit. For the complete protection of the child, DPT injections should be given at the interval of 1½, 2½ and 3½ months.

To be borne in mind

(i) If, due to some reason, the child is not immunised in time, it is vital to have the child immunised at the earliest possible thereafter;

(ii) There should be at least a gap of one month between two doses of immunisation;

(iii) It is essential for the infants to complete full course of immunisation. If the prescribed repeat doses of immunisation are not taken, the child will not have full protection from killer diseases;

(iv) Vaccination against measles is recommended at nine months of age, because, for the first few months of the life, the child has natural protection against it inherited from the mother. After about 9 months the natural protection comes to an end and the child must be immunised against the risk of measles as soon as it attains the age of 9 months.

Is it safe to immunise a sick child. Yes, it is safe to immunise a child suffering from minor illness or malnutrition. All efforts should be made to get the child immunised even if he has mild fever, cough, cold, moderate diarrhea or some other mild illness on that day. No time should be lost in having him protected from the dangerous diseases before it is too late.

Protection of women against tetanus.

(a) In many parts of our country, mothers give birth in unhygienic conditions. Hence, the mother and newborn are at risk of tetanus;

(b) Tetanus bacilli grow in dirty wounds made by an unclean knife used to cut the umbilical cord during delivery. The knife to be used should be first cleaned, boiled or heated in flame and allowed to cool before use;

(c) If the mother is not protected against the tetanus, the exotoxin liberated by tetanus bacilli in the infected wound may be absorbed in to the mother's body and endangers the life of both mother and child;

(d) Tetanus toxoid (TT) injections at one month's interval are necessary as soon as the mother becomes pregnant. If she is already immunised, then one injection is enough;

(e) As a rule, every woman between the age of 15 and 44 years should be fully immunised against tetanus. Every woman who becomes pregnant should make sure that she is immunised. All infants should be immunised against tetanus during the first year of life.

Where to get the immunisation services. Immunisation services can be obtained free of cost from all health, family welfare, primary health centre and public hospitals throughout the country.

Adverse effects of vaccines. Vaccines for immunisation have no side effects. A child may cry after an injection, develop slight fever, rash or small sore. As with other illness the child may be given plenty of fluid and food and it may be alright soon. If the problem is serious and the child has vomiting, diarrhea, high fever, a pediatrician may be consulted.

Breast feeding is important. Breast feeding is a kind of natural immunisation against several diseases. Mother's resistance to disease is transferred to the child through her milk, i.e., the thick yellow milk (colostrum) which is rich source of antibodies and is produced in the breast during the first few days after birth.

1. *Immunisation* protects the pregnant woman against tetanus and the children against several dangerous childhood diseases, i.e., three killer diseases (diphtheria, pertussis, tetanus (DPT)), tuberculosis and measles;

2. Immunisation is provided through vaccines which are given orally or parenterally;

3. The child's body defence mechanism against diseases is built up by vaccination. If the disease strikes before the child is immunised, then the immunisation is too late;

4. Children who survive the diseases are weakened and may die later from nutritional deficiency and other illness. The diseases may hamper the child's growth and development.

Why Immunisation is of Great Necessity

If the child is not immunised

(a) He is more likely to become undernourished, disabled or to die;

(b) The child is likely to get measles and whooping cough. These diseases can kill the child. Measles is also an important cause of mental retardation and blindness;

(c) The child can be infected with polio virus which can cripple him for life;

(d) The child is exposed to the danger of tetanus which kills most of the people who become infected.

It is the right of every parent to ask for immunisation for the protection of their children.

Immunisation when

- Protection of the child has to begin right after a woman becomes pregnant. This is done by injection of TT to the mother at one month interval at the earliest possible after conception.
- Immunisation is urgent. It is very important to immunise a child early in life.
- All immunisations should be completed within the first year of a child life.
- Half of all deaths from whooping cough, one-third of all cases of polio and one-fourth of all deaths from measles occur before the age of one year.

Adverse reactions following vaccines

Some instructions to field workers

The reactions that follow vaccination are generally mild and of a short duration. Serious reactions are known to occur but they are extremely rare and form a small fraction of similar type of complications that occur as a result of disease itself. Neurological syndromes can also occur spontaneously in infant and vaccination may only be coincidentally related.

The common reactions are mild fever, redness, tenderness and pain at the site of injection. Fever and rash on the sixth or seventh day after measles vaccination have also been reported.

The number of severe reactions and deaths following vaccination are rare.

Measures to minimise risks

The following measures are to be followed to minimise risks of adverse events following vaccination :

1. Vaccination sessions should be held on fixed days. The children should be collected at the subcentre at a central point of a village. Door to door vaccination should not be practised as such a strategy carries a high risk of break in the cold chain and contamination of the syringes and needles.

2. Procedures for sterilisation of syringes and needles should be scrupulously followed and monitored whenever feasible, steam sterilisation should be preferred to boiling :

- Single sterile syringe and a single sterile needle are used for each injection.
- Issue of the vaccine to the field staff should be strictly monitored. Only required quantities of the vaccine should be taken from the primary health centre on the day of the session.
- Vaccines may be taken on the previous day only if these are carried in vaccine carrier with fully frozen icepacks.
- Supervision should include measures to ensure that vaccine vials are not stored in the periphery and reused subsequently. Batch number and expiry date should be recorded before issue.
- Vaccine should be discarded at the end of the session. Opened vials of vaccine should not be reused under any circumstances.
- Potentially harmful injectible drugs should be kept separate from vaccine vials and diluent.
- Field monitoring of the services must be regular so that any deficiencies could be noted and corrected in time. Reporting of abscesses by the health workers in their areas should be made compulsory.
- Measles vaccine should be reconstituted with the diluent provided with the vaccine. The diluent should be cooled before use. The vaccine should be kept on ice while in use. The children should be administrated 0.5 ml of the vaccine in the arm subcutaneously. A separate sterile syringe and needle should be used for each injection. (Extract from "National Immunisation Mission". — Ministry of Health and Family Welfare — 1989, New Delhi, India).

Remember.

- An unimmunised child is more likely to become disabled, undernourished and to die.
- Immunisation is no less important than the mother's love for a baby. It is urgent. It has to begin soon after birth and completed within the first year of a child life.
- The last dose of Tetanus toxoid (TT) injection during pregnancy for protection against tetanus must be had at least thirty days before the expected date of delivery and also for protecting the child to be born against neonatal tetanus.
- For protection against three killer diseases, three vaccines are given together in a single injection called DPT.

COLD CHAIN for vaccine

Vaccines are thermolabile products, hence they require special storage and transportation arrangements to retain their efficiency.

If vaccines are kept at the recommended minimum temperature, they will remain potent for a longer period of time. All vaccines retain their potency at temperature +2 to +8 degree C. The vaccines must be transported and stored at these temperatures at district and primary health centres.

For long term storage, measles and polio vaccines are kept at sub-zero temperature. If freezers are available these vaccines should be kept in a freezer. DPT, DT and TT vaccines should not be frozen. Vaccines should not be exposed to direct sunlight. The cold chain for vaccines consists of three vital elements — the cold storage equipment, transportation and motivated and trained manpower for operating the vital link.

The importance of people in the cold chain can not be overemphasised. Often the cold chain is thought to refer only to the refrigeration of the vaccine. Even if the finest and most modern equipment and transportation are available the cold chain will not be effective, if the people do not handle the vaccine properly. Several steps have been taken over the last few years to strengthen the cold chain for vaccines.

The activities have been directed both at improving the storage and transportation facilities as well as in training manpower in logistics of vaccines and handling of the refrigeration.

(Excerpts from the publication "National Immunisation Programme" published by National Institute of Health and Family Welfare, New Delhi, India).

DISEASES

Tetanus

Symptoms:

- For the first two days of life, the new born does normal suckling but keeps crying;
- The infant is unable to suckle between 3rd and 21st day;
- The child cannot open the mouth fully;
- Facial, neck and trunk muscles of the child get stiff and the child gets convulsions;
- His body bends like a bow due to the contraction of neck and trunk muscles.

Danger:

The survival rate is very low.

Diphtheria

Symptoms:

- Sore throat with or without difficulties in swallowing;
- Mild fever, no appetite;
- The child looks ill;
- Neck is swollen;
- Whitish membrane in the throat;
- The child has difficulty in breathing due to obstruction in airways.

Danger:

- The toxin can affect the heart muscle and nerves;
- Diphtheria has high rate of fatality;
- It is highly infectious, painful and dangerous for the children.

Pertussis (Whooping cough)

Symptoms:

- To begin with, the child has slight fever, running nose, cold and cough;
- Gradually, cough gets worse, child gets fits of cough and struggles for breath;
- Breath is in noisy whoop;
- Spasms are common during cough, the eyes bulge and bleed;
- The child often vomits after or during cough.

Poliomyelitis

Symptoms:

- The child has fever and headache;
- Feels sudden onset of weakness and paralysis generally of one leg or arm or trunk;
- Muscle pain with touch sense remaining normal;
- Wasting of the affected muscles later.

Danger:

- Paralysis of one of the limbs leading to lameness;
- May even lead to paralysis of muscles of respiration.

Measles

Symptoms:

- The disease starts with fever, running nose and cough;
- The child's eyes become red and watery;
- Rash appears on the face between the third and seventh day.

It appears over the whole body.

Danger:

- The child gets weak, becomes prone to secondary infections of lungs, ears, eyes and gastrointestinal tract. It can be fatal due to complications like pneumonia.

Tuberculosis (Childhood)

Symptoms:

— Low grade fever;

— Swelling of lymph glands;

— Loss of weight; cough and weakness, high fever;

— Severe headache, stiffness of the neck and convulsion in the case of tuberculosis meningitis;

— The child becomes hunch-backed;

Danger:

— If not cared, the disease becomes fatal.

Recommended age for BCC vaccination against tuberculosis is just after birth; only one dose is given.

Schedule of Immunisation

For Whom/When	*What*	*Why*
To pregnant woman at the earliest possible after conception.	Two injections of Tetanus toxoid (TT) at an interval of one month. If already vaccinated, only one injection of TT in pregnancy.	Protects the mother and newborn from the tetanus.
To the infant after birth.	One injection of BCG.	Protects the infant from tuberculosis.
When the child is 1½ months old	One injection of DPT and first dose of polio-drops.	Protects the child from diphtheria, pertussis, tetanus and polio.
When the child is 2½ months old	Second dose as above.	—
When the child is 3½ months old	Third dose as above.	—
When the child is 9 months old	One injection of measles.	Protects the child from measles.
When the child is 1½ years	One booster dose of polio drops, and DPT injection.	Protects the child from diphtheria, pertussis, tetanus and poliomyelitis.

— At the age of five years, an injection of DT and one injection of TT at the age of ten and again at sixteen years particularly in the case of girls;

— Interval between two doses of vaccination should not be less than one month;

— Vaccination for immunisation can be got done without hesitation even in the case of minor cough, fever, diarrhea, in consultation with a physician or health worker;

— For the health of the child, it is essential to have the child vaccinated at the right time;

— Polio drops are given orally when the child is brought for DPT. These drops are to be given when the child is 1½, 2½ and 3½ months of age;

— BCG injection is given for protection against tuberculosis to the infant at birth, only one injection is enough.

So little care, so bIgA Protection

(From Centre Calling, November 1989, Vol. XXIV, New Delhi, India).

Application to Nursing

The knowledge of immunology is extremely essential for the professional nurse in her day-to-day practice and is of great importance, particularly, for public health nurse. Public health nursing can be very effective, if the nurse could teach about the basic facts of immunology — why the administration of specific antigens are important to the health of the children and how the epidemics are controlled and how the susceptible individuals can be protected against the dreadful diseases. One of the frequent responsibility of the nurse is the administration of antigens and antibodies (immune sera). While shouldering this responsibility she should be able to understand intelligently what are to be administrated with precaution, their adverse reactions and the expected results of the immunisation.

In conducting the field trial programme of a newly developed vaccine, the nurse is one of the important members of the team to find out the efficacy of the administration of the antigens. Besides this, the nurse has a great role to collect data and to convince the people to participate in the full programme by explaining them in explicit clear local language. Because of her sound knowledge of immunology and immunisation schedule, she will be able to communicate the parents the importance and necessity of repeated childhood vaccination at fixed time interval and about the blood collection for the evaluation of antibody titres in the blood after vaccination.

In public health nursing, since the nurse is always in touch with the public, she will be the first person to recognise the necessity of active and passive immunisation in an individual, family, community, for this important and quick decision, she should be well equipped with the essential knowledge of immunity and she can transmit this information to the higher authority who will be responsible for the immunisation of the public living in that situation.

The nurse is always on the *frontline* and comes in close contact with the patients because of the nature of her work; and she is always at the risk of getting infected with the communicable diseases during epidemics. Therefore, she should maintain the highest degree of protection against all these diseases for her own good health and life by regular immunisation.

SECTION 5

CHAPTER 23

NON-PATHOGENIC (USEFUL) MICROORGANISMS

Microorganisms may be divided into two groups according to their activities : (a) the useful and (b) the harmful.

The first group — the harmless, non-pathogenic microorganisms to man live mostly in the environment. They are called as *saprophytic* or *autotrophic* (yeasts, moulds and bacteria) and are very useful to the industries for the manufacturing of alcohol, lactic acid, butter, cheese, solvents of paints and antibiotics etc. and to the agriculture to improve the soil fertility.

The second group — the harmful, may be called *pathogenic* microorganisms — damages the host and produces diseases in man, animals and plants. Out of 1,700 groups of bacteria, about 70 groups are pathogenic to man and can live only in human body, but they may die in external, unfavourable conditions.

The activities of useful microorganisms.

Decay, putrefaction and fermentation.

Decay is the term used generally to denote the gradual decomposition of organic matter (dead animals, plants and their wastes) on or in the soil.

Putrefaction is the decomposition of proteins(animal matter) under anaerobic conditions and of carbohydrates (vegetable derivatives starch or sugar). These two processes transform organic matter into useful plant foods. When dead animals and plants are buried in the ground, the soil microflora and the intestinal microflora of dead animal enter into the tissue of the animal or plant. Because of their lipolytic, proteolytic and saccharolytic activities, the microbes break fat, proteins and sugars, respectively. The gases (carbon dioxide and hydrogen sulfate etc.) liberated and water formed enter the air or soil. Besides, nitrogen, phosphorus, sulphur, produced from dead animal body combine with water and become soluble and suitable as food for plants. Ultimately, the dead animal disappears. Later, the living animals and men use the plants as food. In this way, the recycle of the elements is continued. Thus, the life would be impossible on earth without microbial activity and the microbes are useful or essential for animal or human life. The colibacillus and other species of microbes in the healthy human intestine produce vitamins (B_1, B_2, B_{12}, K) essential for the human body. Acidophilic microbes are beneficial to the human body as they interfere with the development of pathogenic bacteria which enter into the intestine alongwith food or drink.

It is well known that human beings cannot digest directly the cellulose of the plants and utilise it for their nutrition; but the rumen (stomach) microflora of ruminants (cattle, sheep, goats)can only digest it anaerobically and convert into easily digestible end products like glucose, amino acids, volatile fatty acids, which are excreted through milk or incorporated in animal tissue or muscle. Man drinks milk containing proteins, fatty acids and lactose which are derived from the cellulose of plant or green fodders digested by the rumen microflora as the rumen of cattle is devoid of digestive enzymes. So the rumen microflora are quite useful for human welfare without which milk or meat cannot be obtained from the animal for the human consumption.

Microorganisms in Food

Moist less acidic foods (milk, cooked cereals, custard, soup) are suitable media for the growth of saprophytic and pathogenic microorganisms at warm room temperature and thus we consume large number of saprophytic microorganisms along with the foods every day with no harmful effects. The growth of certain microbes in some kinds of foods is useful. Certain harmless streptococci added to cheese and butter may produce good flavours in them. Therefore, "starters" (materials containing the desired bacteria) are added to the cream before it is churned into butter and they are also added to milk that is used for making the cheese. Flavour producing bacteria (Lactobacillus) can ferment pickles.

Putrefaction is the anaerobic digestion and decomposition of proteins (muscle, egg white, fish) by microorganisms. It is usually accompanied by bad odour due to formation of ammonia, hydrogen sulfate and other volatile odouriferous substances. Mostly, putrified materials are not agreeable, but we consume the putrified milk in the form of cheese and they are dangerous if contaminated. If foods are contaminated with excessive growth of saprophytic microbes, they are *spoiled* foods. This process is known as *spoilage*.

Fermentation. Under anaerobic conditions, the microorganisms (bacteria, yeasts, moulds) decompose, by their saccharolytic activities, the carbohydrates (sugars) into different kinds of acids, such as lactic acid, alcohol, and gases like carbon dioxide. One of the most familiar type of fermentation is the production of alcohol by yeast from the sugar of fruit juices as in wine manufacture. Certain streptococci (*Streptococcus lactis*) ferment sugar of milk (lactose) into lactic acid which causes souring of milk. This harmless streptococcus alongwith other saprophytic bacteria enters into the milk from the dust, splits the milk if it is not refrigerated. The yeasts multiply in the dough and decompose the starch (sugar of the flour) and form alcohol and carbon dioxide. The gas bubbles entangled in the dough raise (leaven) the bread. The bread dries and becomes firm due to the evaporation of alcohol during baking.

The *decomposition* of fat by microorganisms is known as *hydrolysis*. When fats containing butyric and similar volatile fatty acids are decomposed, these acids are liberated and are responsible for the odour and rancidity taste.

Pathogenic (harmful) bacteria may contaminate the foods or milk products, grow and liberate toxin (preformed toxin of *Staphylococcus* aureus and *Clostridium* botulinum) causing food poisoning. *Salmonella typhimurium* (pathogenic to mice), when consumed alongwith the food, may also cause food poisoning in man in whom the illness takes the form of gastroenteritis.

The food should be thoroughly cooked, *kept closed in a* vessel or should not be allowed to stand unrefrigerated and should not remain moist, as the moist food is a suitable medium for the growth of bacteria.

Application to Nursing

Nurse must understand that the food should be protected from the microbes and should serve her patients and her own family with clean food.

Microorganisms of Water

In ancient times and even now, in some back ward community, the people throw the wastes of household out of window in the streets. These wastes and faeces may contaminate the community water supplies and thereby there will be great epidemics due to pathogens of intestinal tract: typhoid, cholera, gastroenteritis, hepatitis etc. Modern microbiology utilises concept of purifying sewage by the activities of certain saprophytic soil and water microbes and is of great importance to the community health in supplying purified water. The microorganisms utilise the organic substances of the sewage as food and turn them into harmless, inoffensive materials which are used as food by plants.

Municipal sewage. Method used for purifying municipal sewage is first straining out extraneous objects by passing the 'raw' (untreated) sewage through metal screens or racks, then allowing it to flow very slowly through large tanks. In such tanks, the solid matter in suspension settles to the bottom. This solid material is slowly decomposed through the hydrolytic action of microbial enzymes of *anaerobic and facultative anaerobic* bacteria. It eventually forms sludge (sort of mud) rich in plant food, which is pumped out, dried and used as fertiliser in garden. This sludge is sterilised before packaging.

The fluid part of sewage is sprayed on the surface of large beds (trickling filters) of coarse gravel. During this process, it becomes fully aerated. On the surface of gravel or sand a slimy film develops. This film consists of the growth of aerobic microorganisms, which get their nourishment by decomposing and oxidising offensive materials in the sewage as the sewage trickles slowly through the gravel. Solid matter (humus) is collected in the final tank and pumped onto the open sludge drying beds. The deodorised, cleaned fluid is collected in drains under the gravel and run out in fields for irrigation.

Activated sludge. In modern activated sludge process, aeration of the sludge is accomplished by violently agitating the sewage with large volumes of the solid matter which is torn into small granules or particles. These particles contain millions of active aerobic microorganisms which use the air to oxidise and decompose rapidly the offensive matter in the sludge. *Aeration* is the key objective in any form of sewage disposal.

Drinking Water

The waters of rivers, lakes, springs and oceans contain many saprophytic microorganisms; and these saprophytes are often present in drinking water and are harmless, since they cannot invade the human body. Man consumes large number of these saprophytes with food, water and milk every day. They are harmless. However, water polluted with sewage usually contains pathogenic microbes (typhoid or dysentery bacilli, cholera vibrios, polio, hepatitis virus, amebae etc.). The only safe way is to boil all water or treat it with chlorine a few hours before use. Tablets of hypochlorite or other chlorine compounds are available for this purpose. The nurse who is faced with the problem of disinfection of water at home can very well remember this method.

Microorganisms of Air

Under ordinary conditions, the spores of numerous microorganisms may be found in air all around us. Many of these are spores of moulds, yeasts, useful conidia of streptomyces and spores of bacteria of the genera clostridium and bacillus. Spores and conidia are excellently adapted to survive floating about on dust in the air for weeks or years. All these spores are harmless except those of Clostridium and bacillus which are pathogenic to man. The number of microorganisms in the air usually depends on the amount of dust since most of the microorganisms are riding around on dust particles. They are usually of the harmless types found in soil and soon die in the dry air and sunlight. However, the air of badly ventilated dark room may contain many pathogenic organisms which are disseminated by the occupants who are carriers of such microbes in the nose and mouth.

In recent years much attention has been paid to the air as a means of disease transmission — especially in hospitals. It is known that every drop of saliva and nasal exudate, even from healthy persons (nurses and doctors) contain microorganisms capable of causing diseases. Among these, are staphylococci, pneumococci, streptococci of scarlet fever, pueperal sepsis, and septic sore throat, diphtheria bacilli, tubercle bacilli and numerous viruses (polio, influenza, adenovirus etc.)

Droplet infection. The air of class-room, theaters and street cars are loaded with microorganisms especially in winter; sneezing and coughing sprays of saliva and mucus are added to the general population of the atmosphere laden by bacteria and viruses. Transmission of diseases by droplets of saliva and mucus is often called droplet infection. These sprays infect the dust and, when dry, this dust carries the bacteria.

Droplet nuclei. The droplets of saliva and dry mucus and the bacteria contaminated in the dried particles float in the air and are inhaled like dust. Such dried particles are spoken as "droplet nuclei". These land on the floor, furnitures, lips, hands, surgical wounds.

Application to Nursing

Knowledge of microorganisms in the air will be useful to take precautionary measures, to protect herself and her patients from the microorganisms which sometimes may be pathogenic to man.

Industrial Microorganisms

It is well established that the microorganisms produce alcohol, lactic and acetic acids during fermentation of carbohydrates; besides these products many other substances of equal importance are also formed. So, the microorganisms are widely used in industry.

The skill and knowledge of microbiologist, engineer and chemist are pooled together in the industrial fermentation to produce the large quantity of butyl alcohol, glycerin, antibiotics, vitamins and other substances of great importance depending upon the species of microorganisms. In the manufacture of rubber, coffee, cocoa, tobacco, linen, spices, leather, pickles, drug and other products, the fermentative, putrefactive, synthetic and other enzymatic powers of microorganisms are utilised. Thus, it can be concluded that the microorganisms have entered in the business and became very useful to mankind.

Nitrogen Fixing Microorganism and Life

Nitrogen is the component of the cytoplasm of the cell and is essential for the life. Though eighty per cent of the atmosphere contain nitrogen, the atmospheric nitrogen cannot be directly utilised by the living cell. But this nitrogen can be utilised from the atmosphere by the microorganisms by combining it with other elements, mainly oxygen, hydrogen and carbon of the atmosphere. The process of combining nitrogen of the atmosphere with other elements is called nitrogen fixation.

The nitrogen of air can be fixed by certain soil microorganisms by two methods : non-symbiotic and symbiotic (living together for mutual benefit) nitrogen fixation.

Non-symbiotic nitrogen fixation. The direct combination of atmospheric nitrogen as part of the protoplasm of a living cell without the cooperation of any other organisms, e.g., atmospheric nitrogen can be built up directly into the protoplasm by the bacteria of the genus Azobacter (*Azo* = nitrogen), the genus *Clostridium* and other microorganisms. These useful microorganisms are plenty in all the fertile soils. Therefore, a farmer permits the Azobaceter, Clostridium and other microorganisms to accumulate nitrogen from the air by allowing a field to lie fallow or unplanted. Nitrogen of the commercial fertilisers are very costly.

Symbiotic nitrogen fixation. The nodules on the roots of leguminous plants (i.e., clover, beans, peas, alfalfa) contain bacteria belonging to the genus Rhizobium. While growing together with the plants, this genus Rhizobium collects nitrogen from the air and combines it into substances essential for the growth of both the bacteria and the plants. The process is known as symbiotic nitrogen fixation method.

Nitrification. Nitrogenous compounds released into the soil by leguminous plants may be taken up by other plants and partly decomposed by putrefaction yielding ammonia (NH_3).

As ammonia, nitrogen is generally useless to most green plants. Ammonia is also produced in small amounts by lightning flashes and is also washed into the soil by the rain. To be most readily available to plants, the nitrogen of ammonia must first be oxidised to nitric acid (HNO_3). This important function is carried out by the soil bacteria of the family Nitrobacteriacae. The nitric acid they form immediately combines with various substances to form nitrates. The process of changing nitrous acid into nitric acid is called *nitrification*. These nitrifying bacteria and nitrogen fixing bacteria are of great importance to agriculture. The nitrogen of the air is useless to many microorganisms. At a depth of four feet (1.2 m), bacteria become less numerous and at 10 to 12 feet (3-3.7 m), there are usually no bacteria.

Microorganisms in and on human beings. The healthy human body harbours millions of microorganisms on the skin, in the mouth, eyes, genitourinary tract and in the intestine and on every surface of the body which comes in contact with the outside of the world (air, food). Under normal conditions, most of the microorganisms do not produce the diseases, but under certain conditions (e.g., in wound or after surgery) gain entrance to the deeper parts of the body and produce the diseases.

The skin carries large number of bacteria. *Staphylococcus aureus* found in the hair follicles and sebaceous ducts causes the boils, carbuncles, breast abscess, infantile impetigo. The organisms lodged in the deeper layer of the skin cannot be removed by thoroughly scrubbing and then by the application of antiseptics, therefore sterile gloves are worn during operation.

Table 23.1 : Microorganisms Found on and in the Human Body

Skin	**Intestine**
Staphylococcus aureus	*Escherichia coli*, coliform
Staphylococcus albus	bacilli
Corynebacterium acnes	Shigella
	Salmonella
Axilla	*Clostridum tetani*
Mycobacterium smegmatis	*Clostridum welchii*
Mycobacterium phlei	*Streptococcus faecalis*
Staphylococcus albus	Klebsiella
	Pseudomonas
	Proteus
Scalps	*Lactobacillus bifidus*
Staphylococcus albus	Poliovirus
Corynebacterium acnes	**Perianal area**
	Mycobacterium smegmatis
Ears	*Escherichia coli* and coliform
Mycobacterium phlei	bacilli
Staphylococcus albus	Enterococci
Corynebacterium Sp.	*Clostridium* Sp.
	Staphylococcus epidermis
Conjunctiva	**Genitalia**
Corynebacterium xerosis	Mycobacterium smegmatis
Staphylococcus albus	Lactobacillus acidophilus
Haemophilus Sp.	(Vagina)
Nose, Mouth and Pharynx	*Trichomonas vaginalis*
Streptococcus pyogenes	*Corynebacterium Sp.*
Streptococcus salivarius	**Hands**
Streptococcus faecalis	Variable
Diphtheroids	(commonly microorganisms
Corynebacterium diphtheriae	of skin, respiratory tract,
Corynebacterium xerosis	faeces, and perianal region)
Neisseria meningitidis.	
Haemophilus influenzae	
Borrelia vincenti	
Fusobacterium fusiforme	
Trichomonas tenax	

NOTES

SECTION 6

CHAPTER 24

PATHOGENIC MICROORGANISMS

Unit A : Pathogens transmitted from the Respiratory tract.

Unit B : Pathogens transmitted from the Intestinal and/or Urinary tract.

Unit C : Pathogens transmitted from the Genital tract.

Unit D : Pathogens transmitted in the blood.

Unit E : Pathogens from the Soil.

Unit A : Pathogens Transmitted from the Respiratory Tract

(A) *Cocci*

(a) Staphylococci;

(b) Streptococci;

(c) *Pneumococcus* (*Diplococcus pneumoniae*);

(d) *Neisseria meningitidis*.

(B) *Bacilli*

(a) *Corynebacterium diphtheriae*;

(b) *Mycobacterium tuberculosis* and *Myco leprae*;

(c) *Haemophilus influenzae*;

(d) *Moraxella lacunata*;

(e) *Bordetella pertussis*.

(C) *Spirochaete*

(a) *Borrelia vincenti*.

(D) *Virus*

(a) Small pox virus;

(b) Measles;

(c) German Measles;

(d) Chicken pox;

(e) Herpes Zoster;

(f) Common cold virus;

(g) Influenza;

(h) Psittacosis virus;

(i) Mumps;

(j) Poliomyelitis virus;

(k) Rabies virus.

Unit B : Pathogens Transmitted from the Intestinal Tract/or Urinary Tract

(A) *Bacteria*

(a) Food borne microorganisms (Food infection and food poisoning);

(b) Salmonella;

(c) Shigella;

(d) *Escherichia coli*;

(e) *Vibrio cholerae;*

(f) Clostridium.

(B) *Enteric Virus*

(a) Poliomyelitis;

(b) Coxsachie virus;

(c) ECHO virus;

(d) Hepatitis virus;

(e) Bacteriophage.

(C) *Parasites*

(i) *Protozoa*

(a) *Entameba histolytica;*

(b) *Giardia lamblia;*

(c) *Trichomonas hominis.*

(ii) *Helminths*

(a) Cestodes;

(b) Trematodes;

(c) Nematodes.

Unit C : Pathogens Transmitted from Genital Tract

(a) *Treponema pallidum;*

(b) Gonococci;

(c) Lymphogranuloma venereum;

(d) *Trichomonas vaginalis.*

Unit D : Pathogens Transmitted in the Blood

(a) Secondary and accidental infections;

(b) Arthropod-borne bacterial infections;

(c) Arthropod-borne rickettsial and viral infections;

(d) Arthropod-borne protozoal and helminthic diseases.

Unit E : Pathogens from the Soil

(a) Bacterial pathogens of the soil :

(i) *Clostridium welchii;*

(ii) *Clostridium tetani;*

(iii) *Bacillus anthracis;*

(iv) Fungi.

Bacteria of medical importance have already been classified earlier according to their shape into three main groups : Cocci (spheres); bacilli (rods); spirochaetes (curved or spiral).

Transmission of Respiratory Tract Infection

Oral and nasal secretions contaminate the atmosphere with pathogenic microorganisms during talking, laughing, sneezing, coughing or by droplet nuclei. Similarly, eating utensils, drinking glasses are contaminated with the ubiquitous pathogens. Thus, we constantly encounter the atmosphere laden with formidable infectious agents. It is very difficult to reduce the atmospheric microbial content as it is in constant continuous process. The health is in constant threat because of the atmospheric pollution.

Control of respiratory infections. The nurse plays a vital role in controlling the spread of respiratory pathogens by her "check posts" in the path of respiratory pathogens.

The following are the effective check posts :

(a) thorough washing of hands known to be soiled with respiratory tract discharges;

(b) adequate sanitisation of dishes and eating utensils;

(c) disinfectant laundering of bedding of patient with any infectious disease (i.e., hot water or soaking in disinfectant, hot ironing);

(d) disinfection of blankets, mattresses by autoclaving or sporicidal vapour or gas;

(e) use of clean handkerchief or tissue paper for sneezing and coughing;

(f) use of proper sputum containers for tuberculosis patients;

(g) use of masks; dust control, ventilation and disinfection.

Masks. They should be thick and cover the nose and mouth completely. They must not be reversed and *never reused after dangling around the neck.* After use, they can be discarded in a closed containers. Routinely, reusable masks can be disinfected in hot (80°C) water and soap. Some modern masks are also available.

Dust control. The disease transmitted by air is mostly by dust and droplet nuclei. The transmission of disease by dust is controlled by treating all floors, window sills and bedding in hospital wards, where the dust accumulates with a film of oil. The dust sticks to the oil and can be easily removed without being disturbed.

The dust control can also be carried out very efficiently by modern vacuum cleaning systems. Devices that combine with wet scrubbing with vacuum systems are also an excellent means of dust control.

Ventilation is very effective method of removing air-borne pathogens.

Disinfection. Air and dust may be disinfected by irradiation with ultraviolet light, surface disinfection and microbial aerosols.

Pathogenic cocci of respiratory tract include staphylococci, streptococci, pneumococci, meningococci. They cause inflammatory process in human beings with the formation of pus. For this reason, they are known as suppurative pyogenic (pyogenic, *pyo* = pus) cocci. There are several types of symbiosis between cocci and the human body. Saprophytic and pathogenic types of staphylococci and streptococci live on the skin, mucous membrane and in respiratory tract. Meningococci may harbour for a long period in the nasopharynx. When body resistance is lowered or the skin and mucous membrane are injured, the bacteria penetrate the body tissue and cause infection. The various pathogenic cocci possess different organotropic affinity pneumococci in lungs; meningococci in meningitis, but staphylococci and streptococci have less affinity.

CHAPTER 25

STAPHYLOCOCCI

Skin and wound infections : Abscess : Osteomyelitis.

Staph. aureus. The most pathogenic staphylococcus has been described as the causative agent of suppurative process.

Morphology. Staphylococci are spherical in shape, 0.8 - 1μ in diameter and form irregular clusters resembling bunches of grapes (Latin, *staphyle*, grapes). Staphylococci are Gram positive organisms; they are non-motile, form no spore, no capsule (Fig. 25.1).

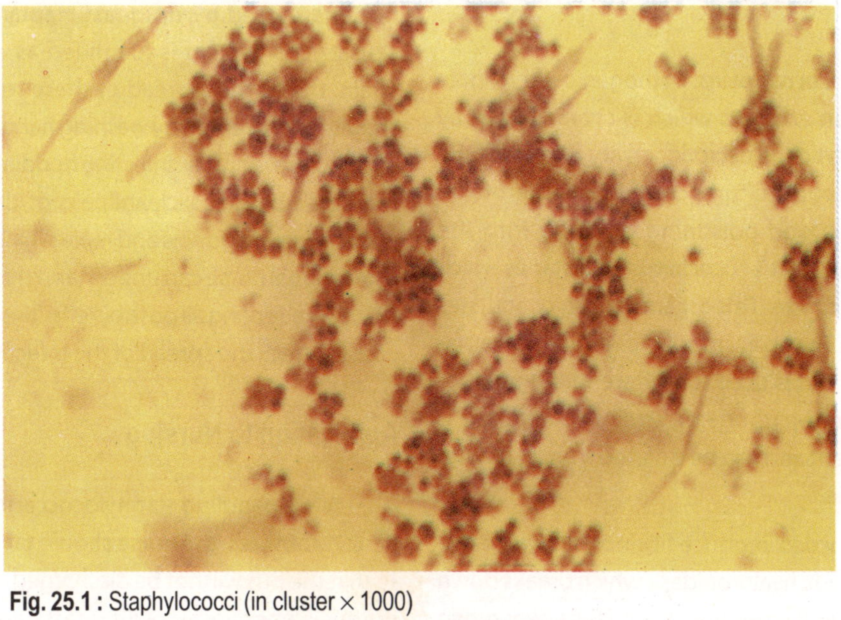

Fig. 25.1 : Staphylococci (in cluster × 1000)

Cultivation. Staphylococci are aerobes and grow well on nutrient agar media (Fig. 62.3) at 37°C and produce three types of pigments (lipochromes) : golden (Latin, *aurum*, gold); white (Latin, *albus*, white); lemon yellow (*citreus*). On the basis of pigment production they are classified into *Staph. aureus*, the most pathogenic; *Staph. albus* (less pathogenic); *Staph. citreus* (least pathogenic). They do not form spores, but they are somewhat resistant to drying; therefore they remain alive for several months under favourable condition in dust or outside the body. They are found in upper respiratory tract.

Resistance. Staphylococci are characterised by a relatively strong resistance to desiccation, freezing, sunlight and chemical substances. After desiccation, they can survive for more than six months. Repeated freezing and thawing do not kill the organisms. They survive for many hours under direct sunlight. They maintain their viability for more than one hour at 70°C. At a temperature of 80°C, they are destroyed within 10 to 60 minutes and at boiling point, they instantly perish. A 5 per cent phenol solution kills the organism in 15-30 minutes. Staphylococci are sensitive to aniline dye (brilliant green) which is used for the treatment of pyogenic skin diseases caused by this organism.

Staphylococcal toxins. Pathogenic staphylococci produce an exotoxin which is characterised by lethal, haemolytic and necrotic activity. Filtrates of staphylococcal broth cultures contain an enterotoxin which causes food poisoning on entry into the gastrointestinal tract. Leucocidin is a substance which destroys leucocytes. This organism also coagulates blood plasma. The ability to coagulate plasma is a stable property and is used for differentiating pathogenic from non-pathogenic strains. Coagulase is thermoresistant and can be isolated from staphylococcal cultures.

Staphylococci produce fibrinolysin which dissolves blood clot; hyaluronidase which breaks down hyaluronic acid (cementing material between two body cells; lecithinase destroys the lecithin; a substance found in the protective membrane of human or sheep erythrocytes. Pathogenic strains isolated from humans produce alpha haemolysin; those pathogenic to cattle produce beta-haemolysin.

Penicillinase or β-lactamase. As a result of genetic mutation, staphylococci acquire the power to produce penicillinase which destroys penicillin, i.e., it is resistant to penicillin.

Adaptive or induced enzyme. Sometimes, staphylococci produce penicillinase by their direct contact with penicillin, not by genetic mutation. Hence, the treatment with penicillin may induce the production of penicillinase. This enzyme produced in response to direct contact of staphylococci with penicillin is known as induced or adaptive enzyme.

Drug-fast Staphylococci and the nurse. Patient visitors, personnels may be carriers of *Staph. aureus* and become sources of the infection. If they carry drug-resistant staphylococci, they will become a dangerous source for the spread of the infection which cannot be controlled by antibiotics. Therefore, the nurse is deeply concerned with this problem as she is in constant contact with patients suffering from infections caused by drug-fast staphylococci. If the causative organism is identified as drug-resistant strain, the further spread of these resistant strains should be prevented by washing hands, disposing of infected dressings, disinfecting bedding, dishes, thermometer, bedpans, cleanliness of the rooms and wards, wearing gowns and masks. Only well trained, professional nurse can understand this problem and tackle by adopting all possible effective control measures to check the spread of the infections.

Application to Nursing

While handling staphylococcal infections, particularly abscess, the nurse should take special care, so that the pus will not be discharged on anything as the pus is an explosive of drug-fast staphylococci and other pathogenic organisms. Dressings of boils and other lesions should be discarded in a disinfectant jar or in a boiling water or tightly wrapped in several thickness of newspaper and fastened securely to prevent the escape of the infected dressings and burnt *completely* in an incinerator. In the hospital, the nurse should pay much attention so that the pathogenic organisms are not disseminated from the bedding soiled with the nasal secretions into the environment and do not contaminate the fomites around the patients.

Pathogenesis and diseases in man, Staphylococci enter the body through the skin or mucous membrane where they overcome the lymphatic barriers and penetrate the blood; staphylococcal septicemia sets in. Both exotoxins and the bacterial cells play an important role in the pathogenesis of diseases caused by staphylococci. So staphylococcal diseases can be considered as toxinfection. Coagulase positive strains of *Staph.aureus* produce six soluble toxins (A-F).

Pathogenic staphylococci are responsible for a number of local lesions in man : abscesses, furuncles, periostitis, osteomyelitis, folliculitis, sycosis, dermatitis, eczema, chronic pyoderma, peritonitis, meningitis, appendicitis and cholecystitis.

Predisposing factors for the formation of pyogenic lesions of the skin and furunculosis are : diabetes mellitus, avitaminosis, excess perspiration, minor skin abrasions and skin irritation caused by chemical substances.

Staphylococcal sepsis and pneumonia in children are particularly severe diseases. Staphylococci play an essential part in mixed infections and are found together with streptococci in case of wound infection, diphtheria, tuberculosis, actinomycosis. Pleuropneumonia may lead to pulmonary abscess. It causes pharyngitis, tonsillitis, sinusitis.

Staphylococcal food poisoning. Ingestion of food stuffs (cheese, curds, milk, cake, pastry, ice-cream etc.) contaminated with *pre-formed toxin* "*enterotoxin* B" liberated by pathogenic staphylococci in these foods may ensue food poisoning. (Enterotoxin refers to an exotoxin that affects the intestinal (enteric) tract (Greek, *enteron* = intestine). The word enterotoxin should not be confused with endotoxin which means a toxin that remains inside the bacterial cell. (Greek, *endon* = inside of). The symptoms of food poisoning are nausea, vomiting, gastroenteritis (diarrhoea). Thorough cooking destroys the organism but not the enterotoxin, so the enterotoxin is resistant to heat.

Prophylaxis of Food Poisoning

1. Prompt refrigeration after cooking;
2. Discarding the stale or spoiled food.

Foods contaminated with staphylococci, i.e., any food that has been handled or exposed to people who are coughing, sneezing or talking may contain large amount of enterotoxin produced by staphylococci, if allowed to stand at kitchen temperature for more than three to five hours. Staphylococcal food poisoning is rarely fatal.

CHAPTER 26

STREPTOCOCCI

Sore throat; Scarlet fever, Impetigo, Bacterial endocarditis, Rheumatic fever, Acute glomerulonephritis.

Several species of Gram-positive cocci (i.e., pneumococci and streptococci found mostly in the throat and staphylococci predominantly found in the anterior nares) have their main habitat in the upper respiratory tract of man. Amongst these groups, there are commensals, pathogens and potential pathogens, but only the last ones affect tissues when the resistance is lowered causing bronchitis, after primary virus infection. The pathogenic haemolytic streptococci or Lancefield group A — *Streptococcus pyogenes* causes acutely inflamed throat (tonsillitis, pharyngitis, septic sore throat), scarlet fever, rheumatic fever, acute glomerulonephritis.

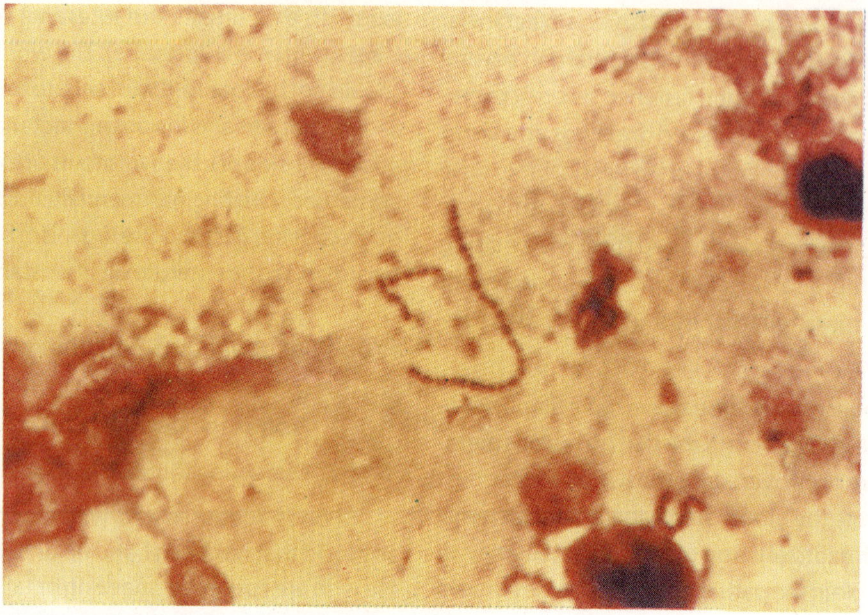

Fig. 26.1 : Streptococcus pyogenes (in chain × 1000)

Morphology. Streptococci are spherical in shape 0.6 to 1 micron in diameter, are Gram-positive and form chains Fig. 26.1. They are non-motile and do not form spores. Some strains are capsulated.

Cultivation. Streptococci are aerobic and facultatively aerobic; some are also anaerobic species and grow well on sugar, blood, serum or ascitic agar or broth. On solid media they produce small (0.5 - 1 mm in diameter) transparent, greyish white colonies. On blood agar media, *Strept. viridans* produce (partial or greenish) α-haemolysis as a result of conversion of haemoglobulin into methaemoglobulin; *Strept. faecalis* cause no haemolysis (i.e., y-haemolysis); *Strept.pyogenes* produce complete β-haemolysis. On sugar broth, growth is granular on the walls and at the bottom of the tube without turbidity.

Serological groups. The beta type haemolytic streptococci were classified by Lancefield (discoverer) into several Lancefield groups A to U except I, J on the basis of carbohydrate antigenic substance. The Group A streptococci are always pathogenic to man and cause serious, acute human disease (scarlet fever, erysipelas, septicaemia). These are called as *Strept. pyogenes. Serological typing of Group A, Streptococci.* Group A streptococci can be divided into some fifty or more types based on the presence of different protein (M antigen) which are differentiated by agglutination and precipitation.

Laboratory Serological Typing Report

Strept. pyogenes.

β - haemolysis on blood agar.

Lancefield Group A (by carbohydrate antigen substance). Serological typing A. 14 (M protein antigen substance).

The knowledge of serological typing of β-haemolytic streptococci is essential for professional nurse to understand the clinical discussion and laboratory report. If streptococci infect brain, respiratory tract, peritoneum or parturient uterus, the nursing procedures can be adopted accordingly.

***Strept. viridans* infection**

Tooth abscess. Streptococci of alpha type (*Strept. viridans*) are found in abscess in the roots of the teeth. The symptoms of these abscesses which are not definite may be found out by dentist X-rays plates; however, the organisms and their toxins may cause severe damage to the heart valve after setting up a focus of infection.

Heart valve injuries. Injured heart valves may be infected by *Strept. viridans* and ultimately these organisms may cause subacute bacterial endocarditis which is fatal. The exact mode of transmission of the organism is not yet well established, but it may, most probably, come via blood from infected teeth and tonsils, chronic sinus infection or from the intestine. The infection via blood is known as *haematogenous* or *endogenous.*

In endocarditis caused by streptococci, there is inflammation of heart valve which is followed by thickening and shrinkage of heart valves causing them to leak. Arthritis may ensue if the joints are infected.

Strept. pyogenes infection. *Strept. pyogenes* produce several exotoxins. Two distinct haemolysins can be recognised; O-streptolysin which is oxygen labile and S-streptolysin which is not oxygen sensitive. These two streptolysins are antigenically distinct and both are toxic to animals. O-streptolysin is found in rheumatic fever. Antibody to O-streptolysin is generally determined; in the patient blood by anti-streptolysin - O titire (ASO titre); whereas S-streptolysin is responsible for β-haemolysis in blood agar medium. Other toxins are leucocidin, fibrinolysin (streptokinase), hyaluronidase, erythrogenic toxin which produces erythema when injected intradermally and plays a role in scarlet faver.

Streptococci gain entrance through injured skin and mucous membrane or enter the intestine with the food. They may be spread by the air droplet route.

When the natural body resistance is lowered down, conditionally pathogenic streptococci normally present in the human body, may become pathogenic. Penetrating deep into the tissue they produce local pyogenic inflammation — streptoderma, abscess, lymphangitis, cystitis, pyelitis, cholecystitis and peritonitis. Erysipelas, inflammation of the superficial lymphatic vessels and tonsillitis (inflammation of the pharyngeal and tonsillar mucosa) are among the diseases caused by streptococci. Invading the blood, streptococci produce a serious septicaemia. They are more commonly the cause of puerperal septicaemia than other bacteria.

Streptococci may cause secondary infection in patients with diphtheria, small pox, whooping cough, measles and other diseases. Chronic tonsillitis is attributed to *Strept. viridans* and adenovirus. Contamination of wounds with streptococci result in wound suppurations, abscess formation and traumatic sepsis.

Cellulitis. Cellulitis is a most dangerous condition in which skin and underlying tissues are infected and it is caused by β-haemolytic streptococci : Group A streptococci (*Strepto pyogenes*) causes a very severe, rapidly spreading infection with much swelling followed by general symptoms due to potent exotoxin. The infection spreads in subcutaneous lymphatic tissue. Erysipelas is another form of acute infection of skin and underlying tissues due to β type streptococci Group A. It is rapidly progressive and frequently fatal.

Like staphylococci, beta type streptococci Group A sometimes invade the blood stream causing septicaemia and are often found in infections of lungs (pneumonia and empyema), meningitis, sinusitis and mastoiditis. Beta type streptococcal infections are controlled by broad spectrum antibiotics or penicillin or erythromycin.

Rheumatic heart disease. Rheumatic fever is very serious and widespread disease with resulting heart disease which often cripples, is frequently fatal and is caused by beta type streptococci Group A. The allergy to *Strept. pyogenes* is, most probably, the underlying cause. "Relapses in rheumatic fever can be treated with sulphonamides or antibiotics".

Puerperal Infection

Haemolytic streptococci gain access into the uterus : (a) from the skin or external parts of vulva that have not been properly cleansed; (b) from the unsterile dressings or instruments; (c) from the hands of the doctor or nurse that have not been sufficiently disinfected, especially if the doctor or nurse is a carrier of haemolytic streptococci, a common situation. The spread of puerperal fever or erysipelas infection can be prevented by the isolation of the infected patients. The discharges, packings, dressings are highly infectious, so they should be discarded into the strong disinfectants or completely burnt. Clean obstetric techniques and antibiotics could prevent post partum mortality due to streptococcal puerperal fever (child bed fever). A pregnant woman should prefer to go to hospital for delivery because of the aseptic technique available than at home. Thus, she can be protected from possible puerperal fever.

Since the open wound in the uterus, vagina and perineum of the recent post-partum patient is a very good portal of entry for streptococci, staphylococci and other microorganisms, the doctor, nurse and other personnels should not be allowed, until and unless they follow all aseptic techniques and observe strict sterility. If these staffs have sore noses or throats, they should be forbidden from entry into the delivery room. Besides, the staffs having infectious lesions on their body are very dangerous to other patients.

Bronchopneumonia. It may be caused by one or variety of organisms (staphylococci, alpha, beta type haemolytic streptococci). The causative agents of bronchopneumonia are usually found in the patient's own mouth or often gain access to the lungs by accidental inhalation of saliva and mucus or by inhalation of microorganisms found in the droplets of sputum of saliva sprayed out while talking, sneezing or coughing. It is evident that the patients likely to develop bronchopneumonia must be protected from both the bacteria in their own mouth and from vomitus. The greatest care to prevent carrying bacteria from patient to patient is to keep the mouth clean. The nursing care adopted for lobar pneumonia should be applied for bronchopneumonia. All persons (including medical and hospital personnel) with respiratory infections should be excluded.

Scarlet fever and Septic sore throat were formerly traceable to the consumption of unpasteurised milk from cows having mastitis due to Group A streptococci introduced by infected milkers. Pasteurisation destroys the streptococci. Septic sore throat and Scarlet fever are different manifestations of the same infection. *Strept. pyogenes* forms an *erythrogenic toxin* that produces rash on the skin which is a common manifestation in scarlet fever. This toxin can be detected by Dick test (Skin test). Dick test is a biological test which determines the immune status of an individual to erythrogenic toxin. A diagnostic skin test, Schultz-Charlton reaction is sometimes made by injecting into the rash of the skin a small dose of scarlet fever antitoxin. If the rash is due to scarlet fever, it promptly fades or is blanched; the blanching reaction.

Persons immunised to the toxin will not have the rash but may still contract the infection with Group A streptococci of other type. The infection may develop without rash and, therefore, it is called by another name—Septic sore throat.

Acute glomerulonephritis is associated with specific serotype or nephritogenic type of Group A streptococci.

Transmission. Scarlet fever transmission from person to person is an excellent model of most diseases of upper respiratory tract. In scarlet fever, saliva or mucus from mouth or nose may contain streptococci; as a result patient's hands and face may be contaminated with these streptococci; so kissing and contaminated handkerchiefs may transmit them and are very dangerous. Convalescents released from isolation may become carriers for a longer period, spread the disease through any discharge from the nose, ears or any other parts of the body and disseminate streptococci. During epidemics in school children, cases of scarlet fever and septic sore throat in amongst school children can easily be detected by the nurses and well informed intelligent school teachers and its further spread can be prevented.

Application to Nursing

It is well established that the discharges from the lesions with streptococci are very dangerous, as these discharges transmit streptococci to clean wounds, scratches, cuts, the post-partum mother, and possibly, to normal mucous membrane of the nose, throat and eyes. Since pathogens fresh from the body are *particularly virulent*, the professional nurse should take care so that dressings from all septic wounds including those infected with staphylococci should be properly wrapped, securely fastened and burnt. Instruments and objects contaminated by the infected wounds should be well disinfected by boiling or with chemicals.

The intelligent nurse must always take into consideration the portal of entry and portal of exit, particularly in streptococcal infections (erysipelas, septic sore throat, scarlet fever and puerperal fever), e.g., the exudate from the erysipelas lesions is very dangerous; the nose and throat secretions of a septic sore throat or scarlet fever patient are highly infectious through only portal of entry. Paper "wipes" or pieces of old linen or gauze can be used to collect all these secretions and ultimately discarded into a paper bag at the bedside. This paper bag should be discarded daily or frequently, according to necessity, after properly securing in a newspaper or it can be incinerated. Dishes and other objects that were in contact with mouth or nose should be adequately disinfected by boiling or with chemicals. Above all, the nurse is responsible for prevention of transfer of the infection to non-professional workers in hospitals (food handlers, dish washers, servants who dispose off trash and garbage).

CHAPTER 27

PNEUMOCOCCI (*Diplococcus pneumoniae*)

Pneumococci are primarily the causative agents of the infections of upper and lower respiratory tract, but are carried in the throat by many healthy persons. They are the commonest primary pathogens in lobar and bronchopneumonia and are frequently associated as secondary pathogens after primary virus infection of the respiratory tract. They are also associated with suppuration as empyema, meningitis, peritonitis and arthritis.

Morphology. Pneumococci are lanceolate cocci occurring in pairs. They are Gram-positive, non-motile and they have no spores. In the human body, they are encapsulated. The capsule can be demonstrated under microscope by India ink method or by capsular swelling reaction (Quellung reaction) by using specific antiserum to capsular polysaccharide. The capsule is responsible for (1) smoothness of colony; (2) antigenic type specificity; (3) virulence.

Cultivation. Pneumococci are aerobes, grow at 37°C, prefer 5 to 10 per cent CO_2 for primary culture. On a blood agar medium around the colony, there is a partial clearing of blood (alpha haemolysis) with greenish colouration like that of *Strept. viridans*. They are distinguished by being capsulated, bile soluble, sensitive to optochin, highly virulent and insulin fermentation.

Toxin production. Pneumococci do not produce exotoxin, but contain an endotoxin and liberate poorly a toxin which is characterised by its hemotoxic and fibrinolytic properties and by its ability to destroy leucocytes.

Serological typing of pneumococci. Pneumococci can be divided into 80 serologic types (Types, I, II, III etc.) on the basis of the type specific capsular polysaccharide Types I, II, III are virulent for human beings, while the rest possesses low virulence. The soluble specific substance or capsular polysaccharide is chemically different in each type.

Resistance. Pneumococci live in dried sputum for two months. They are destroyed at 50-60°C within 10 minutes and in 3 per cent phenol within 1-5 minutes, are sensitive to optochin and bile salts.

Pathogenesis and disease in man. Diplococcus pneumoniae causes *lobar pneumonia* (which derives its name from the fact that one or more entire lungs become infected).

Bronchopneumonia localises in scattered patches throughout the lungs and may be caused by variety of organisms. Sometimes, streptococci or *klebsiella pneumoniae* may cause lobar pneumonia. The pneumococci may invade pleural cavity causing empyema, the meninges, causing meningitis, the peritoneal cavity causing peritonitis. Because of the reduced body resistance (chilling, bronchitis, influenza, overstrain) the disease (lobar pneumonia) develops; use of antibiotics has considerably reduced death due to lobar pneumonia.

Transmission. Saliva or sputum of patients with lobar pneumonia and as well as normal persons may contain *D.* pneumoniae. The following are the main sources for the lobar pneumonia :

(a) the sputum and saliva of lobar pneumonia patients;
(b) convalescent carriers; and
(c) healthy carriers.

Another important vector is infected dust (droplet nuclei). Since pneumococci are quite resistant to drying, they are found in the dust of the houses in which lobar pneumonia cases have occurred. The same mode of transmission is observed in streptococcal, staphylococcal infection, diphtheria, tuberculosis.

Application to Nursing

The nursing care procedure of the patient with lobar pneumonia has been modified because of the widespread use of sulphonamides and antibiotics, ultimately the infectious stage of the disease has been considerably decreased.

The nurse should be very much careful to disinfect the dishes by boiling during infectious stage of the disease.

The linen should be boiled or adequately washed with hot water. Paper 'wipes' used for collection of respiratory secretions and disposable handkerchiefs should be burnt. The patient with lowered body resistance should be isolated from other patients to protect from the disease. In a ward, the nurse should develop barrier technique with adequate screening to protect other patients. She should also follow precautionary measures to prevent the transfer of the infection.

Since lobar pneumonia is frequently transmitted by droplet infection, the nurses and other medical staffs should wear mask for their protection.

CHAPTER 28

MENINGOCOCCI *(Neisseria meningitidis)*

Meningococcus was isolated from cerebrospinal fluid (CSF) of the patient with meningitis.

Morphology. Meningococcus is a coccus 0.6 - 1 μ in diameter resembling a coffee bean and is found in pairs. The organism is Gram-negative. As distinct from pneumococci, meningococci are joined longitudinally by the concave edges while the external sides are convex. Spores, capsules and flagella are not formed. In pure culture, meningococci occur in tetrads (in fours) and in pus they are usually found within and less frequently outside the leucocytes.

Cultivation. Meningococci are aerobes and do not grow on common media. They grow readily at pH 7.2 to 7.4 and at a temperature of 37°C in presence of 5-10 per cent CO_2 on chocolate agar medium and Thayer and Martin medium.

Fermentation properties. Meningococci cannot be differentiated from gonococci morphologically. They are distinguished by their ability to ferment maltose with acid production.

Oxidase reaction. Meningococci produce an enzyme *oxidase* which can be detected by adding fresh 1 per cent solution of an oxidase indicator, tetramethyl paraphenylene diamine. Over the surface growth of meningococci on the medium oxidase producing colonies turn purple in contact with this indicator.

Resistance. Meningococcus is a microbe of low stability and is destroyed by drying in a few hours. By heating to a temperature of 60°C, it is killed in 10 minutes and at 80°C in one minute. This organism is very sensitive to a low temperature, hence the material containing meningococci should be transported in a Stuart's transport medium which protects meningococci from adverse conditions. Meningococci are easily killed by chemicals containing silver and hence silver nitrate is used as drug externally in case of gonococcal ophthalmia.

Antigenic structure and classification. Meningococci were found to contain three fractions : Carbohydrate (C) which is common to all meningococci; Protein (P) which is found in gonococci and in Type III pneumococci and a third fraction with which the specificity of meningococci is associated. Meningococci are classified into group A, B, C and D on the basis of the chemical nature of the polysaccharide capsular substance. Recently, the number of types has increased to several, but only the first two are dominant.

Pathogenesis and disease in man. Persons suffering from meningococcal infection and carriers are the sources of the infection. The infection is transmitted by the air droplet route. The causative agent is localised primarily in the nasopharynx. From here, it enters the lymphatic vessels, blood and causes the development of bacteriaemia. Thus, as a result of metastasis, meningococci pass into the meninges and produce acute pyogenic inflammation in the membranes (meninges) of the brain and spinal cord. The disease usually arises suddenly with high temperature, vomiting, rigidity of the occipital muscles, severe headache and increased skin sensitivity. Later, paresis of cranial nerves develops due to increase in the intracranial pressure. Dilatation of the pupils, disturbances of the accommodation and other symptoms appear. A large number of leucocytes exist in cerebrospinal fluid (CSF) and the latter after puncture escapes with a spurt because of the high pressure. In some cases, meningococcal sepsis develops. In such conditions, the organisms are found in the blood, joints and lungs. This disease mainly attacks children from 1 to 8 years of age. Before the discovery of antibiotics and sulphonamides, the death rate was very high (30-60 per cent). Drug resistance of this organism develops rapidly. Ceftriaxone (cefaxone) intramuscularly once a day is effective against purulent meningitis.

Transmission. Meningitis can also be caused by other pathogenic microbes (streptococci, pneumococci, staphylococci, tubercle bacilli and certain viruses). These organisms, however, cause sporadic outbreaks of the disease, while meningococci may cause epidemic meningitis.

The population density plays an important role in the spread of meningitis. During epidemic outbreaks, there is a large number of carriers for every individual affected by the disease.

Diagnosis. Meningococci can be demonstrated in smear from centrifuged CSF obtained by the lumbar puncture. This is of great importance for immediate diagnosis and therapy.

Application to Nursing

In dealing with epidemic meningitis, the nurse should follow the same precautions adopted for infections transmitted by the oral and nasal secretions (lobar pneumonia and scarlet fever).

CHAPTER 29

DIPHTHERIA BACILLI (*Corynebacterium diphtheriae*): Diphtheria

Corynebacterium diphtheriae, the causal agent of diphtheria (G.*diphtheria*-skin, membrane) is usually confined to the respiratory tract. It is rarely found in any part of the body. In general, it is a good example of respiratory tract pathogen.

Diphtheria bacilli was first discovered in 1883-84 by German physicians (Kleb and Loeffler) in bacterial specimens from the throats of patients. These bacilli are sometimes spoken of as Klebs - Loeffler or K-L bacilli.

Morphology. *C. diphtheriae* (L. *Coryna*-club) are pleomorphic, Gram-positive, club shaped bacilli looking like Chinese letters. When they are stained by polychrome methylene blue or a selective stain (Neisser or Albert-Laybourn stain), the volutin (metachromatic granule) stains very darkly purple in contrast with the brown or green colouration. So the rods show 'beaded' or 'barred' appearance. *C.diphtheriae* are non-motile, non-sporing and non-capsulate. These morphological and staining peculiarities are very useful in the immediate bacteriological diagnosis of diphtheria.

Cultivation. Corynebacteria are aerobes, grow best at 37°C on Loeffler serum slopes, on blood potassium tellurite (KTe) agar media on which three types of colony have been recognised as characteristic of different biological types designated *C. diphtheriae gravis*, and *mitis* have been applied in virtue of the association of these types with severe and mild forms, respectively, of the disease. The gravis type produces relatively large greyish black, flat, lustreless colonies exhibiting often "daisy head" formation. The *mitis* type yields a convex, small, translucent colony. The intermedius type is represented by relatively small, black, lustreless colonies with domed centre and flat, irregular margins like a "poached egg".

Toxin Production. Diphtheria bacilli produce a powerful exotoxin with specialised toxic properties, while they remain localised at the site of infection, the diffusible toxin is absorbed into the blood stream and leads to various systemic disturbances of diphtheria (in particular myocardial damage) and to such sequelae as post-diphtheric paralysis. All strains of diphtheria bacilli produce the same toxin but it has been claimed that two distinct substances designated by A and B enter into its constitution. Substance A is toxin which is lethal to guinea pig; whereas the substance B is not definitely toxic *per se* but acts by promoting the spread of substance A in the tissues. This toxin is unstable and its potency diminishes on exposure to sunlight. The toxin has two components : toxic and antigenic components. When toxic component is removed, it has only antigenic property which can be used for immunisation. The conversion of toxin into toxoid can be carried out most effectively by adding 0.3 per cent of formalin and incubating the toxin with formalin for two to three weeks at 37°C. The detoxified or converted toxin is known as "toxoid". The toxoid is a valuable immunising agent for active immunisation.

Test for toxigenicity. It is important to determine whether diphtheria bacilli isolated are virulent, i.e., toxigenic to guinea pig. The virulence test is usually done by intradermal injection of pure culture into guinea pig.

Gel diffusion test. The production of toxin by a virulent strain of *C.diphtheriae* can be determined by the line of precipitation formed, when toxin meets antitoxin in the agar gel diffusion technique **(Elek test)**. Diphtheroids non-pathogenic corynebacteria (*C.pseudodiphtherieum* and *C. xerosis*) are frequently found in the normal throat and nose and often mistaken for *C. diphtheriae*. The pathogenic activity of *C.diphtheriae* can be determined by toxigenicity and gel diffusion tests.

Resistance. C.diphtheriae are relatively resistant to harmful environmental factors. They survive for one year on coagulated serum, for two months at room temperature and for several days on children's toys. They remain viable in the membrane of diphtheria patients for long periods, particularly when the membranes are not exposed to light. They are killed at a temperature of 63°C for 30 minutes (Pasteurisation) and by a one per cent phenol solution in ten minutes.

Transmission of diphtheria. Patients suffering from the disease and carriers are the sources of infection in diphtheria. The disease is transmitted by an air droplet route and sometimes with dust particles. The transmission by various objects (toys, dishes, hooks, towels, handkerchiefs etc.) and foodstuffs (milk, cold dishes etc.) contaminated with *C.diphtheriae* is also possible. The carriers play an essential part in the epidemiology of diphtheria. Infection is spread by close contact, i.e., schools, fomites and institutions but the actual mode of transmission has not yet been clearly defined. Spread of the contaminated dust and fomites play an important part than direct droplet infection. Nasal cases and carriers have been recognised as dangerous sources of infection. The carriers may be segregated and the susceptibles may be protected by combined active-passive immunisation. Carriers and cases of diphtheria have become rare in communities subjected to mass immunisation.

Pathogenesis and Diseases in Man

In human beings pseudomembranes containing a large number of *C.diphtheriae* and other bacteria are formed at the site of entry of the causative agent (e.g., nose, throat, pharynx, trachea, conjunctiva, skin, vulva, vagina and wounds). The exotoxin is of greatest importance in pathogenesis of diphtheria. *C.diphtheriae* is capable of producing hyaluronidase and invading the blood and tissues of patients. For this reaction, diphtheria is considered to be toxinfection. The toxin produces diphtherial inflammation and necrosis in the mucous membrane or skin. On being absorbed, the toxin affects the nerve cells, cardiac muscle and parenchymatous organs and cause severe toxaemia. Deep changes take place in the cardiac muscle, blood vessels, adrenals and in the central and peripheral nervous system.

According to the site of the lesions, faucial diphtheria and diphtheric croup occur most frequently and nasal diphtheria somewhat less frequently. The incidence of diphtheria of the eye, ears, genital organs and skin are relatively rare. Faucial diphtheria constitutes more than 90 per cent of all the diphtheria cases and the nasal diphtheria takes the second place. The infection becomes more severe in the presence of the pathogenic streptococci and staphylococci. Sometimes, non-toxic diphtheria corynebacterium (diphtheroid) and anaerobic corynebacterium may be responsible for some cases of diphtheria.

Therapeutic use of Diphtheria Antitoxin

The unit of antitoxin. The potency of diphtheria antitoxin is stated in units. The unit of antitoxin is the amount that counteracts strictly over 100 minimal lethal doses (MLD) of diphtheria toxin. An MLD of toxin is the least amount of toxin necessary to kill a guinea pig in four to five days. A unit of antitoxin, therefore, neutralises a little over 100 MLD of toxin. The unit is used to express the dosage of antitoxin just as milligrams are used for ordinary medicines. A strong artificially concentrated diphtheria antitoxin contains 2,000 to 2,500 units per ml. Dosage may range from 20,000 to 100,000 units, depending on age, weight, severity of the attack and time after onset. The same basic principles are applicable for the use of other antitoxins (tetanus, gas gangrene etc.), though units and dosages are somewhat different for each kind of antitoxin.

Necessity for Early Diagnosis and Therapy

Any uncomplicated infectious disease caused by toxin producing bacteria can be cured by administration of sufficient quantities of specific antitoxin in early (first day after onset) stage. The serum therapy is said to be effective if it can neutralise the toxin before it could damage the body cells. Even few hours' delay in administrating the antitoxin may create a problem between life and death.

Immunity to Diphtheria

(a) *Passive immunity.* A small dose of antitoxin (500 to 2,000 units) will usually prevent the development of diphtheria in those exposed to the disease. This is called a prophylactic or preventive dose. The immunity lasts for two to three weeks only. This is a good representative of the temporary nature of passive artificial immunity. This type of preventive measure is usually undertaken to those immediately exposed to a case of diphtheria, e.g., public health nurse and doctor.

Serum Sickness may sometimes develop after the administration of antitoxin, because of the manifestation of allergy to the foreign protein in the horse serum containing the antitoxin. The use of horse serum sensitises the patient, usually for life time, to other antisera derived from horses (e.g., tetanus antitoxin), hence it can be used judiciously for prophylaxis until unless it is indicated.

Active immunity. Individuals having little or *no antitoxin in the blood stream*, e.g., *as indicated by a positive Schick test,* may be actively immunised by the injection of one of the following preparations :

1. Formol-Toxoid (FT) diphtheria toxin is rendered non-toxic by formalin. The recommended dose is three intramuscular or deep subcutaneous injections, each of 1 ml, at four weekly intervals. Recent studies proved it is a poor antigen.

2. Toxoid-Antitoxin floccules (TAF). A suspension of the precipitate floccules formed when toxoid and antitoxin are mixed in appropriate"neutralising" amounts. Its tendency to cause reactions is slight and a good immunity follows the injection of three doses, each of 1 ml given at intervals of four weeks. TAF has been recommended for immunisation of adults or adolescents.

3. Alum Precipitated Toxoid (APT). A suspension of washed precipitate produced by the addition of small amount of aluminium hydroxide to toxoid is gradually liberated from the site of injection. Reactions are negligible in children under eight years, but in older children and adults they may be somewhat more severe than with TAF : Two doses, each of 0.5 ml., are given at an interval of four weeks, but the interval may be lengthened, e.g., to 3-8 months without any loss of antibody response to the second dose.

4. Another alum containing prophylactic is a suspension of purified toxoid absorbed on hydrated aluminium phosphate (PTAP) and this preparation is more potent and more reproducible antigen than APT. However, with alum-absorbed antigens, there is slight risk of provocation poliomyelitis in susceptible individuals.

When an outbreak of diphtheria has occurred in a school or institution, the susceptible contacts should, after preliminary Schick testing, be given passive immunity by the injection of a small dose of antitoxin (500-1,000 units) followed by active immunisation which may be given immediately or after two weeks.

Triple vaccine or triple toxoid (DPT). It is more common practice to combine diphtheria and tetanus toxoids with pertussis (whooping cough). So the vaccine is a triple vaccine (DPT) or triple toxoids (refer to chapter 22 on immunisation). The three mixed antigens, tetanus, diphtheria and pertussis, act together than any one of the three above antigens. One product, which includes also Salk, (killed) poliovirus vaccine, has been introduced. All are very effective.

Primary and Secondary stimulus. The two or three initial doses in infancy constitute a *primary stimulus.* Antibodies formed due to primary stimulus may circulate in the blood and disappear with time. The person who had primary stimulus may respond *quickly* to *secondary stimulus* which may be due actual infection : tetanus, diphtheria, pertussis or polio. The previously immunised person is usually able to respond quickly with the production of specific antibodies. Immunised persons may rarely get diphtheria, pertussis, tetanus, poliomyelitis, even though they did not have a booster dose at all. Therefore, every child receives at least *primary stimulus* with multiple antigens early in life and a second or"booster"stimulus a year later and again at the time of entering the school.

Antibodies derived from immune mother's blood may protect the infant up to 2-4 months of age against many diseases (including diphtheria). Therefore, children are naturally protected against diphtheria by mother antibodies against diphtheria; but it is essential to immunise artificially after this period.

Schick test. For the first time Viennese physician put into practice the Schick test. This test can be used to detect the presence or absence of significant amount of diphtheria antitoxin in the blood and can be carried out by injecting a minute quantity of diphtheria toxin (1/50 MLD — minimal lethal dose) intradermally. If the person has no antitoxin in the blood (i.e., is not immune), a red area or wheal appears at the site of injection within 24 hours and spreads for a centimeter or more. This reaction is due to irritating effect of the toxin on the cells of skin. In five days, the area becomes slightly pigmented and later scale is formed and it falls off. This test should not be read earlier than fifth day of the injection, because a temporary irritation (pseudoreaction), caused by foreign substance present in the toxin, persists. An area that persists after five days and undergoes the changes is a positive reaction (i.e., the person has insufficient antitoxin in the blood and may be susceptible to diphtheria if under fifteen years of age).

If an individual has antitoxin in his blood, this antitoxin will neutralise the toxin injected in the Schick test and the skin remains normal. This is a negative Schick reaction and it indicates that the individual has sufficient antitoxin (about 0.01 ml. unit per ml. of blood) to protect him from diphtheria. This test is harmless, painless and leaves no scar.

Immunisation of Nurse. At the beginning of the training, every student nurse should be protected compulsorily against diphtheria by active immunisation, though her first year training does not mainly involve with the nursing care of the contagious disease patients.

Application to Nursing

The nurse should know very well that she may get infected while caring for a diphtheria patient. Therefore, she must wear the mask for her own protection from this highly infectious disease. The respiratory secretions and saliva are highly infectious, so all these materials and contaminated objects should be destroyed or completely burnt.

The professional nurse should have knowledge that no antiseptics (e.g., in the form of gargles etc.) must be applied within twelve hours before the collection of samples. The lesion in the throat can be clearly viewed by depressing the tongue with tongue depressor or table spoon, then to obtain a specimen of the throat secretion or lesion, she must rub with a sterile throat swab over the affected area in the faucial region of the throat or where there is no definitely localised lesion, over the pseudomembrane of the pharynx and tonsils. She should label the throat swab test tube with the patient's name, the date and the time. If the patient has been on antibiotic or sulphonamides within five days, this information should be sent to the laboratory with the throat swab since these drugs may inhibit the growth in the culture. If the diphtheria patient is admitted in a special or isolation ward of the hospital, and whenever the same patient is discharged, the *terminal disinfection* of the room should be carried out under the observation of the well trained intelligent knowledgeable nurse. This technique is always followed in the hospital. School nurse should assist the school doctor in the segregation, isolation and immunisation procedure during an epidemic of the diphtheria in the school or other institution. Besides she should be very careful to see that the nasal secretion and saliva are properly disposed off.

CHAPTER 30

TUBERCLE BACILLI (*Mycobacterium tuberculosis*)

Order Actinomycetales, family Mycobacteriaceae, genus Mycobacterium, include bacteria which are characterised by their ability to branch and by their acid-alcohol-fast properties.

The genus Mycobacterium consists of organism responsible for tuberculosis and leprosy and number of acid fast saprophytes.

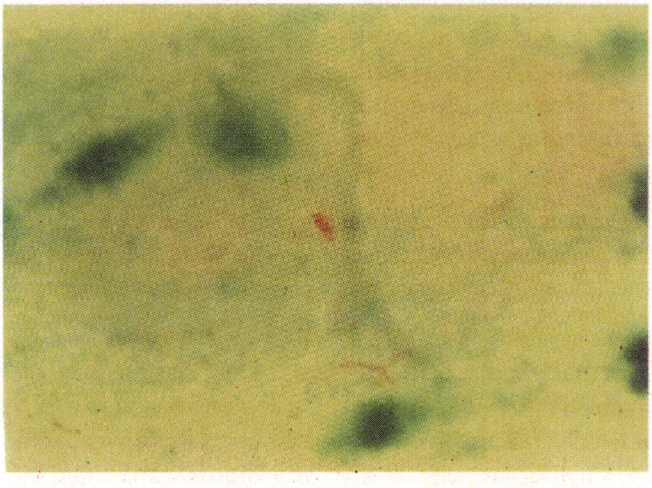

Fig. 30.1 : Mycobacterium tuberculosis (Tubercle bacilli × 1000)

Mycobacterium tuberculosis, causing tuberculosis in man, was discovered by Robert Koch in 1882.

Morphology. Myco. tuberculosis (G . *mykes* — fungus or mould) is a slender, straight, or slightly curved pleomorphic rod, 0.5 - 4μ in length and 0.3μ in breadth. These organisms are non-motile and do not form spores or capsules (Fig. 30.1).

Though they are Gram-positive, they cannot be readily stained by Gram method, but they can be easily stained by Ziehl-Neelsen method, as they resist decolourisation with 20-25 per cent sulphuric acid and alcohol, they are described as acid-alcohol-fast bacilli or acid-fast bacilli (AFB).

The acid-fastness is due to the fact that *Myco. tuberculosis* contains *mycolic acid* and lipids. This organism consists of three fractions : (1) phosphatide which is soluble in ether; (2) fat which is soluble in ether; (3) wax which is soluble in chloroform and ether. There are four main serological groups : mammalian (human, bovine, murine), avian, reptilian and saprophytes.

Cultivation. Myco.tuberculosis human type is aerobic, grows well at 37°C as late as 6-8 weeks (average 4 weeks) on selective media containing glycerol, whole egg or egg yolk (Dorest egg or Lowenstein Jensen medium — in screw capped bottle, because screw cap can prevent the dehydration of these media during the long incubation period). The growth is luxuriant (eugonic) and wrinkled at first while, later, buff coloured. As compared to *Myco. tuberculosis* human type, the growth of bovine type is less luxuriant (dysgonic) thin, whitish and smooth. Glycerol favours the growth of human type, but has no effect on the bovine type.

Toxin production. Myco. tuberculosis does not produce an exotoxin. It contains toxic substances which are liberated when it is lysed.

In 1890, Robert Koch isolated a substance known as "tuberculin" from tubercle bacilli. The tuberculin is an extract containing the specific protein of tubercle bacilli. The tuberculin reaction is due to the development of tissue hypersensitivity — or bacterial allergy — and is used in men and animals to find if they have or have had tuberculosis in an active or latent form.

Tuberculin is originally obtained from a six week old culture in glycerol broth evaporated to one-tenth of its volume, sterilised by heat and filtered (old tuberculin — OT). Various other methods have been employed in its preparation. The specific tuberculin protein can now be separated from other constituents and products of culture in a synthetic medium and then purified. This purified protein derivative (PPD) is preferable to old tuberculin as it is consistant in composition. It is used in dry state, from which it can be diluted by addition of a borate buffer solution.

It should be noted that the tuberculin prepared from the human and bovine types are indistinguishable as they contain the same specific substance.

Tuberculins are standardised in such a way that a dilution of 1 : 10,000 of OT is equivalent to 1 tuberculin unit (TU), while 0.000028 mg of PPD equals 1 unit. A common practice in using tuberculin is to test first with 3 or 5 TU and if the individual gives no reaction, retest with a dose of 100 TU.

Tuberculin Test. Tuberculin test in man is carried out on the skin by different techniques; those most commonly used are Mantoux, Heaf and jelly tests. Mantoux test is performed by injecting intradermally 0.1 ml of the appropriate dilution of tuberculin, the test is positive when there is an area of induration measuring 5 mm in diameter in 2-3 days after injection. In Heaf test, a multiple puncture spring release gun is used to prick the previously applied tuberculin into the skin. A positive reaction may range from 4-6 discrete papules to solid induration. These two tests are usually done on the forearm. In the jelly test, a tuberculin jelly is applied in a form of "V" in the intrascapular area of the back and covered with a plaster; the control is required only for this jelly test, but not with other two tests.

Only Mantoux and Heaf tests were found to be reliable and acceptable to large scale epidemiological investigations, when compared to these tests and Von Pirquet scarification test; Heaf test is generally preferred to Mantoux test. The tuberculin test may be used in epidemiology to determine the incidence of tuberculous infections in a community. A positive reaction in a young child may also be useful for case finding among the family contacts; in immunisation campaign in order to separate the positive and negative reactors and to assess the response to vaccination by simple testing afterwards.

The 38K Da protein of *Myco. tuberculosis* induces B and Tcells response with high specificity for infection with *Myco. tuberculosis* and is a prime candidate for development of new diagnostic reagent for tuberculosis.

Resistance. Tubercle bacilli are most resistant to external effect as compared to other non-spore forming bacteria as a result of high lipid content (25-40 per cent).

These organisms survive in the flowing water for over a year; in soil and manure up to 6 months; on the pages of books over a period of 3 months; in *dried sputum for 2 months*; in distilled water for several weeks and *in gastric juice for 6 hours*. They are rendered harmless at temperature ranging from 100 to 120°C. The thermal death point is 60°C for 15-20 minutes. Pasteurisation (62°C for 30 minutes or 80°C for 15-30 seconds) also kills these organisms. Many individual bacilli die when desicated, a proportion of them may survive for several weeks or months, if protected from sunlight.

They are sensitive to exposure to sunlight and ultraviolet radiation; and ordinary daylight, even through the glass, has a *lethal effect*. They can resist 5 per cent phenol for several weeks in putrifying materials and in sputum. *Myco. tuberculosis* is sensitive to streptomycin, rifampicin, viomycin and cycloserine among the antibiotics and to Para amino salicylic acid (PAS), isonicotonic acid hydrazide (INAH or isoniazid thiosemicarbosone, methionamide and pyrazinamide among chemotherapeutic agents.

Pathogenesis and Disease in Man

It has been shown that tuberculosis in human beings is caused by two types of Mycobacteria — the human type (*Myco. tuberculosis*) and the bovine type (*Myco. bovis*). The human type is responsible for 90 per cent of the cases and the bovine type for remaining 10 per cent. The avian type may also be the cause of human tuberculosis in some cases on ingestion of insufficiently cooked chicken meat and eggs contaminated with *Myco. avium*.

Infection with tuberculosis takes place through the respiratory tract by the droplets dust and sometimes per os through contaminated food stuffs and through the skin and mucous membrane. Intrauterine infection via placenta may also occur.

The most common form of primary infection with tubercle bacilli is a pulmonary lesion known as the primary complex or Ghon focus (not more than 5μ in diameter) in the terminal bronchioles or alveoli and the primary lesion may occur in any part of the lungs. From it, the organisms are carried by lymphatic drainage by the regional mediastinal lymph glands in which there may be progressive enlargement and involvement, followed by caseation and later calcification.

More generalised infection may follow the spread of organisms either by blood stream or the bronchi, resulting, respectively, in miliary or bronchopneumonic tuberculosis, usually with lesions in other organs besides the lungs, e.g., brain and meninges (tuberculous meningitis), spleen, liver. Primary infections may also occur via the intestine with the involvement of the mesenteric glands or via the tonsils with secondary cervical adenitis, usually from ingestion of infected milk. These forms of tuberculosis have become much rare now, as most milk supplies are pasteurised. Primary infection of the skin (Lupus *vulgaris*) is now a rare condition. Infection of skin lesions sometimes occurs from handling infected materials (laboratory workers and veterinarians) while intracutaneous Bacille Calmette-Guerin (BCG) vaccination may produce a form of primary complex with local skin lesion and an associated adenitis.

While tuberculous meningitis occurs characteristically as a complication of the primary lung lesion in very young children, it may also develop in older children and young adults as an apparently primary infection. Renal, bone and joint tuberculosis may be due to "seedling" of blood borne tubercle bacilli from the primary lesion in the lung or elsewhere.

The post primary (or adult) form of pulmonary infection is the most common form of clinical tuberculosis in which one or more lung lesions progress to caseation and cavitation and after involving the bronchial tree create a case of open tuberculosis. Tuberculous ulcerations in the larynx and intestine, if they occur, are usually sequelae of pulmonary tuberculous spread of infected sputum; similarly secondary infection of ureter, bladder, epididymis may follow renal tuberculosis.

Transmission

This organism is expectorated in sputum and expelled in droplets during coughing and speaking and there have been instances of explosive outbreaks of tuberculosis in school children and others exposed to an infective teacher or singer. But, since very small droplets that can be inhaled directly from the infective patient are less likely to carry tubercle bacilli than larger droplets or sputum, infection may occur more often indirectly from the dried dust particles than directly from moist droplets or droplet nuclei.

The tubercle bacilli can survive slow drying for days or weeks, if protected from the bactericidal day light or sunlight. The spread of infection from infected cases to susceptible contacts by contaminated dust or fomite would be facilitated in overcrowded, badly lit rooms or buildings. Primary infection may occur at any stage, if it occurs in early life (0-3 years) it is often associated with signs and symptoms of the disease.

At school age (5-15 years), infection usually occurs in an inapparent form, but, in adolescents or young adults, it is again more likely to result in clinical disease.

Infection occurs earlier and is more likely to result in clinical disease among susceptibles living in close contact with open cases, but many personal and environmental factors (age, malnutrition, other respiratory diseases, hormonal dysfunction, pregnancy, stress, genetic constitution etc.) may contribute to overt tuberculosis.

Workers exposed to the inhalation of dust containing silica have a high incidence of tuberculosis. Nurses, medical students, doctors and workers in the pathology laboratory and in the hospital are more exposed and tend to have a higher than an average rate of infection.

In lung tuberculosis, the sputum is the main source of infection; in tuberculosis of kidneys and bladder, the bacilli may be excreted in the urine in plenty; in intestinal tuberculosis, faeces may contain tubercle bacilli and similarly, the pus in the tuberculous abscess may also contain tubercle bacilli. It has been estimated that a patient may discharge in 24 hours 500 millions to 3 billions bacilli in his sputum. A spray of sputum from a coughing or sneezing tuberculous patient may contain tubercle bacilli may get infected with tuberculosis by coming in contact with the patient.

A careless person with active pulmonary tuberculosis may kiss a child, contaminate the floor or furniture with sputum or expectorate into the street or other public place which is a *very common practice in under-developed countries.* So, children playing in the street or room, creeping on the floor may get the tubercle bacilli on their hands and ultimately into their mouth. The hand to mouth transmission is very common among the children. In ancient times, children were also infected by drinking unpasteurised milk from tuberculous cows. While handling food, the fingers soiled with the sputum may contaminate the food. Flies which crawled on the tuberculous sputum may contaminate the food. Improperly washed spoon, plate or common drinking cup may also carry the tubercle bacilli.

Tubercle bacilli are ubiquitous in nature. Particularly in urban area they are widespread in city streets, theatres and other public places and may result into an imbalanced urban health. Everything that keeps one person in good conditions (good food, sufficient rest, and recreation alongwith the chemotherapy) may pave ways towards the recovery and good health of the tuberculous patients. Measles, whooping cough, influenza, frequent child bearing, continuous strain and fatigue, poor living and unhygienic conditions, alcoholism and malnutrition are the predisposing causes of tuberculosis. Only the public health nurse can educate and influence the public to lead an healthy happy life.

Socio-economic conditions are also related to tuberculosis in a community. Tuberculosis is very common amongst the poor people than among the rich people. Low standards of living are : lack of isolation, rest, sunlight, fresh air and cleanliness; lack of medical, nursing care and lack of sufficient nutritious food.

Tuberculosis and Nurses. In the developed countries, there is an accumulated evidence that the nurses are more frequently infected with tuberculosis than women of same age in other occupation, which may be as a result of breakdown of resistance of the individual who had already been heavily infected in childhood. Tuberculin test carried out on a group of student nurses indicated that the primary infection is often acquired during the period of training, most probably from patients.

It has been shown that the incidence of tuberculosis among nurses is higher in general hospitals than in tuberculosis hospital and it seems that the nurses acquire the infection most frequently from unknown cases than from known cases as they take all possible precautions including the use of masks during nursing care of the tuberculous patients.

Before admission into the school of nursing, each candidate should undergo the physical examination which is followed by the intradermal tuberculin test; if the test is positive, an X-ray chest is essential. This study may help the candidate to divert into less arduous occupation. Besides, the tuberculin test should be conducted at six months' interval on nurses who were previously negative for tuberculin test and at the same time intervals chest plates should be done on all nurses who were tuberculosis negative.

Since overwork and excessive stress may break down the body resistance, the work load should be within the permissible limits and the general health condition should be supervised. For the safer side, all tuberculin negative student and nurses should be immunised with BCG before the commencement of the training.

Laboratory Diagnosis. Direct microscopy of smears from sputum, pus, spinal or pleural fluid, urine, faeces, lymph nodes etc. stained by Ziehl-Neelsen method can reveal the presence of tubercle bacilli.

Tubercle bacilli are plenty in lesions of rapid caseation. In miliary tuberculosis, they are relatively rare.

Smears stained with auramine can be examined by Fluorescence microscopy. Coughing may be induced by passing a swab onto the posterior pharynx, the expectoration on it can be used to prepare a smear.

Urine, pleural, peritoneal fluid are centrifuged, films are made from the deposit and stained by Ziehl-Neelsen method. In examining the urine, it is advisable to obtain the sediment from a 24 hours specimen because of intermittency of excretions of tubercle bacilli. Alternatively, three consecutive morning specimens may be examined.

"Spider web" coagulum obtained from an hour longer standing CSF in a stoppered tube can be easily transferred to a slide, dried, fixed by heat and stained by Ziehl-Neelsen method. Recent Polymerase Chain Reaction (PCR) is 95% sensitive and 93% specific when compared to culture, direct microscopy and gas chromatography. Very recently, molecular biological technology — DNA probe and polymerase chain reaction (PCR) — can detect even a single *Myco. tuberculosis* in clinical specimen with 100% sensitivity and specificity. Complement fixation test (CFT), agar gel precipitation test, modified haemagglutination (HA) test had fallen behind Enzyme Linked Immunosorbent Assay (ELISA) in term of specificity and sensitivity. ELISA has become the method of choice. Radio-immunoassay (RIA) also gives promising results.

Isolation of the pure culture can be done on Dorset egg or Lowenstein Jensen medium.

Chemotherapy. The most effective and least toxic chemotherapeutic agents against tuberculosis are streptomycin, para amino salicylic acid (PAS) and isonicotinic acid hydrazide (Isoniazid). It is essential to have a combination of two or three antituberculous drugs, because of the appearance of resistant strains of tubercle bacilli after the commencement of treatment.

Vaccination. Killed vaccines of tubercle bacilli give no protection against tuberculosis. In 1921, two French scientists, Calmette and Guerin, introduced a living vaccine prepared from a bovine strain that had been cultured for many years on a bile potato medium. This "Bacille Calmette-Guerin" (BCG) vaccine is given intradermally. It has been demonstrated conclusively that BCG vaccination may give a protection of 80 per cent against clinical infections.

The dose of BCG vaccine is a single intracutaneous injection of 0.1 ml containing 0.05 to 0.1 mg moist weight of the constituent bacilli (= 1-2 million viable organisms). A small inflammatory lesion develops at the site of inoculation and usually goes on to superficial ulceration after some weeks. Adenitis of the regional lymph nodes may follow in infants (rarely in older children). Except in case of babies of 0-3 months old, all children must first be tuberculin tested and only the negative reactors should be given vaccine.

Anonymous Mycobacteria

Acid-fast bacilli which cannot be identified as either human or bovine type tubercle bacilli and which may be associated with human diseases have attracted considerable attention in recent years and have been given the name *anonymous* or *atypical mycobacteria.*

These mycobacteria were originally divided by Runyon into four groups according to their morphology, colonial texture, production of pigment in the presence of light (*photochromogens* or in the darkness) *scotochromogens*, rapidity of growth and growth at different temperatures (25°C = *psychrophiles*; 37°C = *mesophiles*; 42°C = *thermophiles*), production of catalase, resistance to certain anti-tuberculous drugs, e.g., thiosemicarbosone, isoniazid and paraaminosalicylic acid (PAS) and the niacin test.

Later these four groups were further expanded to seven provisional groups of which Group I (Photochromogens) are in most common association with respiratory diseases, Group II (Scotochromogens) are found in neck abscess, Group IV is similar to *Myco. avium* and Group VII is associated with cases of pneumoconiosis.

Application to Nursing

Well trained professional nurse should have a profound knowledge of the localisation of the lesion in the lungs, intestine, lymph nodes which is discharging living organism, so that she may be able to determine the types of preventive measures to be adopted according to the different situations. All patients with copious secretions should be regarded as possible causes of pulmonary tuberculosis. The nurses in tuberculosis hospital who are responsible for the prevention of the transmission of infection from the infected materials (e.g., linens, thermometers, dishes, dust) to other people and to themselves should bear in mind that *Myco. tuberculosis* is very resistant to chemical disinfectants and drying.

The patient with active tuberculosis should be kept well informed by the nurse of the fact that he is a dangerous source of infection to others. Hence, he should remain isolated from other persons and should also he instructed not to cough or expectorate openly; if he moves out of the house, he should carry a pocket sputum flask, have separate set of dishes which should be washed in boiling water after use, should sleep isolated; if his hands are soiled with sputum, he should not forget to wash his hands; while coughing or sneezing, he should cover his nose and mouth. Besides, the nurse must instruct that he should not come in contact with children under 5 years of age and other persons. In the public health nursing, the nurse gives training, care and encouragement to the patient in his own home. The sputum coughed up from the lungs of the patient in active stage of the infection must be completely disinfected or destroyed. If the tuberculous patient has copious pulmonary secretions, he should be directed to cough into a bag tied to the bedside stand or pinned to the bed. If this bag is full to certain extent, it should be folded at the top so that the paper wipes will not spill out, wrapped in the thick newspapers, placed into the trash cans; at last it should be taken to the incinerator when it should be completely burnt. The sputum cup, if used, can be disinfected satisfactorily, and special care should be taken to destroy all materials (sputum and secretions) in a close incinerator system to avoid the spillage.

The professional nurse in the tuberculosis hospital ward should be able to differentiate that *Myco. tuberculosis* causes tuberculosis and atypical mycobacteria cause other respiratory diseases which are less serious and should know how to interpret the report from the diagnostic microbiological laboratory and inform the doctor immediately if it is *Myco. tuberculosis* causing a serious communicable disease — tuberculosis.

CHAPTER 31

LEPRA BACILLI (Myco. leprae)

The organism, *Myco. leprae*, responsible for leprosy (Hansen's disease) was discovered in 1874 by the Norwegian doctor; Hansen. Hence, it is called as Hansen's bacillus.

Morphology. Myco. leprae have many properties common with tubercle bacilli. They are straight or slightly curved bacilli and have club-shaped swellings. They measure 1 to 8μ in length and 0.3 to 0.5μ in breadth, occurring in groups resembling packets of cigars or clusters. They are decolourised more easily than *Myco. tuberculosis.* They are non-motile, they produce neither spores nor capsules and are Gram positive.

Myco. leprae is similar to *Myco. tuberculosis* in chemical composition. Their lipid content ranges from 9.7 to 18.6 per cent. Besides mycolic acid, they contain laeprosinic oxyacid, free fatty acids, wax (leprozine), alcohols and polysaccharides.

Cultivation. Many workers have made attempts to cultivate *Myco. leprae*, but ultimately they became unsuccessful. However, successful results have been claimed by inoculating the armadillos and the foot pad of mouse.

Pathogenesis. Leprosy is a disease of great antiquity and is infective granuloma developing as 1. *Lepromatous* or *nodular type* in which granulomatous nodules (lepromata) form in the skin, mucous membrane and various organs (e.g., lungs, liver, spleen, testes); 2. *tuberculoid type*, when the granulation tissues infiltrate certain nerves and lead to motor and sensory nerves paralysis with characteristic trophic change (e.g., anaesthetic skin areas — maculae). Both types of the lesions may occur in the same patient.

IMMUNOLOGY OF *MYCO. LEPRAE*

Many million people encounter *Myco. leprae*, yet only a small proportion may develop clinical disease; the majority develop protection immunity.

1. Protection antibody develops in most individuals after a sub-clinical infection with *Myco. leprae*. It may be from self-healing or with indeterminate or tuberculoid disease:

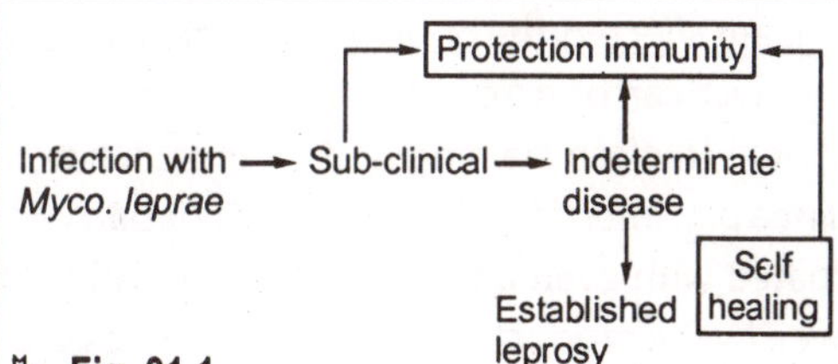

Fig. 31.1

2. Inside the macrophages, *Myco. leprae* are broken down and processed, with mycobacterial antigens then being displayed on the cell surface together with Human Leucocyte Antigen (HLA), class II antigen. This antigen complex is recognised by and interacts with T cells through T cell receptors and T cell proliferation results from this antigen stimulation. The activated T cell also produces cytokines which are polypeptides that act as molecular regulators by stimulating other components of the immune system. The growth and activation of T cells is enhanced

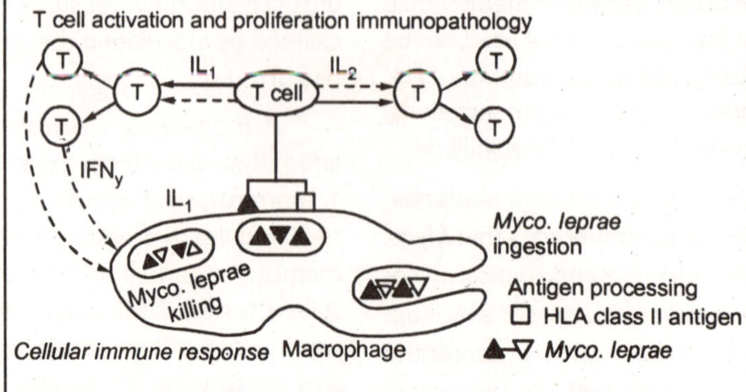

Fig. 31.2 : Cellular immune response to *Myco. leprae* infection

by the cytokines inter leukine (IL) 1 and 2 while other cytokine interferon gamma (IFNy) activate macrophage so that *Myco. leprae* are killed. Ultimately the immunological memory is established to encounter *Myco. leprae* subsequently. Based on this, there is possibility to discover a vaccine against leprosy.

Laboratory diagnosis. Films of lymph exudate from the ulcerated nodule on the skin or non-ulcerated nodule as well as from scrapings or secretions from nasal mucosa can be stained with Ziehl-Neelsen method with *5* per cent sulphuric acid. The characteristic acid-fast bacilli are present in the films. When lungs are affected, the bacilli may be seen in the sputum which can be differentiated from tubercle bacilli by Ziehl-Neelsen staining and by inoculation into guinea pig. Infection of the mouse foot pad can be initiated with even a few leprosy bacilli and is followed by the production of characteristic lesion.

The production of *Myco. leprae* antigens lead to hopes that a serological test for leprosy could be developed.

Myco. leprae synthesizes a unique species specific lipid, phenolic glycolipid (PGL) which is found in substantial amounts in tissues surrounding foci of infection. PGL is an important antigen and high titers of antibodies directed against PGL are only found in leprosy patients. Serological test, which is not specific and sensitive and cross reacts with *Myco. tuberculosis* antigen, is not useful to detect antibody, yet is under experimentation.

As PCR method develops, it will be undoubtedly be useful in the diagnosis of paucibacillary leprosy and early disease, when few bacilli are present.

PCR to amplify part of a *Myco. leprae* protein antigen (36 K Da) was able to detect *Myco. leprae* with a detection limit of one bacterium when using purified *Myco. leprae* DNA and a limit of 1,000 bacteria when using armadillo liver. This is more considerably sensitive than other methods for direct detection of *Myco. leprae* such as microscopy. It will be exciting to use PCR as a tool for epidemiological studies.

Transmission. Leprosy is often acquired in childhood or early adult life and is most common among the lower social classes. Males are more often affected than females. Infection is probably spread by direct contact through the skin abrasion or may be acquired by inhalation of infected dust via the nasal mucosa. Blood sucking insects also may possibly act as carriers. Patients with lepromatous lesions are much more infectious than tuberculosis cases. The incubation period is variable (weeks to years), but it is most commonly 2-4 years.

Because of its chronicity, crippling disabilities and social barriers, leprosy presents very large public health and economic problem in many developing countries.

Lepromin and BCG Vaccination

Lepromin, as ordinarily used, is a boiled unstandardised extract of leprous tissues, which when injected intracutaneously, produces an area of nodular infiltration reaching its maximum in 3 to 5 weeks (Mistuda reaction) in cases of tuberculoid leprosy and in apparently healthy people. The reaction is usually negative in cases of lepromatous leprosy.

Recently an antigen containing 160 millions lepra bacilli per ml has been recommended as "standard lepromin" of which 1 : 4 dilution containing 40 million bacilli would, on intradermal injection, be adequate to produce a nodule of 3 mm or more after 4 weeks as a criterion of positivity. The positive reaction indicates the resistance to leprosy and the negative reaction is related to cell mediated immunity deficiency.

Chemotherapy and Chemoprophylaxis

Oral administration, in particular dapsone (4-4' diamino-diphenylsulphone or DDS) has become the most practical chemotherapy for mass campaign against leprosy. The recommended dose ranged from 6.0 to 10 mg per kg. body weight per week over a period of 3-5 years or more depending upon the nature and extent of the infection.

Long term chemoprophylaxis of leprosy with dapsone among child contacts of infective cases has given encouraging result in India.

WHO multiple drug treatment regimens for Leprosy

Patient classification*	Rimfampicin 600 mg once daily	Dapsone 400 mg daily	Clofazimine 300 mg once monthly + 50 mg daily	Duration (months)
Multibacillary	+	+	+	> 24⁺
Paucibacillary	+	+	–	6

*Any patient whose skin smears are positive for AFB should be treated as multibacillary.

+ Wherever possible until the skin smears show no AFB.

Application to Nursing

Public health nurse has a very important role to play in the control of programme of leprosy, she should have a main objective of creating in the minds of the community, the patients and their families a reasoned attitude towards leprosy. She should also educate in clear explicit language that the leprosy is a curable disease, if diagnosed early and the treatment started early. Children can get the infection by contact with infective cases, which can be prevented by chemotherapy with dapsone. Successfully she should also advise the community so that their children should not be allowed to come in contact with the infective cases and she should also take all possible steps to rehabilitate the lepers in the society through mass community education.

CHAPTER 32

MYCOPLASMA

Mycoplasma is the smallest prokaryotic organism to grow in cell free culture medium. Out of 8 or 9 species, *Mycoplasma pneumoniae* is the only pathogen.

Clinically *M. pneumoniae* infections take the form of a febrile bronchitis or pneumonia with generalised symptoms — malaise (which may overshadow the respiratory symptoms), myalgia, sore throat, headache, cough, which starts around the third day, is characteristically troublesome. Coryza is unusual, but nausea and vomiting may be a feature. It is also an important cause of otitis. Complications are — rashes, urticaria, maculopapular rash, erythema multiforme (vesicular and bulbous lesions on mucocutaneous junctions), meningitis, encephalitis, sometimes haemolytic anaemia. In 5 to 15 years age groups and in both sexes, *M. pneumoniae* may be the major cause of (20-40%) of all non-bacterial pneumonia.

Treatment. Tetracycline is the drug of choice. The spread of the disease can be prevented by proper disinfection and disposal of sputum.

CHAPTER 33

ACTINOMYCOSIS

Actinomycosis occurs as a chronic granulomatous infection in men and animals. In man, the infecting species is *Actinomycosis israelii* which occurs commensally in the buccal cavity.

Morphology. Actinomyces are intermediate between bacteria and fungi. They have non-septate mycelium with aerial sporangia. They grow as colonies in the tissues, called as" sulphur granules" which are macroscopic. If these granules are crushed between the two slides, stained by Gram method and examined under microscope, the central filamentous mass is Gram-positive and the surrounding zone of radiating clubs is Gram-negative. These clubs represent lipoid material derived from the host tissues to prevent further invasion by filamentous growth.

When such smear preparations are stained by Ziehl-Neelsen, by replacing 20 per cent sulphuric acid by 1 percent for decolourisation, the peripheral clubs are stained acid-fast and the central mycelial mass is non-acid-fast. Club formation is less frequent in human than in animal lesions.

Resistance. Actinomyces are very resistant, withstand a temperature of 60°C for 1 hour and remain viable for a longer period when dried; their spores are particularly resistant.

Clinical Infection. Actinomycosis may result from endogenous infection when actinomyces penetrates from the digestive tract. The chewing of the grain, skin and mucosa injuries and particularly carious or worn out teeth facilitate the infection. The causative agents spread gradually in the connective tissue and between the muscles and are circulated in the blood or lymph. The infectious process is accompanied by the formation of suppurative foci and fistulae which open within or outside the body. The disease is characterised by chronic inflammation with subsequent development of suppurative process. Hard infiltrates or granulomas form at the site of localisation of the organism. The skin becomes purple blue and the infiltrates soften, necrotise and discharge pus which has an offensive odour and contains sulphur granules made of threads of actinomyces. Affection with pathogenic actinomyces is mostly accompanied by secondary pyogenic infection.

According to clinical manifestations, actinomycosis of the face and neck, *pulmonary actinomycosis*, abdominal actinomycosis, actinomycosis of internal organs, skin actinomycosis, skin and muscular actinomycosis, bone and muscular actinomycosis, actinomycosis of the nose, ears, larynx, pharynx, eyes, central nervous system etc. can be differentiated. The involvement of lungs is followed by pleuropneumonia or kidney metastases, skin abscess.

Laboratory diagnosis. The sulphur granules in the pus can be harvested by shaking the pus with water in a test tube; after standing for few minutes, the granule sediments may be collected with a capillary pipette. A granule would be crushed between two slides, fixed and stained by Gram stain method and by modified Ziehl-Neelsen technique.

Treatment. Before the advent of penicillin, the surgical treatment was adapted. Penicillin is the drug of choice. Other antibiotics were also prescribed in combination with iodine, X-ray therapy and surgery.

Human actinomycosis includes Madura disease (Madura Foot or maduromycosis) which is caused by *Nocardia madurae* and other actinomyces. It is a chronic foot infection, the foot becoming swollen and deformed. At times, the process may be localised in the shank, hands, abdomen etc. Following penetration of the organisms, nodules are produced at the site of entry, the skin becomes red violet or brown, the nodules soften and break through the skin forming fistulae which discharge pus. Patients are treated with penicillin in combination with sulphonamides. Chlortetracycline and oxytetracycline are also used.

Respiratory Fungus Disease

Histoplasmosis and coccidioidomycosis are important and widespread infections of respiratory tract caused by fungi. They are not transmitted from person to person, but mainly from soil (refer to chapter "pathogenic fungi of the soil").

CHAPTER 34

LARYNGOTRACHEITIS, WHOOPING COUGH, CONJUNCTIVITIS AND TRENCH FEVER

Genus Hemophilus, Morexella and Bordetella belong to the family Brucellacae as they have common properties of this family.

Properties of the Brucellacae. Brucella are very small Gram-negative bacilli (0.3 - 0.6 micron in width and 3-8 microns in length). They are non-motile, non-spore forming. They are killed by common disinfectants, pasteurisation and boiling and grow at 37°C in presence of 5-10 per cent carbon dioxide in media containing blood or serum and meat extract and they are parasitic in the human body.

Genus Hemophilus

Hemophilus influenzae (Influenza bacilli) was originally described as the causal organism of epidemic influenza, now this theory has been completely disproved. The modern concept is that *H. influenzae* is a secondary pathogen on respiratory mucosa that has become susceptible to bacterial attack of the primary influenza virus infection. The genus name is derived from its requirement for blood (Greek, *haima,* blood; *philus,* loving). It is particularly adapted to live and grow in the body. Outside the body, it grows in the media containing whole blood or blood derivative *hemin* or X-factor and a *coenzyme* L or V factor. V factor is also produced by *Staph. aureus.* Becuase of this factor, enlarged colonies of *H. influenzae* around colonies of staphylococcus (Satellism) are observed.

H. influenzae is inhabitant of nose and throat of normal persons, it is a typical respiratory tract organism and is transmitted in droplets by sneezing and coughing. It causes many inflammatory conditions of the respiratory tract (bronchopneumonia, sinusitis). It may sometimes cause meningitis and endocarditis. It also causes secondary infection.

Application to Nursing

The nursing precautions and isolation techniques are same as those of upper respiratory tract.

Genus Morexella

Moraxella lacunata (Bacillus of Pink eye) closely resembles and has the general character of *H. influenzae,* but it does not require X or V factor. It is the cause of acute conjunctivitis or inflammation of the lining of the eyelids commonly called as "Pink eyes". Virus, pneumococci, streptococci, staphylococci and influenza bacilli may also cause acute conjunctivitis.

Pink eye due to *H. influenzae* is very contagious and spreads rapidly in families, institutions and schools. The transmission may be by direct contact with the infected eyes or by fingers, towels, wash clothes, handkerchiefs contaminated with secretions of the eyes. As *M. lacunata* is very resistant to drying, it can be transmitted by dust. The disease is not serious, as it can be treated early and it may last for 3 days or 2 weeks.

Application to Nursing

The infection and inflammation of the eyes can be reduced by bathing the patient's eyes with mild disinfectant solution. The school or institution nurse should know that a child with pink eye may be kept away from other children. She should also segregate the child, his bed linens, handkerchiefs, wash clothes, towels etc. which may be soiled with the infected eye discharge. Conjunctivitis due to *M. lacunata* may clear up spontaneously, if it is lasting, the treatment and care should be as in gonorrheal ophthalmia.

Genus Bordetella

Bordetella pertussis (whooping cough bacillus) was discovered and isolated in pure culture from patients by J. Bordet and O. Gengou in 1906. These organisms are small, oval shaped, non-motile rods, produce no capsules, no spores and are Gram-negative; they grow best at 37°C on glycerine potato or blood agar medium. They are very sensitive to environmental factors. They withstand exposure to direct sunlight for one hour and a temperature of 56°C for 10-15 minutes. They are destroyed in 3 per cent solution of phenol and lysol.

Pathogenesis and disease in man. Whooping cough is transmitted from the patient to a healthy individual by the air droplet route. Patients are most contagious in the catarrhal stage. Various objects in the vicinity of the patient are insignificant in relation to the transmission of the infections, as *Bord. pertussis* cannot withstand external environmental factors.

Whooping cough is a severe infectious disease of childhood and is characterised by typical symptoms and cyclic course (3 stages):

(a) Catarrhal stage, lasting about 2 weeks.

(b) Paroxysmal (convulsive) stage which is accompanied by a paroxysmal cough and lasts for another 4 to 6 weeks.

(c) Final or convalescent stage, lasting for 2 to 3 weeks.

Bord. pertussis enter the body through the upper respiratory tract and multiply in its mucosa. The blood is not invaded. These organisms liberate toxin which causes inflammation of the trachea and bronchial mucosa. This toxin stimulates the receptors in the mucous membrane and gives rise to a continuous flow of impulses to the central nervous system thus forming a stable focus of excitation. The attacks disappear when the patient changes his surroundings or residence, when the patient is taken on an air trip or when he is occupied in the games.

Children are treated with antibiotics (streptomycin, oxytetracycline, chlortetracycline), gamma globulins and vitamins and they should be exposed to fresh air.

Prophylaxis is ensured by early recognition and isolation of children with whooping cough. Specific prophylaxis is performed by vaccinating children with triple vaccine (Diphtheria, Pertussis, Tetanus — DPT vaccine).

Application to Nursing

Since the child with whooping cough expels large number of organisms by sneezing and coughing from the nose and mouth and infects other susceptible children. The nurse should apply all strict measures to check the transmission of the organisms from the infected ones to others. Even in outdoor, the close contact should be prohibited. All fomites of the patients contaminated with the sputum or vomitus should be thoroughly disinfected, as *Bord. pertussis* survive longer to be effectively transmitted by droplets, saliva etc.

Oral Spirochaetes

Borrelia vincentii is commonly present in the normal mouth in small numbers. It is anaerobic and is very difficult to grow in the laboratory. It is implicated in a painful, ulcerative disease of the gums, cheeks, and throat called "Trench Mouth", because it was common amongst military troops in the trenches during World War I. It is also known as "Vincent's angina". It is believed to be infectious disease causing a superficial gangrenous ulceration or stomatitis often with an offensive odour (oral fetor). It may be that certain vitamin deficiencies are the basic cause of the lesions in Vincent's angina and the spirochaetes then multiply in the lesion as secondary invaders or opportunists. They are always found in large number in the ulcers, associated with fusiform bacilli (*Fusobacterium fusiformis*). They can be seen under microscope as Gram-negative spirochaetes and fusiform bacilli.

The disease can be transmitted by sneezing, speaking by improperly disinfected drinking glass, eating utensils, kissing and articles that pass undisinfected from an infected mouth to another. Vigorous mouth washing with disinfectant may cure the infection. The ulcerations may cause great discomfort. In some cases, *Treponema pallidum* may occur in mouth of primary syphilis.

CHAPTER 35

RESPIRATORY VIRAL INFECTIONS

Small Pox

Small pox was known in Egypt in 3,000 B.C. In China and India, people have suffered from small pox from time immemorial. The disease swept throughout the world, becoming pandemic and it is now completely disappeared from the world. Person, reporting at present the small pox in any part of the world, will be suitably rewarded.

Morphology. Pox viruses (small pox; vaccinia; *Molluscum contagiosum*) are large enough to be seen under the light microscope. They can be cultivated on chorioallantoic membrane (CAM) (Fig. 35.1) of chick embryo and produce eosinophilic intracytoplasmic inclusion bodies. When dried and negatively stained films are examined under electron microscope, they are seen as brick-shaped particles with a dense central area.

Pathogenesis and disease in man. A source of infection is the patient. The infection takes place by the air droplet route and through contact with the infective material. The causative agent is spread by dust particles and certain objects (clothes, bed clothes and dishes) and also when the patient talks, coughs and sneezes.

Small pox virus enters the body through the upper respiratory tract; first it infects the mucosa and soon afterwards it reaches the regional lymph nodes. At this stage, the patient is not infectious. A transient viremia may follow with the infection of reticuloendothelial cells throughout the whole body. During the first 3 to 4 days of the fever, the virus multiplies in the epithelial cells of the skin, because of skin "low ceiling temperature" for growth; focal lesions are produced which give rise to the rash and progress to popular, vesicular and pustular stages. The skin rashes appear on the face, trunk and extremities. The vesicles appear as pearls. The small pox pustules have a crater-like depression at the top. From the time of appearance of the rash until all crusts disappear, the patient may be the source of virus.

Clinical small pox (variola major) is fatal, whereas variola minor (alastrim) in much less severe.

Sometimes, small pox is confused with chicken pox with its severe form with a confluent rash and the chicken pox may have some of the features of variola minor.

Immunity. Small pox leaves a lasting immunity and reinfections are extremely rare.

Vaccination. Jenner, a British physician, introduced small pox vaccination in 1798 by inoculating a boy on the arm with exudate obtained from a cow pox lesion on the hand of dairy-maid. The same principle is followed even today.

For mass vaccination, the *vaccine lymph* is usually obtained by inoculating the shaved skin of a calf or a sheep with pustular material from the skin of rabbit similarly inoculated. After 5 to 7 days, the contents of skin vesicles are harvested, homogenised and finally suspended in 50 per cent glycerol. The bacterial content is further reduced by addition of 0.4 per cent phenol.

Egg vaccine. Small pox vaccine can also be prepared by inoculating the vaccinia virus on the chorioallantoic membrane of chick embryo. This procedure can be done under sterile condition.

Tissue culture vaccine. The vaccinia virus for small pox vaccine production is propagated on the bovine or chick embryonic tissues. The sterility and potency of these vaccines are still in the process of development.

Technique of Vaccination

The *multiple pressure method* is as follows: First, the skin is cleansed with soap and water and then with alcohol and allowed to evaporate iodine solution should not be used as it kills the virus. A drop of lymph is then placed at the site of inoculation and with the help of Hagedorn needle, multiple pressures are made to the skin through the lymph. This method gives a higher success rate compared to scratch method.

Single scratch method. A single scratch method is made through the drop of lymph, the bleeding should be avoided. The lymph should be allowed to dry *in situ* and no dressing is required.

In a person *lacking immunity* a papule forms at the site of inoculation in 3 to 4 days and this becomes vesicular in 5 to 6 days and in 8 to 10 days, the vesicle becomes pustular with a zone of surrounding inflammation; finally the pustule heals with the formation of crust leaving a depressed scar.

In an immune person, there may be no reaction or a papule may appear more rapidly than in non-immune subject.

Vaccination provides a powerful defence against the risk of contracting small pox and gives a high degree of protection from the death. Generally, protection lasts for 5 to 7 years.

Application to Nursing

Small pox vaccine is essential for the protection of nurses, since they may have to care the small pox patient. When a case of small pox is diagnosed, the patient should be removed to the hospital or isolation ward. After admission, strict isolation precautions should be observed. The patient's clothings, bedding and his house should be disinfected with steam or formaldehyde vapour. All persons who were in contact with the patient during the feverish phase may be traced, vaccinated and placed under strict observations for 16 days. With the result of the microbiological laboratory investigations the first notified case may be followed back. The pustules, the oral and nasal exudates, bedding and fomites of small pox patients are highly infective, so they must be handled carefully so as to avoid the spread. Since the discharges may have a very disagreeable odour, the disinfectants (saponated solution of cresol or chloride laundry bleach which have deodorant properties) are used.

Molluscum contagiosum. Their lesions are copper-coloured waxy papules on the trunk, buttock, arms and face. This disease is spread by direct contact or by contaminated fomites. These virus particles are morphologically similar to the vaccinia virus. The acidophilic inclusion bodies crowd the host cell nucleus to one side.

CHAPTER 36

MYXOVIRUSES

Myxoviruses received their name because of their special affinity they have for mucus and they cause a variety of diseases in men and animals.

Myxoviruses are classified into

(a) *Orthomyxoviruses* (with their types A, Band C) cause *true influenza* in man.
(b) Paramyxoviruses which cause *mumps, measles* and respiratory diseases in man.

(a) Orthomyxoviruses (Influenza virus type A, B, and C) Influenza

Description. These viruses are spherical or filamentous. From the viral envelope project spikes or haemagglutinin which are protein molecules. Between these spikes, there is neuraminadase. Influenza viruses of type A were recovered from men, pigs, horses. All the strains of type A share the common antigen (S antigen), while strains of Type B share a different one. Influenza Type C is distinct from both A and B.

They remain viable in a dried state and at low temperature for longer period. They withstand exposure to glycerin for 3 months and they are killed at 65°C in 5-40 minutes. They are sensitive to drying, rapidly destroyed in both alkaline and acidic media and they are inactivated by all disinfectants and destroyed by ultraviolet irradiation.

Pathogenesis and disease in man. The virus is inhaled and penetrates the cells of the surface epithelial layer of the respiratory tract mucosa.

Influenza virus is strictly pneumotropic and multiplies only in the cells of the respiratory tract epithelium. As the virus multiplies and the infection develops, the trachea, bronchi, bronchiole and alveolar epithelial cells gradually become involved in the process. The injured ciliated epithelium loses its cilia and as a result of this becomes deprived of its defence function. It serves as a favourable medium for the penetration of secondary bacterial flora (streptococci, pneumococci, *Haemophilus influenzae* etc.) which give rise to complications (pneumonia, encephalitis, influenzal meningitis and otitis media).

Immunity. After an attack of influenza, the ensuing immunity persists for a year or more and confers resistance to the virus strain concerned.

Treatment. Recent findings indicate that L-amantadine hydrochloride is useful because it can block the entry of influenza virus and if given very early after exposure to the virus can prevent viral replication.

Transmission. Influenza virus is spread by the air droplet route. The source of infection is the influenza patient who may infect healthy people when sneezing, coughing and talking.

Influenza is highly contagious, it causes epidemics and pandemics.

Prophylaxis. Spread of infection is prevented by isolating the patient, regularly ventilating the room and cleaning the room with a damp cloth (soaked in chloramine solution). Physical exercise and sports serve to strengthen the body.

A vaccine prepared from various strains of given types of influenza is used. Liquid and dry vaccines are available as monovalent or polyvalent forms. The vaccine can be introduced intranasally or into the upper respiratory tract with a pulveriser.

(b) Paramyxoviruses (Respiratory infection; Mumps; Measles)

Although the paramyxoviruses resemble orthomyxoviruses in morphology and symmetry, they are, as a rule, larger and more pleomorphic. This group includes the parainfluenza viruses types 1 to 4 which are responsible for respiratory illness, mumps.

Resistance. They are quickly killed by heating and exposure to the action of disinfection.

Pathogenesis and disease in man. Parainfluenza virus Types 1, 2 and 3 are more frequently recovered from children suffering from upper respiratory tract lesions (rhinitis, pharyngitis and bronchitis) which are accompanied by a rise of temperature. They produce mild disease in adults.

It has been proved recently that other viruses (over 70 in numbers) may also produce acute respiratory diseases. They include the reoviruses, ECHO (Enterocytopathogenic Human Origin) viruses, rhinoviruses, coxsachie A and B viruses.

CHAPTER 37

MEASLES (RUBEOLA)

Measles is *extremely infectious and contagious* of the common fever. It is diagnosed by the development of a characteristic macular rash after a prodromal period of fever with catarrhal symptoms, conjunctivitis and the appearance of Koplik's spots on the buccal mucosa.

Morphology. Measles virus can be grown on the most suitable continuous line of amnion or chorion cell culture. It resembles the para influenza virus but it has *no neuraminadase.*

Resistance. The causative agent is very susceptible to high temperature and is quickly destroyed at

58°C outside the body it survives for not longer than 30 minutes. It is extremely sensitive to the exposure to sunlight. *Because of these properties, the disinfection is not carried out in measles.*

Pathogenesis and disease in man. Man is the only source of infection. He becomes infective from the first day of prodromal period till the fifth day after the appearance of eruption. The contagious period is 8 to 10 days. The discharged infected particles are inhaled by the new victim and enter the upper respiratory tract where it grows silently for some days in lymphoid tissue. After the maximum multiplication, many infected cells break open, the virus floods into the circulation (Viraemia) and causes the prodromal illness. During the following two to three days the virus is localised in the skin and there produces the rash. The rash often appears on the fourteenth day after exposure. Measles may attack the adults who have not had the disease previously. Children who have been given prophylactic injections of anti-measles serum or gamma globulin (human immunoglobulin) acquired a mild form of the disease.

Immunity. Measles produces high grade immunity for long duration. Reinfection hardly occurs. Individuals who had measles harbour antibodies in their blood for life.

Treatment. There is no specific treatment. In the case of complications, antibiotics (penicillin, chlortetracycline, streptomycin) are prescribed.

Prophylaxis. Sick children are not normally sent to the hospital, but they are treated at home. Only those living in the hostels or suffering from severe forms of the disease are transferred to the hospital. Children who have been in the vicinity of a measles focus and have not given gamma globulin are isolated for 17 days, while those who have received gamma globulin are isolated for 21 days. If the patient has not been isolated, segregation of healthy contacts is prolonged for a further 5 days.

Room occupied by measles patients should be well ventilated and the hygienic conditions should be maintained.

Passive immunity can be conferred on contacts by subcutaneous inoculation of human immunoglobulin. The protective effect is complete, if an adequate dose is given within 5 days of exposure; after this time, the disease may not be prevented. Immunoglobulin prepared from pooled normal human adult sera is effective in a dose of 15 mg per pound body weight.

Active immunisation. The adaptation of *Edmonston* strain of measles virus (named after the patient from whom the strain was originally isolated) to grow in chick embryo tissue culture has decreased its pathogenicity for man but retained its antigenicity (i.e., capacity to stimulate the production of antibodies). There are two types of vaccine.

(a) *Live virus vaccine.* It is similar to Sabin oral poliovaccine, but it differs from Sabin poliovaccine in that the measles live virus vaccine must be injected instead of being given orally. It is advocated to susceptible children or after the complete disappearance of maternal antibodies, but not to pregnant women or those with leukemia and other malignancies. Use of this attenuated live virus vaccine is frequently followed by such clinical reactions — fever and rash characteristic of measles. However, such reactions can be significantly reduced by simultaneous injection of measles human immunoglobulin. The immunity produced by this live virus vaccine is durable and very effective.

(b) *Killed virus vaccine.* Measles virus is grown in tissue culture and inactivated by formalin. This killed vaccine is analogous to Salk killed polio virus vaccine. This vaccine can be used when live virus vaccine is injected in three doses at 3 months intervals followed by a booster dose. It may also be used to provide a partial immunity, before giving the live virus vaccine and human immunoglobulin. Neither vaccine should be given to persons allergic to eggs if the vaccine was prepared in avian embryo.

Application to Nursing

The occurrence and spread of the infection can be prevented by good nursing. To ward off the infections of ears and lungs, the mouth and nose should be kept clean. If measles patients are treated in the wards, the most rigid precautions must be taken to prevent the spread of measles through infected droplets, saliva and other materials. Complete isolation of the patient is preferred. In an open ward, it is practically impossible to prevent the spread of measles. Since measles virus is short lived, the rigid terminal disinfection is not necessary, but for secondary invaders (streptococci, pneumococci) the terminal disinfection is of great importance. Bedding and clothings should be sterilised and the room should be cleaned with soap water and then disinfected.

CHAPTER 38

GERMAN MEASLES (RUBELLA)

Rubella or German measles is a common and mild infectious disease characterised by fever, a generalised macular rash and enlargement of the sub-occipital, post-occipital and cervical lymph nodes.

Pathogenesis and disease in man. The source of infection is man from whom the virus is transmitted in nasopharyngeal secretions borne in air or in dust. The virus is inhaled and multiplies in the mucosa of the upper respiratory tract. After an incubation period of 16 to 18 days, there is a viremic phase with fever and the localisation of the virus in the lymph nodes and skin lesions. In adults, complications are uncommon, but arthralgia and arthritis may occur.

In pregnant women, during the viremic phase of the illness, the virus is able to cross the placenta and multiply in the embryonic cells. In the first month of pregnancy, the infection of the embryo occurs most frequently; but less often in the second, third and fourth month resulting in the congenital abnormalities (deafness, congenital heart disease, persistent ductus arteriosus, venticular septal defects, chorioretinitis and cataract; mental defect; microcephaly). Deafness is most frequent. The incidence of prematurity and still-birth is also increased in women who contracted rubella during the first trimester of pregnancy. The children of mothers exposed to but not contracted clinical rubella during pregnancy show no increased frequency of malformation. One attack of the disease confers lasting immunity.

Active immunisation against rubella can be conferred by a single subcutaneous (or intranasal) inoculation of live attenuated vaccine.

The vaccines available are :

(a) *Cendehill vaccine* which was developed in Belgium by passage in primary cultures of rabbit kidney cells.

(b) The *RA 27/33 virus vaccine.* The vaccine prepared from the virus grown in the human embryonic cell line.

The Cendehill vaccine has been licensed for use in many countries, because it is more attenuated than most other virus strains, rarely produces arthritis in adult or reaction in children.

Passive immunisation of non-immune woman during the first four months of pregnancy to protect the unborn child has been recommended. Gammaglobulins (antibodies) from the blood of immune persons are used.

VARICELLA-ZOSTER

Infection with varicella-zoster (v-z) virus takes two forms. Primary infection or *chicken pox* presents a generalised skin eruption with typical vesicular lesions and occurs most often in children, whereas Zoster or shingles is a localised vesicular eruption confined to one or a few areas of skin surface and affects adults.

Morphology. Both viruses are biologically and serologically identical. They produce Cowdry Type A intranuclear inclusion bodies. Human amnion and embryonic lung cultures are now most frequently used for the detection of the virus.

Resistance. Chicken pox virus is unstable in the external environment and dies quickly and for this reason the disinfection is not carried out.

Pathogenesis and disease in man. Varicella is common in children. It is characterised by a vesicular skin eruption.The earliest manifestation is a maculopapular rash that progresses in a few hours to a vesicular stage. The vesicles are characteristically surrounded by a red rim, the lesions then rupture and crust on may become secondarily infected and pustular before healing. The lesions are most frequent on the trunk, neck and proximal areas of the limbs. Crops of vesicles appear over 2-5 days.

Varicella may vary from a mild disease with only a few scattered skin lesions to a severe febrile illness with a widespread skin rash particularly in adults.

In large proportion of adult patients with varicella a primary atypical pneumonia follows the rash. The patient is infectious from the last day of incubation to the time the crusts fall off. Since the virus is extremely sensitive to the action of environmental factors, the infection takes place only in closed premises (apartments, child and medical institutions).

Before the appearance of rash, the following symptoms are observed; rise of temperature; chills; loss of appetite; sometimes vomiting and diarrhea, uncomplicated cases of chicken pox normally terminate in recovery. Some cases become fatal due to secondary infection.

Immunity remains for life and reinfection is rare. *Treatment and Prophylaxis.* There is no specific therapy. Antibiotics are prescribed for prevention of secondary infection. The lesions are treated with a 1 per cent alcoholic solution of brilliant green or with 10 per cent potassium permanganate solution. The patient is not hospitalised but isolated at home, until the crusts fall off. In medical institution, all child contacts are injected with human immunoglobulins. Individuals who have not suffered from chicken pox in the past should not be allowed to go to the children's institutions for three weeks.

Zoster is localised disease, usually unilateral and confined to one or more areas of skin surface and affects mostly adults. The vesicles are usually distributed along the course of intercostal nerves and eruption is accompanied by a burning sensation, pruritus, neuralgia and sometimes by a rise of temperature. The vesicles contain clear fluid. Eruption is of variable size. In a number of cases, the lesions may become confluent and resemble a continuous girdle (thus the term zoster which means a girdle or encircling structure).

The clinical picture is diverse. There can be an extremely severe complication when the eyes are involved (iritis, ulceration, keratitis, retinal detachment etc.).

No age group is free from herpes zoster, particularly children younger than 10 years of age are vulnerable.

The disease leaves high grade and lasting immunity and reinfection is rare. Treatment is symptomatic. The affected areas are treated with an alcoholic solution of brilliant green. Novocain, morphine etc. are prescribed for releiving pain. Antibiotics (tetracycline, penicillin) are recommended for the prevention of the secondary infection. Acyclovir (ACV reduced the morbidity and mortality associated with herpes virus infection particularly Herpes Simplex (HS and Varicella-Zoster (VZV) virus infection. This discovery has opened a new chapter on antiviral chemotherapy.

Prophylaxis is ensured by isolation and by observing quarantine requirements.

CHAPTER 39

EPIDEMIC PAROTITIS (MUMPS) VIRUS

Mumps is an acute contagious disease characterised by a large painful swelling of one or both parotid glands. Mumps is known from ancient time and was one of the first infections described by Hippocrates. The name is derived from the numbling speech which is result of the pain on moving the jaw. Usually, there is a constitutional reaction and other glands (testes, pancreas, parotids) are involved.

Pathogenesis and disease in man. The parotitis virus causes fever and inflammation of the parotid, sublingual and submandibular glands. The disease is prevalent amongst children. Mumps is a very contagious disease. Severe cases are accompanied by viremia. In addition to parotitis, the virus penetrates other organs and produces orchitis and meningitis. Complications are polyneuritis, paresis of facial and auricular nerves, impairment of hearing and visual disturbance.

Immunity. It is life long immunity after the disease is produced.

Treatment. Drugs (corticosteroids and gamma globulins) are prescribed for symptomatic treatment. These drugs reduce the severity of the disease but do not prevent the development of meningitis and orchitis.

Prophylaxis. Isolation of patients until they recover. Patients are discharged from the hospitals only when all clinical manifestations of the disease have disappeared. The disinfection is not required. Specific prophylaxis is by injection of gamma globulins and a vaccination with a live vaccine prepared from a strain of Mumps virus which has lost its pathogenicity as a result of passage on chick embryo. It is inoculated intracutaneously in a single dose.

Rhinovirus

The viral nature of contagious rhinitis (common cold) was known more than 50 years ago. Rhinovirus can be cultivated in human kidney culture. It is identical with enterovirus in size, resistance to ether and in the non-pathogenicity for suckling mice.

CHAPTER 40

ANTERIOR POLIOMYELITIS (Infantile paralysis)

Although poliomyelitis is primarily an infection of gastrointestinal tract (i.e., one of the enterovirus), poliomyelitis virus is also present in the respiratory (pharyngeal) secretions of many patients for several days before the onset of the symptoms. The respiratory (pharyngeal) secretion of patients in early stage is highly infectious.

Application to Nursing

Precautions described for diseases of respiratory tract are also applicable for proper handling of respiratory secretions.

CHAPTER 41

PSITTACOSIS OR ORNITHOSIS

Previously called Psittacosis — Lymphogranuloma venereum — Trachoma group (PLT organisms) or the TRIC group (Trachoma — Inclusion Conjunctivitis organisms) are included in the family chlamydiae.

Morphology. These organisms are small, non-motile, Gram negative, obligate, intracellular parasites which have two forms of cells : Small and large forms.

Cultivation. They can be cultivated in chick embryo or in mice and tumour cells.

Psittacosis (Gr. *Psittakes*, Psittacine) or Ornithosis (Gr. *ornis*, bird) is acquired by inhalation of infected aerosols or dust from birds during handling chickens, pigeons, geese, turkeys etc., while killing, plucking or cleaning for the table. The incubation period is ten days and the illness ranges from influenza-like syndrome with general malaise, fever, anorexia, rigor, sore throat, headache, photophobia to a severe illness with delirium and pneumonia with consolidation similar to bronchopneumonia and the sputum is scanty. Pneumonia foci are accompanied by dyspnoea, cough and pain in the chest and characteristic of Ornithosis. X-ray reveals lobar pneumonia.

In short, the clinical picture of Ornithosis is similar to that of atypical pneumonia, influenza, typhoid fever, typhus fever, lobar and catarrhal pneumonia and Q fever. Infection from person to person by air droplet route is also possible.

Resistance is very high. They survive for longer period in desication state and at low temperature. At - 70°C, they remain viable for two years. They are killed by heating at 60°C - 70°C in 10-15 minutes. They are sensitive to common disinfectants.

Immunity is of short duration and the reinfection is possible.

Treatment. Chortetracycline, oxytetracycline and streptomycin are effective.

Application to Nursing

Just after early diagnosis by the physician, the patient should be sent to isolation ward and hospitalisation. Nurses should wear masks and regularly wash hands with 0.5 per cent chloramine solution; patients should be discharged only after complete recovery. Premises and patients' clothings should be disinfected. The patients' sputum should be disinfected with 4 per cent chloramine solution; 5 per cent calcium chloride; 0.5 per cent potassium hydroxide or sodium hydroxide and 5 per cent solution of lysol.

RABIES (Hydrophobia)

Rabies may also be included in this section on diseases transmitted via respiratory tract, since it is transmitted like Mumps via respiratory secretions in saliva.

Rabies is primarily a disease of animals caused by neurotropic virus. It is dreaded viral zoonotic disease known to mankind since antiquity before 2,300 B.C. It has been reported that over 3 million persons are bitten annually by dogs in India. Over 30,000 Indians die of Rabies every year. It is incurable but preventable by immunoprophylaxis.

Rabies virus is bullet shaped. It forms eosinophilic intracytoplasmic inclusion bodies in the nerve cells of the hippocampus — known as "Negri bodies", which are specific in rabies infection and enable a diagnosis of rabies. Rabies virus is more resistant to disinfectants : 0.5 per cent formaldehyde fails to kill in two months at 4°C; but 1 per cent formaldehyde, 3 per cent cresol and 0.1 per cent mercuric chloride inactivate in 15 minutes; also it is inactivated at 60°C in 10-15 minutes. It is destroyed by a 5 per cent phenol solution and other disinfectants.

Pathogenesis and disease in man. The portal of entry is the bite and the rabies virus in the infected saliva is introduced into the wound or scratch or abrasion contaminated by saliva. The virus multiplies locally in the tissues, invades the damaged nerve fibres and spreads centrally to reach the brain and spinal cord.

The incubation period is ten days to two years after the bite of rabid animals, its duration depends on the distance between the point of entry and the brain; bite on the legs, 60 days; on the arm, 40 days on the head, 30 days. It is short in children than in adults.

The first symptoms of the disease are headache, fever, a profound sense of apprehension and a feeling of irritation at the site of the bite. The patients complain of a dry throat, but they will not drink. High fever, difficulty in swallowing and a fear of water (hydrophobia) become dominant symptoms and the patient passes into delirium with generalised convulsion. The outcome is invariably death.

Vaccine

Passive immunisation. In case of severe bites, anti-rabies serum or hyperimmune horse serum is injected for passive protection of around the bite wounds.

Active immunisation, various vaccines are used to confer active immunity.

1. *Semple Vaccine* which contains a 4 per cent suspension of the brain of sheep infected with the "fixed virus" inactivated by 0.5 per cent phenol. This vaccine has a drawback that it may contain nervous tissue which may sensitise a small proportion (1 : 4,000 to 1 : 10,000) of person who may develop an allergic type of encephalitis.

2. *Avianised Vaccine* contains no nerve tissue, it avoids the neuroparalytic accidents. The inactivated duck embryo vaccine was first introduced in United

States of America and is mainly used in Britain and is less effective than brain tissue or tissue culture vaccine.

A similar vaccine prepared from Rabies virus grown in primary chick embryo cell culture and purified to remove cell proteins and nucleic acids has been recently made available in India through Hoechst India Ltd., Mumbai. It is given intramuscularly one dose (1 ml) in the deltoid muscle of alternate arms on days of 0, 3, 7, 14, 30 and 90 days. O indicates the day of the first dose.

3. Human diploid cell vaccine (HDCV) is recently used for immunoprophylaxis without side effects. This vaccine is prepared from rabies virus grown in human diploid cells. Chloroquine was found to decrease the immunogenicity of Rabies vaccine when the two are given concurrently.

Hantaan Virus causes the clinically severe form of Hemorrhagic fever with renal syndrome (HFRS) called Korean haemorrhagic fever in Korea and epidemic hemorrhagic fever in the People's Republic of China; while clinically milder disease called nephropathia epidemica, which occurs throughout Europe, is caused by Puumala virus. Multiple species of rodents serve as the natural reservoir of hanta an viruses and humans are primarily infected by respiratory route.

Application to Nursing

All possible precautions should be taken to prevent the entrance of virus, present in the saliva, into the cuts, wounds or scratches on the nurses' or physicians' hands or face by wearing gloves or masks. Affectionate licking of rabid pet dog should be avoided. The wound should be thoroughly cleaned and washed with 20 per cent soap water or painted with tincture of iodine. These measures may not exclude the vaccination.

Unit B
PATHOGENS TRANSMITTED FROM THE INTESTINAL AND/OR URINARY TRACT

Transmission of enteric and food-borne pathogens

Human intestinal tract contains millions of pathogenic and non-pathogenic microorganisms. Thus, the excreta of healthy or diseased individuals

SYMPTOMS, CAUSES AND MANAGEMENT OF UPPER RESPIRATORY TRACT

Condition	*Symptoms*	*Causes*	*Management*
Pharyngitis (including tonsillitis)	Last 5-10 days; painful throat, fever.	70% viral (as in coryza and measles, herpes simplex, infectious mononucleosis); 30% bacterial (haemolytic streptococcus, pneumococcus, haemophilus).	Hot drinks, Paracetamol, Penicillin V, if severe; Erythromycin, if allergic to Penicillin.
Coryza	Last 5-14 days; blocked/runny nose; clear/purulent nasal discharge, headache, fever, sneezing.	Rhinovirus, adenovirus, coronavirus, influenza virus, parainfluenza virus, respiratory syncytial virus.	Paracetamol oral/topical decongestant.
Sinusitis	Last 7-21 days or longer; sinus pain, purulent nasal discharge, fever, headache, other underlying irritable airways.	Coryza virus, haemophilus, pneumococcus, Moraxella catarrhalis.	Steam, Paracetamol, Amoxycillin/Doxycycline short term decongestant, long term steroid spray/ solution if underlying perennial / allergic rhinitis.

constitute the principle source of one or many species of virus, bacteria, protozoa or helminths. Sometimes, some pathogens may be excreted in the infected urine (*Escherichia coli*, Proteus, Pseudomonas) which may be transmitted to others by drinking water polluted by this infected urine. Feces or urine from the infected persons may be the primary source for (a) drinking water to be polluted through the sewage, (dysentery); (b) even *food* can act as vector for food borne diseases (cholera, bacillary and amoebic dysentery).

The following are the food borne pathogens :

(a) Family *Enterobacteriaceae* (Salmonella, Shigella);

(b) Family *Bacillaceae* (Clostridium);

(c) Family *Micrococcaceae* (Staphylococcus, Streptococcus);

(d) Family *Brucellaceae* (Brucella);

(e) Family *Mycobacteriaceae* (*Mycobacterium tuberculosis*, bovine or human type);

(f) *Enterovirus* (epidemic hepatitis virus)

(g) Protozoa (*Entamoeba histolytica*)

(h) Helminths (roundworm)

Pathogenic bacteria may grow in the improperly refrigerated or cooked food and may cause (1) Food infection, and (2) Food poisoning or both.

Food infection is due to the intake of bacteria along with the food (i.e., Typhoid fever due to *Sal. typhi*. The symptoms of food infection usually begin from 18 hours to several days after the ingestion of the infected food. During this time (incubation period), the organisms grow sufficiently to liberate the toxin responsible for the symptoms of the disease (Typhoid fever).

Food poisoning. Persons suffer from food poisoning because of the consumption of preformed toxin by bacteria in food, i.e., toxin already produced outside the body in the food. In true food poisoning, there is no infection. In contrast to food infection, the symptoms of food poisoning generally develop within 12 hours or less, because the toxin which causes the symptoms is *already formed* in the food.

1. Food infection

The principle sources of infection are

(a) Infected animals;

(b) Infected food handlers or cooks; and

(c) Pathogens in the food.

(a) *Infected animals.* Food may be infected by two ways :

(i) animal (rat or mouse) may pollute the food with their excreta.

Sal. typhimurium causes septicaemic lymphoid-like infection in the natural host (rat or mouse). Excreta of the infected mice may therefore infect the food with *Sal. typhimurium* which after ingestion causes in man "typical food poisoning". Characterised by vomiting, abdominal pain and diarrhea.

Flesh from infected animal used as food. Milk and milk products from tuberculous cattle may be highly infectious. Flesh and milk of cattle with brucella infection may cause human brucellosis. *Sal. typhi*, causal agent of typhoid fever, found in oysters and other seafoods from sewage polluted fishing ground may be infected with *Sal. typhi*. If these infected foods are eaten, *Sal. typhi* found in them may cause typhoid fever. Ingestion of larva of *Trichinella spiralis* in the flesh of infected animal can cause trichinellosis in man. Thorough cooking may make these foods safer. Rats can transmit in the urine leptospira which causes leptospirosis or Weil's disease (hemorrhagic jaundice) in man.

(b) *Infected carriers.* The hands or forearms of food handlers or cooks can be soiled by saliva droplets containing the organisms of common colds, influenza, scarlet fever, diphtheria or tuberculosis or by toxin producing staphylococci in the respiratory secretions. Pimples or boils on the forearms of the cooks may contaminate the food. Besides sneezing, talking and coughing over the unwrapped food displayed in open cases in the restaurants and handling foods with soiled hands may infect the food.

Food handlers may be carriers of intestinal pathogens (infectious hepatitis virus, salmonella, shigella, and cysts of *Entamoeba histolytica*) on the hands.

(c) *Pathogens in the foods.* Possible pathogens (*Proteus* sp., *Clostridium welchii, Pseudomonas aeruginosa, Streptococcus faecalis* may grow in the food and decompose it. Some of the products of decomposition of food may cause irritation of the intestine causing gastroenteritis.

2. Food poisoning

Bacterial food poisoning is due to toxin liberated in the food during their growth in the food, *not in the patient*:

(a) Staphylococcal food poisoning due to *preformed* enterotoxin produced in the food.
(b) *Botulism* caused by *Cl. botulinum.*
(c) *Cl. welchii* food poisoning due to toxin of some strain of *Cl. welchii.*
(d) Ptomaine poisoning.

(a) *Staphylococcal food poisoning. Staph. aureus* are Gram-positive cocci arranged in clusters. They are most pathogenic and produce an enzyme called coagulase which causes citrated blood plasma to coagulate. In addition to this enzyme, they produce also a *potent toxin* in the improperly precooked food outside the body. Later, it is called enterotoxin as it acts on the intestinal mucosa.

Enterotoxin is an intestinal toxin formed by 30-50 per cent of strains of *Staph. aureus.* It is heat stable and withstands an exposure at 100°C for a few minutes; when ingested the food in which *Staph. aureus* was growing profusely and producing toxin; this enterotoxin causes nausea, vomiting and diarrhea within 6 hours, which is called *Staphylococcal food poisoning.* Five types of enterotoxin — A to E — are produced. Staphylococcal food poisoning is rarely fatal.

(b) *Botulism* is caused by *Cl. botulinum.* This causal agent is strictly anaerobic, Gram-positive bacillus. It bears oval, subterminal bulging spore. It is motile and has no capsule. It is widely distributed saprophytic organism in the soil, on the vegetable fruits, leaves, produces preformed toxin (*neurotoxin* in food). Its spores withstand moist heat at 100°C for several hours. Insufficient heating in the process of preserving foods is an important factor in the causation of botulism. Thus sufficient heating should be achieved in all parts of the can or tin food in canning factories. The appearance, taste, odour of the food is often deceiving.

Human cases of botulism originate after ingestion of variety of preserved spoiled foods (ham, sausage, home canned meat, fish, vegetable etc.). The intoxication follows absorption from the intestine of toxin preformed by this bacillus in the food, but there may be also some formation of a powerful exotoxin by the organism after ingestion. This toxin is destroyed at a temperature of 80°C for 30-40 minutes. The estimated lethal dose of this potent toxin for one mouse is 0.000000033 mg. In other words, one kilogram of this potent toxin may kill the world population. It appears that this toxin interferes with the mechanism of acetylcholine release from the endings of the motor nerve cells of parasympathetic system.

The early clinical symptoms may suggest a coronary thrombosis. The neurotoxic signs and symptoms are vertigo, oculomotor and pharyngeal paralysis, difficulty in speech, swallowing and breathing, loss of voice (aphonia). Death due to respiratory failure occurs a few days after the onset of symptoms, because of the thoracic muscle involvement.

(c) *Cl. welchii food poisoning. Cl. welchii* is Gram positive bacillus and bears subterminal spore. In contrast to *Cl. botulinum,* it is non-motile and is capsulated. It is distributed in soil, faeces. Strains of *Cl. welchii* conforming in most respects to type A, but producing non-haemolytic or feebly haemolytic colonies on horse blood agar and strains which do not produce *theta toxin* are associated with a mild form of food poisoning. The exact mechanism of *Cl. welchii* food poisoning is not well understood, but it depends upon the ability of the food poisoning producing strains to produce an enterotoxic exotoxin. Ingestion of large number of viable organisms in the contaminated food is necessary for the production of typical food poisoning in man. Typical symptoms are abdominal cramps starting after 8 to 12 hours after ingestion, followed by diarrhea. Fever and vomiting are not typically encountered. The condition is usually transient and normally subsides within 24-48 hours.

Cl. welchii food poisoning may be avoided by clean preparation of food and by prompt eating, or refrigeration of freshly prepared foods. In preparing canned foods, the same precaution should be taken as in the prevention of botulism.

Ptomaine poisoning. Ptomaines are products of protein decomposition that liquefies the food, which is offensive to sight, taste and olfactory sense. Such putrified matter is never accepted as food. Acute gastroenteritis associated with ptomaine poisoning does not simulate the symptoms of botulism.

Prevention of food infection and food poisoning

Cooking. Cooking may or may not prevent food infection and food poisoning, because vegetative cells of *Cl. botulism, Cl. welchii, Staph. aureus,* Salmonella, Shigella, *Vibrio cholerae* and *Cl. welchii* are all inactivated by boiling (100°C) for 10 minutes. Spores of *Cl. botulinum* will survive oven baking and steam pressure cooking (autoclaving) unless prolonged at high temperature. Spores of *Cl. welchii* are also very thermostable. *Staph. aureus* enterotoxin will resist boiling for one hour or more.

Because of the variable effect of cooking on bacterial cells and spore, food to be eaten uncooked should be selected with care. Never eat or serve food kept open or handled in warm place for more than 4 hours. The organisms will not grow in acid foods, dry foods (salted nuts and cookie) but will multiply in gravies, in cheese, cream, bread or rice pudding.

Refrigeration. Efficient and prompt refrigeration of foods just after preparation prevents the bacterial spoilage and growth of harmful bacteria which entered into the food during handling. Sterilised babies' bottles can be refrigerated with complete safety.

Freezing is another method of inhibiting the growth of microorganisms. Frozen foods are not necessarily sterile; but most will keep for months or years; because all the metabolic activities of microorganisms are stopped. Medicines in solution are liable to deterioration or microbial spoilage are preserved by freezing and refrigeration (caution : Aqueous fluids may break glass containers on freezing).

Supervision of food handlers. Before appointing food handlers or cooks in hotels, restaurants, they should be examined for general cleanliness, enteric infections, the presence of boils or sores due to staphylococci or diphtheria, tuberculosis or syphilis. The person harbouring infectious disease organisms should not be allowed to handle the food in the kitchen or drinking place. The hands should always be washed thoroughly before preparing or serving the food. After blowing the nose and after using the toilet the hands should be well washed.

Proper dishwashing. The method of proper dishwashing has great bacteriological importance and it is of no use from the standpoint of preventive medicine and public health, but it is too common a practice. Washing dishes in a pan of lukewarm water with a dirty mop with a detergent or soap water merely distributes the bacteria over them, but it will not destroy them.

Hand dishwashing. The proper hand dishwashing of spoons, forks, cups and glasses with plenty of *scalding water* with detergent is essential. After hand dishwashing, the dishes should be rinsed in a basin of cool, clean water containing 50 parts per million of free chlorine. Alternatively, the dishes can be dipped in boiling water for 5 minutes. Organisms associated with pneumonia, diphtheria, tuberculosis, Vincent's angina, scarlet fever, sore throat, influenza can be transmitted from one person's mouth to another's by poorly washed hands or forks.

Machine dish washer is a very effective method and much hotter water can be used. Dishes and utensils of the patient should be *boiled* so to prevent the transmission of the disease by saliva and sputum.

Milk-borne disease. Tuberculous cows excrete *Mycobacterium tuberculosis* bovine type through their milk. Rabies virus, *Coxiella burnetti* and Brucella organisms are disseminated through the milk of infected cows. *Strept. pyogenes* causing septic sore throat and scarlet fever may gain entrance into the milk directly from the infected persons who handle the milk or indirectly by means of cow's udder infected by infected milker. Since cows are not normally infected by shigella, salmonella, and diphtheria bacilli, these bacilli may find their way into the milk after it has been drawn. Milk kept in warm place is the best medium for the growth of microorganisms except *C. burnetti* and possibly *Mycobacterium tuberculosis* bovine type. Milk from mastitis (infected udder) cases due to *Staph. aureus* may contain preformed toxin (enterotoxin) causing severe food poisoning in man, in spite of pasteurisation, since staphylococcal enterotoxin is heat stable.

Pasteurisation. Both holder method (62°C for 30 minutes) and flash method (80°C for 15-30 seconds) or high temperature, short time (HTST) process can kill all pathogenic microorganisms in dairy products. Many harmless bacteria may survive, so pasteurisation disinfects but does not sterilise. So, after pasteurisation, the milk should be refrigerated promptly and bottled under hygienic conditions.

CHAPTER 42

SALMONELLOSIS, SHIGELLOSIS AND ESCHERICHIA COLI

Family Enterobacteriacae include many interrelated bacteria; few are saprophytic and found in soil and water; some of which are common inhabitants of intestine of men and animals, while others are the causative agents of salmonellosis (typhoid and paratyphoid fever - enteric fever); shigellosis (bacillary dysentery); gastroenteritis in children or infantile diarrhoea and urinary tract infection (*Escherichia coli* and Proteus). All of which are Gram-negative rods, either motile with peritrichous flagella or non-motile. They are non-sporing and grow on ordinary media; all ferment glucose rapidly with or without gas production and reduce nitrates to nitrites.

The family can be divided into the following genera :

(a) Genus Salmonella

Species			
1. S. *typhi* — causes typhoid			enteric fever (Salmonellosis)
2. S. *paratyphi* A	cause paratyphoid		
3. S. *paratyphi* B			
4. S. *paratyphi* C			
5. S. *typhimurium*	causes bacterial food poisoning.		

(b) Genus Shigella

Species	
1. *Sh. dysenteriae*	cause bacillary dysentery (shigellosis)
2. *Sh. flexneri*	
3. *Sh. boydii*	
4. *Sh. sonnei*	

(c) Genus Escherichia

Species. 1. *Esch. coli*

(d) Genus Proteus

Species	
1. *Pr. vulgaris*	cause urinary tract infection.
2. *Pr. mirabilis*	
3. *Pr. morganii*	
4. *Pr. rettgeri*	

SALMONELLA

It is now well established that the genus Salmonella comprises more than 1,000 serotypes which are mainly parasites of animals (*S. typhi* and its cousin, the three paratyphoid bacilli are essentially parasites of man).

Bacterial food poisoning is more commonly caused by ingestion of foods contaminated with any of the numerous serotypes of the genus Salmonella : *S. typhimurium, S. dublin, S. heidelberg, S. enteritidis, S. newport, S. infantis, S. thompson.* These serotypes cause primarily septicaemic disease in animals (natural host), but they cause food poisoning in man (unnatural host). Symptoms are vomiting, abdominal pain and diarrhea. The severity of diarrhoea varies from the very slight, i.e., passage of one or two loose stools which may be disregarded by the patient, to a violent diarrhoea.

The carcass or animal products, e.g., cooked meat, eggs or milk of naturally infected domestic animals are the commonest sources of food poisoning infection. Flesh may be infected when an ill, septicaemic animal is slaughtered. More commonly uninfected meat or carcass may be infected in the abattoir by a human case or carrier.

Control measures. In an endeavour to reduce the incidence of food poisoning, two basic principles must be followed :

1. raw foodstuffs which are partially contaminated must never have contact, either direct or indirect, with cooked meat;
2. if a foodstuff is contaminated with salmonellae, it should be treated or held under temperature conditions which prevent the organisms growing, i.e., either under refrigeration or at sufficiently high. temperature and then consumed immediately.

ENTERIC FEVER

Enteric fever includes both Typhoid and Paratyphoid which are clinically similar. The word "Typhoid" is derived from "Typhoid Mary"— a cook in a restaurant in England was a carrier of *S. typhi* and transmitted to the community. Typhoid is caused by *S. typhi* and paratyphoid by *S. paratyphi.*

A significant endemic level of infection with *S. typhi* persists in the warm climate. *S. paratyphi* A is frequently endemic in Eastern Europe, America and India; *S. paratyphi* C as a cause of paratyphoid fever in Eastern Europe and Asia.

Morphologically, members of the genus Salmonella cannot be distinguished from each other and from other members of the family.

Enterobacteriacae. They are motile, non-capsulated. On differential or selective media, MacConkey, Desoxycholate citrate agar (DCA) media, the colonies are pale coloured, i.e., they are non-lactose fermenters, similar to Shigella.

Pathogenesis and disease in man. Natural infection in the enteric fever is mostly by ingestion of contaminated water or foods. *S. typhi* penetrates the mucous membrane of the small intestine and submucosa where they are phagocytosed by polymorphs and multiply in them, kill and escape. The organisms pass via the lymphatics to the mesenteric lymph nodes. After a period of multiplication, they invade the blood stream via the thoracic duct; the blood culture is positive; Staphylococcal slide coagglutination test appears to be rapid and simple to diagnose Typhoid fever in the first week when culture facilities are lacking.

Latex agglutination test for rapid diagnosis of Typhoid fever is more useful and sensitive to patients with prior history of antibiotic therapy; the liver, gall bladder, spleen, kidney and bone marrow become infected during the primary bacteriaemic phase in the first 7-10 days of incubation period. After multiplication in these organs, bacilli pass into the blood causing secondary bacteriaemia. During this secondary phase, pyrexia and other clinical signs develop - Widal test (serological test) or slide Salmonella agglutination test is positive in the second week of the infection. In second and fourth week, *S. typhi* may appear in the urine (bacteriuria) and stools; sometimes it may be present in the stool from first to fourth week; from the gall bladder, a further invasion of the intestine takes place as a result Peyer's patches and lymphoid follicles are involved. They become inflammed and infiltration with mononuclear cells followed by necrosis, sloughing and formation of typical "typhoid ulcer" with haemorrhage. In severe complicated cases, there is perforation through a necrotic Peyer's patch leading to peritonitis.

Fever and illness continue for 3-4 weeks. Temperature shows a step ladder rise over the first week of the illness, remains at 39.5 to 40°C for 7-10 days and then falls by lysis during the third and fourth week. The symptoms are headache, body pain, loss of appetite. The bowels may be constipated or loose, abdominal bloating and discomfort may occur. Dry cough and nose bleeding are occasional features. It is important to exclude malaria, tuberculosis and other generalised illness which mimic typhoid. If untreated, the fever rises unabated, and the patient becomes dehydrated. Either delirium or stupor may supervene and the patient may go into coma. In very few cases, bleeding into the gut or perforation of the gut may occur, giving rise to pain, a fall in blood pressure and shock. Otherwise, slowly abate and the fever comes down in a month. Severe weakness during the period of convalesance and temporary loss of hair are feared sequelae. A pregnant woman affected by typhoid may abort in third and fourth month.

Epidemiology. Typhoid remains a disease that is several hundred times more common in India; than in the developed world. It is not notifiable disease in India. It is estimated that during the rainy season, typhoid outbreaks are common.

The reasons for its wide prevalence in India are lack of proper sanitation and effective sewage disposal, faecal pollution of soil and drinking water and improper personal hygiene as well as food and kitchen hygiene.

Typhoid can be contracted from two types of persons — a patient suffering from the disease and from a *carrier* who is healthy but harbours the bacteria in his body.

S. typhi is usually excreted in the faeces. Faecal contamination of food, milk, drinking water or our own hands help the bacteria to enter the intestine and spread into the body. Flies too are potent disease spreading agents as the bacteria survive in them throughout their life time of 20 days. In water, *S. typhi* can live for more than couple of days, whilst in moist soil it can live up to 2 months. Thus vegetables grown in such soil, if improperly cooked and eaten, can lead to typhoid. Milk is another medium in which the bacteria can multiply without altering its taste and appearance. Typhoid bacilli are easily killed by heat, drying, boiling, chlorination and other disinfectants; it however resists the freezing, so ice-cream is a dangerous source of the spread of typhoid.

Treatment. Antibiotics are the corner-stone of typhoid treatment. Chloramphenicol introduced four decades ago still remains the drug of choice though bacterial resistance to it is being reported to now-a-days. The fever takes two to four days to come down, but the drug should be taken for at least two weeks. Because of a rare risk of suppression of blood formation associated with the use of chloramphenicol, some physician prefers ampicillin, amoxycillin or cotrimoxazole (Septran or Bactrim); these drugs however take a longer time to bring down the fever. *S. typhi* resistant to these drugs are sensitive to latest newer antibiotics (floxacin, norfloxacin or ciprofloxacin). Corticosteroids are not advisable except in severe illness with high fever and altered consciousness. Furazolidine is also effective against chloramphenicol resistant *S. typhi.*

A few patients have a relapse of typhoid especially if they use the drug irregularly. Treatment of a relapse is as for the first attack. On the other hand, a few persons, who have recovered from the illness, continue to excrete the bacteria. Such carriers must be detected. Some carriers need removal of the gall bladder which may be harbouring *S. typhi.* Carriers (as cooks, waiters etc.) must not be allowed to come into contact with food and observe routine measures of hygiene and sanitation.

Prophylaxis.

1. Personal hygiene;
2. Proper cooking methods;
3. Disinfection or boiling of drinking water;
4. Avoiding eating out during the rainy season and at the time of epidemics.

Immunity. One attack of typhoid gives fairly lasting immunity. Heat killed TAB (*S. typhi, S. paratyphi* A and *S. paratyphi* B) Vaccine given in two doses, gives a seventy five per cent protection against typhoid for three years, after which a booster dose may be given. Another live vaccine which claims 100 per cent protection is under trial.

"Porin", isolated from the outer membrane of *S. typhi* at Madurai Kamaraj University, Immunology department, India (Chennai) is a protein with immense potential in the prevention and diagnosis of typhoid, which is under experimentation.

The oral live attenuated typhoid vaccine *S. typhi* Ty 21a provides a relatively effective, safe and more expeditions alternative to the traditional parenterally administrated killed *S. typhi* vaccine.

SHIGELLOSIS

Bacillary dysentery. Dysentery or bloody flux, known clinically since biblical time, is characterised by the frequent passage of stools mixed with blood and mucus, pus and caused by the genus shigella. It is also prevalent in many countries with temperate climate.

The genus Shigella (Dysentery bacilli) is one of the several genera in the large family enterobacteriacae. The shigellae are Gram-negative bacilli very similar to other enterobacteria; but they are non-motile and non-capsulate. On MacConkey or Desoxychocolate citrate agar (DCA), they are lactose non-fermenters; hence they form "Pale" colonies similar to the genus Salmonella. They can be differentiated from Salmonella, since Salmonella are motile, produce gas and acid in sugar solution, Triple Sugar Iron (TSI) agar. There are four species of Shigella : *Sh. dysenteriae, Sh. flexneri, Sh. boydii, Sh. sonnei.*

The first species, *Sh. dysenteriae*, was discovered and described by a Japanese physician, Shiga; similar type, later discovered in Europe, was called as *Sh. ambiguae* or Schmitz bacillus. Another type was discovered by American physician, Flexner, in 1906 and named as Flexner dysentery bacillus or *Sh. flexneri.* Still another type common in United States first discovered by Duval and described by Sonne is now called as Sonne dysentery bacillus (*Sh. sonnei*). Later on British worker, Boyd, first discovered *Sh. sonnei.*

Resistance. Dysentery bacilli live in the external environment for a period of 5-10 days (in soil, food stuffs, water, on objects, plates and dishes). Direct sunlight and a 1 percent phenol solution destroy the organisms in 10 minutes. The bacilli are easily killed by treatment with chloramine and calcium chloride solutions. *Sh. dysenteriae* are most sensitive to physical and chemical factors to which *Sh. sonnei* are relatively resistant.

Dysentery bacilli may acquire resistance to drugs (sulphonamides, antibiotics) and to ionising radiations. Dependal, Amicline plus are drugs of choice for treatment.

Transmission. Dysentery bacilli are transmitted by the faecal-oral route as typhoid, that is by faeces, fingers, flies, milk, foods by other objects contaminated with the faeces of a patient or carrier. Waterborne epidemics of bacillary dysentery are less common than those of typhoid. Shigella species are not commonly found in animals.

Pathogenesis and disease in man. People suffering from acute and chronic dysentery as well as carriers are source of infection. Infection takes place through the mouth by ingestion of contaminated food stuffs and water, by contaminated hands, house flies and other objects. Dysentery bacilli are confined to the intestinal mucosa and submucosal layer where they multiply and do not invade the blood. The infected epithelial cells are killed and lamina propria and submucosa develop an inflammatory reaction with capillary thrombosis. Patches of necrotic epithelium are sloughed and ulcers form. There is polymorphonuclear cell infiltration.

Sh. dysenteriae is usually associated with a severe abdominal pain, tenesmus, pyrexia, prostration and, sometimes, convulsions, the stools loose their usual faecal character, are small and frequent and are composed mainly of fresh stool, pus and mucus. The illness associated with *Sh. sonnei* is mild and confined to the passage of few loose stools with abdominal discomfort. The illness due to *Sh. flexneri* and *Sh. boydii* is more severe than the Sonne dysentery. Death due to bacillary dysentery is uncommon.

Laboratory diagnosis. Diagnosis of bacillary dysentery in the laboratory is similar to that of typhoid, except the blood culture, since dysentery bacilli do not invade the blood stream. Repeated stool examination is necessary. Since Shigella are fragile, the responsible nurse should have knowledge that stool specimens should be transported in glycerosaline transport medium.

Control of the disease is ensured by a complex of general and specific measures :

1. Hospitalisation of patients or their isolation at home with observance of the required regimes.
2. Thorough disinfection of sources of disease.
3. Adequate treatment of patients with highly effective antibiotics and use of chemotherapy.
4. Babies should be kept away from the patient of bacillary dysentery.
5. A person caring for a child with summer diarrhea should not cook the food for other children or adults.
6. The diapers of infants suffering from diarrhoea should be disinfected at once by placing in a bucket of full of 2 per cent saponated cresol or other good disinfectant.
7. Old linen should be burnt. The public health nurses connected with baby welfare clinics visit the homes and teach the mothers correct methods of preparing the baby's food and the general care of the child.

ESCHERICHIA

Escherichia coli : gastroenteritis; urinary tract infection.

E. coli as a pathogen is associated with two main clinical syndromes : (1) acute gastroenteritis in infants under two years of age and rarely in adults with lowered resistance; (2) infection of urinary tract, particularly in married women but also in girls and in elderly man with prostate enlargement. *E. coli* may be the causal organism of appendicular abscess, peritonitis, cholecystitis, wound infection etc.

Description. *E. coli* is Gram-negative, motile, non-sporing bacillus, morphologically identical to salmonella and on ordinary media their colonies are very similar. On MacConkey medium, *E. coli* yields rose pink colonies since they ferment lactose in the medium. But they grow poorly on DCA or Salmonella Shigella (SS) medium. They can be differentiated from other enterobacteriacae by biochemical test, $IMV_{(i)}C$ - Indole and MR are positive and VP and citrate are negative.

Resistance. *E. coli* survives in the external environment for months. It is more resistant to physical and chemical factors of the external environment than typhoid and dysentery bacilli. It is killed comparatively rapidly by all methods and preparations used for disinfection. At 55°C the organism perishes in one hour and at 60°C in 15 minutes. *E. coli* is sensitive to brilliant green. Gastroenteritis is caused by *E. coli*. The enteropathogenic strains of *E. coli* seem to belong to a limited number of 0 serotypes. The most common and widely distributed serotypes are 0 26; 0 55; 0 111; 0 127; 128. Outbreaks of acute gastroenteritis occur in infants, nurseries, and pediatric units under 18 years of age. More widespread outbreaks may occur in the general community.

The pathophysiology of infantile gastroenteritis associated with enteropathogenic *E. coli* is characterised by massive fluid loss from the gut, causing acute dehydration, acidosis and hypovolaemic shock. The pathogenesis of infantile gastroenteritis seems to be related to the production of an enterotoxin similar in action to the cholera enterotoxin.

Four groups of *E. coli* responsible for diarrhoea in infants, children and adults are : Enteropathogenic *E. coli* (EPEC); Enterotoxigenic *E. coli* (ETEC); Enteroinvasive *E. coli* (EIEC); Enterohaemorrhagic *E. coli* (EHEC).

EPEC is responsible for infantile diarrhoea. The pathogenic mechanism of EPEC has only recently been developed. They adhere to the intestinal mucosa, cause the loss of microvilli and prevent entry of bacteria into the mucosa. It also produces a shigella-like toxin.

ETEC. Its enterotoxin is now known to produce diarrhoea in children, traveller's diarrhoea in adults and sometimes cholera infantum similar to cholera. ETEC also possesses colonisation factors (pili, K antigen) to enhance its virulence.

EIEC does not produce enterotoxin, but invades the intestinal mucosa like dysentery bacilli. It causes keratoconjunctivitis on instillation in to the eyes of guinea pig *(Sereney test)* which is a diagnostic method for EIEC. Another diagnostic method is its invasion of HeLa cells in tissue culture. It has an antigenic relationship with shigella.

EHEC has been very recently identified and is found to cause colitis with marked haemorrhage and absence of fever, produces *verotoxin* (cytotoxin) which affects the vero cells in tissue culture.

Urinary tract infection. Predisposing factors of urinary tract infection are the urinary retention and stasis in pregnancy and in elderly males.

E. coli is the most common coliform species present in the urine of pregnant woman with significant bacteriuria. Serotypes 01, 02, 04, 06 and 075 are most commonly involved in urinary tract infection.

Transmission. Outbreaks of gastroenteritis occur most commonly in institutions and affect either newborn babies in a maternity nursery or infants up to 18 months of age in paediatric wards or other institutions.

The infection occurs much more frequently in artificially fed babies than in wholly breast fed babies. This may be due to the milk feed; and feeding bottles are the most likely vehicles of infection from a case or carrier. Infantile enteritis may occur during or shortly after weaning.

Control measure. Since outbreaks of gastroenteritis may result in high fatality rate in maternity nurseries and institutions caring for young children, every precaution should be taken to prevent the introduction of infection, particularly by infants coming from other institutions. This may require some system of preliminary quarantine and bacteriological screening of new admission. If the infection becomes established, drastic measures should be taken for its control, including closure of a ward, nursery or institution.

Generally, the prevention of infantile gastroenteritis demands that bottle milk feeds served to infants must be sterilised in hospital that is best effected by terminal heat sterilisation or the fully prepared, sterilised feed in the feeding bottle. In the house, the mother should be encouraged to use domestic pressure cookers for the same purpose. The most effective preventive measure is breast feeding. Nurse should make every effort to encourage mothers to appreciate that breast feeding is best for the babies. In case of acute infantile diarrhoea, mothers should follow Oral Rehydration Therapy (ORT) recommended by World Health Organisation (WHO).

KLEBSIELLA

It is widely distributed in nature occurring both as commensals in intestine and saprophyte in soil and water. It is non-motile, capsulated rod, grows on ordinary media. In MacConkey's agar medium, its colonies are large, dome-shaped, mucoid and pink. It is indole and methyl red negative and Voges Proskarer and citrate positive.

It causes urinary, pyogenic infections (abscess, meningitis), diarrhoea, pneumonia characterised by massive mucoid inflammatory exudate, and nosocomial infection.

CHAPTER 43

CHOLERA

Cholera is an acute gastroenteritis of sudden onset characterised by effortless vomiting, often running a rapid and fatal course; the patient becomes acutely dehydrated and dies of hypovolaemic shock within 12-24 hours.

Vibrio cholerae is the causative organism of cholera or Asiatic cholera. It is comma-shaped rod, actively motile because of single long terminal flagellum; its movement is of "darting" type — likened to fish in a stream. It grows on Thiosulphate Citrate Bile salt Sucrose (TCBS) producing yellow colonies, and in alkaline medium, the optimum pH is 8.2. It is non-sporing and is easily killed by boiling, pasteurisation and disinfectants.

Resistance. Vibrio cholerae survives for a long time at low temperature. It lives in faeces for up to a month; in oysters, crabs; on the surface of fish and in their intestines for 1 to 40 days; in water for several days; on food stuff for 1 to 10 days and in the intestine of flies for 4 to 5 days. It shows a low resistance to sunlight, X-ray, dessication and high temperature. It is destroyed instantly at 100°C and in 5 minutes at 80°C and is easily killed by pasteurisation, disinfection, particularly to acids (e.g., a 1 : 10,000 solution of hydrochloric acid kills them within one minute) and is also sensitive to gastric juice.

Pathogenesis and disease in man. Vibrio cholerae are ingested in drink and food. Those escape the acid barrier of the stomach, multiple in the alkaline medium of the small intestine and produce potent exotoxin, called *enterotoxin*. This toxin is thought to react with a receptor in the membrane of the intestinal epithelial cell, then to activate adenyl cyclase in the membrane and thereby raise the intracellular level of cyclic adenosine monophosphate (CAMP) which induces the increased secretion of water and electrolytes in the intestinal lumen.

Arrows show bicarbonal movement of intestinal fluid across the intestinal mucosa. In resting healthy gut (left) absorption roughly equals secretion. As a result of action of cholera endotoxin (centre) secretion greatly exceeds the absorption with a net loss of large quantity of isotonic fluid. When glucose electrolyte solution is administrated orally (right) glucose facilitates fluid absorption and counter-balances toxin induced fluid secretion and fluid balance is maintained.

The professional nurse should never collect the stool samples from the bedpan because of its contamination or the presence of antiseptic in it, but she should collect the stool passed on to a clean paper or a large leaf and should send to the laboratory in a transport medium (Venkatraman-Ramakrishnan VR fluid) or alkaline taurocholate tellurite medium. Quick diagnosis can be obtained by vibrio-immobilisation test with dark field microscopy using specific hyper immune serum for *Vibrio cholerae.*

Epidemiology of Cholera. Man is the only natural host of *Vibrio cholerae*. The spread of infection is from person to person with contaminated water or food. Cholera is characteristically an infection of crowded poor class community living in low-lying areas and sharing communal water supplies (tanks, ponds, canals, rivers). In Bangladesh, the Cholera season (November to February) follows the monsoon rains and ends with the onset of the hot, dry months; across the Bengal delta, the epidemic wave in Kolkata, India (May to July) rises to its peak in the hot, dry season and ends with the onset of monsoon, but extends in land to neighbouring states during the rainy season.

Prophylaxis.

1. Recognition of the first cholera cases, accurate registration of all cases and information of higher Public Health authorities;
2. Isolation and hospitalisation of patients and carriers;
3. Routine and terminal disinfection of department of cholera patient and disease foci;
4. Protection of water supply sources, enforcement of sanitary inspection of catering establishment and fly control;

5. Strict observance of personal hygiene, boiling or chlorination of water, disinfection of dishes and washing of hands;
6. Specific prophylaxis is by vaccination with killed monovalent or polyvalent cholera vaccine. The immunity lasts for 6 months or less and is not very potent;
7. Recent live Oral cholera vaccine CVD 103 -HgR provides significant protection against cholera due to classical and EiTor *V. cholerae*. Two oral vaccines that have exhibited considerable promise consist of inactivated *V. cholerae* O_1 whole cells; either with cholera toxin B subunits (BS-WC) or without B subunits, each vaccine conferred 50% protection.

   CVD 103-HgR was 100% protective against diarrhoea and significantly reduced the rate of shedding of vibrio after challenging with *V.cholerae* classical Inaba strain.

Application to Nursing in Enteric Infection

In dealing with enteric infection one of the greatest responsibility of professional nurses is to control most efficiently at the bedside the dissemination of *Vibrio cholerae*, typhoid and paratyphoid bacilli, poliomyelitis virus and hepatitis virus, pathogenic protozoa and helminth from the patients or healthy carriers and, at the same time, she should be very vigilant in the proper disposal of the excretions. The faeces and urine must be first disinfected and properly disposed off for the welfare of the other patients, for her own protection and community. Bed pans should be given special attention immediately after use by the patient. The faeces and urine shall be transferred to a covered vessel, then thoroughly disinfected with saponated cresol or chloride of lime. The bed pan should be returned to the patient after it is thoroughly flushed and boiled or soaked in disinfectant solution and the careful nurse should not allow the entry of visitors into the sick room. Cholera, typhoid and dysentery patients should be admitted in the hospital and treated in isolation ward designed to exclude the flies. If the patient is at home, the empty milk bottles should not be returned to the vendors, as the empty milk bottles may carry the infecting agents to the dairy. The patient in an infectious stage, before a diagnosis is made, is a greatest danger of infection. The nurse attending on these patients should not prepare food for herself and for any other person.

Control of carriers. The carrier should wash and disinfect if possible his hands after using the toilet. He should not engage in any work which requires handling of food and milk. His faeces should be disinfected and disposed off so to avoid infections to others. The health authorities should keep in touch with these carriers by visits. In this regard, the public health nurse plays a great role.

Precautions. If water supply is polluted, water should be boiled. If the facility for boiling is not available, commercially available tablet for disinfecting water can be used. Pasteurised milk should always be used.

CAMPYLOBACTER

Genus *Campylobacter* (Greek, '*kampylos*' bent/ curved and '*bacterior*' little rod) is distributed worldwide has now emerged as new recent pathogen causing campylobacter enteritis in children (acute infantile diarrhoea) and consists of *C. jejuni* and *C. coli*. They are small flagellate, Gram-negative curved, coccoid, degenerate bacilli and exhibit the rapid darting type of motility of *Vibrio cholerae*. They grow best at 42°C under 5-10 % CO_2 on Skirrow or Buzzler blood agar medium or on blood free medium - Charcoal Cefazolin Sodium Deoxycholate Agar (CCDA) medium of Bolton and produce typical grey, flat spreading moist colonies, which form an important identification characteristic of campylobacter. They produce oxidase, catalase, H_2S biochemically. *C. jejuni* biotype 1 do not produce H_2S.

The incubation period of Campylobacter enteritis is 1-13 days. It is an acute self-limiting diarrhoeal disease mostly affecting children. It is a zoonosis (disease transmitted from animal to man through contaminated milk, food or water with cowdung). There is general malaise, headache, backache, aching limbs, dizziness, abdominal pain and seldom vomiting.

Laboratory diagnosis. Rectal swabs should be carried to the laboratory in transport medium, Cary-Blair medium. Rapid bacteriological diagnosis can be made by direct dark ground microscopy by characteristic darting motility and by colony characteristics. Isolation of Campylobacter on selective media.

Treatment. Erythromycin, furazolidone, tetracycline, gentamycin are used.

Prophylaxis. Avoidance of contamination of food or drink with cowdung from animals.

CHAPTER 44

BRUCELLOSIS, LEPTOSPIROSIS, AND TETANUS

Since the mode of transmission of these three groups of bacteria is mostly through urine or faeces, they are included under this section.

Genus Brucella

These bacteria were first described in 1887 by Bruce. They cause the disease undulant fever or brucellosis in man, They are Gram-negative cocco bacillary smallest rods; they are non-motile, non-capsulated, non-sporing, microaerophilic. They grow best in a medium enriched with animal serum or glucose at 37°C.

There are three strains of Brucella :

Brucella melitensis infects mainly man; *Br. suis,* pigs and *Br. abortus,* cattle, sheep, goats.

Resistance. Brucella organisms survive in the soil and in the manure, urine for many weeks and remain viable in dried fetal material and ice-cream prepared from the infected milk. They are sensitive to phenol, formalin and other disinfectants to high temperature. At 60°C, they are destroyed in 30 minutes, at 70°C in 30 minutes, at 100°C in few seconds.

Pathogenesis and disease in man. Brucellosis is a zoonotic disease (i.e., the disease transmitted from animal to man).

Man acquires the infection very often through the consumption of milk of infected animal and dairy products prepared from such milk. The organisms enter the body through the abraded skin surface or rarely thorugh intact skin, through mucous membrane of the alimentary or respiratory tract and sometimes through the conjunctiva and reach the blood stream via the regional lymphatics.

The incubation period is from few days to one month. The disease is characterised by increased weakness, backache, stiffness of the joints, loss of weight and variable symptoms. There are usually severe night sweats and remittant fever lasting for several days. Very rarely pregnant women may have miscarriages but it is very common in cows occurring as "Stormy abortion" due to presence of erythritol in their placenta.

Laboratory diagnosis is done by blood culture test or SEROLOGICAL tests (tube agglutination test, Coombs test), Complement fixation test, Enzyme linked immuno sorbent assay (ELISA) test and Milk Ring Test (MRT) for animal brucellosis.

Prevention of undulant fever. The disease may be prevented by using only pasteurised milk and dairy products and avoiding the contact of infected animals.

Vaccine is useful for the prevention of the disease in calves; but there is no vaccine for human beings; however, human beings can respond to a combination of streptomycin and tetracycline.

Application to Nursing

If the undulant fever patients have draining lymph nodes or open lesions, their clothings and dressings soiled with such drainage should be disinfected effectively and not be allowed to touch other articles. If the faeces and urine contain Brucella organisms, they should be disinfected and disposed off as in typhoid stools.

Genus Leptospira

Leptospirae are small, delicate, slender, flexuous organisms. They are composed of tight coils and curved into a hook at both ends like hockey stick. There are many pathogenic leptospirae. They are highly organised than other bacteria. In addition to cell wall and cytoplasm, they contain from one to twelve filaments which are responsible for corkscrew like motility. They may be seen readily under dark field illumination method in the infected urine or tissue, wriggling and twisting. They grow at 22 to 37°C in liquid media containing animal serum.

Resistance. Leptospira withstands low temperature and survives in water over a period of many months. They are very sensitive to dessication and acids. Exposure to 56°C kills the organism in 30 minutes. They are lysed in bile.

Pathogenesis and disease in man. Infected rats, dogs, cattle, pigs are the main source of leptospira. They discharge them into their surrounding environment (water, soil, foodstuffs) with the urine. Contaminated water and foodstuffs are transmission factors. Human beings acquire the disease after swimming in contaminated water, drinking contaminated water or milk from infected cows. Leptospiral jaundice is an occupational disease as a result of which people are in constant contact with water contaminated by rats. The same hazards occur during work in rice fields (Japan, Indonesia).

The pathogenic leptospirae are responsible for the zoonotic diseases which are subdivided into icteric and anicteric leptospirosis. Icteric leptospirosis (leptospiral jaundice, Weil's disease) is caused by *L. icterohaemorrhagiae.*

This organism enters the host body by the gastrointestinal tract and by injured skin and mucous membrane. The disease is characterised by a sudden onset of high pyrexia, headache and pain in the muscles. The disease involves the central nervous system. Jaundice develops and the liver becomes enlarged and painful. Haemorrhagic eruptions, nose bleeding, gastric and intestinal haemorrhages may occur and the spleen becomes enlarged. Nephritis and anuria are also observed.

Bacteriemia developed in the first days of the disease plays an important role in the pathogenesis of leptospirosis. At the end of the first week, the organisms accumulate in the liver, spleen, lymph node and bone marrow. Then they penetrate the kidneys and are discharged in the urine for 4 to 6 weeks.

Anicteric leptospirosis (Water fever) is characterised by a sudden onset, fever, severe headache and pain in the bones and muscles. The patient loses his appetite. Nausea and lassitude are observed. The spleen and liver are enlarged. A typhoid condition, mental depression, delirium, dulled consciousness and insomnia occur.

Laboratory diagnosis can be done — 1. by direct dark field microscopy of blood smear; by blood or urine culture; 2. by agglutination and lysis reactions with convalescent sera (dilution not less than 1 : 400) which are of diagnostic value and by complement fixation test or indirect haemagglutination test.

Prophylaxis can be done by destruction of rats; by general sanitation; by prohibition of swimming pool; prophylactic vaccination with vaccine prepared from a suspension of more common types of Leptospira.

Treatment. Penicillin, chlortetracycline, oxytetracycline are drugs of choice.

Application to Nursing

Urine of patients with Leptospirosis should be considered as infectious; clothes and bedding soiled with such urine should be disinfected. The nurse should instruct the patient to avoid the contamination of his surroundings with urine. The drinking water should be boiled or chlorinated. Food possibly contaminated with excreta of rats should not be eaten.

Genus Clostridium

Tetanus and *Gas gangrene.* The causative organisms of these diseases are always present in the intestine of man and animals and are excreted in the faeces; but when they penetrate the damaged tissues (wounds) they produce severe and fatal conditions. Their spores remain viable in soil for long period of time (for several years). They grow at 37°C anaerobically in Robertson's cooked meat medium.

Tetanus occurs in man and animal when a wound is infected with *Clostridium tetani* under conditions that allow this organism to multiply and produce toxin. Absorption of the toxin leads to hypersensitivity of voluntary muscles. The disease is characterised by increased muscle tones and exaggerated muscular responses to simple stimuli.

Cl. tetani are straight, slender motile rod-shaped organisms. They form spores which are characteristically terminal and spherical, producing "drum-stick" appearance.

If the stumps of the umbilical cords of the neonates are contaminated with soil or faeces, the death of newborn infants may occur due to tetanus. This condition is known as "Tetanus neonatorum".

Since the damaged necrotic tissue is the best medium for the growth of *Cl. welchii* and for the optimal production of toxin which is responsible for Gas gangrene. These two conditions (Tetanus and Gas gangrene) are sometimes confronted in the surgical patients by the nurse, if the unsterilised or improperly sterilised contaminated surgical instruments are used.

CHAPTER 45

ENTERIC VIRAL INFECTIONS

Viruses of poliomyelitis and those of coxsachie and Enteric Cytopathogenic Human Orphan (ECHO) groups are included in Enteroviruses, as they multiply primarily in the human gastro-intestinal tract, produce clinical diseases involving central nervous system (brain and spinal cord).

Respiratory Enteric Orphan virus (REO Virus) is constantly associated with diarrhoea than with respiratory symptoms.

Enteroviruses
- Polio (type 1-3)
- Coxsachie
  - Group A (type 1-5)
  - Group B (type 1-5)
- ECHO (type 1-8, type 9, type 10 - a reovirus ?)

Another virus, *infectious hepatitis* (IH) or *epidemic hepatitis*, present in the intestine which is transmitted by faecal-oral route is not considered under enterogroup virus, as they multiply in the liver, not in the intestine or central nervous system.

POLIOMYELITIS

Though poliomyelitis is known as one of the most ancient contagious diseases, its infectious nature was ascertained only in 1905 by Wickman; later, in 1908-09, it was proved to be of viral aetiology.

Poliovirus ranges from 8-27 nanometer (nm) - nanometer (1 nm = 10 meter) or equal to millimicron (mμ) and forms intranuclear inclusions. It is cultivated *in vitro* in tissue culture of monkey kidney or He La cells.

There are three types of viruses which do not possess common immunogenic properties:

Type I viruses include Brunhilde strains which are pathogenic to man and monkey;

Type II viruses include the Lansing strains which are responsible for diseases in man, monkey and rodents (rats, mice, hamsters etc.).

Type III viruses (the Leon strain) are pathogenic only to man and monkeys and differ immunologically from two types.

Resistance. The poliomyelitis virus survives in sterile water at room temperature for more than 100 days; in milk for 90 days; in faeces in cold for more than 6 months and in sewage for several months. It withstands exposure to 0.5-1 per cent phenol solution and remains viable for several weeks at pH 3.8 - 8.5. It is very sensitive to calcium chloride, formalin, potassium permanganate and hydrogen peroxide. It is rapidly killed on boiling.

Pathogenesis and disease in man. The virus is extremely *neurotropic*. It causes the degenerative inflammatory process in the anterior horns of spinal cord and in the grey substance of the brain. However, the virus circulates in the blood. It may be discharged in the faeces of patients and convalescents for 2-7 weeks and is discharged through the nasopharyngeal mucous membrane secretion and sometimes up to 4 months and during the incubation period. Healthy carriers also excrete the virus with the feces. This virus may be found in the nasopharyngeal mucus and tonsils approximately 3 days before the temperature rises and for 3 days after the onset of the disease. According to the clinical symptoms, three forms of poliomyelitis are distinguished; abortive, non-paralytic and paralytic.

Immunity. There are three immunologically distinct types of polioviruses : I, II and III. Immunity to one does not confer immunity to another. A very stable immunity is produced following the disease. No case of reinfection has been described. Immunity is associated with the presence of virus neutralising antibodies in the blood.

Poliovaccine. In 1949, Enders, Weller and Robbins (Nobel Prize winners) were able to cultivate poliomyelitis virus in tissue cultures, made from human, monkey kidneys, human intestinal tissues, human embryonic tissues and human cancer (Ha La cells). This virus multiplies and kills the tissue cells.

The *Salk vaccine* was prepared by Jones Salk by cultivating poliovirus Type I, II, III in live monkey kidney tissue cells and after an incubation, the dead tissue cells and other debris are removed and the remaining fluid containing poliovirus is collected and formaldehyde (1 : 4,000) is added to kill the virus and allowed to act for one week and excess of formaldehyde is removed. Safety tests were then carried out to determine whether the virus is really killed and the fluid is not contaminated with bacteria. If satisfactory, the preservative is added and the vaccine is ampouled and used.

Use and effectiveness of Salk vaccine. Three doses are recommended; first two doses at an interval of about four to six weeks apart and the third at an interval of 1-3 years or more.

This vaccine does not prevent poliomyelitis, but the incidence is reduced to a very low level, when it is used consistently, because of the antibodies in the blood and the tissues of vaccinated persons which interpose a barrier between the gastrointestinal source of virus and the central nervous system. Thus, the most important effect of the vaccine is to prevent severe *paralytic polio*, e.g., crippling and deadly "spinal paralysis". This vaccine is 90 percent effective in preventing the *paralytic polio*.

Vaccination in Pregnancy. Immunisation of the mother with the vaccine probably gives some passive protection to the infants for a few months.

The Sabin or Oral Polio vaccine. On cultivation, the poliovirus would probably lose its virulence for man and become available as living, attenuated virus vaccine. Sabin and World Health organisation conducted a large scale experiment with this living attenuated virus vaccine and the vaccine was found to be excellent and approved in 1962 for general use. The vaccine is given routinely by oral route to millions of people by incorporating it in candy, food, beverage.

Following the oral administration of the Sabin vaccine, the virus multiplies in the alimentary canal and the virus is discharged in the faeces. No symptoms are observed. In addition to the excellent antibody response, the intestinal infection apparently results in an immunisation of the intestinal tract as well, thus preventing subsequent reinfection.

Triple Living Polio Vaccine. A second type of oral vaccine (Orimune) containing all types of live, attenuated poliovirus was licensed in 1963 by the United States Public Health Service. This vaccine yields a high degree of immunity if given in only two doses two months apart.

Polio and Surgery. The injury or wound due to tonsillectomy, adenoidectomy or tooth extraction and other surgical procedures during the season of epidemic of poliomyelitis is open door for the entry of the virus through the damaged tissues. Therefore, such procedures should be avoided during the season of poliomyelitis. However, the paralysis of the legs and arms may frequently occur at the site of injection of vaccine or penicillin during the epidemics of poliomyelitis. Thus, the risk of paralysis and also infection may be increased due these injections.

Epidemiology. Faeces provide a rich and persistent source of the poliovirus. Sewage in urban areas contain this virus. Water supply may be contaminated by sewage and in rural areas this may be a means by which the infection is spread. Fly may carry the virus on their feet or by regurgitating after feeding on the exposed faeces or sewage.

Application to Nursing

A professional nurse shall be vigilant in proper disposal of all respiratory secretions during the first two or three weeks from the onset of the infection. The nurse's hands, objects and dishes used by the patient should be well-disinfected to prevent the spread of the disease. Since boiling and adequate exposure to chloride of the lime will inactivate the poliomyelitis virus, these procedures should be applied by the nurse while dealing with poliomyelitis.

COXSACKIE AND ECHO VIRUSES

Diseases caused by Coxsackie and Echoviruses were discovered by Dall dorb and Sickles in 1948 in Coxsackie (New York State) from children suffering from paralysis and other infections resembling poliomyelitis. ECHO virus (enteric cytopathogenic human orphans) virus were discovered by Melnick and others.

Coxsackie virus is extremely small and resembles poliomyelitis virus. They are grown on tissue cultures (human and monkey kidney cells) and pathogenic to newborn mice. The majority of ECHO viruses are *non-pathogenic to newborn mice.*

Resistance. Coxsackie and ECHO virus possess relatively high resistance. They survive for a long time at -70°C. In the refrigerator, they survive for more than a year. They survive at pH 2.3 - 9.4 for 24 hours and at pH 4.0 - 8.0 for 7 days. At temperature of 50 - 55°C kills these viruses in 30 minutes and they are extremely sensitive to hydrochloric acid and formaldehyde.

Pathogenesis and disease in man. There are several forms of the diseases : (a) aseptic serous meningitis; (b) pleurodynia; (c) aseptic meningitis; (d) three day fever; Both these viruses are responsible for a number of other disease; non-diphtheric croup; influenza like disease.

Application to Nursing

The methods adopted for the prevention of urine or faeces-borne diseases should be applied by the nurse for the control of the disease.

HEPATITIS VIRUSES

There are five major types of primary hepatotrophic acute hepatitis viruses. Besides, other viruses are also responsible for acute viral hepatitis.

Classification

HEPATITIS TYPE	PREVIOUS DESCRIPTION
Hepatotrophic viruses	
1. Hepatitis A (HAV)	Infectious hepatitis.
2. Hepatitis B (HBV)	Serum hepatitis (a) Wide type (b) African HB_sAg — anti HBC + mild disease course (c) Mediterranean HBC Ag- HBV-DNA + aggressive liver disease.
3. Hepatitis C (HCV)	Parenteral non-A, non-B hepatitis.
4. Hepatitis D (HDV)	Delta hepatitis (agent).
5. Hepatitis E (HEV)	Enteric non-A, non-B hepatitis.
Others :	
Cytomegalovirus (CMV) Epstein-Barr Virus (EVB) Herpes simplex virus Coxsackie B virus Echovirus Yellow fever virus	All these viruses cause acute hepatitis in which involvement of other organs is more common and more prominent then evidence of liver involvement.

HEPATITIS A VIRUS (HAV)

In 1973, Feinstone *et al* first discovered HAV in feces of infected patients by immune electron microscopy. World Health Organisation (WHO) considered that this infection is prevalent worldwide, particularly in countries where over-crowding, poor hygiene and sanitation are common. Recent outbreaks in 1988 in China involving 1.2 million persons were presumed due to over-crowding, poor hygienic condition.

HAV was classified as picornavirus. However, there is now more evidence to support that HAV is different from well-studied four genera of this virus family.

Two HAV cell systems have been very recently described in which replication of HAV seemed to be paralleled by virus specific cytopathology.

The pathogenic mechanism of liver cell damage in acute HAV infection is not yet well understood.

There are two recent studies which strongly proved that the cytotoxic T cells capable of lysing HAV-infected target cells developed in the course of HAV infection.

Usually, HAV causes a minor or unnoticed illness in children and young adults and high mortality in patients over 60 years of age.

Laboratory findings. In HAV infection, elevated serum transaminases are often accompanied by non-specific rise of Ig M, Ig G, antismooth muscle antibodies and acute phase proteins. The raised Ig M is mainly polyclonal and only a small proportion is directed against HAV antigen. The extent of serum transaminases elevation does not appear to be of diagnostic significance.

Immunisation

High titer serum immunoglobulin preparations have value in the prophylaxis against HAV infection. HAV infection is an important source of morbidity and economic losses, although it does not lead to chronic hepatitis and cirrhosis. Killed HAV vaccine has been found to be safe and efficient in animals and it is under clinical trials.

HEPATITIS B VIRUS

World Health Organisation (WHO) estimated that in 1988 there are about 300 million chronic HB_SAg carriers in the world and suggested that 40 per cent of them will eventually die of chronic liver disease and/or hepatoma.

HBV genome has been well-characterised and consists of 4 overlapping open reading frames designated S, C, P and X.

HBV Polypeptides

HBV Genome	Polypeptides
S	HB_SAg (major protein)
pre S_2 + S	pre S_2 peptide (middle protein)
pre S_1 + pre S_2 + S	pre S_1 peptide (large protein)
C	HB_c Ag and HB_e Ag
pre e + c	pre core peptide
P	FNA polymerase
X	X protein

Both HB_c Ag and HB_e Ag are encoded by C gene. The presence of HB_eAg in the blood is, therefore, an indication of ongoing viral replication. The X protein presence may also be suggestive of HBV replication.

Liver Damage

In the natural host, man, HBV is not cytopathogenic because there is existence of HBV carriers state for many years without evidence of parenchymal liver damage and it may not be the same in the animal experimentation. Recently, it has been shown that HBV itself can inhibit interferon production in an *in vitro* system thus explaining the decreased interferon production in a group of patients.

SEROLOGICAL FEATURES OF VIRAL HEPATITIS

Form of infection	Serologic markers	Interpretation
Hepatitis A	Ig M anti-HAV	Acute disease
	Ig G anti-HAV	Remote infection
Hepatitis B	HB_sAg	Acute or chronic disease
	HB_cAg	Active replication
	Ig M anti-HB_c (high titre)	Acute disease
	Ig G anti-HB_c	
	HB_sAg positive	Chronic disease
	HB_sAg negative	Prior exposure
	Anti-HB_s	
	Ig G anti-HB_c positive	Past infection and immunity
	Ig G anit-HB_c negative	Immune response from vaccination
Hepatitis C	Anti-HCV	Acute, chronic or resolved disease
Hepatitis D	HB_sAg and anti-HDV	Acute disease
	Ig M anti-HB_c positive	Coinfection
	Ig M anti-HB_c positive	Super infection
Hepatitis E	None	

There is serological evidence showing that the acute HBV infection progresses to chronic HBV infection. Reverse passive Hemagglutination (RPHA), Counter-immuno electrophoresis (CIEP) and ELISA Tests can detect HB_cAg.

Aniviral Therapy

At present, interferon-alpha is the only promising mode of therapy. Further studies are still conducted to evaluate the role of new drug combination therapy and continuous low dose interferon-alpha therapy in the interferon-alpha resistant patients.

Agents that have been studied in the treatment of chronic HBV infection.

Antivirals	Immunosuppressive	Immunostimulators
Interferon	Corticosteroids	BCG vaccination
Alpha		Levamisole
Beta		Interleukin-2
Gamma		Interferon gamma
Adenine arabinoside (Ara-A)		Thyamosin
Acyclovir deoxyacyclovir		
Zidovudine		
Suramin		
Ribavirin		
Phosphonoformate		
Quinacrine		
(+) - Cyanidanol-3		
Phyllanthus amarus (Plant extracts)		

Active Immunisation

In 1981, the first generation plasma derived HBV vaccines were licensed. There was limitation regarding their acceptance and use, because of their high production cost and the fear of the possible transmission of blood borne disease. Much more rapid progress had been done by the vaccination of the high risk group (health personnels and babies born to HB_s Ag seropositive mothers) with the second generation yeast derived recombinant HBV vaccine launched in 1986. Routine HBV vaccination was recommended by WHO for countries that possess the economic capacity to purchase the vaccine.

Now, the third generation synthetic peptide vaccines have been developed; their safety, immunogenecity and protectivity against HBV infection are under evaluation and these vaccines may become cheap and efficient.

Hepatitis B vaccine consists of purified hepatitis B surface antigen (HB_SAg). The vaccine induces neutralising HB_SAg antibodies which confer protection against Hepatitis B virus.

Plasma derived HBV vaccine is no longer available in USA, but the two yeast derived recombinant vaccines are qualitatively similar to plasma derived vaccine.

Engerix - B, the only genetically engineered Hepatitis B vaccine, is at present available in India. Engerix - B is supplied in a 20 μg dose and Recombivax in a 10 μg dose.

HEPATITIS C VIRUS

There was a proportion of cases clinically viral hepatitis without defined etiology, after the isolation of HBV in 1960s and HAV in 1970s. The majority of these cases occurred after blood transfusion of intravenous drug users and led to chronic hepatitis. The term non-A non-B hepatitis (NANB) was carried to describe these cases. The clinical diagnosis of NANB hepatitis was imprecise. There are two blood borne NANB hepatitis agents; NANB hepatitis virus was between 30-60 nm. diameter.

Identification of Hepatitis C Virus

Because of the recent advances in molecular cloning technique, non-A non-B virus has been recently identified and termed as HCV.

Half of the patients with presumed chronic NANB hepatitis become positive when recent polymerase chain reaction (PCR) was used to detect HCV RNA in tissue and serum.

Recent Serology

It has been very recently shown that the anti-HCV antibodies appeared only several weeks after the infection, but persisted for more than 10 years in most patients.

A recombinant immunoblot assay (RIBA) was established by utilising the western blotting technique and was found to be more sensitive and specific. Serum HCV RNA was successfully detected by employing the polymerase chain reaction and molecular hybridisation. All these newly developed techniques need to be confirmed for their specificities.

HEPATITIS D VIRUS (Delta agent, Dane particle)

A new viral antigen was observed by Rizzitto *et al* in the nuclei of hepatocytes in patients suffering from HAV infection. Later studies showed that this antigen was related to a new virus, now named as HDV.

HDV is an incomplete single stranded circular RNA virus that depends on the helper function of HBV to replicale. It is uncoated in HB_s Ag and RNA genome. Thus, it appears that HDV requires HB_s Ag for its hepatotropism and propagation, but it does not depend on HBV for replication.

Epidemiology

HDV infection is endemic in Italy, Middle East, Africa and South America. The major route of transmission in non-endemic areas is the intravenous drug use. Placental transmission may not be always important route.

Liver Disease (Hepatitis)

Replicating HDV appears to be mostly associated with liver damages suggesting that HDV may be directly hepatotoxic.

The possible similarity in the pathogenic mechanisms of HBV and HDV may be due to the similar pattern of T cells infiltration in chronic HBV and HDV infection.

Clinical Features and Laboratory Diagnosis

In chronic HB_SAg carriers, infection with HDV may occur simultaneously with HBV infection (co-infection) or as a superinfection; but these two infections have two different clinical courses and outcomes. As acute HBV infection, coinfection is usually self-limiting, although morbidity may be higher. A massive infecting dose may be associated with a more severe outcome.

Superinfection of HB_SAg carriers with HDV may cause severe acute hepatitis and lead to chronic hepatitis and cirrhosis in over 70 per cent cases. Chronicity in HDV superinfection is usually accompanied by a decrease in HBV replication markers. A subacute, rapidly progressive form of HDV superinfection has been reported.

The diagnosis of different forms of HDV infection relies in detection of HD Ag in liver biopsies and serum HDAg, HDVRNA and Ig M, Ig G and anti-HD antibodies. In acute HDV infection, HDVRNA and HDAg appear transiently in serum of about 25% cases. Ig M and anti-HDV occurred in 93% lasting for about 2-10 weeks. In those patients who develop chronic HDV infection, serum HDVRNA and Ig M anti-HDV usually persist and HDAg can be found consistently in the liver.

In chronic HB_SAG carriers with HDV superinfection, the suppression of HDV replication may lead to a transient absence of HDV markers in the serum and liver.

Antiviral Therapy and Immunisation

Interferon-alpha has an inhibitory effect on HDV replication but beneficial effect is transient in most cases.

Fulminant HDV infection may respond to treatment with trisodium phosphonoformate. Control of HDV infection is by vaccination against HDV.

HEPATITIS E VIRUS

In 1983, virus-like particles (VLPs) measuring 27-32 nm. were demonstrated by immune electron microscopy in the stools of three of nine cases of HEV infections in Taskhent of the-then, USSR. A volunteer developed an acute hepatitis with anti-bodies detectable to the VLP by immune electron microscopy IEM after ingesting a dilute suspension of stools pooled from patients. In the liver of experimentally infected macaques an antigen related to HEV (HEV Ag) was detected. In the early phase of experimental infection, there is a granular distribution in up to 90% of hepatocytes.

Clinical Features and Laboratory Findings

In the well-characterised Indian epidemics, many clinical cases were detected. The incubation period was between 3-9 weeks. The attack rate was higher in young adults (2.9%) than children (1.4%) or in those aged over 40 (2.0%). A prodrome illness with anorexia, nausea, vomiting and abdominal pain is followed by jaundice. The disease is usually benign and self-limiting with no chronic sequelae. Fulminant hepatic failure has been reported in 2.8% of men and 22% of pregnant women in whom it is usually fatal. It may cause severe form of the disease during third trimester of pregnancy.

An antibody blocking assay was developed with the development of fluorescent linked anti-HEV Ag, as a prototype test for identification and titration of specific anti-HEV Ag antibody in the serum samples. The immune electron microscopy (IEM) findings have confirmed this test which is available only in specialised countries.

Epidemiology

The first and most massive outbreak of an enteric non-A, non-B epidemic was reported in 1955 when drinking water was contaminated by the overflow of an open sewer in Delhi (India). A total of 29,000 residents developed an acute hepatitis which ran a benign course in the majority and was self-limited. However, 10% women, affected in their third trimester of pregnancy, died of fulminant hepatic failure. These reports confirmed the existence of fecal-orally transmitted type of non-A non-B hepatitis with completely different characteristics to blood borne NANB hepatitis of 10 Indian hepatitis epidemics subsequently investigated. None has been found to be due to epidemic of enteric NANB hepatitis HEV.

Treatment and Control

The treatment is purely supportive as in the case of HAV.The supply of clean water and adequate sanitation can control the disease. Viral antigen obtained by recombinant technology may be used for the diagnostic test and for the development of vaccine.

Following the initial report of HEV epidemics in India, similar epidemics were also reported in Asia, Africa, America. A reservoir of HEV infection is therefore required to perpetuate the infection in the absence of the carrier state.

Recently, Russian research workers were able to transmit HEV to pigs with the hepatitis illness. Besides, they have also found anti-HEV antibody in rats from areas where the disease is endemic.

SERUM HEPATITIS

Immunoglobulins can be administrated for passive immunity against hepatitis B virus.

Development of Vaccine

A vaccine has been prepared by purifying HB_SAg associated with the 22 nm. particles from healthy HB_SAg - positive carriers. Fortunately, protection is conferred by antibody to the "a" antigen, an antigen that is common to all subtypes.

Control and Prevention

1. Clothes of jaundice patients should be washed separately in boiling water;
2. Jaundice patients should be kept in isolation wards;
3. All syringes, needles and equipments should be autoclaved to prevent the entry of hepatitis B virus in the body;
4. Australia antigen test should be conducted by the most sensitive method to detect HB_SAg in :
   (a) Jaundice patients;
   (b) Blood donors;
   (c) Persons to be operated;
5. Cleanliness and hygiene should be maintained at all public eating places;
6. Drinking water should be chlorinated;
7. Laboratory investigators should wear gloves, while testing sera of patients;
8. Used materials and glasswares should be discarded in formalin (1 : 4,000);
9. Laboratory and hospital wards should be fumigated.

IMMUNOPROPHYLAXIS OF VIRAL HEPATITIS

Virus	Pre-exposure prophylaxis	Vaccine available	Post-exposure prophylaxis	Perinatal prophylaxis
Hepatitis A	IG	No	IG	?IG
Hepatitis B	Hepatitis B vaccine	Yes	HBIG	HBIG
Hepatitis C	No	No	IG	?IG
Hepatitis D	Hepatitis B vaccine	Hepatitis B vaccine	No	No
Hepatitis E	?IG	No	?IG	?IG
Non-A; non-B hepatitis	No	No	IG	?IG

HBIG, Hepatitis B Immunoglobulin

SECTION 7

CHAPTER 45A

HUMAN IMMUNODEFICIENCY VIRUS (HIV)

In 1981, virus was believed, hypothetically, to be responsible for Acquired Immunodeficiency Syndrome (AIDS). AIDS was first detected in homosexuals at USA. All victims suffered a depletion of a specific subset of T-cells (T_4 cells). As a result they were susceptible to pathogens that will be controlled by a healthy immune system.

In 1983, it was observed that Human T-Lymphotropic Virus (HILV) had affinity for T_4 lymphocytes *in vitro* and *in vivo.*

In USA, Gallo (Chief of the Laboratory of Tumour Cell Biology at the National Cancer Institute, USA) hypothetised that AIDS is caused by HTLV virus or related virus. The two agents known in human pathology at that time (HTLV — I and II) induced leukaemic lymphoid proliferation, while in case of AIDS, lymphocyte depletion was observed.

Montagnier (Professor of Virology, Pasteur Institute, Paris) discovered a new retrovirus known by him as Lymphadenopathy Associated Virus (LAV) from a patient affected with chronic lymphadenopathy. Later, LAV was found similar to HTLV III. Gallo (1984) isolated HTLV III similar to be morphologically and immunologically identical to LAV after molecular cloning.

In 1985, it was confirmed that AIDS was caused by virus as shown by serodiagnosis or isolation of virus, serodiagnosis for LAV was also made compulsory.

In 1986, HIV was well-established as etiological agent of AIDS. Montagnier has also isolated a new virus, HIV-II. The source for a new focus of AIDS in West Africa was HIV-II. In 1987, it was realised that HIV may be a mutant — dating to 20-40 years — of a human virus not much pathogenic or of a simian virus. Existence of vector of this disease was also demonstrated. HIV and HTLV-III are the same. To eliminate the confusion, an international commission had changed its name to HIV. It is isolated from blood, semen, cerebrospinal fluid, urine, saliva, tears, vaginal secretions, milk, cerebral nervous tissue and spinal marrow. It has tropism for cells (1) Tropism for T_4 lymphocytes, (2) for macrophages—hence it is isolated in CNS.

HIV is 110-120 nm particle. Its envelope is external part. It has small core (nucleotide) which contains viral RNA. HIV is a RNA retrovirus. It has 9,200 nucleotides in length.

Its genome contains 3 genes of retrovirus respectively coding for :

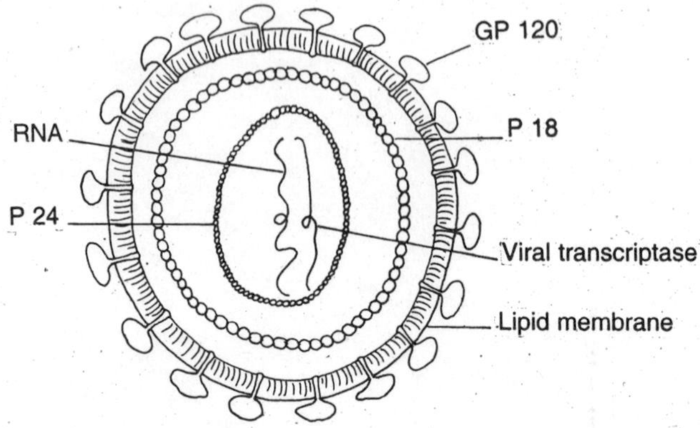

Fig. 45A.1 : Structure of HIV

(a) internal protein in core,

(b) inverse transcriptase necessary for replication,

(c) glycoprotein on the envelope.

HIV genome also contains :

1. gene coding for small protein known as 'tat' (for transactivation),

2. gene coding for small protein 'art' which has same role as 'tat',

3. gene coding for 2 proteins Q and F whose role is unknown (Fig. 45A.1).

AIDS in 1988 (Retrovirus). Few years ago, Retrovirus was found in human beings. Like other viruses, retroviruses cannot replicate without taking over biosynthetic apparatus of the cell. Unique role of retrovirus is their capacity to reverse the ordinary flow of genetic information from DNA to RNA to proteins (which are the cell's structure and functional molecules). The genetic material of a retrovirus is RNA. In addition, it carries an enzyme called reverse transcriptase which can use viral RNA as a template for making DNA. The viral DNA can integrate itself into genome genetic information. Having made at home among the host's gene, the viral DNA remains latent till it is activated to make a new virus particle. The latent DNA can also initiate the process that leads to tumour formation.

No human retrovirus was found. Most animal retroviruses were easily found out, as they replicate in large quantities and the new virus particles were readily observed under electron microscope; no such phenomenon was found in human being. However, Gallo isolated the first human retrovirus Human T-Lymphotropic Virus Type-I (HTLV-I).

HTLV-I infects T-lymphocytes, white blood corpuscles, which play a role in immune response, it causes also malignant cancer (adult T-cell leukaemia-ATL). Two years later, a close relative — HTLV-II, was isolated which causes (a) hairy cell leukaemia, (b) T-cell leukaemia and lymphoma. It spreads by blood, sexual intercourse, from mother to child. Both types I, II cause disease or have latency and infect T-lymphocytes.

New virus, lymphadenopathy associated virus (LAV) grew in T_4 cells, not in related T_8 cells. Later LAV were identified as HTLV-III and were found to be the best cause of AIDS. LAV, HTLV-III, HIV are the same.

HIV is the cause of AIDS and is now firmly established. It could affect T_4 cells and macrophages. HIV binds with CD4 marker for T_4 cells, infects and kills T_4 cells.

Genetic make up of the virus (HIV) is highly variable from strain to strain, hence vaccine preparation is difficult.

Virus related to HIV. HIV-II is closely related, in evolutionary forms, to HIV-I which is mainly responsible for AIDS. The two viruses are similar in their structure, both can cause AIDS, but the pathogenic potential of HIV-II is not well-established as that of the first AIDS virus (HIV-I). However, HIV-I is common in Central Africa and other regions of the world. The finding of HIV-II suggests that other undiscovered HIV may be in existence to fill up the gap of related pathogenic viruses.

HIV-II may have come into human beings relatively recently from another primate species, because Simian Immunodeficiency Virus (SIV) — which is the first virus found in macaque monkey — has been shown to be closely related to HIV-II. No such close simian relative has been found for HIV-I, hence the origin of HIV-I still remains mysterious. HIV infected human beings live for more than 20 years but less than 100 years, because, possibly, it was present in small isolated groups in Central Africa or elsewhere for many years. In such groups, the spread is limited and these groups may have little contact with the outside world. People migrating from remote areas of Central Africa to cities brought with them HIV and transmitted through sex. Sexual acts in urban centers were different from what they had in villages. Blood transfusion is common in urban and the generalised exchange of blood products can carry HIV to every corner of the world. HIV infection can cause fusion of infected cells called as 'Syncytia' which are not functional. Infected cells may send out protein signals that weaken or destroy other cells of Immune system besides HIV fragments. As virus particle leaves its host's cell, a molecule called gp 120 (glycoprotein of the envelope) frequently falls off the virus outer coat. gp 120 can bind with CD_4 molecule of uninfected cells and this complex is recognised by the immune system. Cells with this marker CD_4 may be destroyed.

HIV is diagnosed by Ig G to viral protein — not to virus or antigen :

(a) *ELISA* is an immunoenzymatic technique, rapid, sensitive, reproducible, less specific, less costly. This test can detect antibody against viral protein.

(b) *WESTERN BLOT* or Immunoblot. Denatured viral protein is the basis for this test. This technique can detect antibody against denatured viral protein or antibody against fragments of gp 120 (glycoprotein of the envelope).

(c) *RIPA test* (Radio immunoprecipitation test) can detect antibody against glycoprotein and also native viral protein by radio isotopic technique. This test is more specific, less sensitive, more costlier than ELISA test.

(d) Polymerase Chain Reaction (PCR) is useful.

PCR and HIV culture are comparable and detect 90% of all positive serum samples, whereas plasma antigen capture (associated HIV p. 24 core antigen) technique detects 3/4 th of all cases. HIV 2 was detected in central nervous system using PCR *in situ* hybridisation and immunopathology PCR can also detect HIV type 1 RNA.

Seropositivity is observed between 1 to 4 months after contamination.

Many AIDS surveillance centres have been set up at various places of India (including one at Microbiology department, B. J. Medical College, Ahmedabad) and are well in progress in detecting AIDS. Since 1989, in India, blood products used for vaccine are to be compulsarily tested for AIDS. Nepal banned import of blood products from India. In 1989 two cases of AIDS—one villager and his son, were detected by ELISA test and were confirmed by other tests. Although it is well-established that AIDS was imported to India from abroad and it is an exotic disease. Now it is spreading into villages and it may become a devastating disease in villagers because of their ignorance of this new disease. Ultimately, AIDS may, possibly, become a Rural Health Hazard in India.

Epidemiology of AIDS in India is from cities to villages, which is quite reverse to that first observed in Central Africa. Thus, there is an urgent need for education about HIV infection in clear, explicit language among village folk through primary health center, block development office or Panchayati Raj. Since there is no vaccine or drug available at present, the education about AIDS infection is one of the best methods to prevent the dreadful disease in rural areas.

Anti cancer drug (AZT) is the first drug to be effective. Another agent, CD4, this molecule serves as viral receptor. This soluble CD4 can bind to the virus and prevent it from infecting nerve cells. In future, drug or vaccine against AIDS may, possibly, be produced by scientific research. The drug called U-90. 152 has been shown to sterilise cell culture that has been infected with HIV causing AIDS. The action of new drug in stopping HIV is different from AIDS drugs now licensed. Currently there are three antiviral agents licensed to combat HIV : (1) Zidovudine (AZT). The use of probenecid with Zidovudine reduces the cost in AIDS treatment. (2) Didanosine (DDI); (3) Zalcitabine (DDC). Each of these drugs combats HIV by blocking the action of reverse transcriptase that HIV uses to reproduce. It is a recent observation.

ACQUIRED IMMUNODEFICIENCY SYNDROME

An Indian medical scientist, Dr. M.G. Sarngadharan, Director of the Department of Cell biology in Maryland, USA, had characterised the virus responsible for Acquired Immunodeficiency Syndrome (AIDS) in USA. Besides, Dr. Robert C. Gallo of the US National Cancer Institute, who was heading a team of scientists, had also characterised an infectious virus called HTLV-III (Human T-Lymphotrophic retrovirus Type III) which attacks the body's important cells known as Lymphocytes, i.e., helper T-cells. WHO recommended to call the virus causing AIDS disease by the term human immunodeficiency virus (HIV). This term will replace other names such as Lymphadenopathy associated virus (LAV) and Lymphotrophic human T-cell Type III virus or the combined abbreviations LAV or HTLV-III.

Dr. M. G. Sarngadharan disclosed that his contribution was also related to the prevention of transmission of HTLV-III through contaminated blood to unsuspected blood recipients. He also discovered the virus infected individuals, even without clinical symptoms of AIDS, carry specific antibodies, antigens of the virus just as clinically ill AIDS patients. Based on his finding, he developed a sensitive and accurate test to screen blood so as to identify these antibodies. He had tested more than 17,000 AIDS patients in the United States since 1981. Three-fourths were homosexual males. Another major category of transmission was intravenous drug abusers who shared contaminated needles.

In United States, by law, all the blood donated to blood banks is screened now by using the test developed by Dr. Sarngadharan. For his contribution, he was given the Advanced Technology Achievement Award of 1985.

In a second international conference on AIDS, sponsored by WHO, held at Paris, among 900 scientific papers presented, the United States AIDS specialist, Dr. Robert Gallo, said that in new future scientists should have a full understanding of the AIDS virus and be ready to develop practical ways of arresting the disease. There may be possibility of a vaccine against this disease in future.

Dr. James Curram, head of the AIDS Task Force at Atlanta's centre for Disease Control said more than 3,00,000 persons worldwide would have AIDS by 1991, if the trend in the United States continued.

A vaccine against AIDS tested on animals (rabbit, guinea pig and mice) had produced immunity through the formation of antibodies. No results are available on tests conducted on chimpanzee, the only animal other than man known to contract the infection. This is the first step. The next step is to see whether the chimpanzees reject the virus.

Dr. Halphand Mahler, Director General, WHO, said that between 5 to 10 million people worldwide are infected and are potential carriers of AIDS virus.

He estimated between 30,000 and 1,00,000 persons worldwide are suffering from AIDS. It takes an average of 4 years for an infected person to develop the disease. Scientists reported that little progress has been made on the treatment of AIDS victims, 50 per cent of whom die within a year after diagnosis.

The United States reported 21,517 cases of AIDS and 11,713 deaths. The US Government predicted total of 2,70,000 cases and 1,70,000 deaths by the end of 1991. In Africa some 2 million people are infected and out of these, 50,000 are suffering from AIDS. In Europe, 2,423 cases had been reported, including 878 in France where 14 new cases are being reported each week. Seventy per cent of homosexual or bisexual males now account for AIDS patients. Dr. Jonathan Mann, head of the AIDS programme for WHO, pointed out that the disease is showing clear signs of spreading in areas where it already existed.

According to Jean Baptiste Bernard, Paris, the virus has spread very rapidly among drug abusers in European capitals. This is very surprising compared to United States cities, where the prevalence is very low.

AIDS is not exclusively a disease of homosexuals or drug abusers, but a sickness principally transmitted sexually, that woman or man can contract. One drug, Suramin, was ruled not effective.

National Seminar on AIDS held at All India Institute of Medical Sciences focussed the attention of medical profession, organised national surveillance strategy and created a greater awareness about this disease.

The effects of AIDS on human body are devastating. Because of immune deficiency the patients are unable to resist the infection and cancer. AIDS virus attacks helper T-cells, is transmissible through lesions caused by anogenital sex or by dirty hypodermic needles. There is clear evidence that man can infect female sexual partners and there is tentative evidence that woman can pass the virus to man. There is no guarantee that the disease will be largely confined to groups at specific risk like homosexuals, haemophiliacs and people who inject drugs.

As regards to the attitude of society towards AIDS victims, he further stressed that AIDS victims and members of high risk groups are shunned by their communities. The drug addicts were ten times more likely to catch AIDS than sexual partners of an AIDS carrier.

AIDS is an avoidable disease. It is estimated that 40 lakhs people world over have been infected by AIDS virus. Out of these, the disease has appeared in nearly 25,000 cases. Although the detection of only six persons with AIDS antibody in Madras appears quite small. AIDS is a disease with a long and variable incubation period extending for a few months. With the introduction of a national strategy for the control of AIDS in India and large scale screening of high risk groups for AIDS in India and large scale screening of high risk groups for AIDS virus antibody, it will be possible to know how the disease is widespread in India. One thousand full blown cases were reported currently in the world (1992).

The transmission of AIDS virus does not take place through food, mosquitoes or casual contact. There are no cases of infection occurring in health care personnel attending on AIDS patients, except for a British nurse who developed antibodies 45 days after a needle prick while handling an AIDS patient.

The incidence of AIDS is increasing day by day in USA according to data upto 30 June 1986 and the society should fight against the disease.

In India, according to the Director, National Institute of Virology (NIV), Pune, there is possibility of transmission from infected mother to foetus. Enzyme Linked Immunosorbent Assay (ELISA) test has been conducted at NIV to diagnose AIDS. AIDS virus has been cultivated in lymphocytes.

According to the Professor of Medicine, All India Institute of Medical Sciences, New Delhi, the main signs of AIDS are chronic diarrhoea, loss of weight and sweating at night.

In 1986, only two full blown cases of AIDS had been detected in India. These were detected at Mumbai and Pune. In all 18 cases of confirmed AIDS infection were detected by serological test in

Maharashtra, Andhra Pradesh, and Tamil Nadu. National Programme has been launched to combat the spread of the infection. Some of the important steps taken included imposing restrictions on import of blood and blood products without AIDS clearance certificate. Blood banks are being asked to screen professional donors (Report 24-7-1986).

All persons who have undergone coronary by pass surgery abroad during 1980 and 1985 would be asked to get their blood tested for AIDS virus antibodies, because U.K. and U.S.A. passed the legislation for compulsory screening of blood only in 1985. The screening of blood became necessary after the patients had a blood transfusion. The condoms were effective in curbing the transmission of virus during sex.

Middle-aged woman with AIDS Related Complex (ARC) had been admitted in the J.J. Hospital, Mumbai (India). The patient was positive for the test and was suspected to have got AIDS through blood transfusion. This is second case in Mumbai. The first AIDS case was reported from Jaslok Hospital, Mumbai, who had apparently contracted the disease through blood transfusion in USA during an operation.

It is well established that HIV type 1 (HIV_1) is responsible for most of the AIDS epidemics in North America, Europe, Central Africa and other countries. HIV_1 epidemic was reported in India in 1986. In 1992, sporadic cases of AIDS have been genetically different from HIV_1. HIV_2 infection was first reported in India, in 1991. In the same year, HIV_2 was reported from two persons of two different port cities, by ELISA test and confirmed by Western Blot.

On World AIDS day 2000 (i.e. 1, Dec. 2000), National AIDS Control Organisation (NACO), Ministry of Health, Govt. of India, reported about 3.7 million adult were infected with HIV / AIDS in India; 89 per cent of the reported cases are in sexually active and economically productive age groups of 18-40 years, with over 50% of new infection taking place among the youth below 25 years. HIV prevalence has reached over 1% among women attending antenatal clinics.

Eighty per cent of new infection are through the sexual transmission, 6% through injecting drugs and another 4% through blood transfusion and blood products infusion.

There are mainly two types of Human Immunodeficiency Virus (HIV) : HIV type 1 (HIV_1); HIV type 2 (HIV_2); within HIV_1, there are various subtypes.

In India, the most common type of HIV seen is type 1 and subtype C which are more virulent, subtype C virus spreads faster and if not controlled, kills faster. As HIV_1 subtype 0 and C are common in Inda, more research has to be conducted on these subtypes.

However, HIV type 2 is generally less common as well as less dangerous and it does not spread as fast as the other in India.

HIV type 1 virus is more common and consists of innumerable other subtypes; within these there are subtypes M, N, O. Within the subtype M which is the most common type in the world, there are two subtypes B and C.

As per VACO figures, in India, around 80% have HIV type 1; 1.8% have HIV type 2 and 1.5% have HIV type 1 and 2 combined. HIV type 1 subtype C is more dangerous as it spreads faster and if not controlled properly it can cause early death.

In rich development world (North America, Europe) HIV type 1 and subtype B virus are more common.

As per Manorama year book, 2002, figures : In 2000, people living with HIV/AIDS 36.1 million, new HIV infections 5.3 million, deaths 3 million for more update report (24.02.03).

Brisborne, California based company said that HIV killed 25 million people around the world and has infected 40 million more. Experts agree that a vaccine is the only hope for controlling HIV. Vaccine maker Vax Gen says that the only waited result for the human test of a vaccine against AIDS virus will be announced today Monday, 24.2.2003. (Times of India, Washington report, 24.2.03).

Vaccine maker Vax Gen Inc. President Dr. Donald Francis said that, on Monday (24.2.03), the first attempt to develop a vaccine to prevent AIDS has failed (Times of India, 28.2.03).

The most important groups of skin conditions associated with HIV infection.

Viral infections	Herpes zoster Herpes simplex Oral hairy leucoplakia (Epstein-Barr Virus)
Bacterial infections	Recurrent folliculitis abscess cellulitis Pyomyositis, multiple lesions Chancroid, Syphilis
Fungal infections	Candidiasis
Non-infective conditions	Pruritic papular eruption-of HIV infection Seborrhoeic dermatitis Atopic dermatitis Acquired Veroderma — dry skin Facial hyperpigmentation
Drug reaction	Tubercular drug-thiace- tazone (+ INH)
Neoplasm	Kaposi's sarcoma

FEVER

Fever is caused by a disturbance in temperature regulation. Normal body temperature varies between 36.6° to 37.2°C. With acute fevers the skin blood vessels are constricted and shivering or rigor results. When a higher temperature is attained the blood vessels dilate. The body surface begins to feel warm.

Fever may be occasional or regular. Terms like intermittent, remittent and continued are used to describe the periodicity. Malarial fever, for instance, is characteristically intermittent. Fevers may worsen in the afternoon or night — as in amoebic abscess, typhoid fever or malaria. Sometimes the exacerbation may be in the morning as in tuberculosis. It is helpful to keep a daily record of the temperature chart, morning and evening.

To take the temperature properly, the thermometer must be in the mouth for at least two minutes. In young children the thermometer may be placed in the fold of the groin with the thigh flexed on the abdomen. Rectal temperature may also be taken by a specially made rectal thermometer. Rectal temperatures are usually half a degree higher than that in the groin or axilla.

Fever is frequently accompanied by chills (rigor). In infants and children there may be convulsions. Various types of skin rash and spots in the mouth may be present — as in measles. Skin rash breaking into pustules suggests chicken-pox. Swelling of the jaw on both sides and testicular swelling indicates mumps. Neck stiffness, delirium and high fever indicate meningitis. Thus, the various signs and symptoms associated with fever give a clue to the diagnosis.

It is worthwhile to remember that many fevers are viral in origin and may be self-limiting. The glycolipid portion of cell wall of Gram-negative bacilli *(S. typhi)* is responsible for fever, similarly Malaria toxin in Malaria.

A word of caution regarding treatment. Indiscriminate swallowing of antibiotics is to be decried. It confuses the clinical picture, causes emergence of resistant organisms and can lead to unnecessary complications of antibiotic therapy. Indeed, drugs themselves can cause fever.

Paracetamol is a useful home remedy for fever. Other home remedies include sponging with ice-cold water and the use of ice-packs.

If the child has fever which does not settle down with the usual home remedies within a day or two the public health nurse should inform the doctor. Today, with the aid of a few investigations like blood count, urine examination, sputum test, X-ray chest or abdominal ultra-sonography, the cause of most fevers can be quickly arrived at. Fever is one of the most useful warning signals of the body. Fever can result in unpleasant complications — death. Thus, the fever should not be ignored.

COMMON CAUSES OF FEVER

Cause	*Signs and Symptoms*
Pneumonia	: Cough, chest pain, expectoration.
Tuberculosis	: Cough, loss of weight, bloody sputum, enlarged lymph glands, pleurisy.
Throat Infection	: Throat pain, enlarged tonsils, cough.
Ear Infection	: Discharge from ear, earache.
Sinusitis	: Facial pain, headache.
Gall bladder inflam-mation	: Pain in the upper part of the abdomen, chills, jaundice.
Hepatitis	: Chills, jaundice, loss of appetite.
Liver Abscess	: Chills, pain in liver region.
Meningitis	: Headache, neck stiffness, mental confusion.
Malaria	: Fever with periodicity, chills.
Typhoid	: Malaise, abdominal discomfort, intestinal bleeding or perforation.
Urinary tract infection	: Chills, burning urine, pain in the flanks.
Rheumatic fever	: Painful joints preceded by sore throat, heart murmur.
Osteomyelitis	: Bone pains, chills.
Collagen disorders	: Rash, muscle pain, kidney involvement, fever responding to steroid therapy, not antibiotics.
Tumours	: Depends on location.
Bacterial endocarditis	: Heart murmur, rash, chills, embolic phenomenon.
Veneral diseases	: Depends on causative organism fever, rash, discharge, swelling of glands in the groin.
Heat Hyperpyrexia	: Exposure to high temperature.

BACTERIOPHAGE

Bacteriophage *(phage = to eat)* is dealt in this chapter as it is commonly found in the intestine of man and the nurse should have a clear concept of bacteriophage. Bacteriophage resemble tadpole having large head and tail. It is a virus of bacteria. Twort (British) in 1915 and d'Herelle (French) in 1917 independently observed the phenomenon of the transmissible lysis of bacteria. If feces from dysentery patients are emulsified in water and filtered through Seitz filter which arrests the bacteria, the bacteria-free filtrate contains a living agent visible under electron microscope, which will dissolve young, growing bacteria, dysentery bacilli. This is called "Twort-d'Herelle phenomenon".

Varieties of bacteriophages. There are many bacteriophages each of which attacks one or more species of bacteria. Usually a given phage will attack only a single kind of bacterium. They have general properties of other viruses. They can be cultivated only in contact with living bacteria.

Bacteriophages are also recognised by their ability to produce a clearing of an area when spotted on to a confluent growth of the host bacterium on an agar plate. The clear zone is known as "*Plaque*".

Thus, the lytic phage has been used in the detection and identification of pathogenic bacteria. The laboratory procedure is termed "*Bacteriophage typing*. In this way phage serves as a tool for medical diagnosis and for tracing the source of the disease spreading in the community.

INTERFERON

Double infection of cells does not always result in complimentation or cooperation; more commonly interference occurs with bacterial viruses previous viral infection may alter the cell surface so that it cannot adsorb other viruses (lysogenic conversion).

The mechanism with viruses and eukaryotic cells depends on a unique substance — *Interferon.*

Interferon. Among animal viruses, interference of one virus with replication of another may be mediated by a protein called interferon which is produced by the cell after infection with the first virus. The ability to produce interferon seems to be a property of vertebrate cell; both DNA and RNA viruses stimulate interferon, but there is considerable variation in inducer efficiency.

Interferon is a protein with molecular weight of about 30,000 dalton. As a result of its size, interferon has been readily released from cell, and in the body it can diffuse throughout the extracellular fluids. It is also a very stable protein which can be extracted by treatment at pH 2.0. This extraction does not reduce its activity although it inactivates the inducing virus. Interferon is sensitive to Actinomycin D and Puromycin. If interferon is produced in human cells, it can be used for human infection. Interferon causes the cell to manufacture the proteins which have direct effect on virus multiplication.

CHAPTER 46

INTESTINAL PROTOZOA

I. Rhizopoda — *Entamoeba histolytica, E. Coli, Acanthamoeba, Castellani, Naegleria fowleri.*

II. Mastigophora — *Giardia intestinalis, Trichomonas hominis*

III. Sporozoa — *Isospora belli, Cryptosporidium, Toxoplasma gondii*

IV. Ciliata — *Balantidium coli*

E. histolytica is cosmopolitan, occurs in three forms : Trophozoite (Fig. 46a.1) precystic (Fig. 46a.2) and cystic (Fig. 46a.3-5) forms and passes its life cycle in one host only, i.e., man. When the fully developed cysts containing four nuclei are swallowed by man, they pass down the intestine where the excystation of oocysts takes place at alkaline pH, hence the trophozoites (Vegetative amoebae) are formed and invade the intestinal mucosa, multiply, cause flask shaped ulceration of the intestine; few enter the blood stream, are carried to other organs (i.e., liver, lung, brain) where they give rise to *amoebic abscess*, some are discharged into the lumen of the gut and are transformed into small *precystic* forms from which

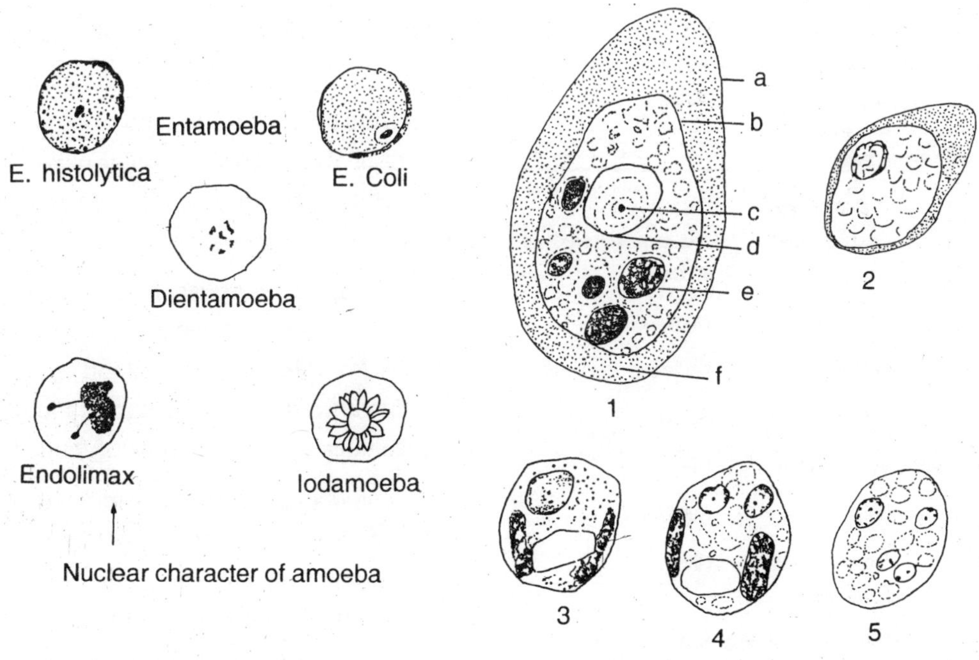

Fig. 46a.1-5 : E. histolytica

Fig. 46a.1 — a - pseudo podium; b - endoplasm; c - karyosome; d - nuclear membrane; e - ingested red blood cells; f - ectoplasm.

the adult *cysts* are developed and passed in the faeces. Thus the life cycle is repeated.

Clinical features. The incubation period is 4-5 days. *E. histolytica* causes *amoebic dysentery* or amoebiasis which is characterised by the passage of blood and mucus in the stool.

The macroscopic and microscopic differences between the stools of amoebic and bacillary dysentery are described below :

	Amoebic dysentery	*Bacillary dysentery*
Macroscopic differences		
Frequency	6-8 motions per day	Over 8 motions per day
Quantity	Relatively copious	Small
Odour	Offensive	Odourless
Colour	Dark red	Bright red
Nature	Blood and mucus mixed with faeces	Blood and mucus only, no faeces
Reaction	Acid	Alkaline
Consistency	Not adherent to the container	Adherent to the container
Microscopic differences		
RBC	In clumps; yellow green in colour	Discrete or in rouleaux, bright red in colour
Pus cells	Scanty	Numerous
Macrophages	Very few	Large and numerous
Eosinophils	Present	Scarce
Pyknotic bodies	Very common	Nil
Ghost cells	Nil	Numerous
Parasites	Trophozoites of *E. histolytica*	Nil
Bacteria	Many motile bacteria	Non-motile bacteria
C.L. Crystals*	Present	Nil

*Charcot-Leyden crystals. In saline preparation, they appear as diamond shaped crystals, clear and refractile.

In intestinal amoebiasis a definite diagnosis can be done by 1) Stool examination in which the cysts (in formed stool), and the trophozoites (in diarrhoeal stool) are identified; 2) Sigmoidoscopy, in which scrapings from any lesions in the rectum are examined for trophozoites.

In extra-intestinal amoebiasis, the following procedures are followed :

1. Clinical diagnosis of amoebic liver abscess (ALA) by (a) hepatomegaly, pain, fever and sweating, which is later confirmed by the presence of cysts and trophozoites in the tissues, (b) X-ray or ultrasonography of the abdomen. (c) Immuno-diagnosis tests. The haemagglutination, complement fixation, gel diffusion; recent cellulose acetate precipitin (CAP), dot immuno binding assay (DIB) and sandwich enzyme linked. *Immunosorbent Assay (ELISA) tests.* Western blot of *E. histolytica* may become one of the very recent more accurate methods for the successful immunodiagnosis of acute intestinal amoebiasis.

Treatment. Amicline is a complete current amoebicide used for eradication of extra intestinal and intestinal amoebiasis. Amicline plus is effective for amoebic and bacillary dysentery. Tinidazole is useful.

Prophylaxis. Personal prophylaxis consists of (1) use of boiled drinking water, (2) protection of food and drink from flies, cockroaches and rats, (3) avoiding eating unwashed raw vegetables and fruits and (4) personal cleanliness while taking food.

Community prophylaxis comprises (1) effective sanitary disposal of faeces, (2) protection of water supplies from fecal pollution, (3) avoidance of the use of human excreta as fertiliser, and (4) detection and isolation of carriers.

E. coli are worldwide and live in the large intestine of man. They are similar morphologically and in their life cycle to *E. histolytica* and are commensal.

TROPHOZOITES AND CYSTS OF E. histolytica AND E. Coli

	E. histolytica	*E. coli*
TROPHOZOITES		
Fresh Preparation		
Size	20-30 microns	20-40 microns.
Motility	Very active	Sluggish.
Cytoplasm	Clearly defined into cytoplasm	Not defined Cytoplasm scarcely seen.
Cytoplasmic inclusions	Red blood cells leucocytes and tissue debris but no bacteria.	Bacteria and other materials but never red blood cells
Nucleus	Not visible in unstained preparation	Visible in unstained preparation
Stained with Iodine		
Nuclear material	Central Karyosome, fine chromatin granules line the delicate nuclear membrane	Eccentric Karyosome, coarse chromatin granules line the thick nuclear membrane
CYST		
Fresh preparation		
Chromatoid bodies	Rounded bars	Filamentous, thread like with square or pointed ends.
Stained with Iodine		
Size	10-15 microns	15-20 microns
Nucleus	1-4; central Karyosome.	1-8; eccentric Karyosome
Glycogen mass	Visible in uninucleate stage	Large and visible in the binucleate stage (Fig. 46b.6, 7, 8, 9).

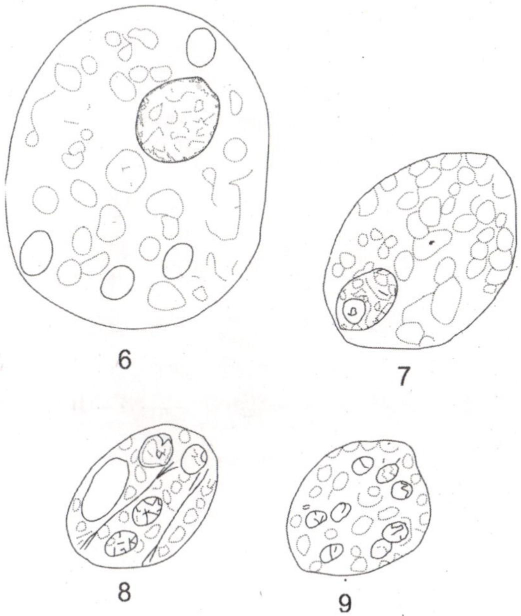

Fig. 46b.6-9 : Entamoeba coli

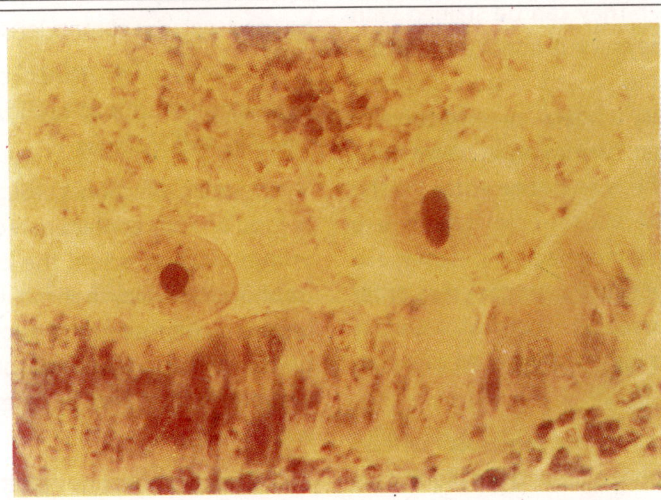

Fig. 46c : Balantidum coli 1. Trophozoite (right); 2. Cyst (left) × 400

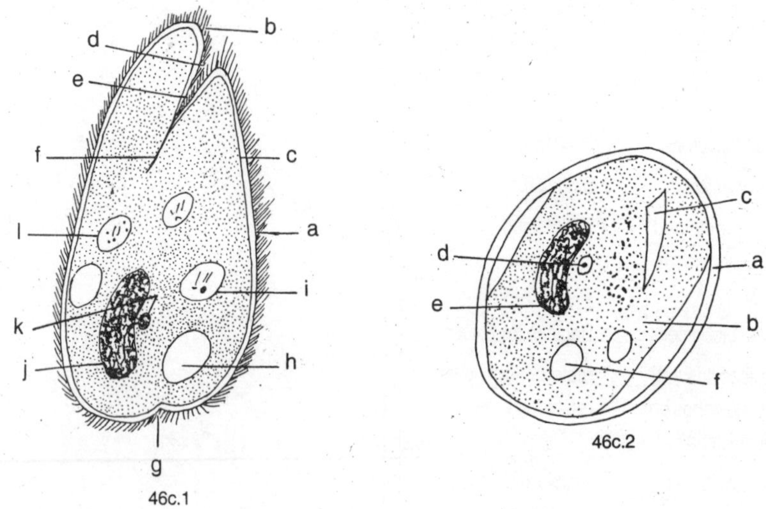

Fig. 46c. 1-2: Balantidium coli

Fig. 46c.1 — a - cilia; b - adoral cilia; c- thin layer of ectoplasm; d - peristome; e - cytostome; f - cytopharynx; g - cytopyge; h - vacuole; i - food vacuole; j - macronucleus; k - micronucleus; l - granular endoplasm.

Fig. 46c.2 — a - double layered wall; b - granular cytoplasm; c - refractile body; d - micronucleus; e - macronucleus; f - vacuole

Naegleria fowleri (Free — living amoeba), *Acanthamoeba castellani*, elongated, 10-22 × 7 microns, are rapidly motile. Their cytoplasm contains vacuoles and mitochondria (absent in Entamoeba), no red blood cells. They develop flagella after 2-4 hours in distilled water. They can be stained with Giemsa stain. Though they survive transit through the gastrointestinal tract and passed in stool, they are known to cause primary amoebic meningoencephalitis (PAM). In children swimming in warm soil - contaminated pools, these amoebae enter, via the nose and cribriform plate, into the brain tissue where they cause extensive haemorrhage and damage in the cerebrum and cerebellum; even they may enter from skin ulcers. There is report of corneal ulceration or keratitis from contaminated saline used with contact lenses.

Microscopic examination of cerebrospinal fluid (CSF) will show the trophozoites and red blood cells but no bacteria.

Treatment with amphotericin B has been successful. Sulphonamide and α - hydroxystibamide have been recommended for Acanthamoebiasis.

Prophylaxis by avoiding swimming in warm soil contaminated pools. Contaminated saline should not be used with the contact lenses.

GIARDIA INTESTINALIS, causal agent of giardiasis, has both trophozoite (Fig. 46d.1, Fig. 46d.2) and cyst (Fig. 46d.3) stages.

Human infection is brought about by ingestion of food or drink contaminated with cysts. Within 30 minutes of ingestion, the cyst hatches out two trophozoites which then multiply in enormous numbers and colonise in the duodenum. When conditions in the duodenum become unfavourable, encystment occurs and the cysts are passed out along with faeces.

Their trophozoites attach themselves on the epithelial cells of the intestine and disturb the intes-

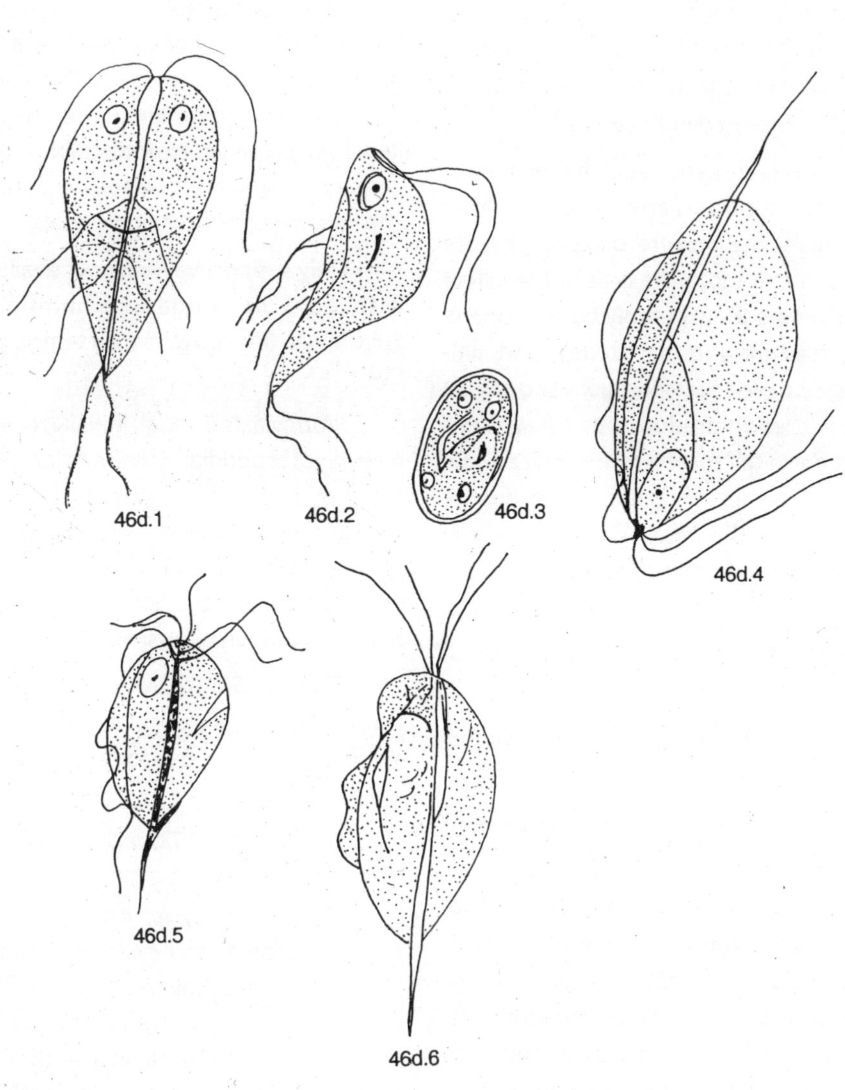

Fig. 46d. 1-6 : Flagellates

tinal function leading to malabsorption of fat. There is mild steatorrhoea (passage of stools with excess fat), loose motions, chronic enteritis and cholecystopathy.

G. lamblia has been shown to induce an intestinal Ig A response against the parasite. This antibody blocks adherance of trophozoite to intestinal epithelium with subsequent removal of trophozoite from the intestine by peristalsis.

Diagnosis is by (1) microscopic examination of trophozoites in diarrhoea stools and cysts in formed cysts; trophozoites in the duodenal aspirates; (2) fluoroscopy which may demonstrate the hypermotility of the jejunum and (3) X-ray which may reveal mucosal defects.

Treatment. Metronidazole or *Quinacrine* can eliminate the infection. Only by personal hygiene, its spread can be prevented. Albendazole is a current effective antigiardial agent.

TRICHOMONAS HOMINIS, found in ileo-caecal region may invade the vagina; but they are non-pathogenic (Fig. 46d.5), T. tenax (Fig. 46d.6).

ISOSPORA BELLI are parasites of the small intestine of man and form oocysts and sporocysts. After ingestion by man, the mature oocysts liberate sporocysts which enter into the cells of the villi of small intestine where they multiply by schizogony (Trophozoite, schizont and merozoites) and, ultimately, the oocysts develop by sporogony and passed in the faeces. The lesion produced by *I. belli* is unknown in man; but in calf, there is mucous diarrhoea. In man, the symptoms are anorexia, nausea, abdominal pain and diarrhoea. The infection in man is usually self-limited. In immuno-compromised (AIDS) patients, *I. belli* causes severe complications (diarrhoea).

Oocysts of *I. belli* can be demonstrated microscopically in the faeces.

There is no specific treatment for human infection. Rest with bland diet is effective.

Prophylaxis can be done by adopting the methods recommended for amoebiasis and giardiasis.

CRYPTOSPORIDIUM are coccidia related to *Isospora*, have long been known as parasites of fowls, rodents, cattle and have probably been an unrecognised cause of self-limited, mild gastroenteritis and diarrhoea in man. It is distributed in many countries including India. The children are more susceptible than adults.

These parasites are minute (2-5 microns) intracellular sphere found in great number just under the mucosal epithelium of the stomach or intestine. The mature trophozoite (Schizont) divide into arc shaped merozoites which are released from the infected mucosal cell to begin a new life cycle. Oocysts (4-5 microns) containing 4 sporozoites are passed into feces and become infective agents. If stained by modified Ziehl-Neelsen staining, oocysts in the stool appear faintly blue with reddish or purple corpuscles.

Patients infected with cryptosporidim have watery diarrhoea, cramps, upper abdominal pain (exacerbated by food ingestion), weight loss and flatulence, nausea, vomiting, anorexia, myalgia, malaise, dehydration, fever not common. The disease is self-limited. They cause severe intractable diarrhoea in the immunocompromised persons (e.g., those with AIDS) and immunocompetent individuals.

Only supportive therapy is available for those with AIDS or congenital immunodeficiency. Spiromycin (Rovamycin) may temporarily be effective.

Prophylaxis. Though initially recognised in animals, cryptosporidial infection is increasingly recognised as important cause of diarrhoea in both immunocompromised and immunocompetent individuals. Previously, it was thought that the source of infection was in animals but the transmission from human to human is possible.

TOXOPLASMA GONDII is distributed all over the world and is an obligatory, intracellular, *coccidial* parasite. It may occur in two forms : *extracellular* and *intracellular* forms.

The life cycle of *T. gondii* may be (a) enteric and (b) exo-enteric :

(a) *Enteric cycle.* After eating mouse brain containing cysts of *T. gondii*, cycles of schizogony and sporogony develop inside the intestinal mucosa of the cat ultimately liberating oocysts in the infected cat's feces.

(b) *Exo-enteric cycle. P* The oocysts, after ingestion, liberate sporozoites which, in man, penetrate the mucosa of the intestine and are carried by blood and lymph stream to distant organs (brain, eyes, liver, lymph nodes, heart, skeletal muscles and placenta of the pregnant uterus) where they from pseudocysts which multiply causing damage to the central nervous system and musculature.

Toxoplasmosis may be congenital or acquired.

In congenital toxoplasmosis, there is encephalitis, chorioretinitis, hydrocephalus, mental retardation and convulsion.

Acquired toxoplasmosis is very rare in adults, often fatal.

In laboratory diagnosis, complement fixation test of Warren and Sabin; skin test of Sabin and Feldman are often used; ELISA (recent) test is used to assist the diagnosis.

The direct agglutination test with 2 mercaptoethanol (AD, 2 ME) and Immuno fluorescent test (IFAT) are very recently used in the diagnosis of Toxoplasmosis. The former is little superior to the latter Latex agglutination test (LAT) or ELISA can detect *T. gondii* antibody.

Radiological diagnosis is done to show cerebral calcification.

Treatment is unsatisfactory. Sulphonamides and pyrimethamine are currently used.

BALANTIDIUM COLI is the largest cosmopolitan protozoon of the large intestine of man, monkey and pig, where the trophozoites feed on bacteria and mucus and on the cells of the intestinal wall. The pig is the reservoir of infection and does not suffer from the infection.

It has two stages : trophozoite (Fig. 46c.1) and cysts (Fig. 46c.2).

Life cycle. Man gets infected after ingestion of cysts in pig's faeces. Excystation takes place in the large intestine liberating trophozoites which enter into the intestinal mucosa causing ulceration and encyst in the lumen and cysts are excreted in the feces.

In majority of cases, dysentery is characteristic accompanied by abdominal pain, tenesmus, nausea and vomiting. Loss of appetite, headache, insomnia, muscular weakness and loss of weight are also observed.

Laboratory diagnosis depends on the demonstration of trophozoites and cysts in dysenteric and formed stools, respectively.

Treatment. Carbarsone, Diodohydroxyquin and Tetracycline are used in treating human cases.

Prophylaxis is same as that of amoebiasis.

MICROSPORIDIA are ubiquitous obligate intracellular new protozoan parasites found commonly in laboratory animals. They are unicellular Gram-positive organisms with mature spores $0.5 - 2 \times 1 - 4\mu$ in diameter. The spores have an extrusion apparatus consisting of a coiled polar filament and anchoring disk and contain the infective agent known as sporoplasm. The potential of Microsporidia for infecting warm blooded vertebrates is only now being recognised. Significant microsporidiosis in human is increasing in association with the increase in patients with AIDS. There are four genera of microsporidia known to infect human beings :

1. *Enterocytozoan bieneusi*, the most common microsporidian observed in AIDS patients, infects the intestinal mucosa and causes diarrhoea. Its estimated prevalence may be as high as 10% in AIDS patients.

2. *Pleistophora* species was reported in an immuno compromised HIV negative patient with myositis.

3. *Encephalitozoon cuniculi* was reported in AIDS patients with peritonitis, hepatitis. Very recently a new *E. heliun* sp. has been isolated from three AIDS patients.

CHAPTER 47

INTESTINAL HELMINTHS

Cestoda. *Diphyllobothrium latum, Taenia saginata, T. solium, Echinococcus granulosus, Hymenolepis nana, Dipylidium caninum.*

Trematoda. *Fasciolopsis buski, Fasciola hepatica, Gastrodiscoides hominis.*

Nematoda. *Trichinella spiralis, Trichuris trichiura, Strongyloides stercoralis, Ankylostoma duodenale, Necator americanus, Enterobius vermicularis, Ascaris lumbricoides.*

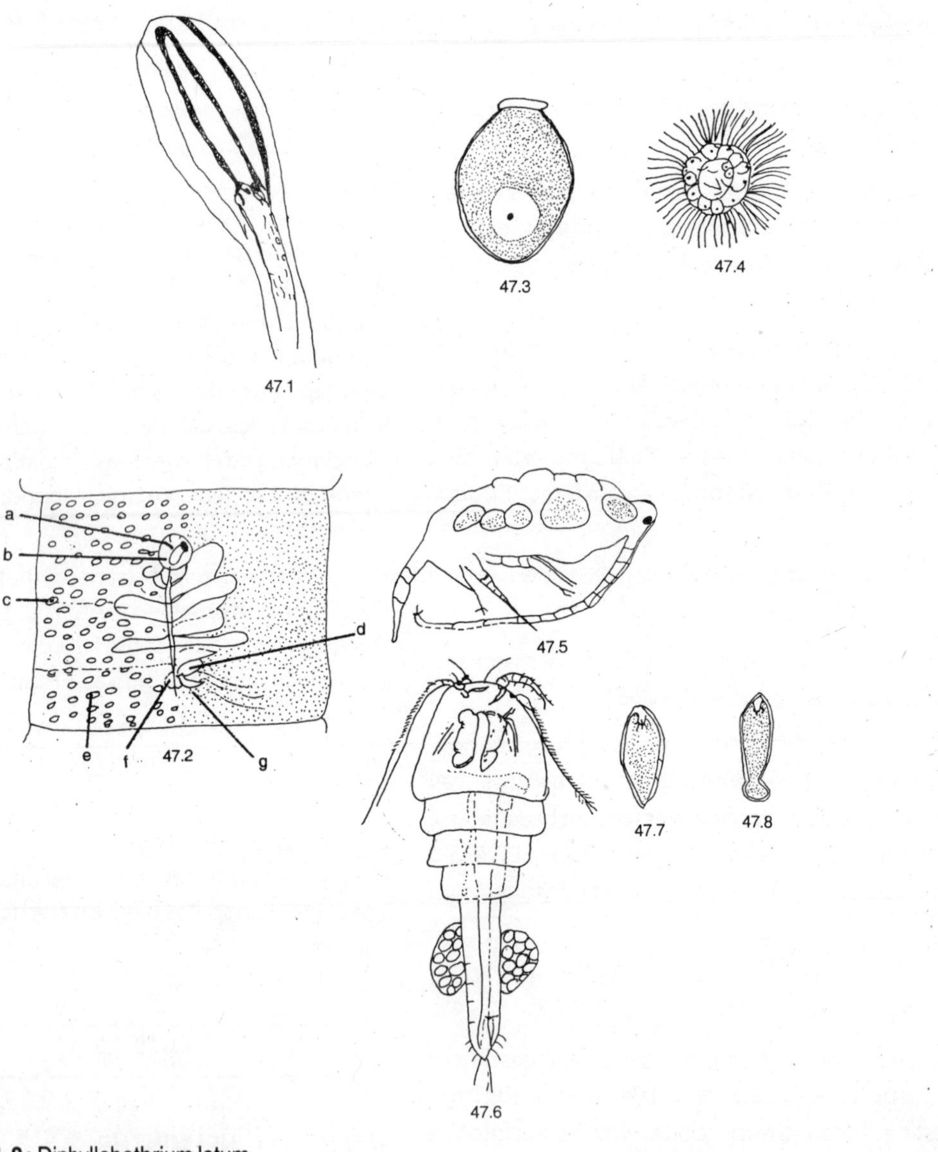

Fig. 47.1-8: Diphyllobothrium latum

Fig. 47.2 — a - male genital sucker; b - uterine pore; c - testis; d - seminal receptacle; e - ovary; f - ootype; g - vittelline gland

DIPHYLLOBOTHRIUM LATUM (Fish Tapeworm)

The adult worm is ivory or yellowish grey in colour, measuring 3-10 meters in length. The head (Fig. 47.1) (Scolex) is small, spatulated or spoon shaped, has a pair of slit grooves (bothria) ventrally and dorsally and has no rostellum (a beak-like projection on the head) and no hooklets. Scolex is followed by "neck" and 3,000 segments (proglottids) (Fig. 47.2). A single worm may discharge as many as one million eggs per day from ootype.

Life cycle. When the egg (Fig. 47.3) of *D. latum* passed out along with the feces of the infected host (man) comes in contact with water, the ciliated embryo (*coracidium*) (Fig. 47.4), escapes from the egg

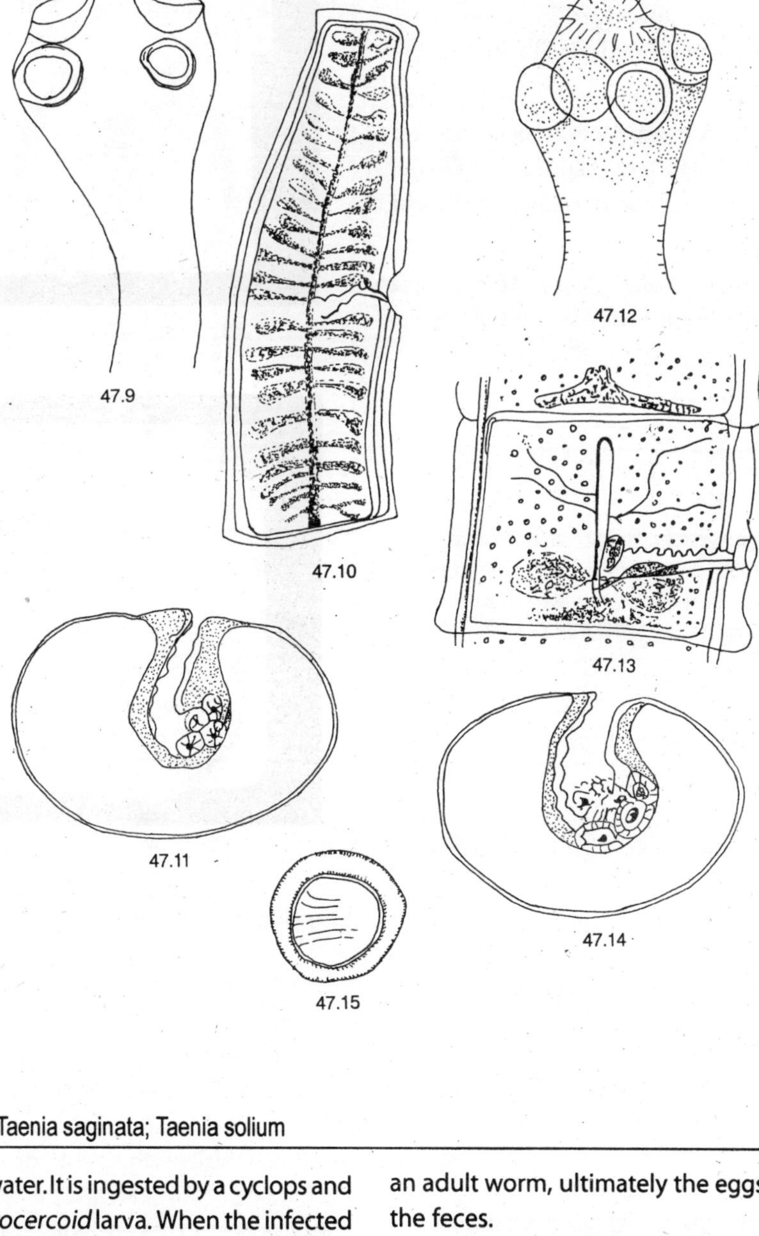

Fig. 47.9-15 : Taenia saginata; Taenia solium

and swims in the water. It is ingested by a cyclops and transforms into *procercoid* larva. When the infected cyclops (Fig. 47.5, 6) is ingested by a fish, procercoid (Fig. 47.7) develops into plerocercoid or sparganum larva (Fig. 47.8) in the fish which is infective to man. On consuming insufficiently cooked fish, man becomes infected. The plerocercoid larva develops into an adult worm, ultimately the eggs are excreted in the feces.

Clinical features. The presence of adult worm in the intestinal tract causes no symptom, but sometimes, non-specific abdominal symptoms have been ascribed. If the worms attach themselves to the jejunum, clinical vitamin B_{12} deficiency develops.

In the *laboratory*, microscopical examination of the faeces will reveal the eggs; sometimes proglottids can be observed in the stool.

Treatment. Quinacrine hydrochloride, niclosamide and paromomycin are found effective. Pernicious anaemia can be treated with folic acid.

Prophylaxis. (1) Thorough cooking of suspected freshwater fish is important; (2) Pollution of water can be prevented by efficient disposal of sewage; (3) In endemic areas of infection, dogs and cats should not be given fish.

TAENIA SAGINATA (Beef Tape Worm) AND T. SOLIUM (Pork Tape Worm) have a cosmopolitan distribution.

Difference between these two worms

	T. saginata	*T. solium*
Length	5 - 10 meters	2 - 7 meters
Head	Large quardrate; without rostellum and hooks; pigmented suckers (Fig. 47.9)	Small globular with rostellum and hooks; suckers not pigmented. (Fig. 47.12)
Proglottid Number	1,000 - 2,000	Under 1,000
Expulsion	Expelled singly (Fig. 47.10)	Expelled in chairs of 5 - 6 (Fig. 47.13)
Uterus	15 - 30 thin lateral branches on each side.	5 - 10 thick lateral branches on each side.
Vagina	Vaginal sphincter present	Vaginal sphincter absent
Ovaries	Two in number without an accessory lobe	Two in number with an accessory lobe
Testes	300 - 400 follicles	150 - 200 follicles
Eggs	Spherical and brown (31 - 43 microns)	Spherical, brown (31 - 43 microns) (Fig. 47.15)
Bladder worm	*Cysticercus bovis* (measly beef), not found in man (Fig. 47.11)	*C. cellulosae* (pork measle, measly pork) occasionally found in man (Fig. 47.14)
Intermediate host	Cattle	Pig

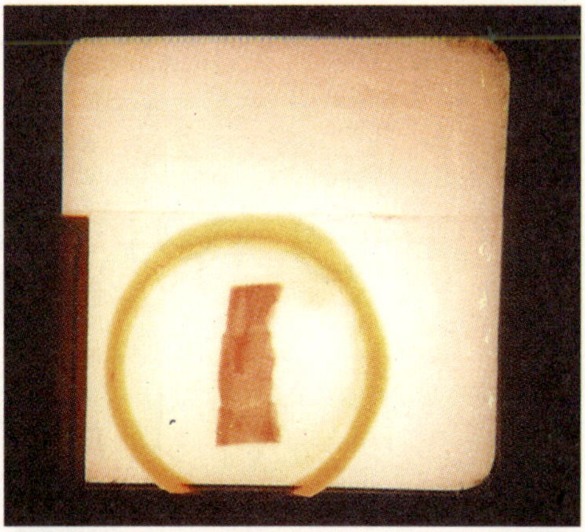

Fig. 47.10 : Taenia saginata — Segment (natural size)

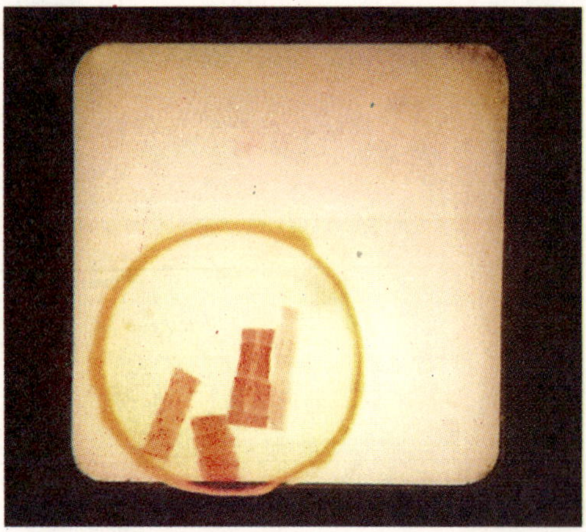

Fig. 47.13 : Taenia solium — Segment (natural size)

Life Cycle of T. saginata

While grazing on the polluted ground, the mature eggs (Fig. 47.15) are ingested by cattle. The onchospheres are hatched out from the eggs in the duodenum. These embryos penetrate the intestinal wall of the cattle, are carried through blood stream and reach the liver, the right side of the heart, lungs, the left side of the heart and the systemic circulation. These oncospheres are filtered out in the striped muscles and transform into bladder worm *(Cysticereus bovis)*. On ingesting infected raw beef, man becomes infected with this bladder worm. The larva is digested out of the beef, the scolex evaginates, attaches itself to the intestinal wall of man and deve-

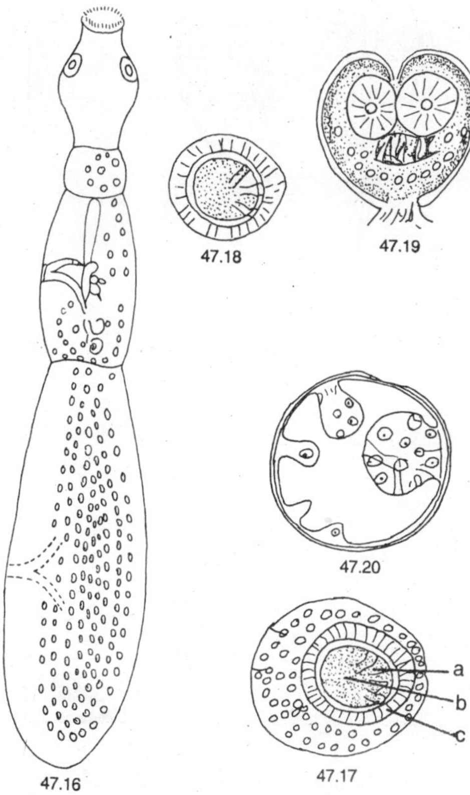

Fig. 47.16-20 : Echinococcus granulosus
Fig. 47.17 — a - hookets; b - oncosphere; c - embryophore

lops into adult worm, which liberates eggs. The life cycle of *T. solium* is similar to that of *T. saginata* but *C. cellulosae* produce *Cysticercosis cellulosae* in man or neurocysticercosis in the brain of man, resulting into epileptiform seizures with a rapidly fatal outcome.

Recent dot-ELISA is very sensitive and quite specific in *the diagnosis of neurocysticercosis.* Magnetic Resonance Imaging (MRI) Ultrasonography and Computed Tomography (CT) scan detect *C. cellulosae* in the brain.

Clinical features. Because of its large size, *T. saginata* is responsible for considerable disturbance in the normal function of the intestine; whereas *T. solium* may cause irritation and less intestinal obstruction, vague abdominal discomfort, hunger pains, chronic indigestion and persistent diarrhoea alternating with constipation are the common symptoms.

Laboratory diagnosis can be done by demonstration of Taenia egg (eggs of both *Taenia sp.* are identical), by recovery of gravid segments. A dot - ELISA test can be used to diagnose neurocysticercosis.

Treatment. Quinacrine, niclosamide, bithionol, mebendazole, are effective. Albendazole is very effective for neurocysticercosis, (*T. solium*).

Prophylaxis. Consist of (1) personal hygiene; (2) general sanitary measures; (3) avoidance of ingestion of raw pork or beef and vegetables irrigated by sewage water; (4) rigid quality inspection of pork and beef in all slaughter-houses; (5) avoidance of fecal contamination.

ECHINOCOCCUS GRANULOSUS (Dog Tapeworm)

The adult worm (Fig. 47.16) is a minute tape worm, has a scolex, neck and strobila comprising three segments and measures 3-6 mm. in length. It has a pyriform scolex provided with four suckers and a protrusible rostellum armed with two circular rows of hooklets. The neck is short and thick. Its egg cannot be distinguished from that of Taenia and is infective to man, cattle, sheep (Fig. 47.17, 18).

Life Cycle. The infected definite host (dog) passes the stool with the eggs onto the ground. While grazing on the polluted ground, the intermediate hosts (sheep, goats and cattle) swallow these eggs, whereas children get infected while playing with dogs. The eggs hatch in the duodenum, the oncospheres migrate through the intestinal wall, en-

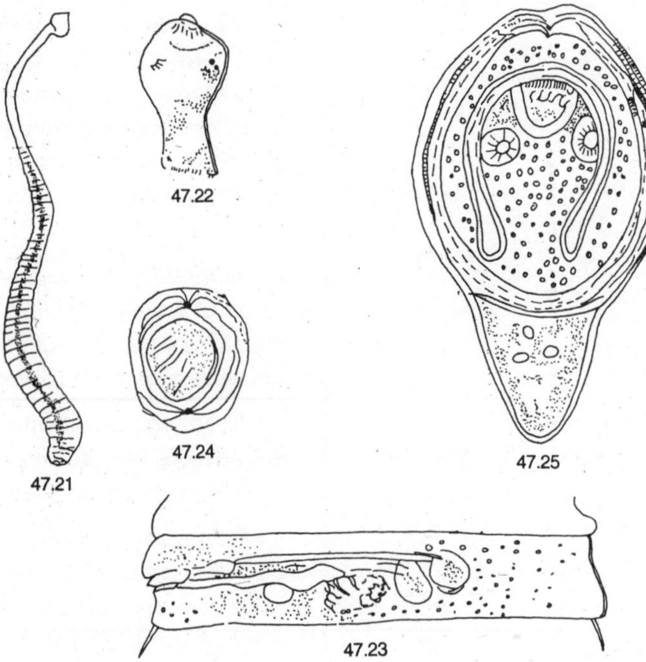

Fig. 47.21-25 : Hymenolepis nana

ter the mesenteric venules and become lodged in the capillary filter beds in various organs and tissues (liver, lungs, various organs) and develop into a cystic cavity (hydatid cyst)(Fig. 47.19, 20). When the organs or tissues containing fertile hydatid cysts are ingested by dog, the cysts develop into adult worms. The eggs are passed out in the dog's faeces.

Clinical features. The damage produced by hydatid cyst of *E. granulosus* is both mechanical and toxic. The young cysts which develop into embryos lodged in the vital centers may interfere with the function of the organs, damage the organ (brain, orbital capillary, heart valve) and even cause death.

Laboratory diagnosis. Casoni's test or intradermal test; precipitin test, complement fixation test; haemagglutination; bentonite flocculation test; latex agglutination test; fluorescent test; ELISA; exploratory cyst puncture; roentgenogram and recent Computed Tomography (CT) scan and Magnetic Resonance Imaging (MRI) are techniques used for the diagnosis of hydatid disease. Immunoblot test is under trial. Hydatid disease can be diagnosed by ultrasonography and is confirmed by Dot-blot ELISA which can detect within 30 minutes the antibodies to antigen B of hydatid fluid.

Treatment. Albendazole is most effective than thiobendazole and mebendazole. Surgical technique is also helpful.

Prophylaxis. This consists of (1) avoidance of handling infected dogs; (2) avoidance of ingestion of

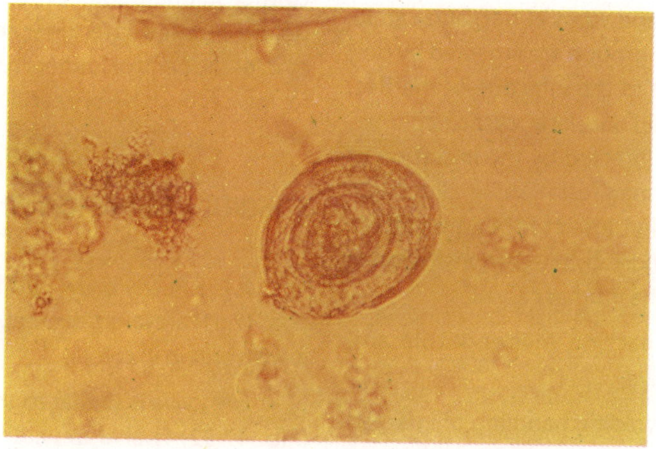

Fig. 47.24 : Hymenolepsis nana — egg × 400

raw vegetable polluted with eggs; (3) personal hygiene (cleaning hands before eating); (4) preventing dogs from eating the carcasses of sheep, cattle and dogs in infected areas; (5) discarding all infected viscera in slaughter houses by dumping them into pits inaccessible to dogs, and (6) educational propaganda in schools.

POLYCYSTIC HYDATID DISEASE (PHD)

It is caused by *Echinococcus vogeli*; the intermediate host is the wild rodent. PHD is mainly distributed throughout America.

Surgical treatment of PHD is not feasible because the multiple cysts involve extensive portion of the liver and other organs and disseminate throughout the peritoneum which are detected by ultrasonography.

Albendazole 10 mg / kg orally is effective in the treatment of patients with PHD.

HYMENOLEPIS NANA

H. nana is a cosmopolitan parasite. It is small and measures up to 25-40 mm in length by one mm in diameter. Its scolex (Fig. 47.21) is minute, rhomboidal and has four suckers and a short retractile (Fig. 47.22) rostellum armed with 20 - 30 hooklets in one single row. The rostellar hooklets are shaped like tuning forks and its neck is long and its segments (Fig. 47.23) are about 200. Its egg (Fig. 47.24) is spherical, contains an oncosphere enclosed in an inner envelope with two polar thickenings from which polar filaments.

Life cycle. When fully embryonated eggs in human feces are ingested by man, only one host, they hatch in the intestine, then the free oncospheres penetrate into the villi of the small intestine and metamorphose into young cercocysts (larvae) (Fig. 47.25) which migrate into the lumen, become attached by their scolices to the small intestine and develop into mature worms which lay eggs.

Clinical features. There is generalised toxaemia due to absorption of the metabolic wastes of the parasite. The general symptoms are headache, dizziness, anorexia, pruritus of nose and anus, periodic diarrhoea and abdominal pain.

In the *laboratory*, the characteristic eggs can be demonstrated microscopically in the patient's stool.

Treatment. Niclosamide, Hexylresorcinol crystalloid, Quinacrine and mebendazole are very effective.

Prophylaxis. This comprises (1) avoidance of ingestion of eggs through contaminated food or drink (contamination may occur from toilet seats, soiled linen or directly from anus to mouth; (2) personal hygiene and (3) a well-balanced diet which reduces susceptibility to infection.

DIPYLLIDIUM CANINUM

It is a common tapeworm of dog and cat. Its eggs deposited on the ground are ingested by dog flea. These eggs hatch in the intestine of the flea, develop into procercoid and, later, cysticercoid larvae. Man or dog gets infected by the ingestion of infected fleas. Clinical manifestations are intestinal disturbances, indigestion, lose of appetite and toxic nervous systems. Diagnosis by the demonstration of characteristic eggs in the mother capsules.

Treatment. Quinacrine, mebendazole and niclosamide are effective.

Prophylaxis by avoiding handling of infected dogs and by dusting of dogs with gammaxene or DDT.

FASCIOLOPSIS BUSKI (Giant Intestinal Fluke)

It is an elongated and ovoidal trematode (Fig. 47.26, 27). The eggs of *F. buski* and *F. hepatica* are large like a hen's egg and are identical.

Life cycle. When immature eggs are discharged in the feces, they mature in water and hatch out the micacidium (Fig. 47.28) which swims in the water, penetrates into the snail (Fig. 47.29) and develops into sporocysts, first, and second generation radiae and cercariae. These cercariae encyst on the seed pods of water caltrop into metacercariae. Man gets infected by swallowing the metacercariae which excyst in the duodenum and ultimately develop into adult worm, which lays eggs in human faeces.

Clinical features. Toxic diarrhoea and hunger pains are the first signs. Heavy infections have symptoms similar to gastric ulcer. Generalised toxic and allergic symptoms appear as edema of the face, abdominal wall and lower limbs.

Specific *diagnosis* depends upon the recovery of the egg of *F. buski* which is similar to that of *Fasciola hepatica.*

Treatment. Hexylresorcinol crystalloids and tetrachlorethylene are very effective.

Prophylaxis. Destruction of snails by 1,50,000 copper sulphate solution, sterilisation of night soil, before it is used as fertiliser and cooking of raw vegetables properly or immersing them in boiling water for few seconds before eating are all effective measures.

FASCIOLA HEPATICA (Sheep Liver Fluke)

It is a fleshy brown fluke (Fig. 47.30). Its eggs (Fig. 47.31) are large, ovoidal, operculated, light yellowish brown in colour.

Life cycle is similar to that of *F. buski.* Cercaria (Fig. 47.32) is also developed but the excysted metacercariae (Fig. 47.33) of *F. hepatica* migrate through the intestinal wall into the peritoneal cavity. From here, they traverse the liver parenchyma to the biliary passages, where they settle down and grow to maturity. Adult worms liberate eggs in the feces.

Clinical features. The clinical manifestations are hepatic and obstructive jaundice with coughing and vomiting, generalised abdominal rigidity, abdominal pain on pressure, urticaria, irregular fever, persistent diarrhoea, later marked anaemia, cholelithiasis is a frequent complication.

Laboratory diagnosis is based on the recovery of typical egg of *F. hepatica* in the stool.

Treatment. Emetine hydrochloride, bithionol, hexachloroparaxylene are effective.

Prophylaxis. (1) Eradication of adult worms in reservoir hosts by adequate chemotherapy; (2) destruction of snails by the use of 1 : 50,000 copper sulphate; (3) education of the local population about the danger in eating raw vegetables.

GASTRODISCUS HOMINIS

The living worm is bright pink in colour and pyriform in outline (Fig. 47.34). Its eggs are ovoidal operculate. Its life cycle is unknown. In man, it produces clinically mucous diarrhoea. In the laboratory it can be diagnosed by the demonstration of the typical eggs in the feces.

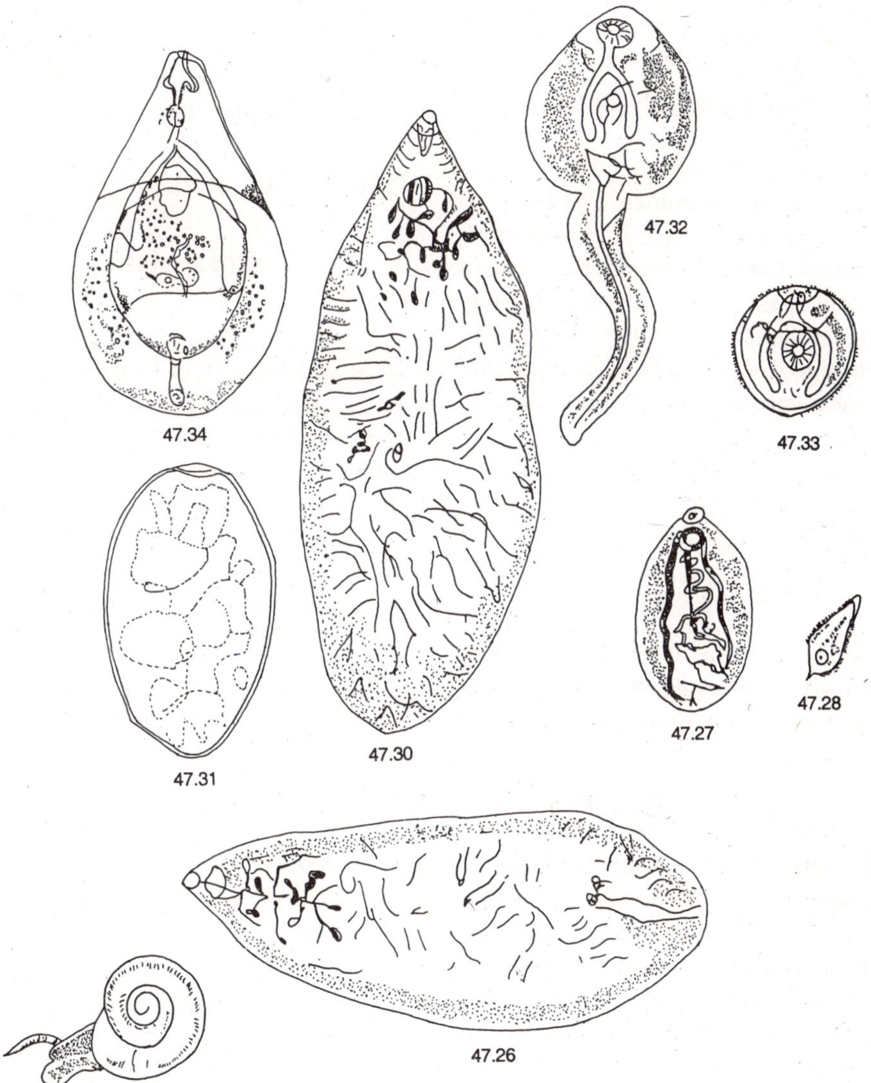

Fig.47.26-34: Gastrodiscoides, Fasciola hepatica, Fasciolopsis buski

OTHER TREMATODES

Clonorchis sinensis (Chinese liver fluke) is flat, transparent, flabby and spatulate. Its eggs are ovoidal, light yellowish and operculated.

Life cycle. When fully embryonated eggs containing miracidium are ingested by snails (Bulimus), the miracidium hatches out from the egg and transforms ultimately into cercariae which escape from the snails and swim in the water. On contact with fresh water fish, these cercariae attach to the fishes and encyst in the skin or in the flesh. Man gets infected by ingestion of infected fish, the metacercariae excyst in the duodenum and enter the common bile duct where they mature and discharge eggs.

Clinical features. There are three stages in the manifestation of symptoms : (1) the mild, symptomless; (2) the progressive stage with irregular appetite, fullness in the abdomen, diarrhoea and hepatomegaly and (3) the severe stage with portal cirrhosis syndrome. Catarrhal cholangitis occurs due to occlusion of bile passages by sticky masses of eggs and by tissue proliferation. Symptoms of systemic toxaemia are palpitation of the heart, tachychardia, vertigo, tremor, cramps and mental depression.

Opisthorchis felineus (Cat liver fluke) is morphologically similar to *C. sinensis* and also its eggs. Its life cycle is too similar, but the cercariae attack fish. Clinical features, diagnosis, prophylaxis are similar to those of *C. sinensis*, but there is no specific treatment.

Paragonimus westermani (Oriental lung fluke) is a reddish brown, plump, ovoidal fluke with rounded anterior end. The eggs are ovoidal and have a flattened operculum.

Life cycle. Eggs escaping through the bronchioles are coughed up, are swallowed and passed out of faeces. They hatch out miracidia in the water which swim in the water and attack the snails in which redia, cercariae produced liberated swim in the water and invade the viscera of cray fish or crab where the metacercariae encyst. Man becomes infected by ingestion of infected crabs. The metacercariae excyst in the duodenum and migrate through the intestinal wall, reach the abdominal cavity and travel through the diaphragm to the pleural cavity and settle in the lungs.

Clinical features. Chest pain, night sweats are common symptoms. Paroxysmal coughing is followed by haemoptysis after physical exertion. The manifestations are severe. Bronchopneumonia, or bronchiectasis with pleural effusion are the physical signs.

Diagnosis by the finding of the characteristic egg in the sputum or feces. The complement fixation test may be positive. Recent Dot-immuno binding (DIB) assay can also be used.

Treatment. Emetine hydrochloride, bithional and hexachloro-paraxylol are found effective.

Prophylaxis. (1) Avoid eating raw crabs; (2) destroy the snails; (3) disinfect the sputum or feces.

TRICHINELLA SPIRALIS (Trichina worm)

It is one of the smallest nematode (1.4 - 1.6 mm in length by 40 -60 mm in diameter (Fig. 47.35, 36).

Life cycle. When man consumes raw meat infected with the cysts of *T. spiralis* (Fig. 47.37) the cysts are digested out of the meat in the stomach. After excystation, the larvae (Fig. 47.38) invade the intestinal mucosa and develop into adults. The males die after fertilising the females which, in turn, discharge larvae. Some of them escape into the lumen of the intestine and the majority enter into the circulation through the mesenteric lymphatics, and settle at last in the striated muscles. Pigs cannot perpetuate the infection.

Clinical features. Symptoms of nausea, vomiting, toxic diarrhoea or dysentery, colic, profuse sweating, muscular pain, edema around eyes, nose and limbs, encephalitis, meningitis, deafness may occur.

Laboratory diagnosis is by the demonstration of Trichina larvae in the muscles, adult worms in the feces, blood or spinal fluid.

Bechman intradermal test; precipitin test; Bentonite flocculation test and fluorescent antibody tests are useful to diagnose Trichnielliasis.

Treatment. Thiobendazole is effective. Supportive treatment by analgesics to reduce muscular pain.

Prophylaxis. (1) Destruction of all carcasses of pigs dying on farm; (2) elimination of raw carbages; (3) extermination of rats and mice; (4) thorough cooking of all pork to be consumed by man.

TRICHURIS TRICHIURA (Whip worm)

The male adult worm is brown in colour and resembles a whip with a handle. Its posterior end of

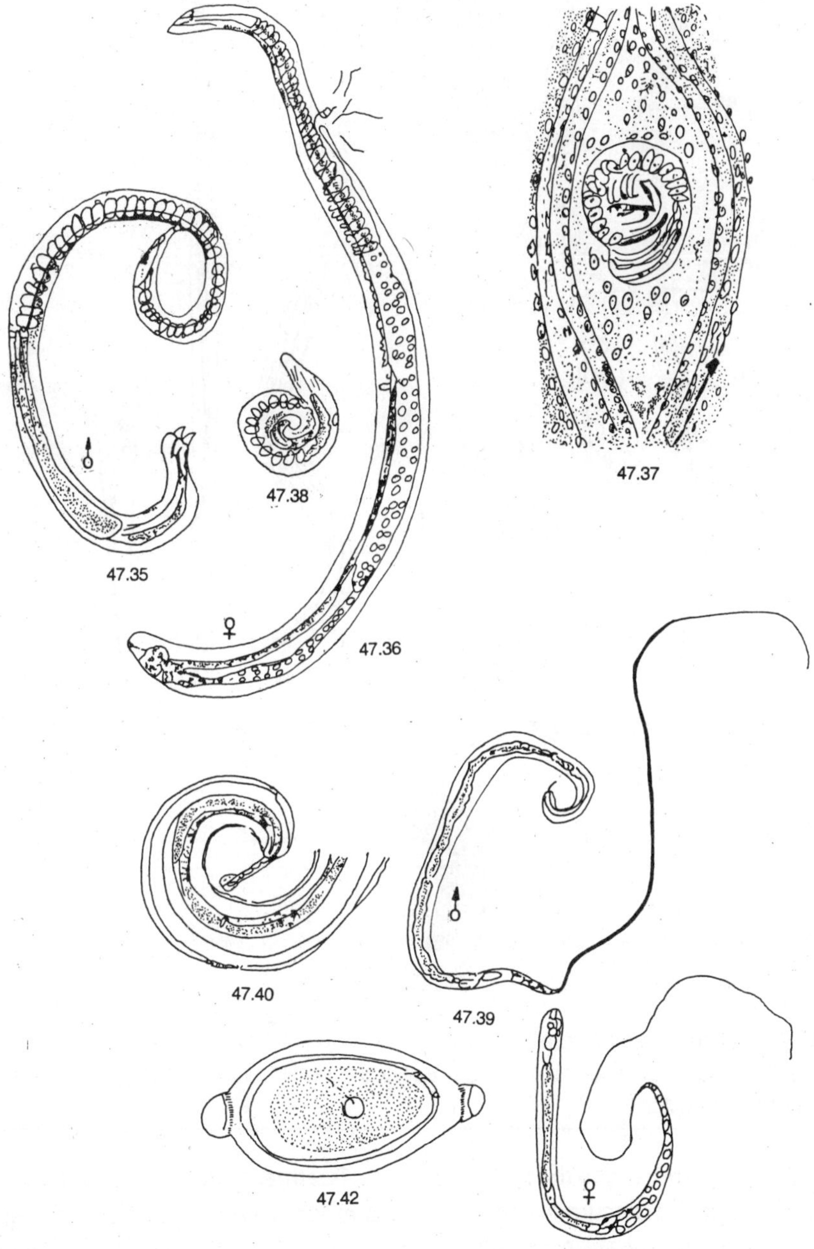

Fig. 47.35-42: Trichinella spiralis, Trichuris trichiura

the male is coiled with protruding spicule (Fig. 47.39, 40), whereas that of female is rounded (Fig. 47.41). The egg (Fig. 47.42) of *T. trichiura* is barrel shaped with mucoid plugs at either pole.

Life cycle. Man gets infected by swallowing the fully embryonated egg containing the rhabditiform larva which is infective to man. The egg shell is digested in the small intestine of man. The liberated

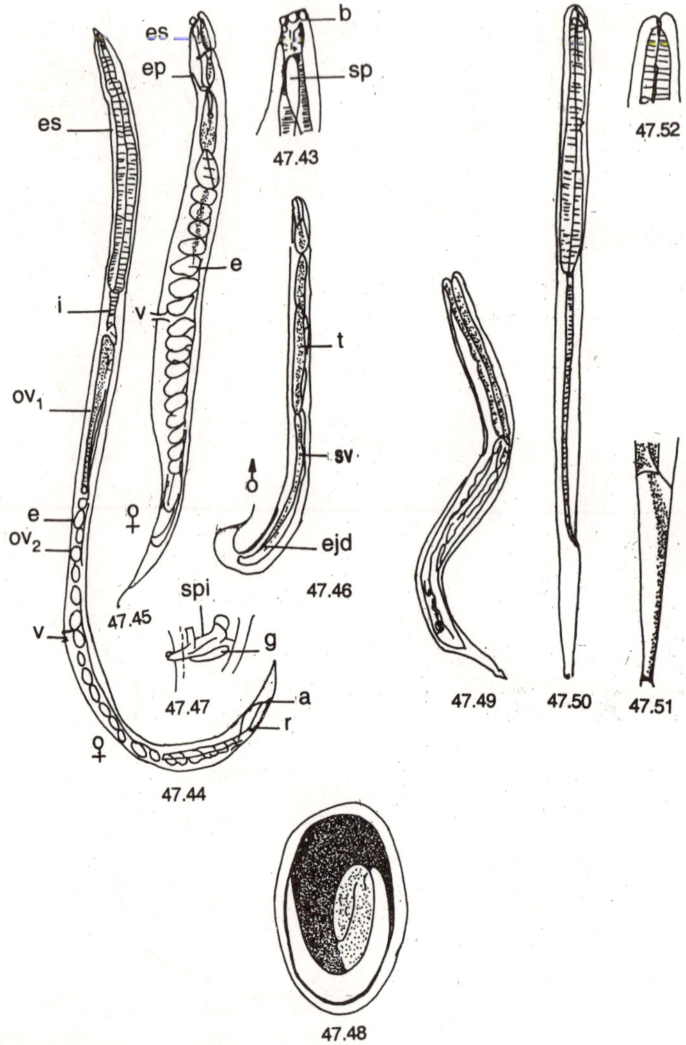

Fig. 47.43-52: Strongyloides stercoralis
es - Oesophagus; i - midgut; ov - ovary; v - vagina; t - testes; sv - seminal vesicle; ejd - ejaculatory duct; spi - spicule; a - anus; r - rectum

larva gets attached for nourishment, to the small intestine and passes down to the caecum to become adult worm which lays eggs, found late in the faeces.

Clinical features. The common symptoms are abdominal pain, vomiting, constipation, abdominal distension and systemic intoxication. The skin is dry and the patient is emaciated. The clinical picture is similar to that of hookworm disease, appendicitis or dysentery. In the *laboratory*, the characteristic egg of *T. Trichuris* can be demonstrated in the patient's stool.

Treatment. Dithiazamine iodide, thiabendazole and mebendazole are effective. Very recent anthelmintic Aldendazole (Chewable single dose) is most effective.

Prophylaxis. Proper disposal of feces, thorough cleaning of hands, before meals, children not allowed to defecate on the ground, avoiding putting dirty fingers into mouth and consumption of properly cooked vegetables are the effective measures.

STRONGYLOIDES STERCORALIS (Thread worm)

The cylindrical muscular esophagus (Fig. 47.43) of the parasitic female (Fig. 47.44, 45) occupies the anterior third of the body, whereas the intestine fills up the posterior two-third. The anus opens mid-ventrally. The parasitic males are similar to the free living males and have two spicules (sp.) and a gubernaculum (Fig. 47.46, 47).

Rhabditiform larva (Fig. 47.49) develops directly from the gravid female and found in the intestine and has short mouth with double bulb of esophagus.

Life cycle. When man walks barefoot on soil contaminated with ovoviviparous eggs (Fig. 47.48) of *S. stercoralis* containing filariform larvae, these filariform larvae (Fig. 47.50, 51, 52) penetrate directly through the skin enter into the circulation and break out of pulmonary capillaries into the alveoli, then migrate to the bronchi, trachea, larynx and epiglottis. They are swallowed and re-enter the intestine. They develop into parasite females and males. The females penetrate the intestinal mucosa and begin to deposit eggs.

Clinical features. There will be petechial hemorrhage at the site of entry of larvae followed by intense congestion, edema, and urticarial rash. There will be broncho-pneumonia with consolidation of the lobules. Frequent coughing, pleural effusion and pyothorax are the symptoms.

Three types of enteritis may occur: (a) Catarrhal enteritis; (b) edematous enteritis; and (c) ulcerative enteritis. There is accompanying diarrhoea with mucus and blood, which may be very painful.

Laboratory diagnosis is by the recovery of active rhabditiform larva from the stool, sputum, duodenal washing. Serology is not quite satisfactory.

Treatment. Thiabendazole, mebendazole and the current albendazole are drugs of choice.

Prophylaxis. (1) The human body must be protected from infective soil and from contaminated feces; (2) constipation should be avoided by use of cathartics; (3) careful cleaning of hands.

ANKYLOSTOMA DUODENALE (Old World hook-worm), *NECATOR AMERICANUS* (New World hook worm).

DIFFERENTIAL FEATURES

	A. duodenale	*N. americanus*
Size	Adult worm, larger, and thicker (Fig. 47.53, 54).	Adult worm, smaller and more thicker (Fig. 47.55, 56).
Anterior end	Bends in the same direction as the body	Bends in the opposite direction of the body
Buccal capsule	Six teeth, four hook-like on the ventral surface and two knob-like on the dorsal surface (Fig. 47.59)	Four chitinous plates, two on the ventral surface and two on the dorsal surface (Fig. 47.60).
Copulatory bursa	Dorsal ray is single, Total number of rays-13 (Fig. 47.61)	Dorsal ray is split from the base. Total number of rays-14 (Fig. 47.62)
Posterior end of female	A spine is present	Spine is absent.
Vulval opening	Behind the middle of the body	In front of the middle, of the body
Pathogenicity	More pathogenic	Less pathogenic

Life cycle. Eggs with four blastomeres (Fig. 47.63) faeces hatch out rhabditiform larva (Fig. 47.57) in soil which develops later into filariform larva (Fig. 47.58), infective to man, enters into the skin causing creeping eruption or cutaneous larva migrans. Blood circulation, breaks out from the pulmonary capillaries, migrate to epiglottis, esophagus, intestine where they grow into adult worm which lays eggs.

Clinical features. In the moderate type, the symptoms are heart burn, flatulence, fullness in the abdomen, and epigastric pain. These are relieved by eating clay, mud or earth (which is known as pica or geophagy). There may be low grade, intermittent fever, lassitude, dyspnea and palpitation of the heart.

In the severe type, there is constipation or diarrhoea. The skin is dry, harsh and pale yellow. Pot belly

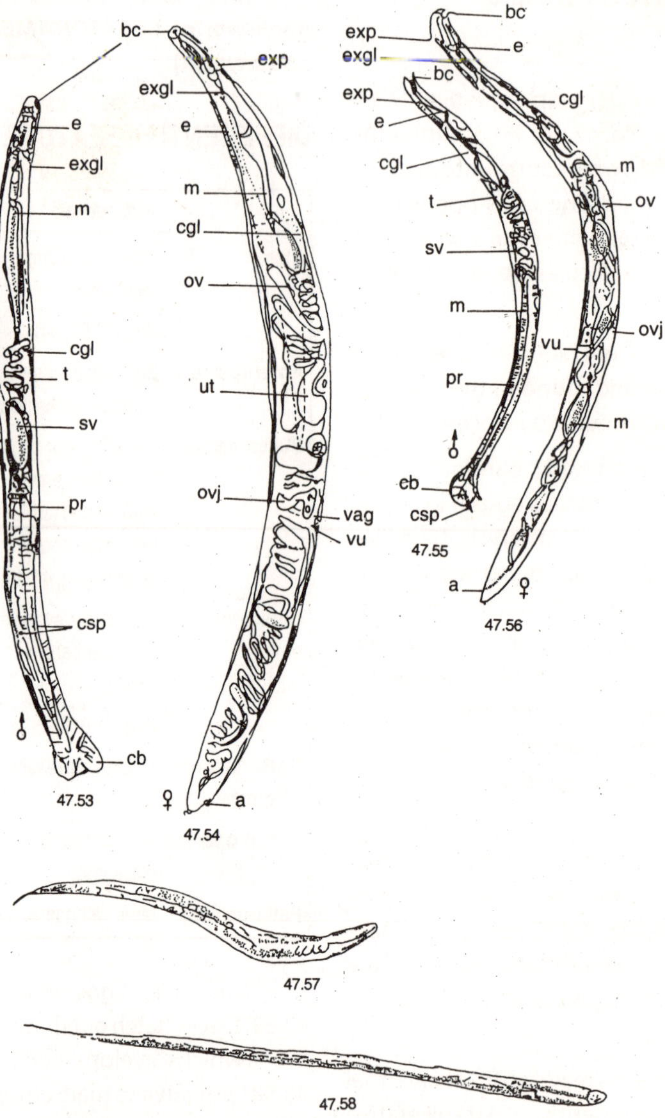

Fig.47.53-58: Ankylostoma duodenale, Necator americanus
bc - buccal capsule; e - oesophagus; exgl - excretory gland; m - mid gut; cgl - cephalic gland; t - testes; sv - seminal vesicle; pr - prostate gland; csp - copulatory spicules; cb - copulatory bursa; ovj - ovijector; vu - vulva; v - vagina; a - anus

is a typical physical sign in children. Finally, there is physical exhaustion, cardiac failure and anasarca.

Laboratory diagnosis. Direct demonstration of characteristic egg in the stool; indirectly, blood examination will reveal the nature of anaemia.

Treatment. Supportive treatment for anaemia. Specific treatment by thiobendazole, mebendazole and current albendazole is very effective. *N. americanus* is cultivated in undefined media based on Chick Embryo Extract (CEE), serum, tissue extract.

Prophylaxis. Personal protection by wearing gloves and boots; disinfection of faeces or soil and prevention of soil pollution; treatment of carrier and whole community is effective prophylaxis.

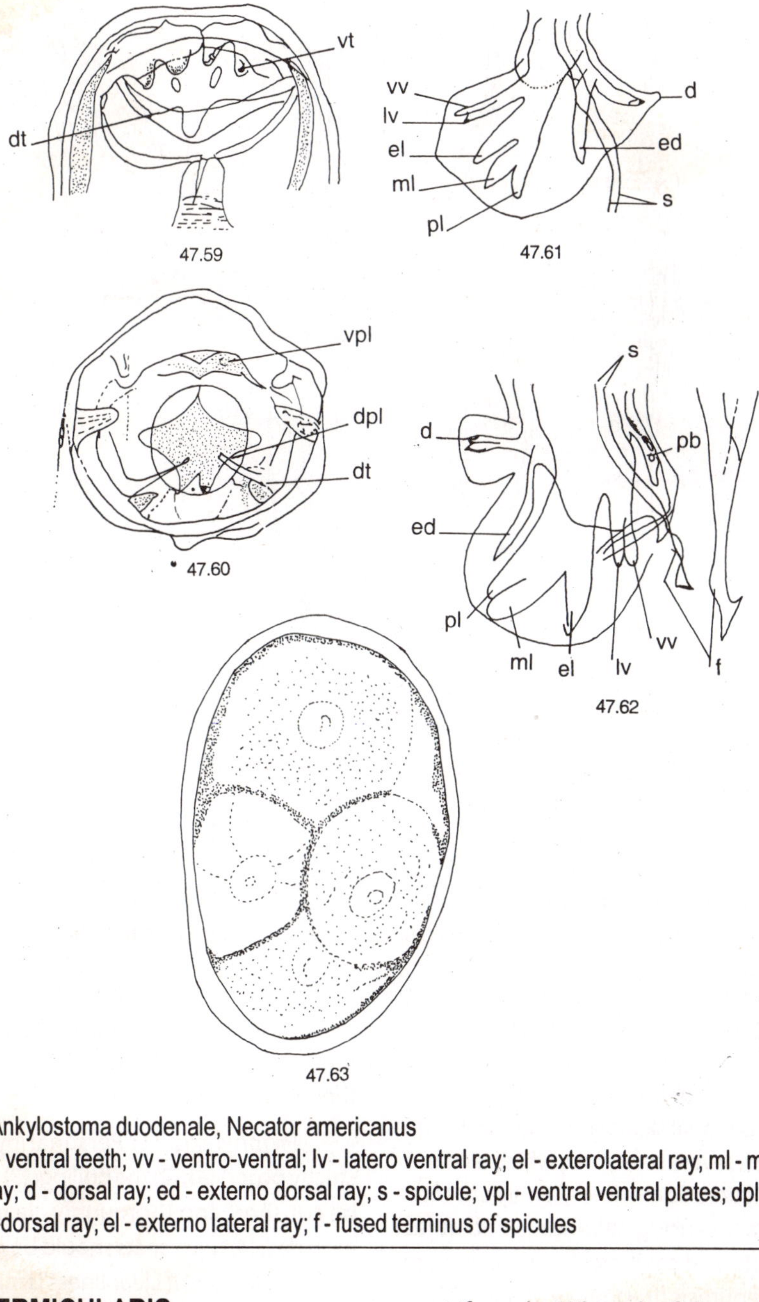

Fig.47.59-63: Ankylostoma duodenale, Necator americanus
dt - dorsal teeth; vt - ventral teeth; vv - ventro-ventral; lv - latero ventral ray; el - exterolateral ray; ml - medio lateral ray; pl - posterolateral ray; d - dorsal ray; ed - externo dorsal ray; s - spicule; vpl - ventral ventral plates; dpl - dorsal cutting plates; ed - externo-dorsal ray; el - externo lateral ray; f - fused terminus of spicules

ENTEROBIUS VERMICULARIS (Pin worm or Seat worm)

The adult worm (Fig. 47.64, 65) is small, white, and similar to a small piece of threat. Posterior (Fig. 47.67, 68) and anterior end (Fig. 47.69) of this worm.

Life cycle. When the fully embryonated eggs (Fig. 47.66), infective to man, are ingested by man, they hatch out the larvae in the intestine, which grow into adult worms which crawl out of the anus during the night and deposit eggs on the perianal skin. The mode of transmission is by anus to mouth (auto-infection).

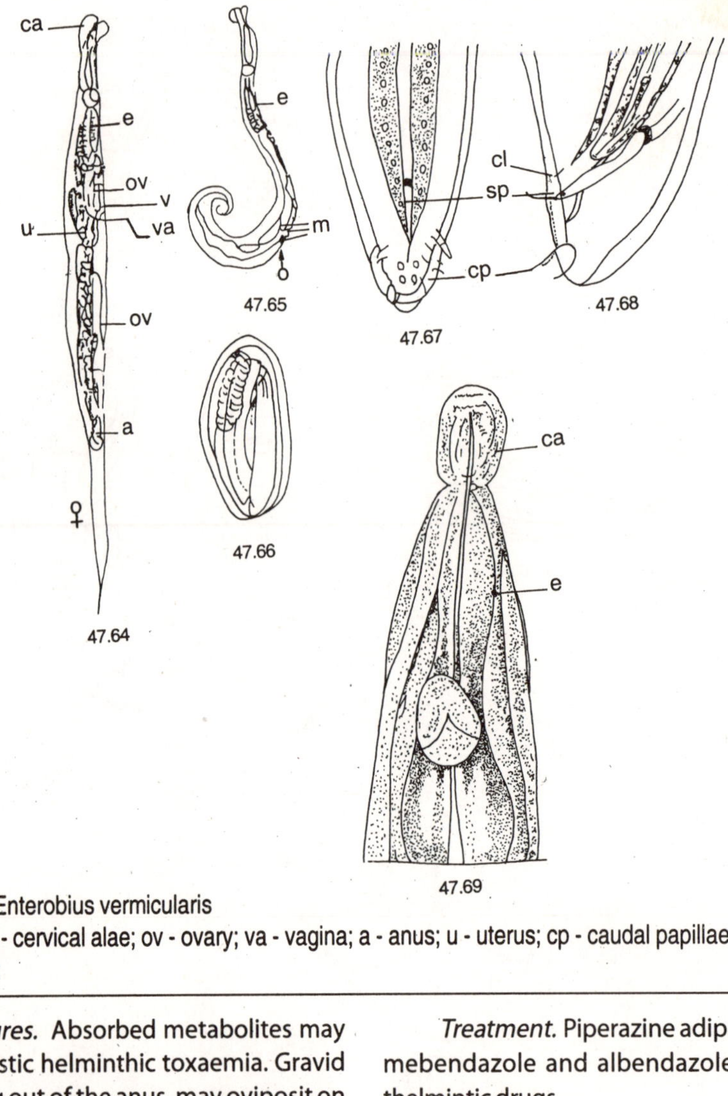

Fig. 47.64-69 : Enterobius vermicularis
e - oesophagus; ca - cervical alae; ov - ovary; va - vagina; a - anus; u - uterus; cp - caudal papillae; sp - copulatory spicules; m - mid gut

Clinical features. Absorbed metabolites may cause a characteristic helminthic toxaemia. Gravid females, migrating out of the anus, may oviposit on the peri-anal and perineal skin of the anus and cause severe pruritus with severe scratching which is characteristic of this infection. Sometimes, it may enter the female genital tract causing salpingitis and at last encyst in the peritoneal cavities. There may be urethritis, nocturnal enuresis (frequency of micturition) and masturbation. Loss of appetite, loss of weight, nervousness, insomnia, nightmare, nail biting, nose picking and grinding of teeth at night.

Laboratory diagnosis can be performed by (1) the identification of the recovered adult worm, and (2) the microscopic demonstration of the characteristic egg.

Treatment. Piperazine adipate, thiabendazole, mebendazole and albendazole are effective anthelmintic drugs.

Prophylaxis. (1) Personal hygiene should be strictly observed; (2) the boiling; (3) finger nails should be cut short and thoroughly cleaned several times each day; (4) toilet seats should be regularly scrubbed and sterilised; (5) if cleanliness is inadequate, chemotherapeutics should be provided.

ASCARIS LUMBRICOIDES (Round worm)

The adult worm is the largest (20-35 cm) of the common intestinal nematodes of man. It is bright pink in colour (Fig. 47.70, 71).

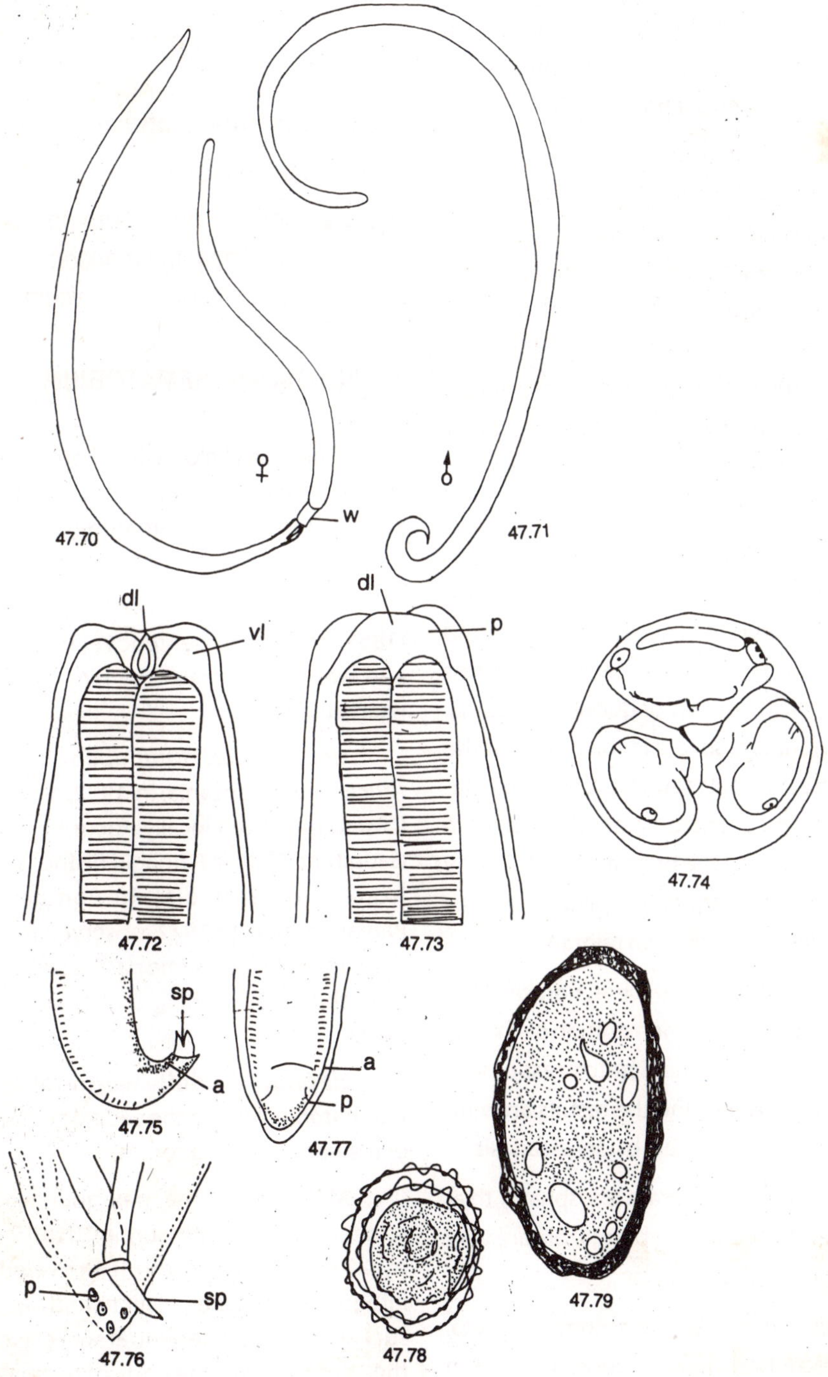

Fig. 47.70-79 : Ascaris Lumbricoides
w - vulvar waist; dl - dorsal lip; vl - ventral lip; p - papillae; sp - spicule; a - anus

The posterior end (Fig. 47.75, 76) of male is curved ventrally with a pair of copulatory spicules without gubernaculum. The female has a vulvar waist (w) situated mid ventrally (Fig. 47.70). Its anterior end (47.72, 73, 74) and posterior end (Fig. 47.77).

Life cycle. When fully embryonated or fertilised eggs are ingested by man, their shells are digested by the digestive juice, the rhabditiform larvae (embryos) are liberated, penetrate into the intestinal wall, carried in the blood stream and break through the pulmonary capillaries into the alveoli. These larvae crawl up the bronchioles, epiglottis and are swallowed. In the intestine, they develop into adult worms, the female is fertilised and lays both fertilised (Fig. 47.78) and unfertilised (Fig. 47.79) eggs.

Clinical features. The most common symptoms are vague abdominal discomfort, acute colicky pain in the epigastric region, poor digestion, diarrhoea and fever. The wandering worms may cause symptoms like acute appendicitis, gastric or duodenal trauma, esophageal perforation, severe involvement of the genito-urinary tract of males and females; and invasion of the heart. Moreover, the larvae which migrate through the capillaries of the brain and eyeball may produce symptoms of meningitis, epilepsy, retinitis and palpebral edema visceral larva migrans.

Laboratory diagnosis : (a) Detection of adult worm in stool or vomit, (b) demonstration of characteristic egg in the stool, (c) the 'Scratch' test or skin test may be found positive and the results are variable. Ultrasonography can detect biliary ascariasis.

Treatment. Piperazine (citrate, phosphate), thiabendazole, albendazole and mebendazole are very effective.

Prophylaxis. Proper disposal of human excreta, treatment of infected individuals, educating children about sanitation and hygiene and avoidance of raw vegatables, food or drink contaminated with the faeces of infected persons.

CHAPTER 48

BLOOD HELMINTHS

Family Schistosomatidae

Genus Schistosoma

Species *Schistosoma hematobium*
Schistosoma mansoni
Schistosoma japonicum

SCHISTOSOMA HEMATOBIUM

(The vesical blood fluke causing schistosomiasis hematobia, vesical schistosomiasis, urinary bilharziasis, schistosomal hematuria). It is not intestinal trematode.

History. This worm was first recovered by Bilharz (1851) from the mesenteric veins of a native of Cairo and was demonstrated by him to be the cause of haematuria.

Geographical distribution. It is distributed in Africa, Egypt, Tanzania. In 1952, an autochthonous (cases contracted locally) focus has been found by Gadgil and Shah in Ratnagiri district about 140 miles from Mumbai (India). In Pondicherry (India), Panjarathinam, in 1972, observed for the first time the eggs of *Schistosoma nasalis* (animal trematode) from the nasal washing of the nasal granuloma of cattle.

Habitat. Adult worm of *Schistosoma haematobium* live in the vesical and pelvic plexuses of the venous circulation.

Morphology. The *male* adult worm is shorter, stouter organism, measuring 10 to 15 mm in length by 0.8 to 1 mm in breadth. It is covered with minute integumentary tuberculations and has two muscular suckers, of which the ventral sucker is larger. Behind the ventral sucker, the body of the male is folded all the way to the caudal extremity to form the *gynaecophoric canal (gc)*, in which the female is held during copulation and oviposition (Fig. 48.1). There is

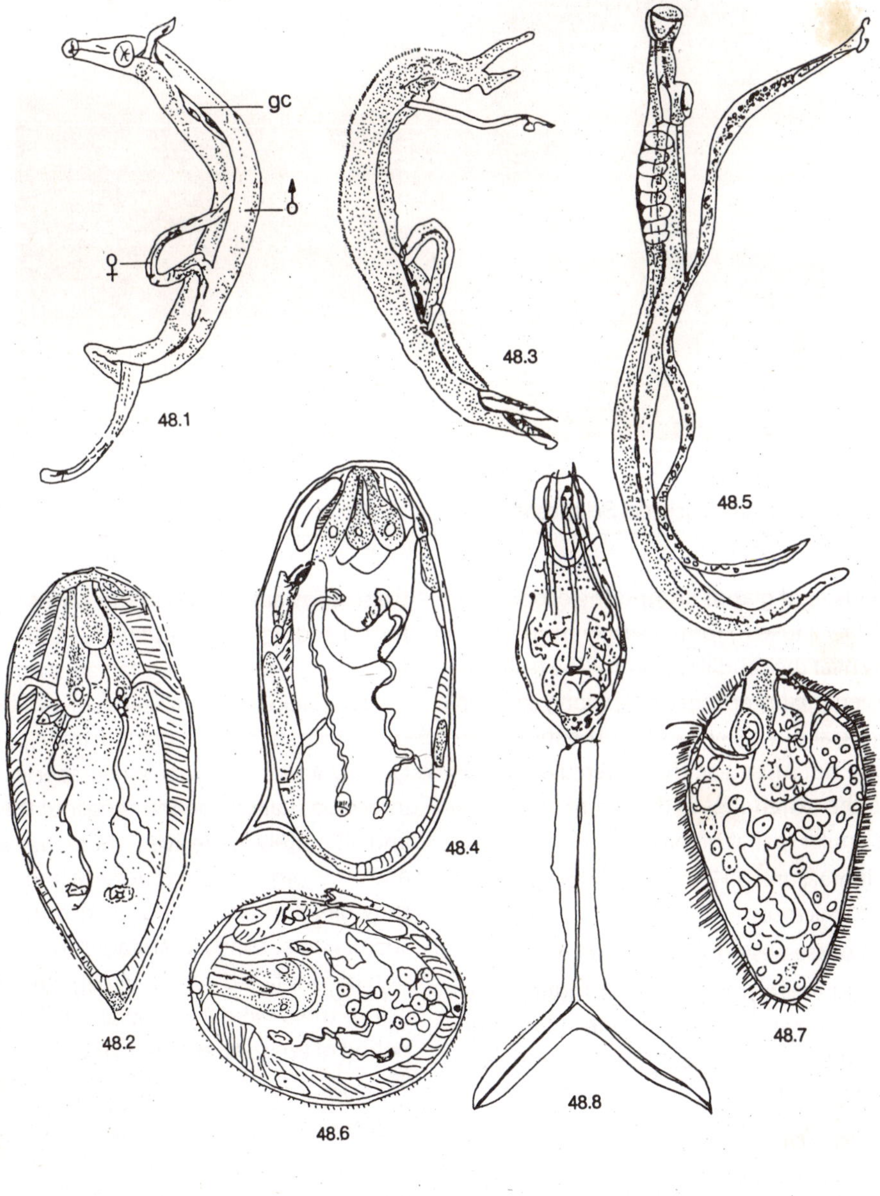

↳ **Fig. 48.1-8 :** Schistosoma

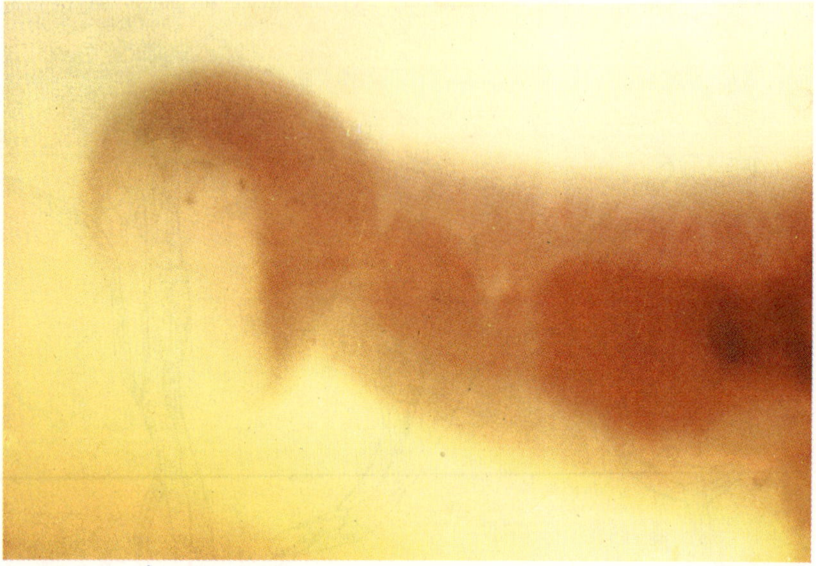

Fig. 48.1a : Oral Sucker of Schistosoma

a bulbous cluster of glands around the esophagus. The paired caeca fuse to form a single trunk which ends blindly near the caudal extremity. The testes are behind the ventral sucker. The *female* is long and slender, measuring about 20 by 0.25 mm. The suckers are small and are not muscular. The tuberculations are confined to the extremities of the worm. The digestive tract is similar to that of the male.

Egg. 1. It measures 112 to 170 microns by 40 to 70 microns;

2. It possesses a distinct terminal spine;
3. Egg shell is transparent and light yellowish brown, every time one sufferer urinates, he releases 20 to 40,000 eggs (Fig. 48.2).

Life cycle. Schistosoma haematobium passes its life cycle in two hosts :

(a) Definite host — MAN;

(b) Intermediate host - Fresh water snail, particularly in India, *Ferrissia tenuis*.

The eggs are discharged in the urine of the infected man, usually at the end of micturition. When these eggs are diluted in the water, they hatch out the ciliated larvae *(miracidium)* — the first larval stage (Fig. 48.7). These ciliated larvae swim in the water with the help of cilia in search of a suitable intermediate host, snail (particularly in India), *Ferrissia tenuis*. On contact with the appropriate species of snails, they infect the snails by penetrating into their soft tissues and ultimately in the liver, where they lose their cilia and other organs and in course of four to eight weeks, they develop into first and second generation of *sporocysts* (second larval stage) and finally a generation of fork tailed cercariae (Fig. 48.8) which break out of the snail daily in swarming in water over a period of ten to twenty five days.

When human beings bathe or wade in cercaria -infested water, the cercariae come in contact with the skin of man and, as the water on the skin evaporates, enter the skin, casting off their tails (cercariae without tails are called as metacercariae or *schistosomules*). Skin (portal of entry) penetration is effected by their anterior ends followed by digestive action of penetration gland secretions and lasts for less than thirty minutes. The metacercariae (infective to man)

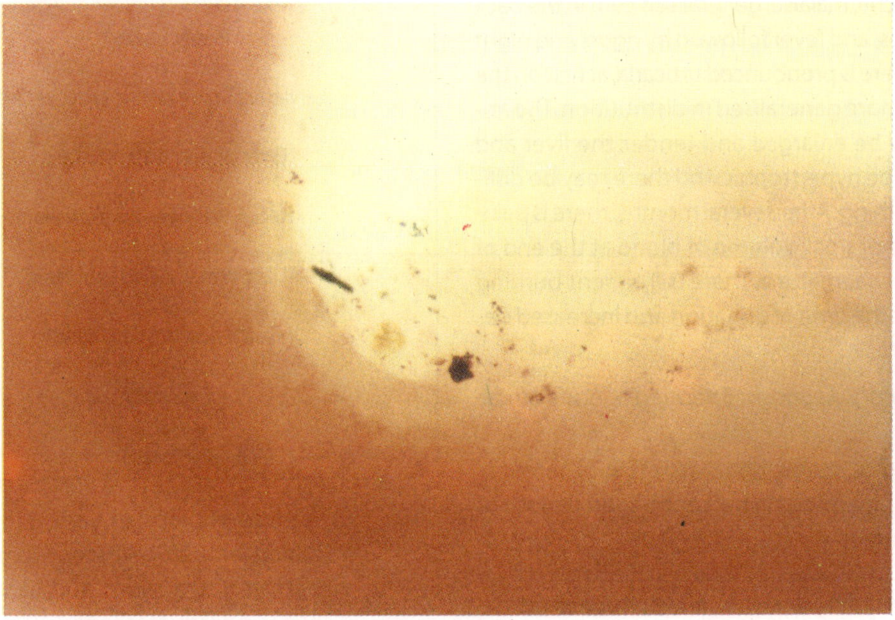

Fig. 48.1b : Gynaecophoric Canal of Male Schistosoma

enter the peripheral venules, are transported to the right heart, pass into pulmonary capillaries, then they are carried through the left heart into the systemic circulation. The majority of them are shunted into the abdominal artery, then gain access to the mesenteric artery, pass through mesenteric capillaries and enter the portal circulation.

In the intrahepatic portal vessels, the larvae begin to feed and grow, become sexually differentiated about twenty days after skin penetration, migrate against the blood stream. They pass through the inferior mesenteric veins, rectal venous plexuses, pelvic veins and, at last, enter the vesical plexus of veins, where they arrive after three months after the initial exposure of the skin. Upon arrival in vesical venules (site of predilection), the worms become sexually mature. Male embraces and holds the female within the gynaecophoric canal, both of them mate and the fertile female begins to lay eggs in the smallest venules by extending its anterior end, one egg immediately followed by another egg after the first. In this way, the venules are filled with eggs which are held in position by their terminal spines. Because of the contraction of vessels, the eggs work their way through the vessels and the mucosa of the urinary bladder, enter into the cavity and are discharged with the urine.

Pathogenesis. During the period of development, the metabolites of *Schistosoma haematobium* are discharged and provoke allergic reaction in the patient. In vesical schistosomiasis, the damage occurs in the wall of the urinary bladder due to escape of the eggs. Infiltration of eggs in the tissues may proceed to fibrosis with resultant miliary pseudotubercles formation. This eventually causes fibrosis of the entire organ. Pathogenic effects of *Schistosoma haematobium* consist of (1) generalised and localised reaction to metabolite of growing and mature worms, (2) trauma with haemorrhage as eggs escape from the venules and (3) pseudoabscess and pseudotubercle formation around eggs lodged in perivascular tissues.

Clinical Features. The incubation period lasts about ten to twelve weeks. The earliest manifestations are irritation and minute haemorrhages at the site of entry of cercariae into the skin. Then there is a gradual onset of toxic symptoms, consisting of anorexia, headache, malaise, generalised pain in the back and the limbs, and fever followed by rigors and night sweating. There is pronounced urticaria, at first on the limbs, later more generalised in distribution. The abdomen may be enlarged and tender, the liver and spleen may be hypertrophic and there may be difficulty in breathing. After several months, there is painless passage of small volume of blood at the end of micturition - *haematuria*. There is frequent burning sensation at the time of urination and increased desire to urinate.

Laboratory diagnosis. Specific diagnosis can be made by :

(i) microscopic demonstration of terminal spined eggs in the centrifuged deposit of urine;

Table 48.1 : Life cycle of *Schistosoma hematobium*

Eggs in urine
↓
Miracidium
↓
Enter in snail
↓
Sporocyst (first generation)
↓
Sporocyst (Second generation) in snail
↓
Cercariae in water
↓
Penetration of human skin
↓
Metacercariae in peripheral venules
↓
Right heart
↓
Pulmonary capillaries
↓
Left heart
↓
Systemic circulation
↓
Abdominal aorta
↓
Mesenteric artery
↓

Table Contd.

Mesenteric capillaries
↓
Portal circulation
↓
Larvae feed, grow in intrahepatic vessel
↓
Enter inferior mesenteric veins
↓
Rectal, pelvic venous plexuses
↓
At last, vesical plexuses of veins
↓
Sexually mature worms develop
↓
Fertilisation
↓
Egg in urine

(ii) A piece of biopsied vesical mucosa obtained through cystoscope is compressed between two slides and examined for eggs under microscope.

Serological tests. Fairley's complement fixation test in which antigens from cercariae and adult worms are used. This is group specific reaction and is sensitive in detecting acute infection.

The intradermal, precipitin, haemagglutination, bentonite flocculation tests are all group-specific for schistosome infection. The precipitin test is more sensititve in chronic than in acute infection. Recent ELISA test can be used for the diagnosis of schistosomiasis.

Treatment. Specific chemotherapeutic agents are potassium antimony tartarate or sodium antimony tartarate. Trivalent antimony compounds : *Neoantimosan* (Fuadin) is better tolerated and less efficatious for *Schistosomiasis haematobia; dimercaptosuccinate* has high cure rates.

Miracil D (Nilodon) has a 55 per cent cure rate in *Schistosoma haematobium* infection. *Niridazole* is effective; *TAC Pomoate* also exhibits activity against *Schistosoma haematobium.* Praziquantal is recently used anthelminthic agents.

Successful treatment is indicated by the disappearance of eggs in urine and absence of haematuria.

Prophylaxis.

1. Eradication of snails by molluscicides;
2. Sanitary improvement of the environment to reduce the pollution of water;
3. Prevent the water pollution by infected persons;
4. Avoid swimming or wading in polluted water;
5. Proper disposal of human excreta.

SCHISTOSOMAL CERCARIAL DERMATITIS (Swimmer's itch, cercarial itch)

There are three types of cercarial dermatitis :

1. *First type of schistosome dermatitis.* It is caused by *Trichobilharzia ocellata*, a non-human schistosome developing in the snail *Lymnaea*. It is prevalent in Oregon, Washington, California, Canada, Germany, Switzerland, France, Burma, India.

Clinical aspects. As the water evaporates from the skin a pricking sensation is experienced, followed by urticarial wheals. After one-half hour the initial dermatitis subsides leaving only a few macules. Several hours later, intense itching of the area develops with edema and the papules transform into pustules grown itch.

2. *The second type of schistosome dermatitis* is caused by the cercarian of avian species of blood flukes, particularly *Trichobilharzia*.

3. *The third type of schistosome dermatitis* results from penetration into human skin by cercariae of mammalian species of blood fluke, *Schistosoma spindalis*. It has been reported in paddy field workers in Malaysia and Thailand.

Treatment. Trimeprazine is given orally.

SCHISTOSOMA MANSONI

(Manson's blood fluke producing schistosomiasis mansoni or Manson's intestinal schistosomiasis often called bilhaziarsis).

History. Bilhaz first observed lateral-spined egg in female schistosoma recovered from a patient at Cairo.

Geographical distribution. Schistosoma mansoni is common in the Nile Delta and is widespread in Sudan, East African coast, United States (New York).

Habitat. Adult worms of *Schistosoma mansoni* are mostly found in the mesenteric veins of the sigmoid-rectal area and live for 26 years. *S. mansoni* may be kept in the laboratory for the study.

Morphology. Adult worms (Fig. 48.3) resemble those of *S. hematobium*; both the male (6.4 to 12 mm long) and female (7.2 to 17 mm long). *S. mansoni* are smaller. The integumentary tuberculations of the male *S. mansoni* are also more conspicuous and

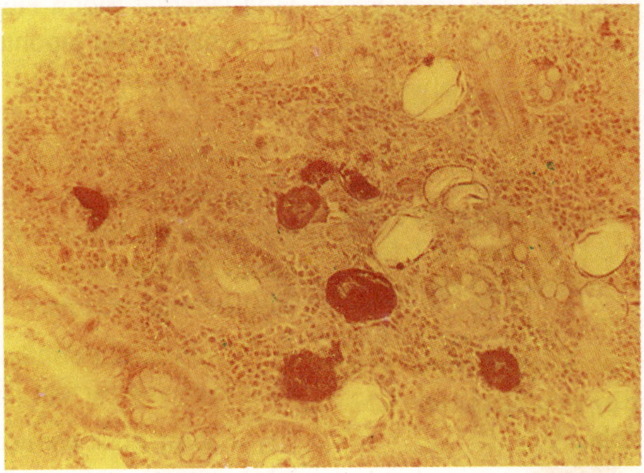

Fig. 48.4 : S. mansoni — egg with lateral spine × 1000

the testes number 6 to 9. In the female, the ovary is situated at the anterior half of the body. The uterus is short and contains only a few lateral spined eggs.

Eggs—They have
(a) a yellowish brown transparent shell;
(b) a characteristic lateral spine;
(c) measure 114 to 175 microns in length by 45 to 68 microns in diameter (Fig. 48.4).

Miracidium. It is larger than that of *S. japonicum* and *S. haematobium* and has larger anterior penetration glands and its life cycle in the snails is similar to that the *S. japonicum* and *S. hematobium.*

Life cycle. It parallels that of *S. hematobium.*

Definite host—Man; intermediate host—Fresh water snail, *Biomphalaria glabrata* in America.

Pathogenicity. The lesions produced by *S. mansoni* are similar to those of *S. haematobium* and *S. japonicum* infections, except that the production of granuloma around the eggs in the tissues is delayed, because of smaller number of eggs produced by *S. mansoni.* The colon and rectum are mostly involved. In the liver, pathological changes are hepatic cirrhosis. A living immature male *S. mansoni* has been recovered from anterior chamber of the right eye.

Clinical features. Initially there is papular rash with pruritus over the skin of the feet. Liver is enlarged and tender accompanied by fever. In classical schistosomiasis dysentery, there are frequent stools with lateral spined eggs and abdominal pain. Dysentery becomes less conspicuous, as the tissue reaction takes place around the eggs in the intestinal wall. The incubation period is 7 to 8 weeks.

Laboratory diagnosis.

1. Diagnosis is readily accomplished by the recovery of the characteristic lateral-spined eggs in the stool, which can be seen under microscope.
2. Microscopical examination of the rectal tissue obtained by rectal biopsy as in *Schistosoma hematobium.*
3. *Serological tests.* Complement fixation and slide flocculation tests are satisfactory and far superior to the intradermal test. ELISA and CIEP are used to diagnose *S. mansoni* infection.
4. *Blood examination.* In early stage, there is leucocytosis with marked eosinophilia, later moderate leucopenia and macrocytosis may develop.
5. Ultrasonography can be useful for the diagnosis.

Treatment. The only effective drug is potassium antimony tartarate or sodium antimony tartarate. Niridazole (Ambilhan) is most effective. Praziquantel is current anthelminthic against *S. mansoni* infection.

Prophylaxis.

1. It is similar to that of *S. hematobium;*
2. Sodium pentochlorophenate has been used with considerable success to control the vector snails;
3. Patients should be treated with tartar emetic;
4. Construction of public bath, laundry tanks and sanitary drainage canals can control the infection;
5. Disinfection of night soil with ammonium nitrate may kill the eggs, before the night soil is used as fertiliser in the field.

SCHISTOSOMA JAPONICUM (The Oriental Blood Fluke, producing Schistosomiasis japonica or Oriental schistosomiasis)

History. This disease was first mentioned by Fujii, a Japanese physician, in 1847 and Fuginami (1904) first found the female worm in the portal vein and Katsurada (1904) first described the adult worm from infected dogs and cats.

Geographical distribution. This infection is confined to areas in Far East, Japan, China, Philippines.

Habitat. Adult worms of *Schistosoma japonicum* inhabit mostly in the radicles of the superior mesenteric veins draining the ileo-caecal region.

Morphology. The adult worm of *S. japonicum* (Fig. 48.5) resembles *S. haematobium* and *S. mansoni*, but lacks integumentary tuberculations. The *male* measures 12 to 20 mm in length and 0.5 to 0.55 mm in diameter. There are seven testes. The female averages 26 mm. in length by 0.3 mm in diameter. The ovary lies behind the mid-plane of the body. The uterus is a long straight tube containing fifty eggs at a time.

Egg. 1. It measures 70 to 100 microns by 50 to 65 microns;

2. is hyaline, oval or biconvex;
3. has an abbreviated spine on the upper right border of the shell (Fig. 48.6).

Life cycle. It is similar to that of *S. mansoni* and *s. haematobium* and takes place in two hosts : (a) Definite host — Man, cat, dog, pig and cattle, (b) Intermediate host — Fresh water snail of the genus *Oncomelania.*

Eggs which are passed out in the feces, require only dilution of the faeces in the water to hatch, allowing the miracidium to escape from the egg and to swim in the water. This miracidium is smaller but similar to that of *S. haematobium* and *S. mansoni.* It enters the soft tissues of the snail (*Oncomelania guadrasi)* in Philippines and produces first and second generation of sporocysts, then fork-tailed cercaria.

On contact with the skin of man or animals wading through the polluted water, the cercariae cast off their tails, penetrate the skin and enter the venous circulation and carried through the right heart to the lungs; and through the pulmonary capillaries they are carried through the left heart into the systemic circulation, reach the intrahepatic portal circulation to feed, grow and migrate into the superior mesenteric venules where the adult worms mate and the females lay eggs which are passed out with the feces of man and animals.

Pathogenicity. *S. japonicum* produces the lesions which are similar to those produced by *S. mansoni* and *S. haematobium.* Intestinal tract and liver are mostly involved. The pseudotubercles around the eggs produce fibrosis and papillomatous growths. The intestinal and hepatic schistosomiasis of the Orient is called as 'Katayema disease'.

Patients with acute schistosomiasis japonicum had disappeared in Japan, but patients with chronic schistosomiasis japonicum are still alive in the previously endemic regions of Japan, they may develop hepatocellular carcinoma with association with hepatitis C virus (HCV) infection.

Clinical features. The manifestations include dysentery, hepatic cirrhosis, splenomegaly, appendicitis, intestinal obstruction, pneumonitis, cerebral syndrome and intoxication, urticarial rashes accompanied by fever may develop into characteristic wheals of varying sizes in the skin.

Laboratory diagnosis. Specific diagnosis rests on the recovery of characteristic eggs in the stools. In proctoscopic aspiration and biopsy, the eggs can be demonstrated.

Complement fixation and slide flocculation tests along with the clinical history will support the diagnosis.

Treatment. Potassium antimony tartarate or sodium antimony tartarate is the most effective drug. Fuadin and anthiomaline are not much effective. Praziquantel (recent anthelminthic) is also very effective.

Prophylaxis.

1. Proper disposal of night soil;
2. Treatment of night soil with ammonium nitrate to kill eggs before it is used as fertiliser;
3. Destruction of snails by molluscicides;
4. Avoid bathing and wading through polluted water;
5. In Philippines, cats, pigs, dogs, water buffaloes and wild rats are commonly infected. These reservoir hosts constitute an important handicap to the control of *schistosomiasis japonica.*

Reference. Panjarathinam R. (1972) Preliminary report on some animal diseases(*S nasalis*) in Pondicherry. Gujvet. *6*:32 - 33.

UNIT C

CHAPTER 49

PATHOGENS TRANSMITTED FROM THE GENITAL TRACT

Spirochaetes

The pathogenic and commensal spirochaetes are slender flexuous spirals 4 - 16μ in length and 0.6 - 0.8μ in thick. They are composed of regular, tight coils or of loose irregular spirals of varying amplitude. They are more highly organised than other bacteria. In addition to cell wall and cytoplasm they contain from one to twelve long filaments applied to their bodies and it is due to these structures that they have their shape, their elasticity and characteristic movements (angulation). Some cells are visible by dark field microscopy, many may be cultivated except *Treponema pallidum* Nichol's strain.

The family Treponemataceae included three genus : Treponema, Borrelia and Leptospira.

Syphilis. The causal agent of Syphilis, *Treponema pallidum*, was first discovered in 1905 by a German scientist Schaudinn in the primary sores (*Chancres*, pronounced shankers, of a syphilitic patient.

In electron micrograph, *Tr. pallidum* is seen to be covered by an outer periplast which covers the whole organism. When the periplast is removed by digestion with trypsin or pepsin, the fine filaments are seen twisted around the organism. It seems likely that they are contractile and maintains the characteristic shape of motility of the organism. *Tr. pallidum* shows rotary cork-screw-like highly characteristic motility (Angulation) which can be easily seen under dark field microscope.

Staining. Tr. pallidum can be stained by Giemsa stain in 1 : 10 dilution over a long period, it appears pink in colour in contrast to the purplish colour of non-pathogenic spirochaete. The organism can be demonstrated by India Ink or by Fontana's silver impregnation method using the exudate from the chancre. In tissues, spirochaetes can be stained by Levaditi's silver impregnation method in which silver salts are allowed to penetrate the inside of the cells. Metallic silver is then precipitated inside the spirochaetes by means of a reducing solution. The organism appears black against a yellowish black background.

Cultivation. Tr. pallidum cannot be cultivated artificially, but the pathogenic strain (Nichol's strain) can be grown in the testicles of experimentally inoculated rabbit. Certain other non-pathogenic strain (e.g., Reiter strain) can be cultivated under strict anaerobic condition in Smith Noguchi medium.

Viability. Outside the body, *Tr. pallidum* cannot live. It is a strict parasite; it dies rapidly in water and is very sensitive to drying. Soap and other detergent quickly destroy it. It is readily killed by heat at 41.5°C in an hour. Secretions containing *Tr. pallidum* are possible source of infection to nurses, doctors and technicians who handle the syphilitic patient. The infections are virtually acquired by direct contact with an infected patient.

Pathogenesis. There are three stages in the untreated cases of syphilis :

(a) *Primary syphilis. Tr. pallidum* gains entrance into the body through the skin and mucous membrane. During sexual intercourse, it infects, generally, genitalia, occasionally the lip during kissing and it is not homosexually acquired. After an incubation period of 4-6 weeks, the initial sore of primary syphilis appears on the genitalia. This lesion is at first small red purple (chancre), it gradually enlarges, becomes indurated and necrosis in the centre to leave an ulcer; then a generalised lymphadenopathy of the inguinal gland develops. Spirochaetes are present in large numbers in the exudate of the primary chancre. As the sore heals, the organism becomes less numerous and may not be demonstrated in the exudate, but, at this stage, it may be possible to find them in fluid aspiration by lymph gland puncture.

Secondary syphilis. After 6 to 12 weeks the appearance of primary chancre, the secondary syphilis develops with the invasion of blood stream and widely distributed throughout the body. The clinical manifestations in this stage are fever, a generalised roseolar skin rash, mucous patches in the mouth and condylomata of the anus and vulva. The severity of the lesion is extremely variable. Sometimes the lesions heal up and disappear completely.

Tertiary syphilis. In the tertiary syphilis, the spirochaetes become localised producing low grade inflammatory lesions in the cardiovascular and central nervous systems and in chronic granulomata (gummata) in the skin, bone and internal organs. This is also called *chronic stage*. Thus tabes dorsalis and meningo — cardiovascular syphilis may be detected 5 - 15 years after the appearance of primary chancre.

The late symptoms of syphilis depend on the organ that is attacked by the spirochaetes. The most frequent, serious and disabling results of syphilitic infection are diseases of heart, arteries, causing sac like dilatation called *aneurysm*. These may burst and the patient may die of the haemorrhage. Syphilis is one of the principle causes of aneurysm of the aorta, of diseases of the *aortic valves*, but not responsible for *arteriosclerosis* and cerebral haemorrhage may occur in young person.

In untreated cases, *Tr. pallidum* lodges in the central nervous system (brain and spinal cord) where they cause a chronic inflammation and destroy the nerve tissue. Various forms of insanity result. These lesions results in paresis (general paralysis) and locomotor ataxia or tabes. In paresis, spirochaetes are present in the tissue of the brain; in tabes, in the spinal cord.

Congenital syphilis. Tr. pallidum can cross the placental barrier and a syphilitic mother — especially in secondary syphilis — may transmit the infection to her foetus. The lesions of congenital syphilis are similar to those already described when the infection is massive, the child may be still born or survive for a short time. The most important defects of late congenital syphilis are mental deficiency, chronic meningitis, blindness and deafness.

Laboratory Diagnosis

Syphilitic exudate. In primary and secondary lesions, it is possible to find and identify *Tr. pallidum* by dark field microscope.

Serology. A specimen of 5-10 ml clotted blood is needed. It should be collected in a sterile dry container without any preservative. If *Tr. pallidum* immobilisation test is required, information must be provided about recent antibiotic treatment, because traces of penicillin or other antibiotics in the blood interfere with this test. Specimens from the newborn babies should be taken by heal stab, cord blood from the newborn is not satisfactory.

Tests for Lipoidophil Antibody

Standard Test for Syphilis (STS). These tests made with cardiolipin antigen, are usually the first investigations carried out to confirm the diagnosis of syphilis. A rapid slide flocculation test, such as VDRL test, is often used for screening, although some prefer the Kahn test. A second test, i.e., Wassermann test, is carried out quantitatively, so that, besides confirming previous tests, it also provides a base line in assessing the effect of treatment.

In primary syphilis, Wassermann antibody is usually detectable about one week after the appearance of the primary chancre. In the secondary stage, virtually all cases give positive findings with high titer.

There are many microbial infections and pathological lesions that may liberate lipid antigen in the tissues with the consequent formation of lipoidophil antibody and the occurrence of biological false positive reaction.

Persons who were vaccinated against small pox or were suffering from various infections (e.g., leprosy, typhus) give weakly positive reaction.

Tests for Treponemal Antibodies

When complement fixation test (CFT) is employed to diagnose syphilis, it is called Wassermann test. CFT may be Reiter Protein Complement Fixation test (RPCFT) when the antigen of Reiter strain of treponemes is used.

Tests for Treponemal Antibodies

Absorbed Fluorescent Treponemal Antibody test (FTAABS) or Treponema Pallidum Immobilisation (TPI) is more specific and can be used to verify STS positive reaction.

An indirect haemagglutination test for the serodiagnosis of syphilis has been developed by using the antigen of the Nichol's strain of *Tr. pallidum*. The specific test is claimed to be similar to that of TPI test and its sensitivity is comparable to that of FTA test.

Tr. pallidum antibody. Of all serological tests, the more reliable, highly specific antitreponemal test is Treponema Pallidum Immobilisation (TPI) test in which the patient serum is incubated with living virulent *Tr. pallidum* (Nichol's strain) in the presence of complement. TPI is not useful in the diagnosis of early syphilis. It is able to distinguish between true and false positive STS. TPI is technically difficult and costly — so it is not frequently used.

If the brain or spinal cord is affected by syphilis, a positive serological test is usually given by CSF. The reactions are practically always positive and frequent in locomotor ataxia.

Of the classes of Immunoglobulins that take part in the TPI and FTA ABS, the most important is Ig G though Ig M is detectable in early syphilis.

Chemotherapy. Penicillin is lethal to *Treponema pallidum* in a concentration of 0.003 unit/ml and is the drug of choice.

Application to Nursing

No special preventive measures are necessary if the syphilitic patients are treated with penicillin, as they respond quickly to the treatment. While handling untreated cases of syphilis, the nurse should be aware that the clothing, bed linen, towels and wash cloth are the potential source of the infection; so these materials should be handled separately and disinfected.

The handkerchiefs, eating utensils, toothbrushes are also potentially infectious; if they are used by persons with primary or secondary lesions of skin, genitals or mouth so these materials should be disinfected. Dressings of any open lesions must be burned or hygienically disposed off. However, the nurse should take her own decisions while working in different conditions.

After the primary and secondary lesions have healed up and as long as no gummas or other lesions are draining to the exterior the syphilitic is no longer infectious in the ordinary relation in his life. This is an important point to be remembered by the nurse. Rash, external gummas and mouth ulcers are, however, infectious at any stage.

Syphilis and Public health. From the preventive medicine point of view, an infectious patient with an open lesion, at any stage, may be made non-infectious by prompt treatment. Thus the patient should be treated immediately in order to prevent the spread of the disease. Mere suppression of the infectious state does not mean a cure.

Syphilis and Family. If a person of the family is found infected with syphilis, there is possibility of the spread of syphilis to other members of the family. So all members should be examined for syphilis. If they are found positive for syphilis, they should be treated immediately. Thus, so to avoid the disease among the members of the family, the public health nurse has a great role to play in this situation.

CHAPTER 50

GONORRHEA AND CHANCROID

Neisseria gonorrheae (gonococci) (Fig. 50.1) is the causative organism of gonorrhea which is a venereal disease spread by sexual intercourse. It is mainly an infection of the cervix (in the female) and urethra (in the male) and of adjacent reproductive organs of both male and female.

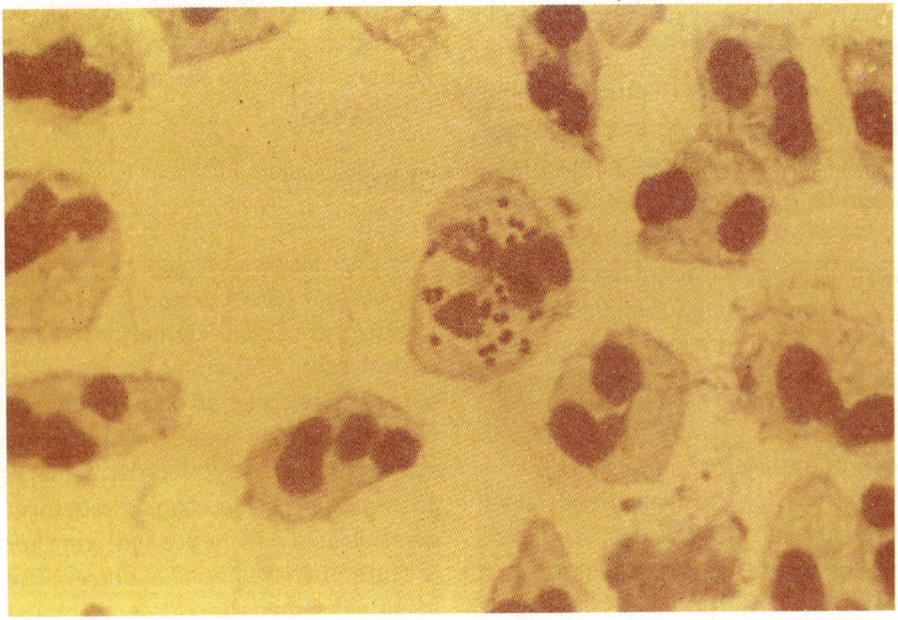

Fig. 50.1 : Neisseria gonorrhoeae in urethral discharge (pus) × 1000

N. gonorrheae is Gram-negative cocci, morphologically identical to *N. meningitis* occurring in pairs. It is oxidase positive. In inflammatory exudate, the intracellular position of the organism is characteristic and some pus cells appear to be almost filled with diplococci. It can be grown on chocolate agar, Thayer Martin or New York city modified medium.

N. gonorrheae can be distinguished from *N. meningitidis* (meningococci) by its fermentative activity of maltose only. It (gonococcus) does not ferment maltose. It has pili or fimbriae (organs of attachment) and is a strictly human parasite. In the male, it infects the mucosa of urethra and produces a suppurative inflammation (urethritis) with purulent discharge with numerous gonococci at early stage, later they diminish and are associated with secondary infecting organisms (e.g., pyogenic cocci, coliform bacilli). Infection may spread backward to the prostate, seminal vesicles and epididymis and may invade the periurethral tissue (producing a periurethral abscess and subsequent stricture). This condition requires surgical treatment.

In the adult female, the urethra and cervix are infected, but rarely the vaginal mucosa, because vaginal mucosa of the sexually mature female is thicker and more resistant to infection, so *N. gonorrhoeae* cannot get attached with their pili (organ of attachment) to the thick vaginal mucosa. Infection may extend to the vestibular glands, the endometrium (endometritis) and the fallopian tubes (salpingitis, Greek, *salphinx*, tube) and even the peritoneal cavity may be invaded.

The mucous membrane lining the vagina and covering the vagina of the immature girls is thin and delicate which favours the initiation of the infection by *N. gonorrhoea*, causing *vulvovaginitis* in girls.

After blood invasion, ulcerative endocarditis, purulent conjunctivitis may sometimes occur as complication. In newborn infants, *gonorrhoeal ophthalmia* (acute purulent conjunctivitis) may result from direct infection at birth. Doctors, nurses and students may acquire this ophthalmia, while caring for patients without much precautions. Gonorrhoeal ophthalmia neonatorum was formerly most frequent cause of blindness in infancy. This condition was prevented by putting of silver nitrate immediately after birth.

Inclusion blennorrhoea. (The name blennorrhoea is derived from Greek *blenno*, mucus and *rhoia*, flow). The causal agent of this type ophthalmia are TRIC-LGV subgroup-A chlamydia. They sometimes cause mild urethritis or cervicitis in adults, possibly of *venereal origin*. The eyes of newborn infants may be infected while passing through the infected birth canal; it develops after 5 to 7 days which may be confused with gonorrhoea ophthalmia which develops within 3 days.

Diagnosis of inclusion blennorrhoea is confirmed by the microscopic examination of stained scrapings of from the inflamed conjunctivae. Typical intracellular inclusions are seen in the epithelial cells (not in pus cells).

Sulphonamide is the drug of choice.

Laboratory Diagnosis of Gonococcal Infection

Films are made from the discharge. In the *male*, from the urethral discharge, the meatus should be cleansed with sterile gauze soaked in saline solution. The specimens are taken with a wire loop or directly on slides. If they are collected with swabs, they should be transported to the laboratory by Stuart transport medium as Neisseria are fragile. In the female, from the urethra and cervix uteri with a wire loop or swab and with the aid of vaginal speculum. The films are stained with methylene blue or by Gram's stain (with neutral red as counterstain).

In acute stage, both in male and female gonococci occur as intracellular diplococci which is strongly suggestive.

In *chronic infection*, in the *females* these gonococci are scanty in film and difficult to identify. In the male, "morning drop" secretion and in the female the secretion from the cervix should be confirmed by cultivation on chocolate agar medium and by biochemical characters. Recently penicillin resistant strains of gonococci were developed, because of the production of penicillinase or β-lactamase enzyme. Resistant strains are sensitive to streptomycin and tetracyclines.

CHANCROID

Chancroid or soft chancre is a severe ulcerative and necrotic (Greek word for deadness, tissue destructive) disease of external genitalia and adjacent parts. It is common among unclean people. This disease is more common and severe in man than in women. It is transmitted primarily by sexual intercourse and very rarely by contact of the genitalia with articles (clothing, bedding, towels, toilets) recently contaminated with the pus and serum from lesions. It is caused by *Haemophilus ducreyi*. The causative agent was named after Ducrey, a famous Italian physician.

A macule and then a soft, necrotic, shredding ulcer process spreads over the surfaces and into the deeper tissue and erodes the tissues of the genitalia and adnexa. It produces inguinal, painful buboes or adenitis (swollen inguinal glands). Diagnosis is by microscopic examination of the exudate and by cultural studies of the organism. Preventive measures are (a) through disinfection of the affected parts, and (b) attention to personal hygiene. Tetracyclines are very effective.

Application to Nursing

Gonorrhea. If, by chance, the nurse gets information from the patient regarding his sexual contacts or otherwise with persons infected with gonorrhoea this information should be passed on to the doctor treating the patient and contacts. Besides, the treatment, the transmission of urethral or vaginal discharge should be prevented by keeping all towels, toilet articles and personal wearings away from those belonging to others. No one should be allowed in the bedroom of the patient and the patient should sleep alone. The bed linen and underwears should be boiled and disinfected. After each toilet, the patient should wash his hands thoroughly and he should not fondle children. Prompt and adequate antibiotic treatment quickly reduce the infectivity.

Gonorrheal and other ophthalmia. Dressings from the infected eyes should be discarded and later incinerated. If only one eye is infected, the healthy eye should be protected; the infected eye should be cleaned by irrigation and washing. Thus the transmission of the infection from the one eye to other can be prevented.

Chancroid. Professional nurse should be careful in preventing the transmission of the organism in the exudate from the patient lesion to others' genitalia. Bandages and dressings should be incinerated. Other belongings should be disinfected.

CHLAMYDIAL INFECTION

The genus chlamydia includes organisms previously called as Psittacosis-Lymphogranuloma venerum Trachoma group (PLT) organism. The generic name Bedsonia has also been used in recognition of Bedson; but by the rules of nomenclature chlamydiae has priority. It is now clear that the chlamydiae are small prokaryotic that have evolved to a highly parasitic existence in the cytoplasm of cells. These organisms are small, non-motile, Gram-negative obligate intracellular parasites. They occur in two forms :

(a) There is a small, 300 nm diameter form, which has a compact electron dense nucleoid which is highly infectious, stable, extracellular form or elementary body.

(b) There is a large form, 800 - 1200 nm in diameter, without a dense nucleoid, the 'initial body' which is intracellular, replicating form. The organisms grow in the cytoplasm of their host cells forming characteristic micro colonies or inclusion bodies which are made up of a mixture of the larger and smaller cells. Both forms stain well with Castaneda or Giemsa stain.

Chlamydiae have 2 sub-groups - A, B :

(a) Sub group-A has compact inclusions with a glycogen matrix. Sub-group-B have no glycogen matrix. These two groups also differ in their susceptibility to suphadiazine.

Chlamydial infection of man takes two main clinical forms : (a) organism of psittacosis-ornithosis causes respiratory illness with fever; and

(b) trachoma-inclusion conjunctivitis (TRIC) - Lymphogranuloma venereum (LGV) organism of sub-group-A causes the clinically quite dissimilar occular, *genital infection. TRIC-LGV sub-group-A chlamydia* contains a group of infections transmitted by contact, mainly sexual in developed countries but also eye to eye in underdeveloped countries where trachoma is endemic.

LGV is more invasive; it starts as a small painless papule or ulcer (Lymphogranuloma chancre) on the external genitalia or internally some 5 to 10 days after exposure. The infection spreads to the regional lymph nodes (inguinal, perirectal) with suppuration in many cases and, sometimes, a generalised infection with fever and rash, arthritis, conjunctivitis and meningo-encephalitis. In late stage of the disease chronic inflammation around lymphatics in the genital and rectal area leads to fibrosis with elephantiasis of the genitalia. Rectal strictures are common in women and male homosexuals. The treatment of genital infections is by 21 days course of tetracycline, 250 mg 4 times a day.

Genital Tract Infection

Recently, more interest was focused on chlamydia because of its involvement in genital tract infection, this infection was known since the first decade of the 20th century. Most of the ophthalmologists who worked on patient with ocular disease traced the infection chain from the genital tract. In 1959, Chlamydiae were isolated from cervix and by 1964 they were recovered from men with urethritis and women with cervicitis.

LGV. Usually, the inguinal lymph nodes of males are involved in LGV. Fistula or anogenital disease may occur in travellers (having sexual exposure) returning from South East, Africa or Central America or South America.

Diagnosis is not easy by physical examination but the serological test (CFT or micro-immuno fluorescence test) may be useful.

Frei test, a delayed hypersensitivity skin test, is not useful as it was once, and is no longer available in United States.

Therapy. Tetracycline or sulphonamides are not very effective.

Erythromycin with full systemic doses is very useful in patients allergic to tetracyclines.

Mycoplasma— are small prokaryotic cells probably the smallest organism to grow in cell free culture medium. The first members of this group *Mycoplasma mycoides* was isolated in 1898 from bovine pleuropneumonia. The most popular group is Pleuropneumonia Like Organism (PPLO). This term PPLO is replaced by Mycoplasma. The human Mycoplasma consists of 8 or 9 species. *M. pneumoniae* is the only unequivocal pathogen, although *M. hominis* may act as a low grade pathogen. T strain Mycoplasma (T for tiny colony) splits urea, requires cholesterol, low pH optimum for growth than classical Mycoplasma.

M. hominis and T strain may cause genitourinary tract infection. Vaginitis, cervicitis, urethritis, puerperal ovarian abscess, salphingitis, pueperal sepsis, haemorrhagic cystitis are caused by *M. hominis.*

Laboratory Diagnosis

Swabs should be collected and sent to the laboratory by transport medium. It should be inoculated into diphasic medium. The best known character of Mycoplasma is the "fried egg" colony in solid medium. Mycoplasma grows best at 35°C - 36°C. Most species are aerobes or facultative anaerobes.

Isolates are identified by glucose fermentation, β haemolysis, haemadsorption and growth inhibition by specific antiserum.

Serum is collected as soon as after onset of illness as possible again after 3 weeks. Sera are tested for CFT.

Treatment. Tetracycline is the drug of choice, less sensitive to erythromycin, chloramphenicol, streptomycin.

Application to Nursing

The nurse should be aware that the most effective method of preventing the venereal disease is to instruct the uninfected healthy persons to avoid sexual contact with the infected persons. Of course, this method is very difficult to adopt. The prevention of venereal disease is one of the most urgent public health problem. The persons in most infectious stages of venereal disease are not usually incapacitated; but they continue in their daily routine work though they are sometimes secretive and may not reveal the truth out of the fear. The most important difficult and immediate problem is to prevent the spread of the disease. Though it is difficult to trace out the source of the infection; if, by chance, traced out and treated immediately the patient may become non-infectious.

During the infective period, the patient should remain away from other family members. He should have a *separate* bed, clothing, towels, eating utensils. All articles contaminated by the patient should be disinfected. If possible, he should have separate bed room.

The public health nurse can assist the diagnosis of the disease by collecting the samples from suspected persons in the community and sending them immediately to the laboratory for microbiological investigation. Every pregnant woman should have a blood test for venereal disease and treated accordingly so that she may not transmit the infection to the fetus.

The chlamydial infections (both by TRIC and LGV subgroup-A chlamydiae) can be treated by the improvements in the environmental hygiene and social circumstances coupled with topical and systemic use of sulphonamide or broad spectrum antibiotics (tetracyclines). The public health nurse should educate the community about the transmission of venereal diseases by means of literatures, notices, talks, lectures and by exhibition or by film shows. She must explain accurately, clearly in simple explicit language.

Genus TRICHOMONAS

These flagellates (Fig. 46d) exist only in the *trophozoite* stage, they are provided with a cytostome (a cleft-like depression) at its side, 3 to 5 free flagella, an additional flagellum on the margin of an undulating membrane, and an axostyle which usually protrudes through the posterior end of the body.

Genus Trichomonas has been classified according to their habitats into :

1. *Trichomonas hominis* — Ileo - caecal region (Fig. 46d.5)
2. *Trichomonas tenax* — oral cavity (Fig. 46d.6)
3. *Trichomonas vaginalis* — Vagina and urinary tract (Fig. 46d.4).

TRICHOMONAS VAGINALIS

History. Donne (1836) observed this species in female and male genital organs.

Habitat. This flagellate is mostly found in human vagina and prostate gland.

Morphology. It exists only in trophozoite stage. It is considerably larger (13 microns), its undulating membrane is shorter and its cytostome is much less conspicuous (Fig. 46d.4).

Biology and Life Cycle. In the female, this parasite feeds on the mucosal surface of the vagina, ingesting bacteria and leucocytes. It grows in the more acid condition than that of the healthy vagina. The infected female is the reservoir of *T. vaginalis* and the infection is acquired by male in extra-marital intercourse.

Pathogenicity and Clinical features. T. vaginalis causes degeneration and desquamation of the vaginal epithelium, followed by leucocytic inflammation of the tissue layer. Very large numbers of trichomonads and leucocytes are now present in the vaginal discharge which is greenish or yellow. The vaginal secretions are extremely irritating, almost unbearable.

Diagnosis:

1. In the female, *T. vaginalis* may be found in the centrifuged urine, vaginal secretions or scrapings. Care should be taken to distinguish it from *T. hominis* which is present in the feces.
2. Indirect haemagglutination test is considered to be highly specific.
3. Serum anti-trichomonal antibodies in urogenital trichomoniasis can be detected by immuno-fluorescence (latest test).

Treatment. Metronidazole is effective drug.

Prevention. The infections in symptomless males must be diagnosed.

UNIT D

CHAPTER 51

PATHOGENS TRANSMITTED IN THE BLOOD

1. Secondary infection;
2. Accidental infection;
3. Arthropod borne bacterial infection.

1. Secondary Infection

Secondary endogenous infection may occur as a result of invasion of blood by pathogenic microorganisms after their primary infection through their usual portals of entry. Infections of various parts of the body by microorganisms transmitted through blood from other infected sites, are called as *haematogenous* infection (e.g., *Salmonella typhi*) enter primarily the body through the consumption of contaminated water or food and invade secondarily the blood via lymphatics and, ultimately, cause the infection in various parts of the body; similarly *Tr. pallidum* penetrates primarily the body through the mucosa of the genitalia during sexual act and spreads via the blood stream to other parts of the body manifesting the symptoms of secondary syphilis.

2. Accidental Infection of Blood Serum Hepatitis

Hepatitis virus B is present in the blood, saliva, semen, urine of cases and carriers. It is transmitted by accidental or artificial tissue penetration — the splashing of blood on the skin, oral mucosa or conjunctiva. Dental operation, vaccine inoculation, tattooing, intravenous injection of blood, blood products during blood transfusion, shaving may transmit Hepatitis B virus (HBV). As little as 0.0001 ml of the carrier's blood can transmit the disease. Hepatitis-B virus infection has been reported in nurse, physician, surgeon by their close contact with the patient.

HBV can be transmitted by the inadequately sterilised syringes and needles used for the laboratory investigations and blood transfusion. Autoclaving is one of the safest method of sterilisation, as HBV cannot withstand the autoclave temperature. The transmission of HBV can be avoided by the use of disposable syringes and needles.

Acquired Immunodeficiency Syndrome (AIDS)

A British nurse developed antibodies 45 days after a needle prick while handling AIDS patient. There is clear evidence that the man can infect female sexual partners and there is tentative evidence that the woman can pass the virus to man. The drug- addicts are more likely to catch AIDS, than the sexual partner of an AIDS carrier. Homosexuals, haemophilia and people who inject drugs are at high risk. AIDS virus can be transmitted through the lesions caused by anogenital sex or by hypodermic needle.

Blood Sucking Arthropods (Natural Vectors)

Only female anopheles mosquito can transmit malarial parasites directly into the human blood stream during their blood meal, because of their well-developed strong stout needle proboscis (mouth parts of mosquito).

Arthropod Borne Infections

Arthropod (insect with jointed leg) can transmit viral, bacterial, protozoal, helminthic diseases. The diseases transmitted by arthropod are called as arthropod borne (ARBOR) diseases. Arthropods can act as vectors.

The most important classes of the vectors are man biting and animal-biting arthropods. Based on the mode of the transmission of the disease, arthropods may be divided into two groups :

1. *Mechanical means.* Those arthropods, which do not bite, are notorious vectors of diseases, as they transmit the diseases mechanically, e.g., house flies walk on feces, boils or sores, soiling their bodies, feet and then they contaminate the eatables. Man acquires the infection by consumption of contaminated food.

Many saprophagic (feces-eating) arthropods, flies, ants, cockroaches may ingest intestinal pathogens while eating infected human faeces. These arthropods deposit *these pathogens* (disease agents) *with their faecal droppings* on the food or wounds, eyes, lips or skin of human beings.

Some insects may also regurgitate (*vomit*) content of their gut when they bite; subsequently the man gets infected by the pathogens of vomitus.

2. *Biological means.* Malarial parasites multiply by *sexual* reproduction in the gut wall and body of mosquito and, ultimately, transform into sporozoites (infective forms) which accumulate in saliva of mosquito. Only the sporozoites are infective to man. Similarly, biologic means is involved in elephantiasis (filariasis).

Vectors and Diseases Transmitted

A. *Mosquito :*
 Malaria (Protozoa)
 Yellow fever (Virus)
 Dengue (Virus)
 Encephalitis (Virus)
 Filariasis (Helminth).

B. *Tick :*
 Rocky mountain spotted fever (Rickettsia).

C. *Flea :*
 Endemic, typhus (Rickettsia)
 Bubonic plague (Bacterial).

D. *Mite :*
 Scrub typhus (Rickettsia)

Many arthropod-borne diseases are transmitted to man from animals which are very far away from human dwellings. The diseases transmitted to man from animals are called "Zoonoses".

CHAPTER 52

Arthropod Borne Bacterial Diseases

Genus YERSINIA (Pasteurella)

The genus Pasteurella is named after Pasteur who worked extensively on this organism. Later it was realised it should be called as Yersinia in honour of Yersin, first discoverer of this agent.

The genus Pasteurella contains 3 species :

(a) *P. multocida* (killer of many) causes, haemorrhagic septicaemia in animals, rarely transmitted to man by dog bite.

(b) *P. tularensis* (derived from Tulare area near San Francisco where it was first discovered) causing tularaemia or rabbit fever.

(c) *P. pestis* causes plague which is one of the major pestilence of the world. This organism is Gram-negative, short, oval with rounded ends or coccobacillary occurring singly or in pair. When stained with methylene blue, both ends are deeply stained (because of metachromatic granules) showing bipolar staining which is an important feature for identification. It is capsulated in the tissues. It grows best at 27°C. If cultured in a flask of broth with drop of sterile oil on the surface, a characteristic growth develops consisting of "Stalactites" hanging down into the fluid from oil drops.

It causes Oriental Plague which occurs in two forms : the severe form of illness (*Pestis major*) occurs either as *bubonic plague* or *pneumonic plague*. In these cases, there is sudden onset with high fever, great prostration delirium and septicaemia. There is also ambulatory form (*Pestis minor*) in which the patient has mild pyrexia with vesicle or papule at the site of the rat flea (*Xenopsylla cheopis*) bite. Plague has, at present, almost disappeared from the world.

Tularaemia caused by *P. tularensis*, often occurs in persons (hunters, marketmen, housewives) handling wild rabbits. It may be also transmitted by ticks (arthropod). Rabbits died of tularaemia on the banks of stream, may contaminate the water which may cause an outbreak of tularaemia characterised by prolonged illness with glandular lesions and ulcers of skin. It is much less fatal than plague.

Tetracyclines can be used in the treatment of the infection.

Application to Nursing

In plague, the nurse should adopt all measures to keep away the biting arthropods from patient and other healthy individuals. She should disinfect and dispose off all dressings soiled with blood or exudates from primary or secondary *bubo* (inflamed lymph node). Plague vaccine (Haffkine's vaccine) — prepared from heat killed bacterial suspension — can be used for prophylactic purposes. It is given subcutaneously in two doses of 1 ml and 2 ml at an interval of 7 days. Its protective value is doubtful.

During the outbreak of Tularaemia, the public should be advised to drink chlorinated or boiled water; infected rabbits should not be handled. Nurse and physicians should wear complete gowns and rubber gloves while treating bubonic plague. When handling with pneumonic plague, they should not forget to wear masks and head coverings in addition to gowns and gloves.

Genus BORRELIA

Borrelia was first studied by a famous French microbiologist "Borrel". It is a spirochaete that infects man and animals and is transmitted by two arthropods; Louse and tick. It is thicker and less regular curved than treponemes. It causes relapsing fever in man.

B. recurrentis is transmitted by louse; but *B. duttoni* by tick.

(a) *Louse borne relapsing fever* (European relapsing fever) caused by *B. recurrentis* is common in America, Africa and Europe.

(b) *Tick borne relapsing fever* (West African relapsing fever) caused by *B. duttoni* is prevalent in Africa and Western states of America and is transmitted by the bite of tick.

Relapsing fever is characterised by the frequent and regular recurrences of the fever and has got its name by this characteristic feature. Relapses of fever, chills and pain are observed for 5 to 15 days and last for several days. Usually 5 to 8 relapses of diminishing severity occur. Dark field microscopy examination will reveal the presence of spirochaetes in the fresh blood during febrile relapse.

These organisms are sensitive to penicillin and tetracyclines.

Application to Nursing

Nurse should take maximum care while collecting blood from the patient in the febrile stage, because these organisms can infect through the cuts or scratches on the hands or very rarely through the unbroken skin. She should take suitable precautions to prevent the arthropod vectors (louse, tick) from biting healthy persons or patients. Blood-engorged ticks, lice or other man-biting arthropods should be removed very carefully with forceps and incinerated immediately.

CHAPTER 53

ARTHROPOD-BORNE RICKETTSIAL INFECTIONS

Rickettsiae occupy a biological position which is intermediate between the smallest bacteria and the largest virus. Rickettsiae are small prokaryotic cells that have an obligate intracellular existence. They resemble bacteria as they are visible under light microscope and are known to divide by binary fission. They have cell walls containing the amino sugar (muramic acid) and are susceptible to the action of antibiotics.

Like viruses, they are obligate intracellular parasites except *Rickettsia quintana* which grows extracellularly in the louse gut and has been cultivated on modified blood agar medium. Under natural conditions, they are present in the alimentary canal of blood sucking arthropods (lice, ticks, flea, mite) but when they are transmitted to man they cause the disease "Typhus"— characterised by fever and rash.

Diseases arranged according to the arthropods vectors

1. *Louse borne typhus*
   (a) Epidemic typhus — *Rickettsia prowazekii*
   (b) Trench fever — *R. quintana*
2. *Flea borne typhus*
   Murine endemic typhus — *R. mooseri*
3. *Tick borne typhus*
   Rocky mountain spotted fever — *R. rickettsii*
4. *Mite borne typhus*
   (a) Scrub typhus — *R. tsutsugamuchi*

Rickettsiae are coccobacillary. Though they are Gram-negative, they can be stained with Castaneda or Giemsa stain. In general, they are easily destroyed by heat, drying and chemical disinfectants.

Rocky mountain spotted fever, first recognised by Ricketts in America, is caused by *R. rickettsii* and is transmitted by a tick (*Dermacenter andersoni*). Fresh tick feces are infectious.

Louse borne typhus fever (epidemic typhus fever) is caused by *R. prowazekii* and is spread by the human body louse (*Pediculus corporis*). Though it is worldwide in distribution, it is confined to Middle East, Asia, Africa and Mexico. Lice become infected while biting infected patients or carriers, when the infected blood reaches the intestine of the louse, rickettsiae invade the epithelial cells until the host cells distend and rupture. As a result, the feces of louse become heavily laden with the organisms and when they are discharged on the skin, they enter the blood stream through the abrasions or fresh bite wounds, causing rickettsiaemia.

Typhus is characterised by an onset about two days during which there are nausea, headache, dizziness and high fever, then appears a *rash* which may cover the whole body. The patient is lethargic and delirious. The blood of the patient is infectious to the louse. The organism cannot be demonstrated microscopically in the blood, but it can be cultivated in yolk sac. However, complement fixation test (CFT) is most accurate and specific as the antigen is derived from the rickettsiae cultivated in yolk sac.

Q fever is an acute systemic infection usually characterised by an interstitial pneumonia clinically resembling Influenza; unlike other rickettsial infections, it has *no rash*. There is only high fever. The name of the disease is derived from the letter "Q" in Query as its aetiology was uncertain, though it was recognised in Queensland (Australia). The causal agent, named as *Coxiella burnetti*, was first recognised by Cox and Burnett. Q fever is quite widespread in Europe and Egypt. It is an obligate intracellular parasite. It can be cultivated in animals and chick embryo. It remains viable for several days in water or milk or butter, Pasteurisation at temperature 145°F or 62.7°C kills *C. burnetti*.

C. burnetti differs from other members of rickettsiae by the following properties : it is filterable, highly resistant to heat and disinfectant, does not produce rash in infected patients and does not elicit the agglutination to the non-motile Proteus strains which is characteristic to typhus fever (Weil Felix test is negative for *C. burnetti*) hence it is not considered as the true member of rickettsiae and has been designated as a new member Coxiella.

Q fever is spread throughout the world, mostly in animals. Infected animals may excrete coxiella in the milk and also during parturition; hence plenty of the organisms are present in the placenta and birth canal. Man may be infected by drinking contaminated milk or by inhalation of infected dust from the straw or dried placenta. *C. burnetti* is conveyed from animal to animal by the bite of tick. Ticks rarely transmit the infection to man. The risk of person to person transmission is small; so the strict isolation procedures are not needed.

Laboratory Diagnosis

Isolation of causative agent is done in animals or chick embryo. Laboratory workers may easily get infected, so they should be careful.

Serology. Some non-motile strain of proteus and rickettsiae are antigenically similar. Proteus organisms can be grown artificially in plenty. Therefore antigens from Proteus OX_2, OXK OX19 are used in Weil-Felix test which is positive for Typhus Fever, except Q Fever. This test is useful but not reliable as it is strongly positive in patient with Proteus infection than Typhus fever. CFT is accurate and specific.

Treatment. Tetracyclines, Chloramphenicol and para aminobenzoic acid exibit a rickettsiostat effect; but in Q fever chloramphenicol and tetracycline are effective therapeutically.

Application to Nursing

Nurse should take due care while collecting blood during febrile stage of Typhus fever, as the blood is highly infectious. The syringes and needles should be sterilised in autoclave. Steps should be taken to destroy all kinds of arthropods.

CHAPTER 54

ARTHROPOD-BORNE (ARBOR) VIRAL INFECTIONS

The term arbor viruses is an abbreviation used to denote a large group of viruses transmitted by arthropods. The name "ARBOR Viruses" has been proposed for these viruses. Members of this group infect man and many other mammals and birds. Arthropods take in the viruses when they feed on the blood of an infected animals and transmit to a new host when they take next meal. The virus multiplies within the body of arthropods, without damaging their tissue or producing the disease.

The tropical heat and rain encourage the breeding of arthropods. So arbor viruses are most prevalent in tropical countries.

In aqueous suspension arbor viruses are unstable at room temperature; at 20°C they survive better. In solid CO_2 at –79°C, the viruses survive for several days.

Formaldehyde at low concentration inactivates the virus; heat at 60°C for 10 minutes or ultraviolet light for 10 minutes kills them. Sodium desoxycholate in 0.1% concentration inactivates arbor viruses. After an incubation period of 4-21 days there is a sudden onset of fever with signs resembling those seen in aseptic meningitis. Marked drowsiness or stupor is characteristic and the mortality is 5-25% It is much high in elderly people.

Viruses Associated with Pyrexia

YELLOW FEVER

It is primarily a disease of monkeys and forest animals. In nature, the infection is transmitted from monkey to monkey by forest mosquito. Man is only accidentaly bitten by an infected mosquito (*Aedes aegypti*). The human disease may vary from symptomless infection to a severe jaundice with haemorrhage and death.

The disease consists of three periods of infection (viraemia); of remission; of intoxication. The dangerous aspects of the disease are intestinal haemorrhage (black vomit blood altered by the gastric juice), albuminuria, liver damage etc. The fatality rate is about 5%.

Laboratory diagnosis. Inoculation of patient's serum into suckling mice intracellularly is a successful method of isolation of yellow fever virus. Yellow fever antibody titre of acute and convalescent sera can be compared.

Prophylaxis. Under rural condition, it is possible to control mosquito; but it is impracticable in jungle cycle of virus maintenance. Two live attenuated vaccines are available.

DENGUE

Dengue virus is widely distributed in the tropics and subtropics and transmitted by the genus *Aedes*. In most cases, the infection is inapparent or clinically mild but it may be a severe diphasic fever; the first stage of fever is characterised by myalgia and arthralgia, photophobia, conjunctivitis; the second stage by rash, sometimes lymphadenopathy. Multiple dengue viruses cause the classical dengue syndrome — haemorrhagic fever.

CHIKUNGUNYA

Chikungunya, the name of the virus, is derived from African word meaning "the thing causing bending up" from the contorted position of patients induced by the joint pain.

Chikungunya virus causes an acute dengue like pyrexia of sudden onset associated with intense joint and muscle pain and a rash.

O' NYONG - NYONG

O' nyong-nyong.- O' nyong-nyong virus is related to chickungunya and produces practically identical clinical symptoms except that lymphadenopathy may also occur. The name of the virus has the same meaning as chickungunya. It is prevalent in Uganda.

WEST NILE (WN)

West Nile virus occurs in Africa, Egypt, France, Asia, Israel, Mostly children are infected. The infection is clinically mild. Symptoms are fever, sore throat, lymphadenopathy and, sometimes, rash.

RIFT VALLEY FEVER (RVF)

RVF virus is endemic in sheep and cattle in Africa. Man is most commonly infected by handling sick and dead animal but sometimes by mosquito bite.

KYASANUR FOREST DISEASE (KFD)

KFD virus appeared as a new disease in the Kyasanur forest in Mysore, South India, in 1957. The clinical infection is often mild, characterised mainly by fever, conjunctivitis, vomiting, diarrhoea. However, severe haemorrhagic cases occur with alimentary tract haemorrhage and epitaxis. Recovery may be slow. The fatality is 10%.

The disease is transmitted from dead monkey by a tick (*Haemophilus spinigera*).

OMSK HAEMORRHAGIC FEVER (OHF)

OHF virus occurs in Russia. Clinically, the disease resembles RFD and is transmitted by rodents (musk rats) and ticks. Man has been infected by handling the musk rats.

COLORADO TICK FEVER

Colorado tick fever is an inapparent or mild infection in man, but it may be a severe diphasic fever with haemorrhagic and encephalitis complications in children. It is transmitted from ground squirrels by the wood tick.

SAND FLY FEVER (SF)

SF virus occurs in Russia. The infection in man may be mild or severe fever characterised by myalgia, conjunctivitis.

Incubation is 7-10 days. Only man has been shown to be infected. Two serological types of virus are known : Naples and Sicily strains. They are transmitted by sand fly.

ARGENTINIAN AND BOLIVIAN HAEMORRHAGIC FEVER (LASSA FEVER)

The South American haemorrhagic fever is caused by Junin and Machup virus of Tacaribe group. Their main clinical pictures : pyrexia, nasal, intestinal and uterine haemorrhage, petechial and purpura with a fatality rate of 20 percent. It is doubtful if this virus is, in fact, arthropod-borne.

LASSA FEVER is characterised by severe muscular pain, a haemorrhagic rash and a high case fatality which appeared in 1969 in Americans living at Lassa, Nigeria. Lassa Fever virus also belongs to Tacaribe group.

VIRUSES ASSOCIATED WITH ENCEPHALITIS

Western Equine Encephalitis (WEE)

WEE occurs in Western states of USA. Most human infections are mild, only some show clinical symptoms. Mild cases are characterised by fever with headache and vomiting, sometimes stiffness of neck and back. More severe cases progress to stupor and coma; convulsions may occur particularly in children. Mortality rate is 3 per cent. Recovery is usually complete without sequelae.

Eastern Equine Encephalitis (EEE)

Occurs in eastern USA and Canada; mild infection is rare, mortality is high as 75 per cent. Symptoms are similar to that of WEE but more severe headache to death. Mental deficiency and paralysis are common sequelae.

Venezuelan Equine Encephalitis (VEE)

Resembles WEE and is usually mild infection. In occurs in America.

Japanese Encephalitis (JE)

JE virus occurs over a wide area of Asia, Malaysia and Japan. Most infections are mild; some develop encephalitis which is of a severe type similar to that caused by EEE virus with a high mortality of 90% and mental impairment, personality change and paralysis as sequelae. The virus is transmitted among vertebrate host, birds by mosquitoes, Aedes and Culex. Pigs are also infected and the infection is mild. Man is also in close contact with the pigs than he is with wild birds, so pigs act as "link host" for the infection of man. Only in man, the "dead-end" host, does clinical disease occur. CT scan appears to be of little use in making the specific diagnosis of Japanese encephalitis in India.

ST. LOUIS ENCEPHALITIS (SLE)

SLE virus occurs in America. Most infections are mild and transmitted by *Culex*.

MURRAY VALLEY ENCEPHALITIS (MVE)

MVE virus occurs in Eastern Australia in New Guinea and is closely related to JE virus and induces a severe disease with a high mortality like JE virus.

Ilheus virus is the cause of mild encephalitic disease in Central or South America and in Trinidad.

CALIFORNIA ENCEPHALITIS (CE)

CE virus was first recognised as a cause of encephalitis in man in the valley of California. It is shown to be the cause of Central Nervous System (CNS) disease in the USA. The clinical disease varies from a mild undifferentiated febrile illness to acute CNS disease, even fatal.

Tabyna. Tabyna virus is the cause of mild illness mainly of respiratory type in Czech republic. Wild vertebrate host and mosquito are involved in the transmission of virus to man.

TICK BORNE ENCEPHALITIS (TBE)

TBE virus occurs widely in USA and in central America. It is cause of encephalitis and transmitted by hard tick, Ixodes. The incubation period is 8-14 days. Onset is sudden, pyrexia with signs of cerebral involvement, photophobia, coma and paralysis. The bulbar centres and cervical cord may be involved. Mild infections may occur. Mortality is highest (30%); paralysis may be permanent.

LOUPING ILL

Louping (= Leaping) ill is an encephalomyelitis of sheep occurring in England, Scotland border. The disease shows typically two phases :

(a) First, viraemia accompanied by high pyrexia, and
(b) Second, neurological incoordination, paralysis, even death.

The second may be absent and the infection may be inapparent. Human cases may derive from contact with infected sheep or from laboratory. Hard tick, Ixodes, may transmit virus to sheep.

Powassan

Virus first isolated from a child with encephalitis in USA, Canada and also isolated from ticks. *Dermacenter* and *Ixodes.*

Application to Nursing

While dealing with arbor viral infections, nurse should strictly adopt all measures to destroy the arthropods and to protect patients from arthropod bite. She should promptly intimate the doctor as soon as she is detecting symptoms like pyrexia and encephalitis.

CHAPTER 55

ARTHROPOD BORNE PROTOZOAL DISEASES MASTIGOPHORA

Genus TRYPANOSOMA

Trypanosoma is blood flagellate protozoon, is an elongated spindle shaped body with tapering ends. Its nucleus is central and anterior to the kinetoplast. The undulating membrane is proceeding forward as free flagellum (Fig. 55.1).

Human pathogenic trypanosomes are :

1. *Trypanosoma brucei - rhodesiense - gambiense* group (the human strain is *T. rhodesiense* (Fig. 55.2).

   T. gambiense (Fig. 55.3) causes African trypanosomiasis.
2. *T. cruzi* causes South American trypanosomiasis (Chagas' disease) (Fig. 55.4).

TRYPANOSOMA GAMBIENSE

T. gambiense occurs in three forms (long, short and intermediate) in the blood and lymph nodes. It appears in cerebrospinal fluid (CSF) after cerebral symptoms development.

Life Cycle. In man, the definite host, *T. gambiense* lives in the blood and multiplies by longitudinal binary fission. In the intermediate host (tse-tse fly), after ingestion, the trypanosomes reach the intestine and reproduce in the lumen, migrate back to the salivary gland where they multiply and fill the cavity of the gland. These metacyclic trypanosomes, infective to man, are introduced into man by the bite of the tse-tse fly. The development in the fly is known as "development at the anterior station".

Clinical features. At the site of the 'bite' of the fly, there is an elevated, indurated, painful initial trypanosomal chancre. The lymph nodes, spleen and liver are enlarged and congested, where they are invaded by the trypanosomes.

The chronic or "sleeping sickness" stage of infection is initiated when the nervous system is invaded. The headache in severe and there is progressive mental dullness and apathy. There is disinclination to work, the patient becomes morose or excitable. The sleepiness becomes so pronounced that the patient falls asleep while eating, standing or sitting. The patient sleeps continuously and cannot get up even to take food and, ultimately, death follows.

In the *laboratory,* (A) Trypanosomes can be demonstrated microscopically in (1) peripheral blood, (2) lymph node aspirate, (3) bone marrow smear and (4) cerebrospinal fluid.

(B) Cultivation in suitable media.

(C) Animal inoculation.

(D) Serological tests : Agar gel precipitation; indirect fluorescent antibody test; complement fixation test; Enzyme linked immunosorbent assay (ELISA) test. Besides ELISA, capillary passive haemagglutination (HA), a card agglutination test (CATT) has also been very recently introduced. It is simple, specific and sensitive.

Treatment. Tryparsamide, suramin and pentamidine are effective; Melarsen and Berenil are recent drugs.

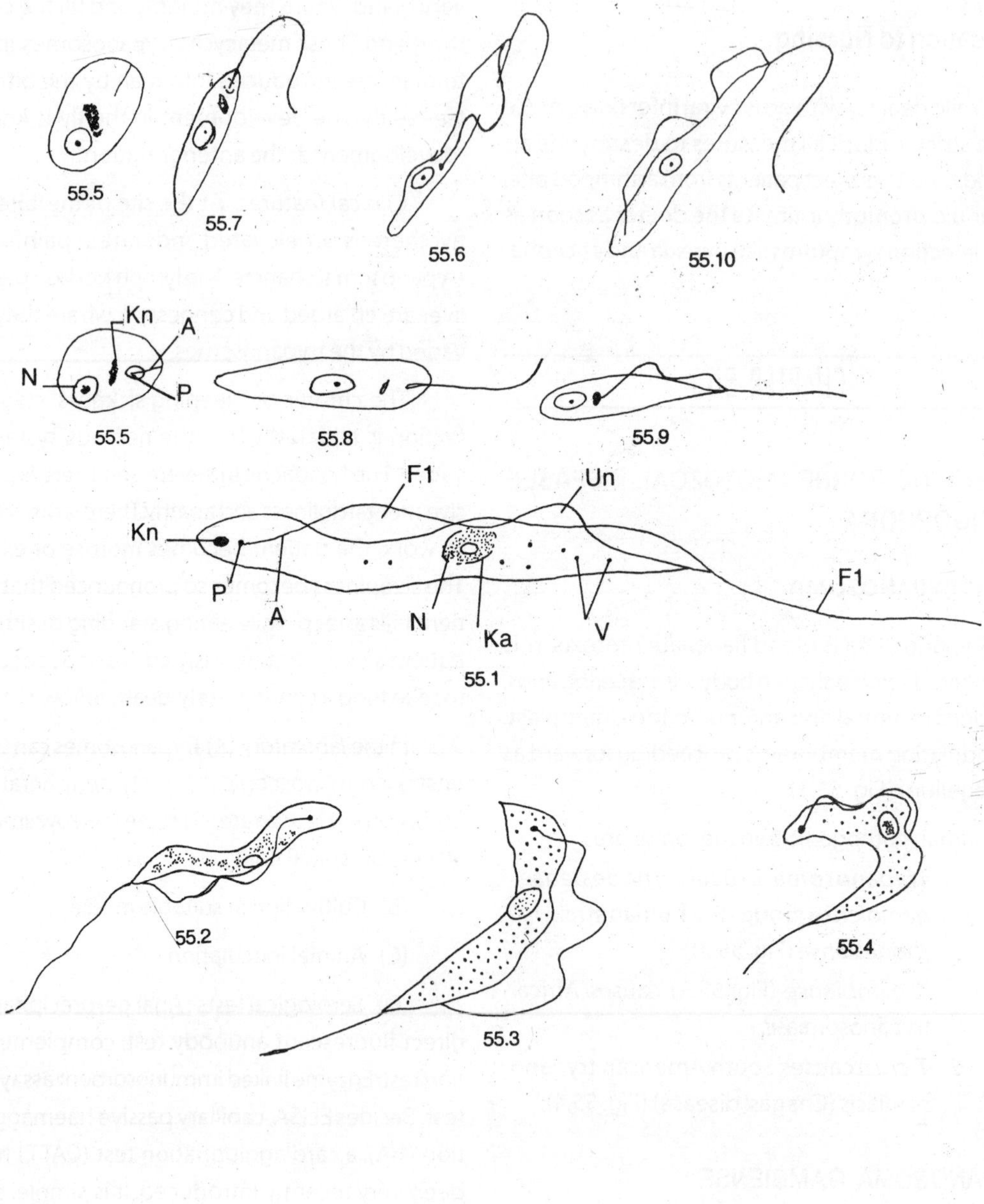

Fig. 55.1-10 : Trypanosoma
Kn - Kinetoplast; P - Parabasal body; A - Axoneme; F1 - Flageltum; Un - Undulating membrane; N - Nucleus; Ka - Karyosome; V - Volutin granule

Prophylaxis. Destruction of vectors, isolation of human population from infected areas and chemoprophylaxis by pentamidine.

TRYPANOSOMA CRUZI

T. cruzi is a pleomorphic trypanosome. In man and animal, the organism occurs in the blood as a typical trypanosome (trypomastigote form) and in the reticulo as endothelial cells and other tissue cells as leishmania (amastigote form) (Fig. 55.5). In insects, it occurs as leishmania (Fig. 55.5) crithidia (Fig. 55.6) and metacyclic trypanosome. It can be cultivated on Novy, MacNeal and Nicolle (NNN) medium. Leptomonas (Fig. 7, 8) in culture.

Life cycle. T. cruzi passes its life cycle in two hosts, one in man and other in the reduvid bug, *Triatoma infestans.*

Development in reduvid bug. The trypomastigote forms are ingested by the bug while biting an infected man. In the midgut (stomach) of the bug they are transformed into amastigote forms which multiply by binary fission and later transform into epimastigote form (Fig. 55.9). These migrate to the hindgut, multiply by longitudinal fission and transform into metacyclic trypanosomes (Fig. 55.10) which are excreted in the faeces of the bug. This type of development in 8-10 days is known as "development in the posterior station".

Development in man. These metacyclic trypanosomes infective to man, when rubbed into the puncutre wound made by the bug or into the abrasion of the skin or on the exposed mucous membranes of the eye, nares or lips, invade the adipose cells of the subcutaneous tissues on nearly muscle cells immediately below the site of inoculation. Then they transform into amastigote forms, multiply by binary fission pass through promastigote forms which are again transformed into trypanomastigote forms and liberated in the blood. (Fig. 55.11)

In Invertebrate Host
↓
Trypanomastigote forms in human blood
↓
Ingested by bug
↓
Amastigote forms in bug
↓
Epimastigote forms
↓
Metacyclic trypanosomes
↓
Excretion in bugs' feces

In Vertebrate Host
Metacyclic trypanosomes in bugs' feces
↓
Enter skin
↓
Amastigote forms
↓
Promastigote forms
↓
Epimastigote forms
↓
Trypanomastigote forms in human blood

Fig. 55.11 : Life Cycle of Trypanosoma Cruzi

Pathogenicity and Clinical features. In the skin, there is a characteristic primary lesion (Chagoma) which blocks the lymphatic capillaries and produces edema of the area. Chagas' disease occurs in acute and chronic forms.

The acute form, which is usually found in children, lasts for twenty to thirty days and is characterised by high fever. The face is swollen, there is marked edema of eyelid (Romana's sign) and Keratitis.

The chronic form follows the acute form in children who survive and is common in adults. The symptoms of the chronic forms are probably related to damage sustained during the acute phase. The chronic infection is characterised by the disturbances of cardiac rhythm. When motor centres are destroyed, there is paraplegia, diplegia and spastic paralysis. Cardiomyopathy may be a complication.

Laboratory Diagnosis

Diagnosis of this infection rests on the demonstration of *T.cruzi* in the blood or tissues and the presence of antibodies. If the blood is negative for *T.cruzi*, inoculation of guinea pigs may be done as a diagnostic measure. If there are nervous symptoms, inoculation of the cerebrospinal fluid (CSF) into susceptible animals is effective in demonstrating trypanosomes. Xenodiagnosis has been employed frequently, allowing trypanosome-free, laboratory bred bug to "bite" the individual suspected to be having the disease. If the infection is present in the blood meal, the trypanosomes multiply in the intestine of the bug and an examination of the intestinal contents in 10-30 days will reveal metacyclic trypanosomes.

The complement fixation test using antigen obtained from cultures of *T.cruzi* is both specific and practical. G-agglutination test is very recent serological method used to diagnose this infection in blood donors in Brazil. ELISA is both specific and sensitive. It is necessary to differentiate Kala azar from Chagas' disease by culture, immunologic tests or Xenodiagnosis. Indirect Fluorescence Antibody Test (IFAT) is also used, but ELISA is the test of choice.

Treatment. Only one case of *T.cruzi* infection in a laboratory attendant was reported successful with nitrofurazone. Few mg of Azardirachtine (a substance present in the seeds of neem tree) is sufficient to block the development or reproduction of *T. cruzi.* Thus its life cycle is broken. It is a very recent, current drug.

Prophylaxis. Consists of (1) destruction of bugs by effective insecticide, BHC (Gammexane); (2) avoiding bug bites by using mosquito nets; and (3) vaccination. An attempt has been made very recently by American scientists to develop a vaccine against Chagas' disease.

Genus LEISHMANIA

There are three species of Leishmania. (1) *Leishmania donovani* which causes Kala azar or Dum Dum fever; (2) *L. tropica* which causes Oriental sore or Delhi boil and (3) *L. braziliensis* which causes mucocutaneous leishmaniasis.

LEISHMANIA DONOVANI

In 1900, Leishman discovered *L. donovani* in the spleen smears of a dead soldier at Dum Dum airport, India. The condition is therefore called Dum Dum fever or Kala azar. Later in 1903, Donovan reported it in Madras — now Chennai (India).

L. donovani is commonly found in America, Africa, Asia (China, eastern India) and Europe and is always present in the reticulo endothelial cells.

Morphology. L. donovani occurs in two stages — the aflagellar leishmania (amastigote) stage in man and reservoir animals, and the leptomonas (promastigote) (Fig. 55.7, 8) in the sand fly and in culture Leishmania is an ovoidal body, 2-3 microns in length and living intracellularly in the monocytes or polymorphonuclear leucocytes of man. In preparation stained with Giemsa's stain, the cytoplasm stains pale blue and the nucleus stains red, there is deep red, rod-like body, known as parabasal body. The kinetoplast is at right angle to the nucleus. Axoneme is a delicate filament extending from the kinetoplast to the anterior tip (Fig.55.5).

Leptomonas are long, slender and spindle shaped, have a single flagellum, possess marked motility, measure 15 microns in length and 1.5 microns in breadth and grow in NNN medium. Amastigote *L. donovani* can be cultivated in a murine tumour cell, dog sarcoma cell, vero cell.

Life cycle. After entry into the human body, the organism is engulfed by the reticulo-endothelial cells, in which it multiplies by binary fission as a leishmania until the host is destroyed. It parasitises the new macrophage cells and the free leishmania and the parasitised macrophage cells enter the circulation.

A blood sucking insect, the sand fly, *Phlebotomus argentipes* (Indian vector Fig. 5.10) draw these circulating leishmania and macrophages cells during blood meal. In the intestine of the sand fly, the leishmaniae become leptomonas (Fig. 55.7, 8) forms and divide by longitudinal fission into two individuals. Enormous numbers of leptomonas are found in the midgut, and later in the pharynx and buccal cavity of the sand fly. The type of development is known as the "anterior station development". The transmission is thus effected through the bite of the infected insect and the cycle is repeated.

Pathogenicity and Clinical features. When an infected sand fly bites a man, the leptomonas stage is inoculated into the victim's skin and nearby macrophages engulf the organisms which metamorphose into the leishmania stage within the cytoplasm of the host cells. Sometimes, parasitised macrophages are set free into the blood stream and are carried from the skin to the viscera where they lodge and develop rapidly. In the spleen or liver, the leishmaniae are taken up by fixed macrophages, such as Kupffer's cells, in the liver and they multiply in these cells and destroy them. These are called as "Kala azar bodies". When the bone marrow is involved, there is diminished production of erythrocytes with ensuing anaemia.

The incubation period is limited to 2-4 months. The first symptoms are malaise, headache and irregular fever, with progressive enlargement of the spleen and occasional abdominal pain. There is edema of the skin, emaciation of chest, dysentery or diarrhoea, bleeding of the mucous membrane of the gums and nares and cachexia, accompanied by a progressive and marked enlargement of the spleen and a lesser enlargement of the liver.

The skin over the entire body is dry, rough, harsh and is often pigmented (darkened). The hair tends to be brittle and falls out. Death frequently occurs from complications (amoebic and bacillary dysentery, pulmonary tuberculosis, pneumonia etc.).

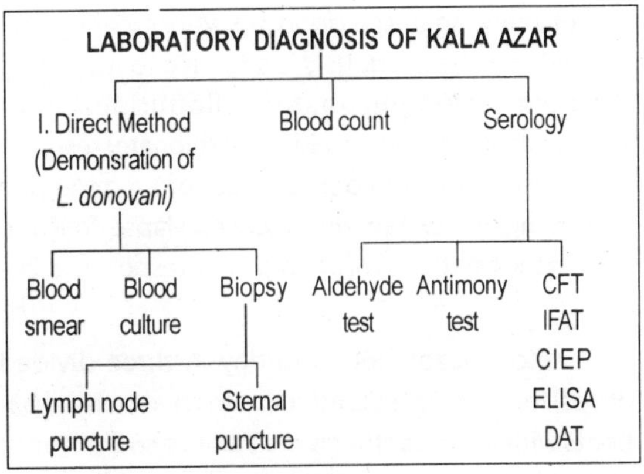

*Basically there are two different kinds of media — monophasic and diphasic.

Senekjie's medium (standard biphasic blood agar medium : 1 liter) similar to NNN medium.

Difco Bacto beef	50g
Bacto agar	20g
Bacto peplone	20g
NaCl	5g
Difibrinated rabbit blood	150 ml.

Several recent serological techniques have been developed to detect and measure specific leishmanial antibodies in patient sera. They are indirect fluorescent antibody test (IFAT), counterimmunoelectrophoresis (CIEP) and ELISA. IFAT is sensitive technique to detect antibody in 93% of patients of visceral leishmaniasis (Kala azar). It becomes positive in early stage. CIEP also become positive in 80% of patients in early stage and in almost all patients with late infection. ELISA is specific and sensitive and is most practical test. As compared to ELISA and IFAT, Direct agglutination test (DAT), which is the most recent technique, was found to be most sensitive, specific and easy to perform at field level and economical enough to be cost effective. The rate of positivity with DAT (96.3%) was comparable and slightly better than that of "splenic smear" examination (94%) the "gold standard" test for Kala azar. DAT appears to be future diagnostic test of Kala azar.

Treatment. In early years, though certain pentavalent preparations of antimony were toxic, they were found to be highly effective. Ketoconazole is also effective against *L. donovani*. Very recently, Amphotericin B intravenously is effective to multidrug (Sodium stibogluconate, allopurinol plus ketoconazole and pentamidine isethionate) resistant *L. donovani* and in low dosage (dose of 1 mg stepped up to 5 mg) it is extremely effective, relapse-free and safer in the treatment of antimony unresponsive Kala azar.

Ketoconazole (600 mg/day in three divided doses) for four weeks is effective in treatment of patients with Kala azar that is resistant to sodium antimony gluconate and pentamidine and should be initial treatment (not just in drug resistant cases) for Kala azar. It is effective *orally* and is relatively less toxic than conventional (parenteral) treatment. It is a recent finding.

Prophylaxis.

1. All human cases should be treated adequately with effective, less toxic drug.
2. Infected dogs should be destroyed, especially in China and Mediterranean countries.
3. Decaying vegetation from the ground which may harbour or breed sand flies would be removed.
4. Adult sand flies should be caught and destroyed each morning and evening.
5. Mosquito nets should be used regularly.
6. Houses should be well lit and ventilated.
7. Sleeping quarters should be above the ground floor because sand flies do not usually fly many feet above the ground.
8. Sand flies should be destroyed by insecticides, e.g., D.D.T.

DERMAL LEISHMANOID

It is a non-ulcerative cutaneous lesion. Usually, it develops in 10% of Kala azar patients after completion of sodium or potassium antimony tartarate treatment and is reported in Africa, China, India and not in the Mediterranean countries. Clinically, they are of three types : (a) Depigmented macules; (b) Erythematous patches; (c) Yellowish pink nodules. It can be diagnosed microscopically demonstrating *L. donovani* in nodular lesion smear. It can be treated with double dose of pentavalent antimony compounds. Post Kala azar dermal leishmaniasis (PKDL) is never fatal and can remain active and potential source of sand fly infection in an untreated patient for at least 35 years.

Recently it has been shown that all cases of (PKDL) can be completely cured if antimonials are given in the correct dosage and for a long enough period, i.e., until the lesion disappears.

LEISHMANIA TROPICA

This parasite was first observed in the tissue of a "Delhi Boil" or "Oriental Sore" in India.

It is distributed in Africa, America, Asia, Europe, Sri Lanka, West Pakistan. In man, it is found in the endothelial cells of the capillaries of the affected areas of the skin.

L. tropica is morphologically similar to *L. donovani* even in the life cycle except that *L. tropica* do not invade the viscera.

Pathology and Clinical features. Lesions are confined to the tissues cells of the corneal layer of the skin; the incubation period of is from few days to several months.

The lesion appears first as a reddish papule which later transforms into a shallow ulcer. The ulcer gradually enlarges and has sharp cut, raised edges surrounded by an indurated area. These ulcers coalesce to produce large ulcers.

Secondary bacterial infection of the sore is common. Then the general symptoms (fever, chills and inflammation) are observed. Varicose, lupoid forms of oriental sore have been described in India.

Laboratory diagnosis. Microscopic examination of Leishman or Giemsa stained smear prepared from the punctured indurated edge of the sore. The flagellates are not found in the blood.

Montenegro reaction (skin test) can also be done.

Treatment. Pentavalent antimony preparation is the drug of choice.

Prophylaxis.

1. The ulcers should be protected from insects with gauze bandage.
2. Transmission to others must be prevented by covering the ulcer.
3. The patient should be warned regarding autoinoculation.
4. Spray of DDT is the most effective method of control of sand flies.
5. Fly repellents can be applied over the skin.
6. Mosquito nets are very effective.
7. All natural reservoirs (dogs, rodents etc.) of *L. tropica* should be destroyed.

LEISHMANIA BRAZILIENSIS

This parasite is found commonly in America and Argentina and causes mucocutaneous leishmaniasis.

Morphology and Life cycle of *L. braziliensis* are similar to those of *L. donovani* and *L. tropica*. The disease is typically endemic. Direct contact may cause infection as the condition is inoculable and autoinoculable.

Pathogenesis and Clinical features. Following inoculation of the leptomonas stages of *L. braziliensis* by an infected sand fly, a small papule appears, this soon transforms into a red, itchy vesicle. Within one to four weeks, the lesion begins to show ulceration, often with a round or oval contour but at times with ragged irregular indurated edges.

Histologically, the elevated circumference shows epithelial hyperplasia and intense dermal inflammation with edema. Beneath the epithelial proliferation, there is a zone of leishmaniae. This primary lesion tends to be self-healing and is mostly found on the ear lobe. The secondary lesions in the mucus membrane may be ulcerative or indurative.

Clinical features. The incubation period is from few days to several days. The primary lesions appear as a papule which develops into a painless ulcer or it may transform into an open weeping sore which is very painful. The first signs usually noted are thickening of the mucosa in the nasal septum. Followed by development of nodules which necrose and form ulcers involving the mucus membrane of the mouth, and hard and soft palates. Constitutional symptoms are fever, anemia, pain in the affected region and malaise.

Laboratory diagnosis is similar to that of *L. tropica* and the skin test is the method of choice.

Treatment is similar to that of Oriental Sore.

Prophylaxis. Consists of avoiding forests where the sand flies breed; protection from sand flies by application of fly repellents; and avoiding direct contact with infected cases.

MALARIAL PARASITES OF MAN

World Health Organisation (WHO), in 1963 recommended that this term 'malarial parasites' be restricted to the family plasmodiiae. The plasmodia normally infecting man are *Plasmodium vivax*, *P. ovale*, *P. malariae* and *P. falciparum* (Fig. 55.12).

Plasmodium vivax causes vivax or tertian malaria.

P. ovale causes ovale malaria.

P. malariae causes malariae or quartan malaria.

P. falciparum causes malignant tertian or falciparum malaria.

History. 1880 Laveran first observed *P. vivax*.

1891 Staining method of malarial parasites by Romanowsky.

1898 Bigmani *et al* worked out the mosquito cycle of human plasmodia, whereas Ross in Calcutta (now Kolkata) demonstrated the same with the avian plasmodium.

1971 MacFie and Ingram first described *P. ovale*.

1949 Short *et al* demonstrated the pre-erythrocytic schizogony of *P. falciparum*.

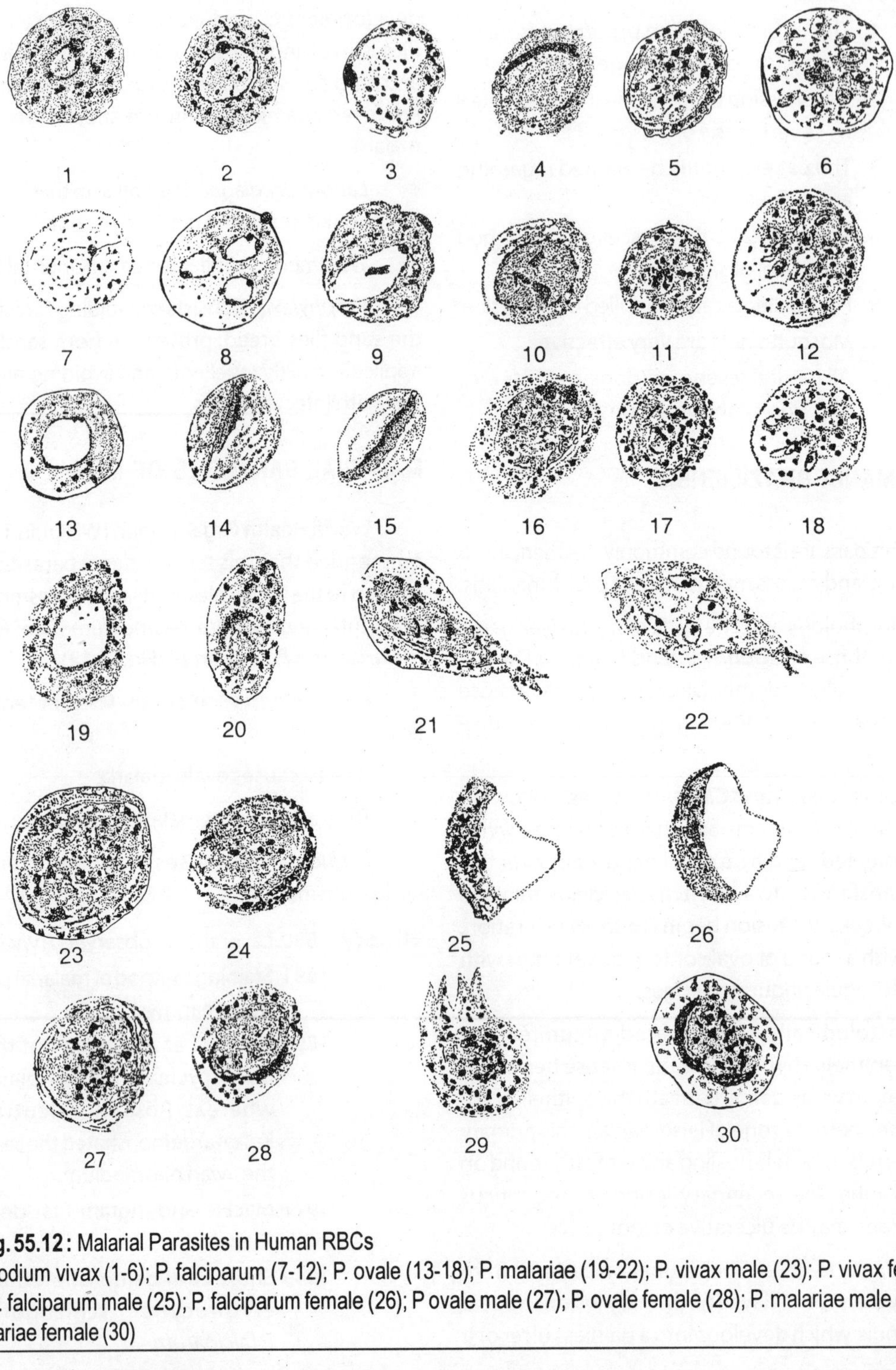

Fig. 55.12 : Malarial Parasites in Human RBCs
Plasmodium vivax (1-6); P. falciparum (7-12); P. ovale (13-18); P. malariae (19-22); P. vivax male (23); P. vivax female (24); P. falciparum male (25); P. falciparum female (26); P ovale male (27); P. ovale female (28); P. malariae male (29); P. malariae female (30)

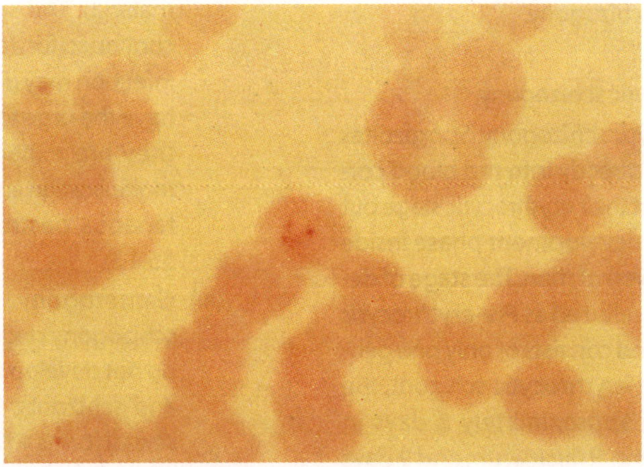

Fig. 55.12.3 : P. vivax trophozoite × 1000

Geographical distribution. Malarial parasites have world-wide distribution. Endemic area of these parasites is the tropical zone. Vivax infections are more common in temperate than in tropical regions. Ovale malaria occurs mostly in tropical Africa. It is endemic in Ethiopia. *P. malariae* is common in Africa, Myanmar, Sri Lanka and India. It is prominent in certain areas of Malaysia and Indonesia. *P. falciparum* is most prevalent in tropics and subtropics.

Habitat. The malarial parasites have a development stage in the parenchyma cells of the liver, reside in the red blood cells of man and are carried through blood stream to various organs.

Life Cycle. The malarial parasites pass their life cycle in two different hosts :

1. MAN (intrinsic phase). Man acts as the *intermediate host* for the malarial parasites. Here, plasmodia reside inside the hepatic cells and red blood corpuscles and reproduce by asexual method (Schizogony). Only in malaria and hydatid disease, man is the intermediate host.
2. Female Anophelene MOSQUITO (extrinsic phase) represents the *definite host* of the malarial parasites, because of the sexual method of reproduction of the malarial parasites. For the initiation of mosquito cycle, sexual forms (male and female gametocytes) are first developed in the human host. Then they are transferred to the definite host (female Anophelene mosquito) where they develop further and transform into "*sporozoites*" which are minute thread-like curved organisms tapering at both ends, measuring 9 to 12 microns in length and having a central elongated nucleus without any pigment. Sporozoites are infective to man. Only female mosquito can transmit the sporozoites to the intermediate host (man); because of their well- developed serrated maxillae and mandibles, they have stout proboscis which can pierce the skin of man as needle. The host specificity is possibly determined by the presence of absence of certain amino acids in the mosquito.

HUMAN CYCLE
(Asexual Cycle of Malarial Parasites)

Human cycle starts with the introduction of sporozoites into man by the bite of infected anophelene mosquito. It consists of the following four stages :

(i) Pre-erythrocytic shizogony,
(ii) Erythrocytic schizogony,
(iii) Gametogony,
(iv) Exo-erythrocytic schizogony,

(i) *Pre-erythrocytic schizogony.* Sporozoites do not enter directly into red blood corpuscles to start their erythrocytic stage but undergo the development phase inside the tissues (liver) of man. The stage of development is referred as *Pre-erythrocytic schizogony* and consists of only one generation of pre-erythrocytic schizont, the cycle lasting approximately 8 days in *P. vivax*, 6 days in *P. falciparum* and 9 days in *P. ovale*. The pre-erythrocytic schizogony occurs inside the parenchyma cells of the liver. The liberated merozoites are called cryptozoites. The smaller ones (micromerozoites) enter the blood stream, bind with glycoproteins of red blood cells membrane and enter into R B cells and the large ones (macromerozoites) reenter the liver cells. During the preerythrocytic schizogony the parasites are not found in the peripheral blood and inoculation of such blood does not produce any infection, i.e., the blood is sterile; when the parasites develop inside the liver, there is no clinical manifestation and pathological damage.

(ii) *Erythrocytic schizogony.* During this phase, the parasite passes through the stages of *trophozoite, schizont* and *merozoites* inside the red blood corpuscles. These asexual forms can be demonstrated in the thick smear of peripheral blood 3 to 4 days after completion of pre-erythrocytic schizogony, i.e., in *P. vivax* about 12 days; in *P. falciparum* infection 9 days after exposure to the mosquito bite. Each erythrocytic schizogony lasts 48 to 72 hours. In *P. vivax, P. ovale, P. falciparum* it is 48 hours but in *P. malariae* it is 72 hours. The parasitic multiplication during the erythrocytic phase is responsible for bringing about a 'clinical attack of malaria' (overt malaria). The schizogony cycle may be continued for a considerable time, but the infection may die out or the parasite may have the urge for sexual multiplication as they are exhausted with the asexual multiplication and as well as with the spontaneous destruction of parasites (Fig. 55.12).

(iii) *Gametogony.* After the erythrocytic schizogony stage some of the merozoites do not develop directly into trophozoites and schizonts, but they transform into sexual forms which are capable of sexual reproduction outside the human host. These forms are known as gametocytes. These gametocytes are produced to propagate and to continue ultimately the life cycle in mosquito. They develop in the red blood cells of the capillaries of internal organs (spleen and bone marrow). Only the mature gametocytes are found in the peripheral blood. The complete maturation takes about 96 hours (4 days), i.e., twice the time taken by an erythrocytic schizont to mature completely. The individuals who harbour these gametocytes are called 'Carriers'.

(iv) *Exoerythrocytic schizogony.* After the micromerozoites infect red blood corpuscles, the preerythrocytic phase disappears completely in *P. falciparum*, whereas in case of *P. vivax, P. ovale, P. malariae*, it persists in the form of a local liver cycle. This tissue phase (liver cycle) is described as 'exoerythrocytic schizogony'. This exoerythrocytic schizogony is responsible for relapse of vivax, ovale and malariae malaria, but there is 'NO RELAPSE' in *P. falciparum*, i.e., there is no exoerythrocytic schizogony of *P. falciparum*. The occurrence of clinical falciparum malaria and parasites persisting in the circulation at a subclinical level following a previous attack is referred as "recrudescence" which is different from malaria relapse.

There is no relapse (hypnozoite) stage of *P. falciparum*. Recrudescence may occur due to inadequate drug therapy, drug resistance or when a person's natural acquired immunity is reduced, e.g., during pregnancy. It may occur within a few weeks or months of a previous attack. Most of the recrudescence die out within a year of the original attack. The merozoites (both micro and macromerozoites) liberated from this exoerythrocytic schizogony are called *Phanerozoites* (Fig. 55.13).

MOSQUITO CYCLE
(Sexual Cycle of Malarial Parasite)

When a female anopheles mosquito bites an infected human host, it sucks blood during its blood meal from the infected person. It ingests both the sexual and asexual forms of malarial parasites, but only the mature sexual forms — which are capable of development — will survive; the remaining asexual forms will die immediately. It has been suggested that a mosquito can transmit the infection to man, if the blood of human carrier contains at least twelve gametocytes per mm^3 of blood; the female gametocytes should be more than male ones to initiate the infection.

In the proventriculus (stomach or midgut) of the mosquito, one male microgametocyte gives rise to four to eight thread like filamentous structures known as *microgametes*. This process of development is called as ex-flagellation; whereas, one female macrogametocyte develops into one macrogamete without forming any flagellation. Its nucleus shifts to the surface where a projection is formed. These gametes are ready for fertilisation. By chemotaxis process, the male microgametes are attracted towards the female macrogametes. One of the male gametes attaches to the periphery of the female parasite at the site of this projection and penetrates through this projection into the body of the female gamete; then there is fusion of their pronuclei, thereby the macrogamete is fertilised, which is called as *zygote*. The zygote formation takes twenty minutes to two hours after the mosquito's blood meal.

After some twenty minutes, the zygote puts out a pseudopodium into which its protoplasm flows to form a fusiform body, the *Ookinete* (a motile zygote) (Fig.55.14)

This mature Ookinete penetrates the brush border of the mucosal cell and its anterior end comes in close contact with the cell membrane of the epithelial cells of midgut of the mosquito. The entry of the Ookinete into the cell is made by the secretion of proteolytic substance, through a slit at the anterior end of the Ookinete, which causes lysis of the cell membrane. Then it is found in the middle of the cell, it secretes a thin wall and grows into a spherical Oocyst, 50 microns or more in size with a single vesicular nucleus and pigment granules.

As many as a thousand sickle shaped bodies — known as Sporozoites — are developed as a result of successive division of nuclear material of the oocyst. The oocyst bursts and sporozoites enter the mosquito's body cavity (haemocele) from which they disperse throughout the mosquito's body, except the ovaries. Those that come in contact with the salivary glands bore into these glands and through acinal cells they lodge in acinal ducts. Therefore, when the mosquito injects saliva while obtaining a blood meal, it also injects sporozoites which thus enter the human host. A single bite of the mosquito is sufficient to transmit the infection. Only female *Anopheles* — not males — take blood meal. Different species of malarial parasites can develop in the same mosquito and may give rise to 'mixed infection', i.e., *P. falciparum* and *P. vivax* (Fig. 55.14).

Ookinete under electron microscope :

1. It is enclosed in a two-layered envelope — inner one is smooth, whereas the outer one is corrugated;
2. Inner layer appears more dense at the anterior end;
3. There are peripheral fibrils under the envelope;
4. There is granular nucleus with nucleolus;
5. There is no micropyle;
6. Cytoplasmic inclusions (mitochondria, lysosome; black pigment granules) are in the vacuoles of the cytoplasm (Fig. 55.43).

Infected Mosquito bite
↓
Sporozoites
↓
enter in liver cells (not in RBCs)
(Preerythrocytic schizogony)

→ macromerozoite
↓
reenter liver cells
(in *P. vivax*, *P. malariae*, *P. ovale* - RELAPSE, not in *P. falciparum*)

→ micromerozoite
↓
enter RBCs
↓
Trophozoites
↓
Schizonts
↓
Merozoites
(Trophozoites → Schizonts → Merozoites: Erythrocytic schizogony)
↓
Gametocytes (Gametogony)
↓
MOSQUITO

Fig. 55.13: Human cycle of Plasmodium

Sporozoites:

1. They are infective forms of malarial parasites to man;
2. They have a complex structure held together by a relatively thick membrane;
3. Their shape varies from narrow, slightly curved (vivax), thick (malariae), to sickle-shaped (falciparum);
4. They measure from about 10 to 14 microns in length;
5. They have peripheral fibrils which may have locomotory function;
6. They possess mitochondria but no pigment;
7. They have deep depression in the surface membrane which is called the micropyle. The micropyle may represent the point of exit of emergent sporoplasm, i.e., the infective material from the sporozite.

Sexual and asexual form of parasites
↓
Ingestion by Mosquito
↓
In stomach (mid-gut)
↓
Sexual forms (asexual forms die)

→ Microgametocyte
↓
4-8 microgametes (male)

→ Macrogametocyte
↓
One macrogamete (female)

↓
Zygote
↓
Ookinete (motile zygote)
↓
Enter into mosquito gut cell
↓
Oocyst
↓
Sporozoites
↓
MAN

Fig. 55.14: Mosquito cycle of Plasmodium

Biochemistry and Metabolism of Malarial Parasites

Plasmodia are complex, obligate intracellular parasites and it has been difficult to determine how they ingest and metabolise their food. It has been suggested that:

1. The parasite feeds on its host's cytoplasm by pinocytosis, i.e., invagination of its plasma membrane to engulf and close around some cytoplasm, forming a vacuole within which digestion takes place.
2. A single food-ingesting organelle resembling micropyle of a sporozoite.
3. A specific cytoplasm that ingests host cell cytoplasm.

In general, the required energy of the parasite depends on phosphorylation of glucose; oxidative processes are maintained by oxyhaemoglobin of the erythrocytes, globin of haemoglobin is split by enzymes into amino acids and peptides that form the parasite's protein, and lipids are synthesised in large quantities. Metabolites of the parasite are derived from haemoglobin of the erythrocytes and from blood plasma.

Effect of Host Nutrition

The host's nutrition influences that of the parasite. When the host is starved the parasite is also malnourished. In primates, restriction of food elements such as thiamine, riboflavin, biotin and coenzyme A seems to inhibit growth of malarial parasites, but in birds opposite effects are observed. West African children restricted to a milk diet remained heavily parasitised by *P. falciparum*.

Glucose-6 phosphate dehydrogenase deficient trait

A genetic deficiency known as glucose-6 phosphate dehydrogenase deficient trait seems to confer some protection against *P. falciparum* infection. Afro-Americans and East Africans inherit this trait. Low activity of this enzyme results in abnormal concentration of reduced glutathione in red blood corpuscles and also in limitation of the hexose monophosphate shunt metabolic pathway. In their metabolism, plasmodia use the hexose monophosphate shunt pathway. Hence, this genetic glucose-6 phosphate trait appears to confer some protection against *P. falciparum*.

Sickle cell anaemia trait is also responsible for resistance to malaria. The sickle cell trait, common in Africa, Asia and Europe, resulting in an abnormal haemoglobin, the molecule of which, when deoxygenated, tend to collect in rigid, rod-like masses which distort the red cells into a sickle like shape. *P. falciparum* schizonts appear to have difficulty in utilizing this abnormal haemoglobin so that their growth and schizogony are stunted.

Thalassaemia haemoglobin and haemoglobin E provide some protection against *P. vivax* and human foetal haemoglobin against all plasmodia. Oocysts develop better when the host mosquito has blood rather than glucose diet. The host specificity is determined by the presence or absence of certain amino acids in the mosquito.

PLASMODIUM VIVAX (Producing Tertian or Vivax Malaria)

The specific name 'vivax' is derived from Latin *Vivere*, to live, and indicates the activity of movement. *Distribution. P. vivax* has nearly worldwide distribution and is more common in temperate than in tropical regions.

Gametes. The microgametocyte of *P. vivax* usually exflagellates six microgametes, each 20 to 25 microns in length. The macrogametocyte becomes a macrogamate. A microgamete penetrates into the small projection of the macrogamete and the ookinete is formed. The process takes from ten minutes to one hour in the mosquito's gut.

Ookinete. Vivax ookinetes are 15 to 22 microns in length and 3 microns in width. They are motile and will penetrate the epithelial cell of mosquito's mid-gut twentyfour to fortyeight hours after the blood meal was ingested.

Oocysts. Their maturing period is 7 to 8 days. Pigment granules are present.

Sporozoites. Vivax sporozoites are narrow and slightly curved, measuring about 14 microns in length.

Exo-erythrocytic (EE) stages. Primary vivax exo-erythrocytic schizogony is completed in from seven and quarter days to eight days. After seven days the schizont is ovoid, 40 microns with blue staining cytoplasm. At maturity, the schizont gives rise to 10,000 merozoites, which are spherical (1.2 micron) and are released to enter the host's circulation.

Secondary exo-erythrocytic schizonts have been observed from fourteen days to nine months after infection.

Erythrocytic stages. Sporozoites leave the blood stream within an hour after injection and a prepatent period of about eight days ensues with the blood stream free of plasmodia. On the eighth day exo-erythrocytic merozoites invade the younger red blood cells. *P. vivax* shows a greater tendency to invade younger red blood corpuscles. The asexual cycle of *P. vivax* usually takes fortyeight hours.

Gametocytes. Vivax gametocytes usually appear on the fifth day.

Morphology. Unstained preparation. The *P. vivax trophozoite* appears within the red blood corpuscles as a small hyaline ring which becomes amoeboid with characteristic movement which justifies its name 'vivax'. In a few hours, it begins to show delicate granules of pigment. At the end of 36 hours, it fills most of the infected cells dividing the organisms into 12 to 24 daughter cells or *merozoites.*

Stained preparation. In blood smears stained by Giemsa's stain, plasmodium cytoplasm stains blue and nuclear chromatin violet colour. While cytoplasm of the infected erythrocytes stains yellowish or salmon pink.

The earliest erythrocytic *trophozoite* is a delicate blue stained ring of cytoplasm with a red chromatin dot. The erythrocyte is stained salmon pink.

As the plasmodium enlarges the ring form becomes irregular and larger and contains dots or threads of red stained chromatin and granules of dark pigment. Orange pink or pink spots known as 'Schuffner's dots' may appear in the cytoplasm of red blood corpuscles.

As *P. vivax* segments, round blue bodies each having a bright red or violet chromatin dot, situated at or near the periphery of the red blood cells, are produced. These bodies are merozoites, typically 16 in number. They are liberated in the blood plasma and enter red blood cells and appear as oval, blue stained bodies having a red dot of chromatin near the center.

The *microgametocyte* cytoplasm stains pale blue while that of *macrogametocyte* stains deep blue. The macrogametocyte of *P. vivax* has a smaller nucleus then the microgametocyte and chromatin is arranged in a complex mass near the periphery. The cytoplasm stains bright blue and the chromatin deep red. Pigment in fine granules is arranged in small masses.

Gametocytes of *P. vivax* appear in the peripheral blood from the first day of fever (16 days after inoculation of sporozoites), i.e., 4-5 days after the initial appearance of the asexual parasites in thick smears. If these gametocytes are not taken up by the insect host, they do not live for more than a week in the human host.

In vivax malaria, severe neurological complications, though rare, do occur. Immunological status, hyperpyrexia and heavy parasitemia are likely causes.

The differences between a microgametocyte and macrogametocyte of *P. vivax* are as follows:

	Microgametocyte	*Macrogametocyte*
Size	9 to 10 microns	10 to 12 microns
Cytoplasm	Stains light blue	Stains deep blue
Nucleus	Diffuse, large; lies laterally.	Small, compact; lies peripherally.

PLASMODIUM FALCIPARUM

The parasite of malignant tertian or falciparum malaria.

The specific name 'falciparum' (*Latin,* falx, a sickle) is derived from sickle shaped gametocyte.

Distribution. P. falciparum is most prevalent in the tropics and subtropics and is also common in tropical and subtropical Asia.

Gametes. Microgametocytes of *P. falciparum* produce 4 to 6 microgametes by exflagellation which begins in the host insect's gut about ten minutes after ingestion, at 37°C. Microgametes are slender and measure about 16 to 25 microns in length. Macrogametes become spherical. Their nuclei approach the edge of the parasite, forming a protuberance into which a microgamete will penetrate.

Ookinetes. Falciparum ookinetes form twelve to eighteen hours after the insect takes its blood meal. These are more slender than those of *P. vivax.* They measure about 2.5 microns in breadth and 13 microns in length.

Oocysts. Falciparum oocysts are generally smaller than those of other malarial parasites of man.

Sporozoites. Falciparum sporozoites are sickle shaped with equally pointed ends measuring about twelve microns in length. They invade the salivary glands of the host mosquito in nine days or more after the insect's blood meal and remain infective up to 40-45 days.

Exo-erythrocytic stages. In *Plasmodium falciparum*, exo-erythrocytic schizogony appears to be limited to a single generation. There is no secondary exo-erythrocytic schizogony and it is completely absent. Hence there is **no relapse.** The exo-erythrocytic schizonts grow rapidly, measure some 60 microns in diameter and may liberate some 30,000 exo-erythrocytic merozoites.

Erythrocytic stages. Falciparum exo-erythrocytic merozoites invade young and old red cells. The schizogony cycle is completed in 36 to 48 hours. Multiple infection of red blood cells is very common in this species.

(a) *Trophozoites.* The early ring form measures 1.5 micron in diameter. It consists of a fine and uniform cytoplasmic ring with nucleus often projecting beyond the edge or lying outside the ring. The parasite often attaches itself to the margin or edge of the host's cell. The nucleus and a small part of the cytoplasm remain almost outside. This is known as form '*applique*' or 'accole'. The nucleus is often divided into two parts which may remain close together or be situated at opposite poles.

The *pigment granules* formed by *Plasmodium falciparum* are dark brown or black in colour and are collected into a single mass at an early stage.

The *infected red blood cells* remain unaltered but the cells containing the large sized rings occasionally show a crenated appearance at the periphery. The colour of the cell is reddish violet. Maurer's dots, staining brick red with Leishman's stain, are seen.

(b) *Schizont.* As the growth continues the nucleus divides into 8 to 32 masses and the cytoplasm forms many segments. The mature schizont measures 4.5 to 5 microns in diameter.

(c) *Merozoites.* Its average number is 18 to 24 and measures 0.5 to 0.7 micron in diameter.

(d) *Gametogony.* At first Falciparum gametocytes are round or ovoid, but become spindle, cigar, or diamond shaped. Falciparum gametocytes appear in the peripheral circulation after 8 to 11 days of parasite patency and by then they have assumed their typical crescentic or sickle shape. The microgametocyte is more banana shaped than crescentic and is more thicker and blunter than the female macrogametocyte, which stains a darker blue and has a more compact nucleus. Gametocytes of *P. falciparum* persist in the blood for weeks after asexual forms have been eliminated. They do not cause the disease, their presence is not due to treatment failure.

The difference between a microgametocyte and a macrogametocyte of *P. falciparum* (Fig. 55.12, 25, 26) :

	Microgametocyte	*Macrogametocyte*
Shape	Broader, shorter, ends blunt	Longer, narrow, ends pointed
Size	8 to 10 microns by 2 - 3 microns	10 - 12 microns by 2 - 3 microns
Cytoplasm	Stains light blue	Stains deep blue
Nucleus	Scattered in fine granules over a wide area	Condensed into a small compact mass at the centre
Pigments	Scattered throughout the cytoplasm	Aggregate like a wreath around the nucleus

PLASMODIUM MALARIAE
(The Parasite of Quartan Malaria)

This species was first studied by Laveran in 1880. The specific name *malariae* was given and still retained.

Distribution. The quartan parasite is common in tropical Africa, Mayanmar, Sri Lanka and parts of India. It is prominent in certain parts of Malaysia and Indonesia.

Gametes. Malariae gametes are smaller than those of *vivax* and *falciparum*. Typically, the microgametocytes form 8 microgametes. The microgamete measures about 16 microns in length.

Ookinetes. They seem to be more dense than those of other species.

Oocyts. P. malariae does not develop easily in mosquitoes and are scanty in malariae infections.

Sporozoites. Malariae sporozoites are thicker and coarser than those of other species that infect man. They measure 13 to 14 microns in length.

Exo-erythrocytic stage. Primary *P. malariae* Exo-erythrocytic (EE) schizogony is probably completed in 13 to 16 days. In secondary EE schizogony relapses are common. Such relapses may occur as long as forty years after infection.

Erythrocytic stage. P. malariae are scanty in red blood corpuscles and show a special tendency to invade mature and older erythrocytes. The cycle of schizogony is completed in 72 hours (3 days) and occurs mostly in the peripheral circulation.

Trophozoites. The characteristic feature of trophozoite of *P. malariae* is that the parasite stretches right across the red blood cells and assumes a band-like appearance. When the parasite is 6 to 8 hours old, coarse pigment granules, dark brown or black in colour, appear in the cytoplasm.

Schizont. It is circular and measures about 7 microns in diameter. When segmentation is complete, the schizonts arrange themselves as 'dairy head' appearance.

Merozoite. It measures 2 to 2.5 microns in diameter.

Gametocyte. : Malariae gametocytes are slow to appear. They appear between tenth and fourteenth day. Peak gametocyte density occurs about six days after that of the asexual parasites. They measure about 7 to 7.5 microns in diameter and are large. The morphological differences between the female and male gametocytes are same as those of *P. vivax*. The host cell is not enlarged.

PLASMODIUM OVALE
(The Parasite of Ovale Tertian Malaria)

Distribution. P. ovale, least common of the species infecting man, occurs mostly in tropical Africa. It is endemic in Ethiopia.

Gametes. Ovale gametes produce upto 8 microgametes somewhat smaller in size than those of *P. vivax*.

Ookinetes. Ovale ookinetes appear eighteen to twenty hours after the mosquito ingests the gametocytes. These ookinetes are smaller than those of *P. vivax*.

Oocysts. Ovale oocysts develop slowly in less than twelve days at any temperature.

Sporozoites. Ovale sporozoites are plump, elongated, pointed at one end, measure 11 to 12 microns in length.

Exo-erythrocytic stage. Primary ovale exo-erythrocytic schizogony is completed in 9 days after the sporozoites enter liver parenchymal cells. The schizont is unusually large and distinctive, confirming the validity of *P. vivax* as a distinct species. Characteristics are relatively enormous nuclei.

Erythrocytic stage. Erythrocytic schizogony in this species requires fortynine to fifty days, a little longer than in *P. vivax*. There may be prolonged latency up to four or more years.

Trophozoite. The ring form measures 2 to 2.5 microns in diameter and resembles more closely that of *P. malariae*, but the band form is not seen. The pigment granules are coarse and dark brown in colour. Even at the early ring stage of the parasite, the infected red blood cells show granules like Schuffner's dots and take a violet tinge; these are named James's dots. The infected red blood cells is slightly enlarged, often oval.

Schizont. It is round or oval in shape, measures 6.2 microns in diameter. The nuclear material is divided into 6 to 12 masses (usually 8).

Merozoite. It measures 2 to 2.5 microns in diameter. The nucleus is crescentic.

Gametocyte. Ovale gametocytes appear on the fifth day of parasite patency. In about 3 weeks they become sufficiently numerous to infect mosquitoes.

Morphology. In quick dried, very thin, stained blood films, the ovale infected red cells is moderately enlarged and presents a characteristic artefact — an oval shape with fimbrination of one or both ends. The artefact is not seen in unstained blood.

Stippling with Schuffner's dots appear earlier and is more prominent than in *P. vivax*. Ovale stipplings which are known as James's dots, are fewer but more prominent and more violet than in vivax infected cells.

Ovale parasites are fairly compact, generally smaller than corresponding stages of *P. vivax*. Mature *ovale* schizonts display fewer and larger merozoites, averaging 8, each with prominent nucleus. Stained ovale gametocytes closely resemble those of *P. vivax*. ovale pigment seems darker than that of *P. vivax*. Diagnostic characters of *P. ovale* are : (1) large nucleus with clear cut borders; (2) absence of much amoeboidicity; (3) large average number of merozoites in primary attack; (4) darker colour; (5) smaller size.

Staining method. Leishman's and Giemsa's stains can be used to study the detailed structures of malarial parasites.

Leishman's stain can be prepared by dissolving the dry powder in acetone free pure methyl alcohol and be used in 0.15 per cent. Giemsa's stain is obtained in a ready made watery solution. Hence the fixation of the film with alcohol is only necessary when Giemsa's stain is used.

Cultivation. It is not fully successful. However, attempts are still made to cultivate successfully malarial parasites in human erythrocytes. Recently *P. falciparum* was cultivated *in vitro* in umbilical cord human erythrocytes.

Epidemiology. Malaria is *endemic* where there is constant measurable incidence of cases and natural transmission over a succession of years. It is epidemic when the incidence of cases in an area rises rapidly and notably above the usual level or when the disease suddenly occurs in an area previously non-malarious. When an epidemic spread far beyond the usual limits, it becomes *pandemic.*

Cases of malaria contracted locally are called *autochthonous*; when acquired outside the area and brought in, they are called *imported.* Cases proved to be locally derived from imported malaria are called *introduced,* in contrast to *autochthonous.* Malaria cases are indigenous if natural to an area. Malaria is *sporadic* when autochthonous cases are few and scattered.

Malaria is *holoendemic* when the spleen rate (frequency of splenomegaly) in children (two to nine years) is constantly over 75 per cent and adult populations have high tolerance; *hyperendemic* where the children's spleen rate is constantly over 50 per cent and the rate is also high in adults; *mesoendemic* when the children's spleen rate is eleven to fifty per cent; and *hypoendemic* when the spleen rate is ten per cent or less.

Animal inoculation. Human species of malarial parasites can now be transferrable to several species of primates.

Reservoir of infection. Lower animals do not harbour human species of malarial parasites. Children in an endemic area act as the only reservoir of infection. In some parts of Africa, chimpanzees may act as a reservoir for *P. malariae.*

Method of transmission. The infection is transmitted by the inoculative method. During the act of biting, the mosquito's proboscis pierces the skin and the salivary secretion is injected into the puncture wound. The salivary secretion carries a large number

MALARIAL PARASITES OF MAN

Table 55.1 : Differential characters of Erythrocytic Phases (After staining)

	P. vivax 48 hours	*P. falciparum* 48 hours or under	*P. malariae* 72 hours	*P. ovale* 48 hours
SCHIZOGONY FORMS IN PERIPHERAL BLOOD	Trophozoites, Schizonts and Gametocytes.	Rings, crescents only.	Trophozoites, Schizonts, Gametocytes.	Trophozoites, Schizonts, Gametocytes.
TROPHOZOITES RING FORM	Size 2.5 μm. cytoplasm opposite nucleus is thicker.	Size 1.25 μm - 1.5 μm cytoplasm fine, regular accole form.	Same as *P. vivax.*	Same as *P. malariae.*
GROWING FORM	Irregular with a vacuole. Actively amoeboid.	Assumes compact form. Pigments collect into a single mass early.	Band-like, slightly amoeboid. Vacuole disappears early.	No ribbon shape. Slightly amoeboid.
SCHIZONT (MATURE)	Size, 9 - 10 μm. Regular, completely fills an enlarged red blood cells.	Size 4.5 - 5 μm. Fills two thirds of a red blood cells which is not enlarged.	Size 6.5 to 7 μm Regular, almost fills a normal sized red blood cells.	Size 6.2 μm. Fills three quarters of red blood cell which is slightly enlarged.
MEROZOITES	12 - 24. Arranged in an irregular grape-like cluster.	18 - 24 or more. Arranged in a grape like cluster.	6 - 12. Arranged around a central mass of pigment like a 'daisy' or a 'rosette'.	6 - 12. Irregularly arranged.
MALARIAL PIGMENTS	Yellowish brown fine granules.	Dark brown or blackish, one or two solid dots.	Dark brown; coarse granules.	Dark yellowish brown; coarser than *P. vivax.*
INFECTED R.B.C.	Enlarged, pale Schuffner's dots present.	Unaltered, crenation reddish violet colour, Maurer's dots.	Not enlarged, not pale and no dots.	Enlarged, oval. James's dots.
GAMETOCYTE	Spherical, much larger than a red blood cell. Schuffner's dots.	Crescentic. Larger than red blood cell. Host cell hardly recognisable.	Round, oval. Size of red blood cell.	Oval. Size of red blood cell. Host cell is slightly enlarged with James's dots.
Female : Cytoplasm blue; nucleus small and compact. Male : Cytoplasm pale blue; nucleus large and diffuse.				

of sporozoites which are directly introduced into the blood stream and cannot be found in the blood after half an hour.

Transmitting agent — Female Anophelene mosquito.

Portal of entry — skin.

Site of localisation — first in liver cells, then in erythrocytes.

Pathogenecity. Infection with *Plasmodium* causes intermittent fevers which are known as 'Malaria'. (The word malaria is derived from two Italian words, *mala* and *aria,* meaning bad air).

Each of the four species causes a characteristic fever and the diseases are named as follows :

Plasmodium vivax : Vivax malaria (Benign tertian malaria).

Plasmodium malariae : Quartan malaria (Malariae malaria).

Plasmodium falciparum : Falciparum malaria (Malignant tertian malaria). It causes also pernicious malaria and Black water fever.

Plasmodium Ovale : Ovale Malaria.

Sporozoites promptly leave the blood stream without having caused apparent harm, and they lodge in the parenchyma cells where exo-erythrocytic schizogony takes place. Destruction of liver cells occurs, but without noticeable host reaction. The exo-erythrocytic merozoites (micromerozoites) invade red cells and pathogenic effects then become significant.

A major factor in malaria pathogenesis is disturbance in oxygen usage caused by the infection. This may occur in two ways :

(1) O_2 supplies may — be reduced below minimum physiological needs - a state of anoxic anemia, and (2) the host may not utilize an adequate O_2 supply because of pathological changes in the metabolising cells — a state of cytotoxic anoxia.

A state of shock may occur in acute severe malaria, e.g., in so called 'algid malaria'. Low blood pressure and cardiac output plus vasoconstriction may result in local anoxic anemia with cellular damage in the liver or kidney.

Incubation period. In *Plasmodium ovale, P. vivax, P. falciparum*, it is 10 - 14 days, and in *P. malariae* it is 18 days to 6 weeks.

Clinical features of malaria. They are :

1. Febrile paroxysm,
2. Anemia,
3. Splenomegaly.

Each febrile paroxysm has 3 stages :

(a) the cold stage (lasting 20 minutes to an hour;

(b) the hot stage (lasting 1 to 4 hours), and

(c) the sweating stage (lasting 2 to 3 hours). The total duration of febrile cycle is 6 to 10 hours.

Paroxysm of malaria occurs at the time of rupture of schizont and is caused by pyrogens and other toxins released from ruptured schizonts although none has been identified to date. Periodicity is produced by synchronised infection in which all the schizonts rupture simultanously. Partial immunity reduces parasitemia and symptoms disappear. This immunity depends upon persistent latent infection known as infection immunity or preimmunition. B lymphocytes produce Ig G and Ig M directed against the merozoites which are coated with these antibodies. Coated merozoites do not enter RBCs and are removed by phagocytes. T lymphocytes release substances that stimulate the phagocytosis and metabolic activities of macrophages.

Diagnosis of a febrile case is important because this can infect mosquito and transmit malaria through blood transfusion.

Types of Fever

(i) Quotidian fever — Fever recurs at an interval of 24 hours, observed in vivax and malariae malaria;

(ii) Tertian fever — Fever recurs every third day;

(iii) Quartan fever — Fever recurs every fourth day.

Anemia. After paroxyms, anemia of microcytic hypochromic type, with iron deficiency, develops due to breakdown of red blood cells during segmentation of parasites.

Splenomegaly. One of the important physical signs in malaria is enlargement of spleen. Initially, the enlargement is slight and by second week, it is much enlarged and palpable.

Symptoms. Onset is usually sudden in vivax; Ovale and Malariae malaria with a shaking chill succeeded by a fever reaching 104° or 105° F (40° or 40.6°C) and accompanied by symptoms of an acute febrile infection such as headache, muscular pains, malaise and increased pulse and respiration. Pernicious symptoms, as coma, convulsions and cardiac failure frequently occur in *falciparum* malaria.

Pernicious malaria. During the course of *P.falciparum* infection which is inadequately treated, a series of phenomenon occurs, it is known as *pernicious* malaria and it may cause death within one to three days. It is characterised by a series of symptoms. Accordingly, it is classified as comatose, algid, bilious, cardiologic, choleraic, delirious, dysenteric eclamptic, hemorrhagic, hemiplegic and pneumonic. The patient may be cold, pulseless and unconscious (algid type), comatose or restless, at times even violent (cerebral type), bleeding from the skin or mucous membrane (hemorrhagic type), vomiting, acute dysentery (gastrointestinal type). Malaria may simulate many other diseases, because of protean manifestations.

Blackwater fever. Blackwater fever appears to be a manifestation of repeated infections with *falciparum* malaria inadequately treated with quinine.

Congenital malaria. It is considered as intrauterine transmission of malaria and is common in non-immune infected mothers than in highly immune mothers whose placentae are more frequently heavily loaded with *P. falciparum* schizonts. It has been reported in each of the four species of plasmodium. Blood examination of mothers, of umbilical cord during delivery and of babies within five hours reveals that malaria is usually connatal, i.e., malaria acquired during parturition.

PATHOLOGY OF MALARIA

The malarial parasites reside in the red blood cells of the human host. The schizogony life cycle is completed within the host cell resulting in the destruction of the red blood cell. During their growth they produce pigment (hematin) from the hemoglobin and also multiply asexually to form daughter individuals (merozoites). On completion of schizogony, merozoites, pigment granules, unused portion of the cytoplasm of the infected red blood cells and 'malarial toxins' are liberated in the blood stream.

Malarial Pigment (hematin). World Health Organisation (WHO, 1963) does not recommend the term 'hemozoin' for malarial pigment. The pigment granules, liberated in the plasma at the time of rupture of segmenting parasites, are filtered out from the circulating blood by the activity of the reticulo-endothelial cells and they may be found in any quantity inside these cells. Therefore, the organs rich in reticulo-endothelial cells become densely pigmented, i.e., slate grey to black, giving characteristic pigmentation of organs in malaria. Although, the malarial pigment contains iron, it does not give the Prussian blue reaction, when stained with potassium ferrocyanide, but stains black. Other pigments which are also found because of the blood destruction, are not specific products of malarial parasites and they are (a) *hemosiderin* (containing iron), (b) *hematoidin* (which is converted into bile pigment — *cholebilirubin*.

During erythrocytic phase, malarial parasites require para-aminobenzoic acid (PABA) for their metabolism. The deficiency of PABA inhibits their growth.

Pathological Changes in Organs

1. SPLEEN

Macroscopic appearance

(a) Spleen is enlarged;
(b) The *colour* is slate grey or black;
(c) The *capsule* is thin and stretched in acute falciparum malaria;
(d) The *consistency* is soft in acute cases and firm in chronic cases;
(e) The *cut surface* has a homogeneous black area.

Microscopic examination

(a) *Hematin* and *Hemosiderin* are scattered throughout;
(b) Sinusoids are congested;
(c) Macrophages are increased in numbers;
(d) The *parasites* appear as black dots in red blood corpuscles, when sections of spleen are stained with hematoxylin and eosin;
(e) Parasites and pigment are not seen in malpighian corpuscles (White pulp);

(f) In chronic cases, *reticulin fibrils* are increased.

2. LIVER

Macroscopic appearance

(a) Liver is enlarged;

(b) The *colour* is slate grey or black.

Microscopic appearance

(a) Parasitised red blood cells fill up the central veins of the lobules and sinusoidal capillaries;

(b) The Kupffer's cells are increased in numbers;

(c) The malarial pigment (hematin) and parasitised erythrocytes fill up the cytoplasm of Kupffer's cells;

(d) There is no increase in fibrous tissue;

(e) Fatty degeneration, atrophy and necrosis are observed in parenchyma cells of liver.

3. BONE MARROW

Macroscopic appearance

(a) In *acute* cases, there is a very little change in the marrow of the long bone; in *chronic* cases, the upper and lower thirds of the long bone are reddish brown in colour or slate grey or black.

Microscopic examination

(a) Parasitised red blood cells are present;

(b) Reticuloendothelial cells are filled with malarial parasites.

4. KIDNEY

The kidneys are congested and may reveal acute or sub-acute glomerular nephritis with hemorrhagic areas.

Urine is usually normal in *P. vivax* or *P. malariae* patients; but in *P. falciparum*, it may sometimes show albumin and hyaline and granular casts.

5. BRAIN

(a) Brain is congested;

(b) The cortex may be greyish or slightly brownish.

6. LUNGS

They may be pigmented and the capillaries may carry free pigments, pigmented leucocytes, phagocytes and infected erythrocytes.

7. STOMACH AND INTESTINE

Stomach and intestine sometimes show marked congestion of mucous membrane with slight pigmentation, while ulceration may be due to blockage of capillaries by pigment, infected erythrocytes and macrophages.

8. HEART

Heart may show fatty degeneration; in *falciparum* malaria, coronary occlusion or thrombosis may occur due to adhesion of infected red blood cells and parasites to capillary walls.

LABORATORY DIAGNOSIS

The only certain method of diagnosis of malaria is the demonstration of the causative organism, *Plasmodium*. It is better to have both thin and thick films on the same slide or on two different slides. Thick film is preferrable for quick detection of plasmodium, if plasmodia are few; the thin film is examined for identifying the species of plasmodium. Acridine Orange (AO) staining technique can be used to detect plasmodium in blood films.

Plasmodium can be detected with difficulties if :

(a) Blood films were taken after an antimalarial drug;

(b) Blood films were taken during apyrexial interval of *P. falciparum* infection;

(c) They were taken during the first 2 to 3 days of primary infection.

(d) Magnetic Resonance Imaging (MRI) is most recently used to diagnose cerebral malaria due to *P. falciparum*.

Serodiagnostic methods for malaria, such as complement fixation, slide flocculation, latex agglutination, indirect hemagglutination, fluorescent antibody tests are still experimental and their use is handicapped by a shortage of antigenic material (WHO, 1968).

Sedimentation, centrifugation, use of fluorochrome stains and of new wide angle microscope objectives are all under study.

The fluorescent antibody test is specially useful in measurement of development, persistence, and specificity of antibodies in human malaria. In recent years, ELISA, ABC-ELISA (new test), Immunoblot, DNA probes are useful epidemiological tools. PCR detects specimens containing *P. falciparum* DNA when parasite densities are below the microscopic threshold Quantitative Buffy Coat (QBC) Malaria test provides marked increased levels of accuracy and sensitivity. It requires not more than one minute. In thick smear films, it requires 10 minutes for 100 fields.

Elevation of plasma Lactate Dehydrogenase (LDH) can be demonstrated in severe cases of malaria with anemia :

(i) *Curative treatment.* Chloroquine, amodiaquine (the drug of choice) and quinine (for drug resistant *P. falciparum*) are potent schizonticidal drugs acting on early erythrocytic phases of parasites. Multi-drug resistant *P. falciparum* can respond to mefloquine. In China, Pyronaridine was found to be highly effective against *P. falciparum* with few side effects.

WHO (1992) recommendation for the treatment of chloroquine resistant *P. falciparum* malaria :

1. *Mefloquine*, 15 mg/Kg. body weight upto 1000 mg. in two doses 12 hours apart. It should not be given if 12 hours have elapsed after completion or parenteral quinine administration. It should not be given to pregnant women in the first trimester of pregnancy.
2. *Halofantrine*, 8 mg. base /Kg. body weight every 6 hours for 3 days. It is not advocated for pregnant women.
3. *Quinine* tablets, 10 mg/Kg. body weight every 8 hours to complete 7 days of treatment.
4. Sulfadoxine/Pyrimethamine (Fansider) single dose following a shorter course of quinine.

Relapse in malaria can be prevented by the use of 8 minoquinoline, primaquine, which acts on the exo-erythrocytic phases of parasites in liver. It also acts on gametocytes but has little action on erythrocytic stages of parasites.

(ii) *Prophylactic treatment.* Unless resistant strains of *P. falciparum* are involved, chloroquine and amodiaquine in weekly doses will prevent acute attack of malaria. These drugs act on pre-erythrocytic phase of parasites in the liver and also inactivate gametocytes which cannot develop further in the mosquito.

Prophylaxis may be (a) Personal prophylaxis, and (b) Community prophylaxis.

(a) *Personal Prophylaxis*

(i) Protection against mosquito by using mosquito net impregnated with insecticide Permethrin, which can deter and kill mosquito;

(ii) Systematic use of antimalarial drugs.

(b) *Community Prophylaxis*

(i) Prevention of carrier by antimalarial drugs;

(ii) antimosquito measures may be;

(a) destruction of adult mosquito; by spraying with insecticides, DDT or gammexane.

(b) antilarval measures consist of destruction of larvae by the use of larvicides (DDT dissolved in oil).

(c) *Biological control.* Adult dragon flies and their larvae feed on adult mosquitoes and their larvae, respectively. Larvicidal fish feed on mosquito larvae.

Vaccination

Very recently, most workers realise that the best approach for human vaccination against malaria is via monoclonal antibody to protective antigen of *Plasmodium*. Once isolated, this antigen may be synthesised, assuming it is protein, mass produced. Then there is possibility of malarial vaccine. Probably, the next decade will see field trials of vaccine against malaria, based on purified antigen. The world first vaccine against malaria developed by Columbian scientist was given in three doses under trial.

Further Reading

Panjarathinam, R. (1986) Hope for malarial vaccine. Current Medical Practice. *30*: 247-249.

World Health Organisation (1963) Terminology of Malaria and Malaria eradication, Geneva.

World Health Organisation (1968) Expert Committee on Malaria. 14th Report. Tech. Rept. Ser. N° 382, Geneva.

Superfamily Filarioidea

Filariform worms have simple mouth. The mouth is circular or dorsoventrally elongated and surrounded by papillae. They have a rudimentary buccal cavity without lips. Males with or without caudal alae. Human representatives are: *Wuchereria bancrofti, Brugia malayi, Onchocerca volvulus, Dipetalonema perstans, D. streptocercum, Mansonella ozzardi, Loa loa.*

WUCHERERIA BANCROFTI

(Bancroft's filarial worm producing Bancroft's filariaris or filariasis bancrofti).

History. Ancient Hindus (Susruta, 600 B.C.) and Persian physicians recognised the dramatic symptoms of filariasis. The microfilariae were first demonstrated by Demarquay in 1863 in the hydrocele fluid of man. Later in 1866 Wucherer found them in chylous urine and in 1972 Lewis, in India, observed them in the human blood. Adult female worms were found in 1876 by Bancroft and the specific name was given as *Wuchereria bancrofti* in honour of discoverers, Wucherer and Bancroft.

Geographical distribution. This parasite is distributed in Europe (Hungary, Yugoslavia, Turkey) Japan, Korea, Central Africa, South America, India, Southern China, Southern Spain, Nile Delta, Tangier, Australia, Philippines, Malaysia, Thailand. In 1990, it has been reported that out of 45 million of filariasis in the world, 20 million were in India.

In India, it is distributed mainly all along the sea coast and banks of big rivers (except Indus). It has been reported from Rajasthan, Punjab, Uttar Pradesh, Delhi and Gujarat. Stoll (1947) estimated the combined infection, Bancroft's filaria and Malayan filaria, to be 25 million in endemic area of India.

Morphology. ADULT WORM (Fig. 55.15. 16) is long minute thread-like and creamy white nematode. The head is slightly swollen and carries two rings of inconspicuous papillae.

The *male* measures 20 to 40 mm in length by 0.1 mm in diameter. Its tail end is curved ventrally and contains two spicules of unequal length and gubernaculum (Fig. 55.17, 18). Caudal alae are lacking. Male is rarely recovered.

The *female* measures 80 to 100 mm by 0.24 to 0.3 mm. The vulva (v) is cervical in position (Fig. 55.19, 20). The short vagina and outer segment of the uterus are single, but the remainder of the female genitalia is paired. The tail end is narrow and abruptly pointed (Fig. 55.21). Though the female is ovo-viviparous (laying eggs with well developed embryo), it liberates active embryo (28 by 25 microns in size). The shell of the embryo becomes elongated to accommodate the active embryo. It is known as 'sheath' of the embryo (i.e., microfilariae). At this stage, the microfilariae escape from the female worm into lymph and blood vessels.

The *microfilariae* measure 244 microns in length and 75 microns in diameter. The anterior end is round and has a stylet, the posterior end is pointed. Their internal structure can be studied only after staining. There is a central column of nuclei extending from

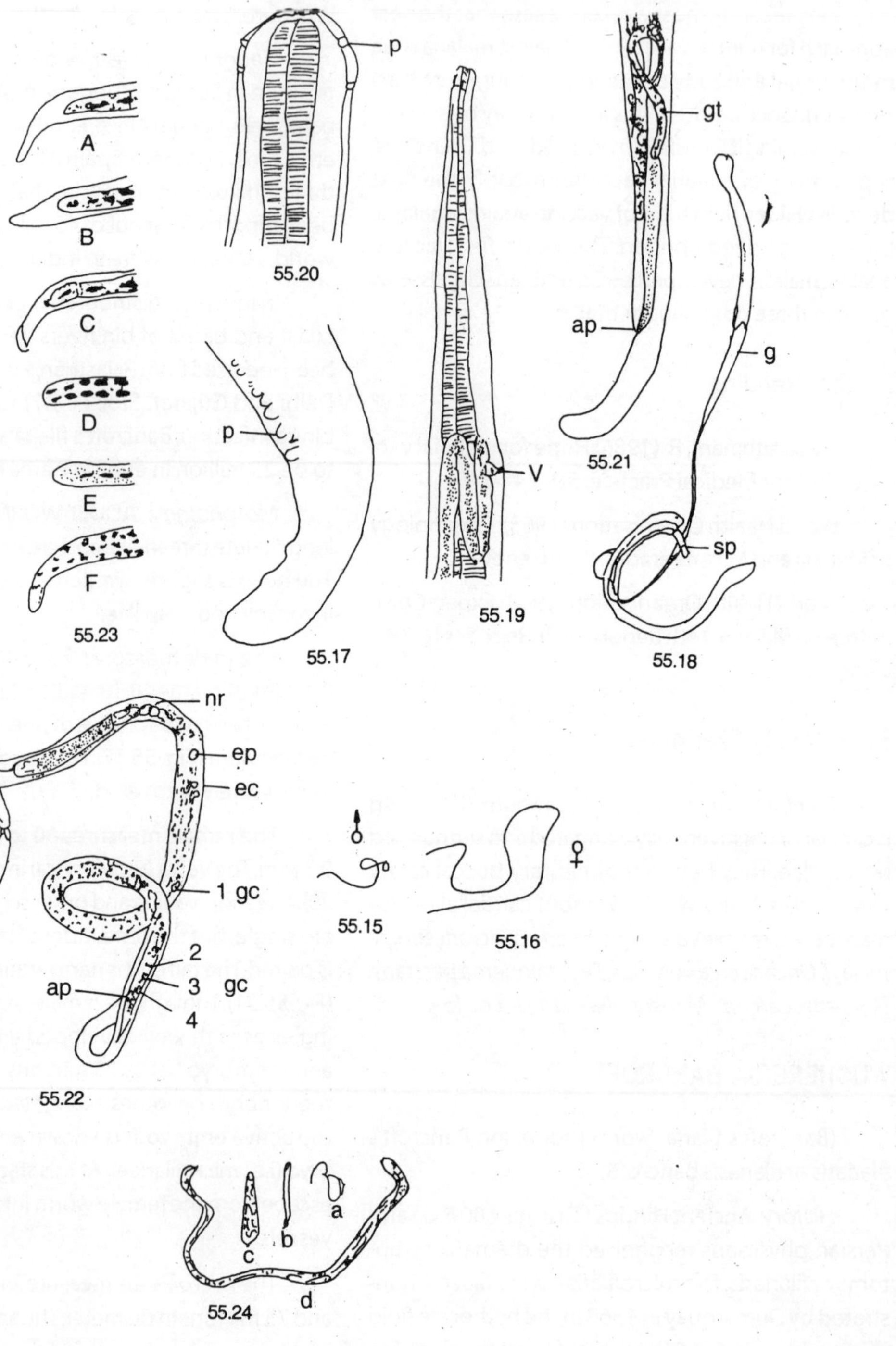

Fig. 55.15-24: Wuchereria bancrofti

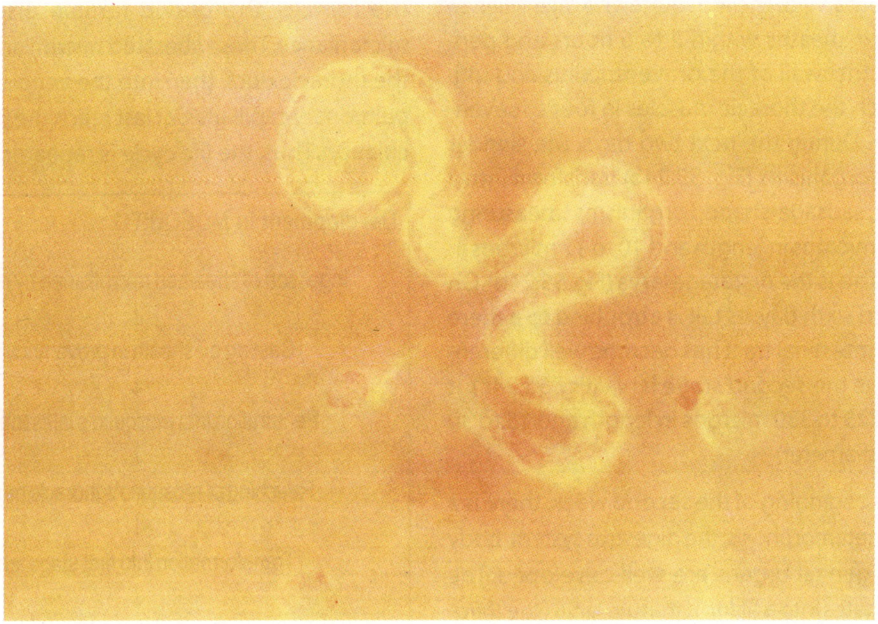

Fig. 55.22: Microfilaria of Wuchereria bancrofti ×1000

the head to the tail. In the column of the nuclei, there are important anatomical 'landmarks' which are used to differentiate this species from other microfilariae — the landmarks consist of nerve ring (nr), excretory pore (ep), excretory cell (ec), anal pore (ap), genital cells (gc), so called G cells. G-cells are in front of the anal pore (Fig. 55.22). *Dipetalonema perstans, Mansonella ozzardi, Onchocerca volvulus* have unsheathed tail (Fig. 55.23DEF).

For further development, the microfilariae require an appropriate intermediate host (mosquito); if they are not sucked up by the mosquito, they may die. The microfilariae are able to pass the placental filter and are reported in the newborn.

Microfilarial periodicity. There is a nocturnal surge of the microfilariae of *W. bancrofti* in the peripheral circulation between 10 PM to 2 AM. Its mechanism is not yet clearly understood. It has been suggested that:

(a) relaxation of the host's body during sleep which may be responsible for the migration of microfilariae to the periphery at night;
(b) there is response to O_2 and CO_2 supply;
(c) the adaptation of the microfilariae to feeding habits of the mosquito, *Culex pipiens quinquefasciatus, C. fatigans* — a night feeder. The non-periodicity type utilised a 'daytime feeder', *Aedes*;
(d) during the daytime, they retire inside the *capillaries of the lungs*, kidneys, heart and carotid;
(e) In Pacific Islands, *Mf. bancrofti* does not exhibit any periodicity.

Life cycle. It requires two hosts : (1) the only known definite host — Man, (2) intermediate host — *Culex, Aedes, Anopheles.*

Development in Mosquito

When mosquito bites an infected man, sheathed microfilariae are ingested during its blood meal. These microfilariae arrive in the anterior end of the proventriculus (stomach) of the mosquito, the microfilariae cast off their sheaths within 2 to 6 hours and penetrate into the wall of the proventriculus and ultimately reach the thoracic muscles in four to seventeen hours. During the next two days, the slender snake - like organisms (Fig. 55.24a) transform into a thick, short, sausage-shaped organisms (measuring 124 to 250 microns in length and 10 to 17 microns in diameter). This is the *first stage* larva (Fig. 55.24b). On the fifth and sixth day, its tail is atrophied to a mere stump, the intestinal tract has become well differentiated. This is the *second stage* larva (Fig. 55.24c). It measures 225 to 330 microns in length and 15 to 30 microns in diameter.

In the beginning of the second week, there is a complete metamorphosis; the digestive system, body cavity and genital organs are well-developed. The worm elongates into a filiform mature larva (*the third-stage larva*) (Fig. 55.24d). It measures 1.4 to 2 mm. in length and 18 to 23 microns in diameter. This third stage larva is infective to man and enters the proboscis of the mosquito on the fourteenth day via haemocele. Only one microfilaria gives rise to one infective larva in the proboscis. So there may be many larva waiting to infect man, when the mosquito bites the man. The complete development of microfilariae in the mosquito require about twenty days. The microfilariae can be kept in an artificial medium (Franke's NI medium).

Development in Man

When a healthy human being is inoculated by the infected mosquito, the third stage larvae (infective forms) are not directly introduced into the blood stream as in malaria, but they are deposited on the skin around the puncture wound. Attracted by the warmth of the skin, the third stage larvae migrate into the wound or puncture the skin. After entering the skin, they reach the lymphatic channels, settle down in certain lymphatic vessels (inguinal, scrotal, abdominal lymphatics) where they grow, sexually mature, become adult and mate. The male fertilises the female, the gravid female discharges the microfilariae. These liberated microfilariae enter into the thoracic duct, then into the venous system and pulmonary capillaries, at last reach the peripheral circulation. Thus, the life cycle is repeated (Diag. 55.4).

Development in MOSQUITO

Ingestion of sheathed microfilariae by mosquito
↓
Casting off sheath in proventriculus
↓
Penetration into mosquito's intestinal wall
↓
Reaching of mosquito's thoracic muscle
↓
Transformation into first stage larva
↓
Second stage larva
↓
Third stage (infective) larva
↓
Entry into mosquito's proboscis

Development in MAN

Deposition of infective larva on punctured skin
↓
Migration of larva and settlement in lymphatics
↓
Growth and sexual maturity in lymphatics
↓
Fertilisation
↓
Gravid female discharges microfilariae
↓
Entry of microfilariae into peripheral circulation

Fig. 55.25: Life cycle of *Wuchereria bancrofti*

Pathogenicity and Clinical Features

If the living microfilariae are lodged in the lymphatic vessels and lymph nodes, the reticuloendothelial cells infiltrate to attack these microfilariae. The endothelial layer of the lymphatic vessels becomes thickened, folded and stratified. There is a fibrin deposition on the endothelial surface and edema of the lymphatic vessel wall.

When the living worms are trapped in the lymph nodes, they are surrounded by eosinophils. The cellular granulation followed by proliferative granulation and fibrocytic repair. The filarial granulation tissue is pathognomonic of this disease. Finally, there is death and absorption (or calcification) of the parasite. The initial tissue responses are stimulated by the filariae and their metabolic products.

The adult worms produce obstruction in the lymphatic vessels, followed by lymph stasis and edema. As the worms die, lymphangitis ensues. The end result is usually lymph varix or elephantiasis.

Lymphangitis. In this condition, the lymphatics of testicle and epididymis (epididymo-orchitis) of the spermatic cord (funiculitis), of the abdomen (retroperitoneal lymphangitis) and lymphatics of the upper and lower extremities are involved. The globus major of the epididymis is the site for the adults of *W. bancrofti*. The lymphatic trunks are red, congested, palpable and painful. When the abdominal lymphatics are involved, the acute abdominal symptoms may result. The Wuchererial lymphangitis may occur periodically once in every month and sometimes it is related to lunar cycle, but the relationship is not well established.

Causes of lymphangitis :

(a) Metabolites liberated by the growing larvae and toxic fluid by fertilised females;

(b) Absorption of toxic products of dead worm;

(c) Mechanical irritation due to movement of the worms in the lymphatic vessels;

(d) Bacterial secondary invasion may cause lymphangitis.

Causes of lymphatic obstruction :

(a) Fibrosis of the afferent lymph nodes draining a particular area;

(b) Obstructive endolymphangitis;

(c) Mechanical blocking of lumen by the dead worm.

Effects of lymphatic obstruction :

(i) Lymph varix — varicosity of lymphatic vessels;

(ii) Elephantiasis — Hypertrophy of the affected part.

Lymphadenitis. It is the inflammation of the regional lymph nodes (lymphadenitis) which preceeds an attack of lymphangitis. It is mostly found in the groin or in the axilla. It is soft and lobulated and is not painful and tender. The skin over the swelling is not adhered.

Elephantiasis is due to the obstruction of lymphatic tracts caused by dead worms or due to recurrent attack of lymphangitis. The affected part becomes enormously enlarged looking like tumour. This is the end result of Wuchererial infection. Elephantiasis of legs is due to the obstruction of inguinal or iliac lymph nodes, whereas the elephantiasis of scrotum results from the obstruction of superficial inguinal lymph nodes. The surface of the skin of scrotum becomes thick, rough, fissured. The hair becomes rough and sparse.

Hydrocele. It results from the obstruction of para-aortic lymph nodes which interferes with lymph drainage from tunica vaginalis, epididymis and spermatic cord. It may also result due to repeated attack of wuchererial orchitis and epididymitis or may exist with or without elephantiasis of the scrotum.

Chyluria. Escape of chyle through the urine after passing through the mucous membrane of the urinary tract.

Urine in chyluria. It is milky white in colour. It coantains (a) fat particles which dissolve in ether, chloroform or xylol; (b) albumin which precipitates on boiling; (c) fibrinogen which forms a coagulation on standing. Microfilariae can be demonstrated microscopically in the sediment of chyluria. Chyluria is rare in India.

Laboratory Diagnosis

It consists of two methods : (1) Direct method; (2) Indirect method.

1. Direct method depends upon the demonstration of (A) sheathed microfilariae (with tail-tip free from nuclei) in the (i) peripheral blood, (ii) chylous urine, (iii) exudate of lymph varix, and (iv) hydrocele fluid. Microfilariae can be demonstrated in thin or thick smear as in malaria (Refer to blood examination chapter 62). Microfilariae are also easily seen by Acridine orange (AO) staining technique.

Microfilariae are not found in the following conditions :

(a) In cases of elephantiasis, due to lymphatic obstruction;

(b) After an attack of lymphangitis, due to the death of the adult worm;

(c) In early allergy;

(d) In occult filariasis;

and the detection of (i) adult worm in the lymph node biopsy, (ii) calcified worm in X-ray.

2. Indirect method (immunological test) comprises (I) Allergic tests, (II) Immunologic tests, (III) Xenodiagnosis.

(I) Allergic tests.

(i) Blood examination will reveal eosinophilia (5 to 15%).

(ii) Intradermal test (an immediate hypersensitivity reaction). *Dirofilaria immitis* (dog heart worm) antigen in the dilution of 1 : 8,000 provides 100 per cent positive intradermal reaction in suspected cases of *W. bancrofti.* The wheal of 2 cm or more appears within 30 minutes in positive cases.

(II) Immunological tests. Complement fixation test was found positive for human filariasis by employing a one per cent alcoholic extract of dried *D. immitis* powdered antigen. A fluorescent antibody technique is not satisfactory. IHA and BF are also used. Dot-ELISA is recent sensitive test.

New diagnostic skin test for filaria. The antigen is specific to filaria alone and does not react with other helminthic parasites. The antigen is very sensitive and the test is quick, cheap and operational in field survey. The results are available within 15 minutes of intradermal injection and does not matter what timing of the day or night it is carried out. It appears that this test will probably play a significant role in monitoring the filaria vector control programme.

(III) Xenodiagnosis. Microfilariae can be demonstrated in the stomach blood of the specific mosquito vector which was allowed to bite the infected person. It is not a very useful method.

Treatment.

The drugs acting on :

1. Adult worm — synthetic arsenical Mel W and antimonial M sb B;
2. Microfilariae — Diethylcarbamazine (DEC, Hetrazan) is the drug of choice. DEC medicated salt is strongly indicated as a simple, rapid, safe, inexpensive, efficient and practical method of filarial control or eradication, as DEC has severe side effects, i.e., fever, chills, nausea, vomiting.
3. Infective larvae and immature adult worms — para-melaminyl phenyl sibonate (MSb). Ivermectin (recent anthelminthic agent) is very effective against microfilariae of *W. bancrofti* in a single dose of 28-200 μg/kg. body weight.

Prophylaxis.

(i) Treatment of carriers by using hetrazan;

(ii) Protection against mosquito bite;

(iii) Destruction of mosquito;

(iv) Biological control programmes were implemented in India using *Bacillus sphaerium*.

BRUGIA MALAYI

(Malayan filarial worm producing Malayan filariasis)

History. This filaria was first observed by Lichtenstein in blood films and was described by Brug (1927) as a new species. Adult females and males were studied and described by Rao and Maplestone (1940).

Geographical distribution. This filaria is a parasite of man in India (Kerala, Hyderabad, Orissa, Madhya Pradesh, Assam), Sri Lanka, Sumatra, Java, Celebes, Malaysia, China, Japan.

Habitat. The adult worms of *Brugia malayi* remain coiled up in the lymphatic system.

Morphology. B. malayi resembles *W. bancrofti*. It is a delicate, whitish, thread-like round worm. The tapering anterior end (Fig. 55.26, 27) is provided with a non-labiate mouth surrounded by two rows of minute papillae and inner row of 6 and outer row of 4 just as in *W. bancrofti*, except that the papillae are slightly larger and more prominent in *B. malayi* (Fig. 55.28). Adult females measure 43.5 mm in length and 130 microns in breadth and adult males 13.5 mm and 70 microns. The anterior end of *female* has reproductive organ. The posterior end of the *female* has cuticular bossing (Fig. 55.29), but that of the *male* has perianal and postanal papillae (Fig. 55.30). These papillae vary from 3 to 4 and are prominent and unequal. At the tip of the tail there are 4 to 6 small papillae. Besides, the posterior end has also copulatory spicules and gubernaculum (Fig. 55.31). Microfilaria malayi (Fig. 55.32) has two discrete nuclei at the tip of the tail and is enveloped in a sheath. It has the following differences when compared to *MF. bancrofti*.

Differences between *MF. bancrofti* and *MF. malayi*

MF. bancrofti	*MF. malayi*
1. Nocturnal periodicity	1. Nocturnal periodicity
2. Anterior end has a stylet	2. Anterior end has 2 stylets
3. Cephalic space is long and broad	3. Cephalic space is broader
4. Length : 244 microns	4. Length : 177 microns
5. Excretory cells : small	5. Excretory cells : large
6. G-cells : small	6. G-cells : larger
7. Tail : tapering to delicate point; no terminal nuclei	7. Tail : often constricted between 2 terminal nuclei
8. Appearance : graceful, sweeping curves	8. Appearance : stiff; with secondary kinks
9. Pathology : in all lymphatics	9. Pathology : confined to lymphatics of extremities
10. Intermediate host : *Culex fatigans.*	10. Intermediate host : *Mansonia* sp, *Anopheles* sp.

Life cycle. it is same as that of *W. bancrofti*. The intermediate hosts are *Mansonia* sp and *Anopheles* sp. The complete larval development in the susceptible mosquito requires a minimum of six days.

Pathogenicity and clinical features. B. malayi causes lymphangitis and elephantiasis (primarily of the lower extremities). Malayan filariasis is characterised by the absence of chyluria and sometimes by the presence of scrotal swellings.

Laboratory Diagnosis

Detection of the characteristic microfilariae in the peripheral blood. ELISA gives 95% positive cases. *Videomicroscopy* of intralymphatic-dwelling *B. malayi* captures on the screen the hidden intraluminal events in the life cycle of lymphatic-dwelling worms and allows direct observation and documentation of interaction between host and parasite. The camera system may also permit direct observation on the effect of filarial drugs to kill the adult worm and its progeny and to speculate that the adult worm feeds on circulatory lymphocytes, thereby averting immunoresponsiveness and its own destruction.

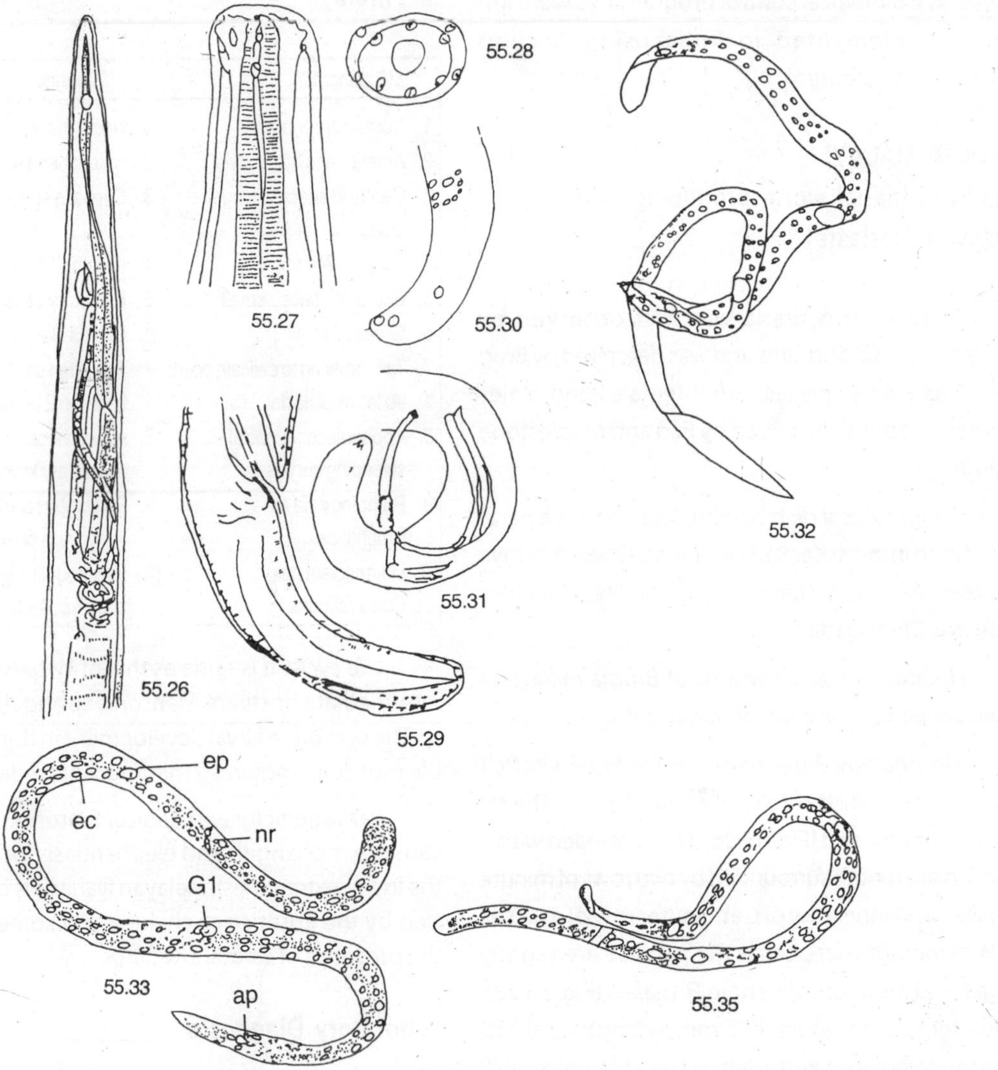

Fig.55.26-37: Brugai malayi; other microfilariae
ep - excretory pore; ec - excretory cells; nr - nerve ring; G1 - genital cells; ap - anal papillae

Treatment. It is same as that of *W. bancrofti* infection, but Ivermectin may prove useful for periodic *B. malayi*, under trial.

Prophylaxis. It is same as in *W. bancrofti*. In addition, certain water plants should be destroyed, as *Mansonia* sp. grows on these plants. In the state of Kerala, India, where *Mansonia annulifera* is the chief vector of *B. malayi*, the destruction of water plant *Pistia stratioides* has greatly reduced new infections. The excretory, secretory antigens of *B. malayi* are effective in inducing resistance against filarial parasites.

Further reading

Panjarathinam, R. (1983). Tropical disease: filariasis. Current Medical Practice. *27*: 63 - 66.

ONCHOCERCA VOLVULUS

(The generic name Onchocerca means 'hooked tail'; the convulated filaria or blinding filaria, producing onchocerciasis, onchocercosis, coastal erysipelas, blinding filariasis, river blindness).

History. This filaria was demonstrated by Brumpt (1919). Simulium was reported as intermediate host by Blacklock (1926).

Geographical distribution. This nematode is prevalent in Africa and America.

Habitat. Adult worms remain tightly coiled in subcutaneous connective tissue tumours (nodules).

Morphology. ADULT WORM. The living worms are white, opalescent and transparent with transverse cuticula. They are wire-like filiform and blunt at both ends. Adult females of *O. volvulus* can live for more than eleven years and produce microfilariae for nine to ten years.

The *males* measure 42 mm in length by 210 microns in diameter. The posterior end of the male is tightly recurved ventrally and has a perianal and caudal papillae.

The *females* measure 50 cm by 400 microns. The vulva opens slightly behind the posterior extremity of the esophagus. *In utero*, the embryos are first ovoidal, but later become elongated, are discharged and escape from their 'sheath'. The microfilariae are of two sizes (368 by 9 microns; 287 by 7 microns). Both ends are nuclei-free. The microfilariae (Fig. 55.33) are unsheathed and rarely appear in the peripheral blood but are mostly found in the lymphatics of the connective tissues and cutaneous layer (stratum germinativum) and corneal conjunctiva.

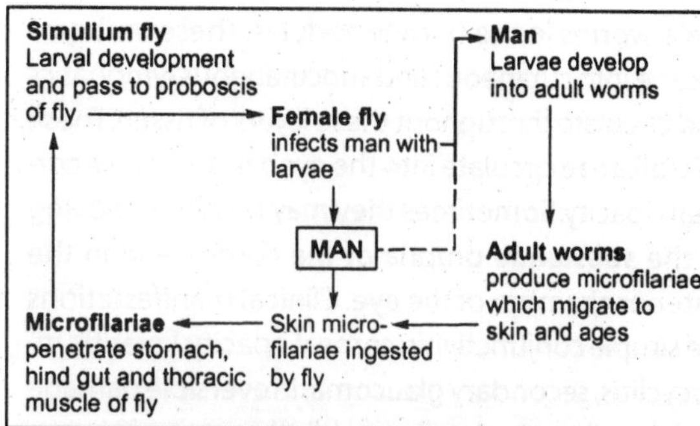

Fig. 55.34 : Life cycle of *O. volvulus*

Life cycle. Man is the definite host, whereas *Simulium* (Fig. 5.12) 'black fly' acts as intermediate host. The complete development of microfilariae of *O. volvulus* in Simulium is the same as that of *MF. bancrofti* in mosquito (Fig. 55.34).

Pathogenicity and Clinical Features

Two pathological processes are involved in Onchocerciasis :

1. The first process is caused by the adult worm. The mature or adult worms in the skin provoke local cellular reaction (eosinophilia) resulting in the formation of a fibrous nodular encapsulation of the worms. The primary lesion is a non-abscessing fibrous tumour. This nodule is hard on palpation, firm, greyish white superficially, yellowish around the worms. Pruritic dermatitis is due to the movement of microfilariae in the skin or to the toxic metabolites of the embryos. The unusual elephantiasis of the external genitalia of males and females, resembling that of Bancroft's filariasis, has been reported in Congo.

2. The second pathological effect is produced by the microfilariae which are discharged by the fe-

male worms in the fibrous nodules. These embryos escape into cutaneous and subcutaneous lymphatics and circulate throughout these layers of tissue. These microfilariae circulate into the eyeball and cause corneal opacity. Sometimes they may be found moving in the substantia propria of the cornea and in the anterior chamber of the eye. Clinical manifestations are simple conjunctivitis, corneal opacity, keratitis, iridocyclitis, secondary glaucoma, irreversible damage to the optic nerve leading to blindness.

Laboratory Diagnosis

1. Demonstration of the microfilariae in the biopsy of the small piece of the epidermis, and
2. The adult worms in the enucleated nodules. Puncture of suspected tumour may produce severe allergic reaction;
3. Microfilariae can be detected in ocular lesion by ophthalmoscopic examination;
4. If the embryos are accidentally found in the peripheral blood, eosinophilia (20 to 75%) is significant;
5. Complement fixation test gives specific reaction, using alcoholic extracts of the worm;
6. Antigens from adult *Dirofilaria immitis* gives satisfactory intradermal reaction in *O. volvulus* infection;
7. Skin test (Mazzotti's test). Within 24 hours after the oral administration of 50 to 100 mg of diethylcarbamazine, there appears a pruritic papular rash suggesting the presence of the microfilariae in the cutaneous tissue. This reaction is due to killed *O. volvulus* by the drug;
8. A fluorescent antibody technique has been adapted using *O. volvulus* antigen. Recent immunoblot can be used for the diagnosis of Onchocercosis.

Treatment

1. The enucleation of the nodules is the simplest method, it may also reduce the ocular complications and infection;
2. Diethylcarbamazine (Hetrazan) kills the circulating microfilariae and *Suramin* kills the adult worms. They are effective drugs in the treatment of onchocerciasis, but they produce side effects, i.e., severe pruritus, urticaria and ocular changes (including temporary blindness). These side effects can be relieved by antihistaminics. Ivermectin (Mectizan) is very effective recent anthelminthic drug against *O. volvulus*.

Prophylaxis. The breeding foci of the intermediate host (Simulium) should be sprayed with DDT emulsifiable concentrate.

DIPETALONEMA PERSTANS

(The persistent filaria, producing dipetalonemiasis)

History. This worm was first found by Daniels (1898); later Manson described microfilariae in the blood smear in Congo.

Geographical distribution. Dipetalonema perstans has an extensive distribution in Africa and America.

Habitat. The adult worms live in body cavities (peritoneal, pleural) and rarely in the pericardium.

Morphology. The adult *male* measures 45 mm by 60 microns. The posterior end of the male has caudal papillae and copulatory spicules. The *female* measures 80 mm by 120 microns. The vulva is situated in the cervical region. The tail end of the female is split and presents cuticular thickening forming two triangular appendages.

The *microfilariae* of *D. perstans* are subperiodic (i.e., they are found in the peripheral circulation in the day time and at night). They are small, measuring 200 microns by 4.5 microns, and are unsheathed. Their tail end is blunt and the nuclei extend upto the tail tip (Fig. 55.35).

Life cycle. It requires two hosts : (a) definite host — Man and (b) intermediate host — *Culicoides austeni.* Like other microfilariae, *Mf. perstans* follows the same larval development in culicoides.

Pathogenicity and clinical features. No definite pathogenicity is known. However, few reported cases showed the following symptoms : fatal pericarditis, local irritation with fibrinous exudate in mesentery, pleura and pericardium where *D. perstans* sew themselves; toxic edema of eyelid, dyspnea, pericardial pain, eosinophilia with allergic dermititis.

Laboratory Diagnosis

1. Detection of the microfilariae of *D. perstans* in the peripheral blood in day or night gives a specific diagnosis;
2. Hemagglutination or bentonite flocculation test can be employed, when the microfilariae could not be demonstrated in the blood stream.

Treatment. Diethylcarbamazine has no action on the *Mf. perstans* and there is no specific drug.

Prophylaxis. The eradication of the intermediate host is not possible as they breed in jungles.

MANSONELLA OZZARDI

(New World filaria, Ozzard's filaria, producing mansonelliasis ozzardi or Ozzard's filariasis).

History. The microfilaria of this species was recovered by Ozzard from Carib Indians of Guyana and was described by Manson as a new species.

Geographical distribution. This worm is distributed in Argentina, America, Venezuela, Columbia, Panama, West Indies.

Habitat. This worm lives embedded in the visceral adipose tissue, mesentery and body cavity.

Morphology. The *male* measures 30 mm in length and 0.2 mm in breadth. The posterior end is strongly curved ventral end has a slightly bulbous termination. The female measures 80 mm in length and 0.25 mm in diameter. The cuticula is smooth, the head is unarmed. The posterior end has a pair of fleshy lappets.

The microfilariae (Fig. 55.36) are non-periodic, unsheathed and resemble *Mf. perstans.*

Life cycle. Man is the definite host and *Culicoides furens* is the intermediate host where the larval development takes place.

Pathogenicity and clinical features. There are no clinical manifestations in infected persons. However, there are some reports of associated hydrocele and enlarged lymph nodes with little tissue reaction.

Laboratory diagnosis. Recovery and specific identification of the non-periodic unsheathed microfilaria in the peripheral blood.

Treatment. Hetrazan has no lethal effect on the microfilaria.

Prophylaxis. This is unstudied.

LOA LOA

(Loa is the native West African name of the worm, the loa worm or eye worm, producing loaiasis, or fugitive swellings).

History. Mongin extracted the worm from the eye of a Negro.

Geographical distribution. This parasite has an extensive distribution in Africa, Sudan, Congo.

Habitat. Adult worms live in the subcutaneous tissue.

Morphology. ADULT WORM. The adult worms are thread-like whitish with tapering cephalic end. The anterior end is unarmed but is provided with three pairs of small papillae. The *male* measures 30 mm. in length by 0.35 mm in diameter. The caudal end of the male curves ventrally with 'cuticular bosses'. There are about 8 pairs of perianal papillae with varying sizes and symmetry. The copulatory spicules are unequal and dissimilar in shape. The *female* measures 50 mm by 0.5 mm. The vulva opens in the cervical region. The life span of the adult worm may be 15 years or more.

The microfilaria (Fig. 55.37) measures 250 microns by 6 microns and is sheathed. It has diurnal periodicity; its excretory cells and G-cells are similar to *Mf. malayi*; its tail is tapering gradually, caudal nuclei are continuous with those of the trunk.

Life cycle. Loa loa requires two hosts :

1. The definite host is Man, and (2) The intermediate host is *Chrysops dimidiata* which is called 'mango or deerfly'. Larval development is same as that of other microfilariae in intermediate host.

Pathogenicity and clinical features. The incubation period is 3-4 years. The adult worms migrate rapidly through the sub-cutaneous tissue of the various parts of the body to reach their special site of predilection for creeping in and around the eye. While wandering, they cause a temporary swelling (fugitive swelling or Calabar swelling) which is a characteristic pathological lesion of the infection. The swellings may develop rapidly, reach the size of a hen's egg, are very painful and last for three days. These are the local reactions to the worm's metabolites. When passing in front of the eyeball or across the bridge of the nose, the adult worms are troublesome, though not very painful. These worms have been removed surgically from the back, groin, axilla, breast, penis, scalp, eyelids, anterior chamber of the eye and bulbar conjunctiva. There is frequent eosinophilia (50 to 70%). Symptoms are reddened giant urticarial swellings of skin and mucous membrane, fever, high eosinophilia.

Laboratory Diagnosis

1. The microfilariae can be demonstrated in peripheral blood during the day;
2. The adult worm can be recovered from the swellings;
3. Immunological tests are same as adapted for *W. bancrofti*, employing *D. immitis* antigen.

Treatment.

(a) The surgical removal of the adult worm may result in complete recovery;

(b) Suramin and diethylcarbamazine are specific chemotherapeutics. They should be administrated with caution as the violent allergic reactions may occur in the allergic individuals. This allergy may be remedied by antihistaminics. Diethylcarbamazine is extremely effective against microfilariae of *Loa loa*. Ivermectin rarely causes serious side effects in heavy infection of loiasis when they co-exist with *O. volvulus.*

Prophylaxis. It consists of :

1. detection and diethylcarbamazine treatment of human cases to destroy circulating microfilariae;
2. antilarval insecticidal campaigns at breeding places of *Chrysops*;
3. protection from *Chrysops* bites by application of fly repellent on the exposed skin.

Two unfertilised female worms of *Loa inquirenda* were described by Maplestone (1938); one of them from the neck of an European women in India.

HUMAN DIROFILARIASIS

Dirofilaria of animals may become adults in man without producing microfilariae. They are :

1. *Dirofilaria immitis* (dog heart worm) is a parasite of dog;
2. *D. conjunctivae* is a natural parasite of animals in USA;
3. *D. tenuis* is a parasite of raccoon in Europe, USSR (CIS), Sri Lanka, India, Asia;
4. *D. repens* is a natural parasite of dog in Europe, Asia, America.

Timor Microfilaria. Clinical features are similar to those of *B. malayi.*

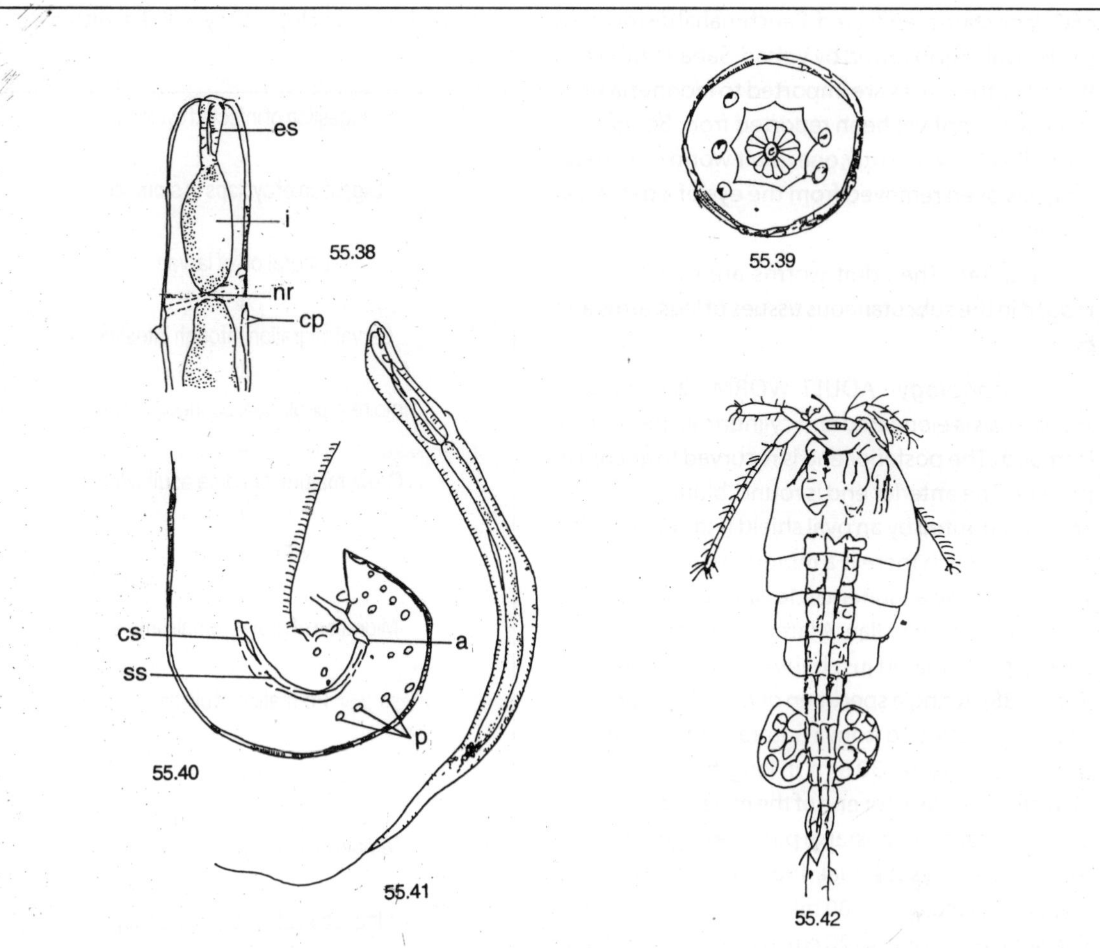

Fig. 55.38-42: Dracunculus medinensis; Cyclops
es - esophagus; i - esophageal gland; nr - nerve ring; cp - cervical papillae; cs - copulatory spicule; ss - spicular shealh; a - anus; p - papillae

Superfamily DRACUNCULOIDEA

Long cord-like worms with simple pore like mouth, surrounded by inner circle of 4 to 6 papillae and outer circle of 4 double papillae; esophagus and intestine rudimentary; females are much larger than males; vulva in middle of the body; uteri divergent; viviparous; larvae typically 'rhabditoid'. Human representative; *Dracunculus medinensis.*

Genus Dracunculus
Species DRACUNCULUS MEDINENSIS

(The medina worm, guinea worm, serpent worm or dragon worm, producing dracunculiasis, dracunculosis or dracontiasis).

History. This worm is known since the days of antiquity. In the Bible, it is called as 'the fiery serpent'; the Arabian physician named this nematode as Vena medina, because it was common in Medina.

Geographical distribution. Dracunculus medinensis is distributed in Africa, Arabia, Burma (Myanmar), Iran, Pakistan, Turkistan, USSR (CIS) and India (Rajasthan — Jodhpur), extensive areas in Mumbai Karnataka, Andhra Pradesh, Chennai, Punjab, Madhya Pradesh, Maharashtra, South India, Gujarat — Panchmahal, highest incidence; 13 out of 19 districts of Gujarat state are affected. Panchmahal district tops the list which is followed by Valsad, Sabarkantha and Banaskantha. Cases are imported to Indonesia from India. It has not yet been reported from Bengal, Assam, Bihar. Very recently, one adult worm one meter long has been removed from the eye of a patient at Orissa, India.

Habitat. The adult worms are mostly found lodged in the subcutaneous tissues of legs, arms and back.

Morphology. ADULT WORM. *Dracunculus medinensis* is elongated and cylindrical. The cuticula is smooth. The posterior end is recurved to anchor in position. The anterior end is round, blunt (Fig. 55.38) and surmounted by an oval shield (Fig. 55.39) in the middle of which there is a minute triangular mouth surrounded by an inner circle of 6 papillae and an outer circle of 4 papillae. A lateral pair of cervical papillae (cp) is situated just behind the nerve ring (nr) (Fig. 55.38). A single specimen of *male D. medinensis* has been recovered from a natural infection of man in India. It measures 30 mm. in length and 0.4 mm in diameter. The posterior end of the male is coiled. There are 4 preanal and 6 postanal papillae (p). The copulatory spicules are subequal, 490 to 730 microns long. The gubernaculum is 200 microns long (Fig. 55.40). The *female* measures 120 cm in length and 1.7 mm. in diameter. It is the largest human nematode. It resembles a piece of long twine thread and is milky white. Its ovarian tubules, oviducts and uteri are paired whereas the vagina is single. There is no vulva in gravid female. Its posterior end is tapering and bent to form a hook. The female worm is viviparous and discharges embryos. Its body fluid is toxic and causes blister if it escapes into the tissues. The life span of the female is one year and that of the male is about 6 months.

Embryos (Fig. 55.41). The rhabditoid larvae are wiry, coiled organisms with round head and long tapering tail. They measure 750 microns long and 25 microns in diameter. When the affected part of the body comes in contact with water, these larvae are discharged and swim in water in search of a minute fresh water crustacean of the genus Cyclops (Fig. 55.42) for their further development. If they are not taken up by the cyclops, they will die within a short time.

Ingestion of infected cyclops
↓
Digestion of cyclops in stomach
↓
Liberation of larvae
↓
Larval migration through intestine
↓
Into retroperitoneal connective tissue
↓
Grow, mature, become adult worms
↓
Fertilisation
↓
Migration of gravid female into skin
↓
Formation of blister
↓
Ulcer
↓
Female discharges embryo in water
↓
Ingestion of embryo by cyclops

Fig. 55.43: Life cycle of *Dracunculus medinensis*

Life cycle. It requires two hosts

(a) Definite host — Man.

(b) Intermediate host — Cyclops.

The human infection results from drinking raw unfiltered water containing infected cyclops (mode of infection). On arriving at the stomach, the cyclops are digested by the gastric juice and the larvae are set free. They migrate through the intestinal wall and reach the loose retroperitoneal connective tissue where they grow, become sexually mature and male and female adult worms in eight months to one year. The paucity of the male worms has not been satisfactorily explained. The males die after fertilising the females and disappear completely. Their copulation takes place only in the deeper connective tissue and not in the intestine. The gravid female migrates and selects only those parts of the skin which come in contact with water, particularly back in case of water carriers, arms and legs of washerman and legs of villagers who fetch water from ponds and 'step wells'. After selecting their sites, the anterior end of the gravid female approaches the skin and a papule is formed in the dermis; the worm secretes a toxin, a histamine like substance which causes 'blister' within twenty four hours. Ultimately, the blister ruptures and forms an ulcer. On contact with fresh water, the worm protrudes out from the centre of the ulcer; a loop of the worm's uterus prolapses through its mouth, bursts open and discharges a milky white fluid containing a large number of motile embryos (first stage rhabditoid larvae). These larvae swim in the water in search of a suitable intermediate host 'Cyclops' and are ingested by the cyclops. On reaching the mid-intestine, they break through the soft intestinal wall, enter the body cavity within 1-6 hours, undergo metamorphosis and increase in size (about one mm in length). It takes about two weeks for the complete development of the embryo. More than 5 to 6 larvae may kill the cyclops in fortytwo days. Heavy infection may kill them within fifteen days. The life span of the cyclops is about three months. (Fig.55.43)

Pathogenicity and Clinical Features

The penetration of the mature larvae into the viscera and deep somatic tissue and the development into the mature worms will not produce any pathological lesions. As soon as the gravid female worms begin to migrate to the skin, there is allergic reaction due to a large amount of toxin of a histamine like nature. When the worm reaches the skin, it produces a cutaneous blister which bursts out by the contact with fresh water. Few hours before the formation of blister, there may be systemic reaction — erythema, urticaria with intense pruritus, nausea, vomiting, diarrhoea, giddiness — due to toxaemia incapacitating the patients and causing much distress. The blister may be on the sole of the feet, ankles, shoulders, hands, arms, trunk, buttocks, scrotum, knee joint (arthritis). Sometimes, the guinea worm emerges out of the breast, tongue, testicles, permanently crippling the patient and even causing the death. *D. medinensis* will come out itself like a long twine thread inch (2.5 cm) by inch daily lasting several days to six months. Extradural abscess (India), abscess cavity in the pericardium, quardriplegia due to the abscess in the spinal cord were caused by *D. medinensis*. A guinea worm was removed from sub-conjunctival space of eye in India. *D. medinensis* has been reported as natural infection in dogs, horse, cattle, wolf, leopard, monkey.

Laboratory Diagnosis

1. Detection of adult worm. The adult female may appear at the centre of ulcer, when the ulcer comes in contact with water;
2. Detection of embryo. When the exposed ulcer is allowed to be bathed with water; the uterus of the gravid female will protrude, rupture and ejaculate a milky white fluid containing active embryo. The embryos can be pipetted off from water and examined under microscope;
3. Intradermal test. In positive case, a wheal appears within 24 hours, if dracunculus antigen is injected intradermally;
4. X-Ray examination. Dead calcified worms may be located by roentgen ray examination. Falcon assay screening test (FAST-ELISA) is most recent serology for diagnosis of dracunculosis;
5. Blood examination — shows eosinophilia.

Treatment. Niridazole is a very effective drug with severe side-effects, but not readily available in India. Hetrazan, orally, kills the adult worms.

Indian barber technique can be adapted with advantage, if the head of the gravid female worm protrudes out from the ulcer. The head of the worm can be tied with a fine silk thread to a matchstick and rolled daily inch (2.5 cm) by inch with gentle traction till the whole parasite is removed. It takes about 15 to 20 days. If the parasite breaks, it may cause allergic manifestations. Thiabendazole or mebendazole or metronidazole marginally reduces duration of emergence and associated pain. Trials with ivermectin are proceeding.

Prophylaxis. The disease can be prevented by:

1. Preventing the infected person from stepping into the water source;
2. Constructing draw-wells;
3. Providing safe water;
4. Boiling before drinking;
5. Sieving contaminated water with a folded cloth;
6. Spraying the insecticides in the step-wells, ponds, tanks;
7. Replacing step-wells by draw-wells.

Further reading

Panjarathinam, R. (1983) Dracunculosis : Rural Health hazard in India. Current Medical Practice. *27*: 302 - 303.

Arthropod borne protozoal diseases. African sleeping sickness (*Glossina palpalis*, tse tse fly); South American trypanosomiasis (Chagas' disease) - *Trisatoma infestans*, reduvid bug; Kala-azar and Delhi boil (*Phlebotomus argentipes*, sand fly); Malaria (female Anopheles mosquito).

Arthropod borne taeniasis. Dipylidium caninum infestation (*Ctenocephalus canis*, dog flea).

Arthropod borne helminthic disease. Filariasis (*Culex, Aedes, Anopheles* mosquito); Onchocerciasis; (*Simulium*, black fly); Dipetalonemiasis (*Culicoides austeni*, biting midges); Mansonelliasis ozzardi (*Culicoides furens*); Loaiasis (*Chrysops dimidiata, mango fly*); Dracunculosis (*Diaptomus vulgaris, cyclops*).

CHAPTER 56

(a) Zoonotic Parasites — Protozoa

Cryptosporidium (Parasite of fowl, rodents, cattle) is unrecognised cause of self-limited mild gastroenteritis and diarrhea in man.

Leishmania identical to *L. tropica* causes oriental sore in dogs of Iraq, Iran, Turkestan, Mumbai, Northern Africa, *L. donovani* is transmitted secondarily from dog to sand fly to man in some endemic areas of China, Mediterranean countries and Brazil. Cat, horse and sheep have been reported infected with Leishmania morphologically similar to *L. donovani*.

T. gambiense. There is no proof any of the game animals of Africa act as reservoirs of *T. gambiense* infection for man, but domestic animals (Cattle, pigs, goats) carry this infection for long periods of time without apparent symptoms.

T. rhodesiense. The reservoirs of infection of *T. rhodesiense* for man are believed to be game animals in Africa.

T. cruzi. In South America, various animals (dogs, cats, armadillos, bats, ferrets, foxes) have been found to be naturally infected with *T. cruzi*. Dogs and cats may be the common reservoirs of *T. cruzi* infection in South America.

Entamoeba histolytica. Animal reservoirs of *E. histolytica* include monkeys, dogs and possibly dogs, but these animals at most constitute a minor source of human exposure compared with man himself.

E. coli. Although monkeys and occasionally the dogs have been found to be naturally infected with *Entamoeba* morphologically similar to *E. coli*, human infection results from the human source.

Isospora hominis. Dogs are suspected to be reseivoir hosts of *I. hominis*.

Toxoplasma gondii infection may occur in man or in any warm-blooded vertebrate animals (cats). Apparent toxoplasmosis is common in reservoir hosts and in man.

Balantidium coli. Man is relatively refractory to infection with *B. coli* of porcine origin. In New Guinea where the pigs are the principal domestic animals, human infection in pig farmers are common to some extent.

Helminths

Nematodes

Trichinella spiralis. Pigs, rats, carnivorous, omnivorous wild hosts are primarily infected with trichinosis, whereas pigs, wild boars, bears, cats, dogs and other mammals which eat flesh become secondarily infected. Polar bears are probably the usual source of human infection in Alaska. Epidemic outbreaks due to consumption of sausage from infected hogs are common.

Strongyloides stercoralis. While man is important host of *S. stercoralis* dogs and chimpanzees have been found to be naturally infected with strains indistinguishable from those in man.

Ankylostoma duodenale. Man is the only normal definite host of *A. duodenale*, although a single female worm from a tiger (Kolkata) and hookworms identified as *A. duodenale* have been reported from the pig, dog and several species of wild animals in captivity.

A. ceylanicum, described from the intestine of a civet cat from Ceylon, parasitises to a lesser extent the dog and man.

A. braziliense. Though first reported from cats and dogs in southern Brazil, it has been incorrectly reported from man in many countries including India and Sri Lanka.

A. caninum is a common parasite of dogs and cats and has been reported once as a parasite of man in Philippine islands.

Necator americanus is a parasite of the small intestine of man (natural host). A hookworm morphologically indistinguishable from *N. americanus* of man have been recovered from several species of simian hosts, rhinoceros, pangolin (indonesia), rodent (Africa).

Trichostroncylus are commonest parasites in the digestive tract of herbivorous animals throughout the world (Egypt, India - Assam, America). The majority of species occur only as accidental infection of man.

Haemonchus contortus is commonest parasite of domestic sheep throughout the world. Human infection is also less common.

Metastrongylus elongatus. Commonly parasitises the respiratory tract of hogs, less commonly of sheep and cattle. Few human infections are on record.

Though *Angiostrongylus cantonensis*, originally described from the rats, is less commonly reported from human infection.

Syphacia muris and *S. obvelata.* These oxyurids are cosmopolitan in rats and mice, their eggs occur rarely in human feces.

Toxocara canis is a cosmopolitan parasite of dogs. Intestinal infection with the adult worm has been reported from the fox and twice from man, although authenticity of the human infection is questionable.

T. catis is the common ascarid of the domestic cat and some of its wild relatives. Some cases of this infection in man have been recorded.

Gongylonema pulchrum. This thread like nematode is a cosmopolitan parasite of ruminant and has been diagnosed from pigs, bears, monkeys and occasionally from man. It was first recovered as a human parasite in Italy, since then additional infections in man have been reported.

Gnathostoma spinigerum has been reported from the domestic cats, wild cat, lion, leopard, mink and the dog in India and in other countries. Human cases are reported from India and countries.

Dipetalonema perstans. Man is the important definite host for this species, although primates in Africa and New World monkeys act as reservoir hosts.

Thelazia callipaeda (Oriental eye worm) is spiruroid nematode of the conjunctiva of dog, rabbit and man.

T. californiensis. In addition to *T. callipaeda*, many species of this genus have a predilection for the conjunctiva of mammals, birds and many human cases have been reported.

Dirofilaria immitis, D. conjunctivae, D. tenuis, D. repens are microfilariae of animals and they may become adults in man without producing microfilaria.

Trematode

Schistosoma japonicum. Dogs, cats, rats, mice, field mice, cattle, water buffaloes, pigs, horses, sheep and goats are naturally infected with *S. japonicum* in many endemic foci.

S. mansoni. Human infection is almost derived from human sources, although monkeys, baboons, gerbil, wild rodents, rats have occasionally been found infected with *S. mansoni* in endemic areas.

S. hematobium. In addition to man, the usual host, the monkeys, baboons and chimpanzees have been found naturally infected.

S. bovis, common parasite of cattle, sheep, goats, and equines have been reported from baboons. Isolated cases of recovery of *S. bovis* eggs from human urine and stools in South Africa, Southern Rhodesia (Zimbabwe) and Congo lack satisfactory proof. In Italy, this species causes cercarial dermatitis in man. Eggs are longer and much narrower than those of *S. haematobium.*

S. mattheei is a natural parasite of sheep, goat, cattle, monkeys and rarely man in South Africa, Rhodesia(Zambia and Zimbabwe). The eggs of this worm were found in the human urine and adults were also found associated with those of *S. hematobium* in two human autopsies. In Rhodesia, over 1 per cent of persons were infected with *S. mattheei*; eggs are found in stool and urine with equal frequency.

S. nasalis is a common parasite of cattle in India (Pondicherry, Panjarathinam, 1972), but there has been no record of human infection.

S. rhodhaini is the parasite of African wild rodents, dogs, cats. Human infection with *S. rhodhaini* has been reported in Congo.

S. incognitum is the natural parasite of Indian pigs and dogs. The eggs were twice recovered from human feces.

Trichobilharzia ocellata, Schistosoma spindale, animal schistosomes, cause cercarial dermatitis in man.

Gastrodiscoides hominis, common human parasites in India and other countries, has been found to infect pigs (common reservoir hosts) and monkeys in India.

Fasciola hepatica. Reservoir hosts (Primarily sheep) play the important role in the propagation of this infection in Nature and, hence, the human infection occurs.

Fasciolopsis buski is a common parasite of man and pig in central and South China and other countries. Dogs are occasionally infected. Other domestic animals, with possible exception of rabbits are probably refractory.

Echinostoma ilocanum (Garrison's fluke). Rats and dogs are reservoirs of *E. ilocanum* infection. Human infection is acquired from the consumption of raw snails containing encysted metacercariae.

Echinochasmus perfoliatus. This echinostome has also been recovered from pig and fox and a human infection has been reported in Japan.

Plagiorchis muris is a natural parasite of several group of birds at Douglas Lake and has been reported once from man in Japan.

Dicrocoelium dendriticum is a common parasite in the biliary passages of sheep, deer, herbivorous and omnivorous mammals. Many genuine human cases have been diagnosed from Europe, Asia and Africa.

Troglotrema salmincola. Human infection is incidental to that in reservoir hosts (dogs, fox, racoon, mink).

Paragonimus westermani. The natural definite hosts are man, tiger, cat, civet cat, leopard, panther, fox, wolf, dog, pig.

Opisthorchis felineus. Man, dog, cat, red, silver and polar foxes, domestic and wild swine, Norway rat, water rat are infected. The definite hosts acquire infection from consumption of infected raw fish.

Clonorchis sinensis. In addition to man, many reservoir hosts (principally the dog, cat) are naturally infected.

Heterophyses heterophyses. In addition to man, *H. heterophyses* has been found as natural infection in the cat, dog, fox and other fish-eating mammals in endemic areas.

Metagonimus yokogawai. Fish-eating mammals and even the pelican are reservoir hosts of the infection.

Cestodes

Diphyllobotrium latum. Man, domestic dog, cat, leopard, mangoose, foxes, seals, sea-lions, bears, minks, domestic pigs have been found infected with *D. latum.*

Dipylidium caninum. Dogs and cats are available sources of infection for man to whom it is uncommon.

Hymenolepis nana fraterna. The variety in marine hosts is infective for man only under exceptional circumstances.

H. diminuta. The tape worm is a common parasite of the rat, mouse, dog (rarely), however, authentic human cases have been reported.

Taenia solium. Man is the usual definite host and gets infected by eating inadequately heated pork. Pigs, less frequently sheep, dogs and cats harbour the cysticercus stage of *T. solium.*

T. saginata. Human infection is acquired by consumption of inadequately cooked beef containing the viable cysticercus larvae.

T. taeniaeformis is a normal, parasite of the intestine of the cat which becomes infected from eating infected rats. A single human infection has been reported.

Multiceps multiceps. Dog, wolf and fox are definite host of this worm. The larval stage is usually found in herbivorous animals (sheep, goats, cattle, horse). Human infection results from the ingestion of eggs passed in dog's feces.

Multiceps glomeratus is reported from the gerbil and man.

Multiceps serialis is a parasite of dog, wolf, fox and rodents. Human infection is also on record.

Multiceps brauni. This cestode was described from the intestine of dog. Infection with the coenurus (bladder worm) has been recorded in man. In 2 patients the parasite was located in the eye.

Echinococcus granulosus. The dog is the optimum definite host, although man, wolf, jackal, fox, domestic cat have been found infected in Nature. Cattle, sheep and pigs are the common reservoirs of the hydatid cyst.

E. multilocularis. Man gets infected sporadically from eggs of *E. multilocularis* infected fox's excreta.

(b) Parasitic Opportunists Associated with HIV Infection

The spectrum of parasitic opportunists found in association with Human Immunodeficiency Virus (HIV) infection or Acquired immunodeficiency Syndrome (AIDS) are protozoa —

Pneumocystic carinii, Toxoplasma gondii, Isospora belli, Leishmania sp. Cryptosporidium and Microsporidia.

Parasites of Radiologic Importance

E. histolytica (X-ray of abdomen is done), *G. lamblia* (X-ray may reveal mucosal defects), *P. falciparum* (recent MRI can be used to diagnose cerebral malaria), *T. gondii* (X-ray of skull to show cerebral calcification — ventriculogram).

Pneumocystis carinii (radiological appearance of pneumocystis pneumoniae), *E. granulosus* (roentgenogram is useful in the diagnosis). *T. solium* (*cysticercus cellulosae* - cerebral cysticercosis can be diagnosed by (CT, MRI or sonography).

S. hematobium (bladder calcification, characteristic feature of urinary schistosomiasis and urinary tract pathology are detected by ultrasonography). *P. Westermani* (chest radiographs early in the disease show patchy cloudy infiltration. Pleural thickening and calcification may be seen late in the disease).

T. solium (In ocular cysticercosis — calcified larvae are detected by roentgenologic diagnosis). Calcified adult worm of *W. bancrofti* can be detected by X-ray.

D. medinensis (X-ray can detect dead calcified worms of *D. medinensis*).

(c) Parasites of Ophthalmic Importance

T. cruzi (edema of eyelids — Romana's sign)

T. gondii (pseudocysts in the eyes).

E. granulosus (hydatid cyst may develop in orbital capillary).

Multiceps brauni was found located in the eye.

T. solium causes ocular cysticercosis.

F. hepatica is seldom found in the eye. During the migration, the larvae of *T. spiralis* cause edema around the eyes, retinal and subconjunctival petechiae and hemorrhages.

Larvae of *T. canis* and *T. catis* are carried into the capillaries of the eyes which is known as ocular larva migrans.

The larvae of *A. lumbricoides* which migrate through the capillaries of the eye ball may cause retinitis.

Microfilariae of *O. volvulus* circulate into the eye ball and cause the corneal opacity. Keratitis, iridocyclitis, secondary glaucoma are irreversible damages to the optic nerve leading to blindness.

The migrating adult worms of *Loa loa* are troublesome while passing in front of the eye ball and they have been removed from the eyelids, anterior chamber of the eye and bulbar conjunctiva.

Thelazia callipaeda (oriental eye worm) and *T. californiensis* have a predilection for the conjunctiva.

D. medinensis (guinea worm) was removed from the subconjunctival space of the eye of an Indian patient.

Parasites of Cardiac Importance

T. cruzi. Cardiac rhythm is disturbed; cardiomyopathy.

P. falciparum. Coronary edema and thrombosis.

T. solium. Cysticercus cellulosae may rarely produce myocarditis or congestive heart failure.

E. granulosus. Hydatid cyst may develop on the heart valve.

C. sinensis produces the symptoms of palpitation of the heart, tachycardia.

In *T. spiralis* infection blood pressure falls rapidly, serious complications are myocarditis.

S. stercoralis larvae may be found in the heart.

Larvae of *T. canis* and *T. catis* may cause cardiac dysfunction.

In *A. duodenale* infection, palpitation of the heart and signs and symptoms of high output congestive heart failure are evident.

The wandering worms of *A. lumbricoides* may invade the heart.

Parasite of Gynaecological Importance

Trichomonas vaginalis causes trichomonas vaginitis (Sexually transmitted disease).

CHAPTER 57

PARASITES OF VARIOUS ORGANS INTESTINAL PARASITES

Intestinal parasites include protozoa, trematodes, cestodes and nematodes. Most of them gain entrance into the intestine by fecal contamination of food, water, or fingers. Some of them may enter the body via skin penetration by the larval stage and after migration through tissue, mature in the gut :

Entemoeba histolytica, Fasciolopsis buski, Schistosoma mansoni, Schistosoma japonicum, Taenia saginata, Taenia solium, Hymenolepis nana, Diphyllobothrium latum, Ascaris lumbricoides, Ankylostoma duodenale, Necator americanus, Strongyloides stercoralis, Enterobius vermicularis, Trichuris trichiura, Balantidium coli.

GENITOURINARY PARASITES

The genitourinary system is not a frequent site of parasitism. However, there are two exceptions which are as follows :

Trichomonas vaginalis, Schistosoma haematobium.

TISSUE PARASITES

The tissue parasites have a common feature of affecting some deeper organ (other than the gut) such as the liver, lungs and central nervous system :

Entamoeba histolytica, Toxoplasma gondii, Paragonimus westermani, Clonorchis sinesis, Taenia solium, Echinococcus granulosus, Trichinella spiralis, Pneumocystic carinii.

VASCULAR PARASITES

The vascular parasites constitute the major group of parasites :

Leishmania donovani, Trypanosoma gambiense, Trypanosoma cruzi, Plasmodium vivax, Plasmodium falciparum, Plasmodium malariae, Plasmodium ovale, Wuchereria bancrofti, Brugia malayi, Loa loa.

CHAPTER 58

SYMPTOMATOLOGY OF PARASITIC DISEASES

The following are important signs and symptoms of parasitic diseases :

ABSCESS, AMOEBIC. The liver is tender and enlarged. There is intense pain, fever, with night sweats when abscess in formed.

ABSCESS, FILARIAL. Along the lymphatics, filarial abscess may appear and the segments of the adult worms may be seen in the abscess drainage which is free from bacteria.

ANEMIA. In malaria, ankylostomiasis, diphyllobothriasis, anaemia is common. Microcytic hypochromic anemia is common in ankylostomiasis, malaria, because of blood loss. In case of hookworm infection, dietary intake of iron may prevent anemia. A macrocytic anemia may develop in diphyllobothriasis, because of vitamin B_{12} deprivation by the worm attached to the jejunal wall. The proliferation of infected reticuloendothelial cells in the bone marrow is responsible for anemia in Kala azar, and Chagas' disease. In trypanosomiasis, schistosomiasis, fasciolopsiasis, systemic toxicity and nutritional defects may result in anemia.

APPENDICITIS. The blockage of the lumen of the appendix by Ascaris and Trichuris causes appendicitis. In amoebiasis, acute appendicitis may occur.

ASCITES. Tissue proliferation around the eggs leading to fibrosis of the liver may cause ascites in *Schistosoma mansoni* and *S. japonicum*.

ASTHMA, BRONCHIAL. Migration of larva of *Ascaris lumbricoides* through the lungs may cause bronchial asthma.

CALABAR SWELLINGS. In loissis, subcutaneous swellings are observed. They are painful and pruritic.

CHAGOMA. A hard, reddened, raised, primary lesion develops on the face, neck, abdomen or limbs in Chagas' disease.

CHORIORETINITIS. Toxoplasma may infect the retina and choroid and there will be disturbance in eye sight.

CHYLURIA. Lymphatic fluid is passed in the urine which is milky white and contains microfilariae of *Wuchereria bancrofti*.

COMA. It is observed in falciparum malaria and in African trypanosomiasis.

CONJUNCTIVITIS. Onchocercal infection produces chronic conjunctivitis.

CONVULSIONS. These may be seen in the malarial paroxysm and in Ascaris infection in children.

DERMATITIS. Strongyloides larvae, hookworm larvae and schistosoma cercariae penetrate through the skin and cause a localised edema and pruritus leading to dermatitis. The cutaneous larva migrans reaction caused by larvae of *Ankylostoma braziliense* is indicated by a red papule at the site of entry and there will be severe itching. Adult *Loa loa* beneath the skin may cause dermatitis. The adult female *Dracunculus medinensis* beneath the skin produces blister. Microfilariae of *Onchocerca volvulus* in the skin may cause pruritis. *Sarcoptes scabei* under the skin causes lesions similar to those of cutaneous larva migrans.

DIARRHEA. Infiltration of the intestinal submucosa by macrophages containing *Leishmani donovania* may cause the mucosal ulceration and diarrhoea in Kala azar. Mucosal capillaries of the intestine plugged with parasitised red blood cells cause profuse watery diarrhoea in falciparum malaria. Mucosal ulceration in amoebiasis or balantidiasis may produce diarrhoea. A mild mucoid diarrhoea caused by Giardiasis may lead to malabsorption of fat 'steatorrhoea' (diarrhoea with fat). Mucous diarrhoea may be caused by the development of cysticercoids of *Hymenolepis nana* within the intestinal villi. Mild diarrhoea followed by constipation or severe diarrhoea may be observed in strongyloides infection. Diarrhoea of toxic origin, characterised by nausea, vomiting, hepatic tenderness and fever is caused by *Schistosoma mansoni* and *S. japonicum* infections. Egg deposition in the intestinal wall may be responsible for profuse diarrhoea or dysentery in Schistosomiasis. Nausea, vomiting and diarrhoea are indicated in heavy hookworm and whipworm infections. In fasciolopsiasis, diarrhoea with much undigested food is observed. Sometimes, there may be diarrhoea in taeniasis and diphyllobothriasis.

DYSENTERY. The passage of six to eight more mucoid blood flecked stools per day is characteristic of acute amebic dysentery. There may be abdominal pain and tenderness.

ELEPHANTIASIS. Filarial elephantiasis is a chronic enlargement of the limb, scrotum, breast or vulva with hyperplasia of the connective tissue and skin. Rarely, the blockage of the lymphatic drainage due to fibrosis caused by eggs deposited by *Schistosoma haematobium* in vesicle plexus of veins.

EOSINOPHILIA. In many helminthic infections, eosinophilia is common. Tissue parasites provoke a higher eosinophilia than the intestinal parasites. It is not characteristic in protozoan infections.

EPIDIDYMITIS. It is seen in filarial infection.

FUNICULITIS. Inflammation of the spermatic cord occurs as an early symptom of filariasis.

HEMATURIA. There may be terminal hematuria in the last few drops of urine in *Schistosoma hematobium* infection.

HYDROCELE. It is common in filariasis.

HYDROCEPHALUS. In congenital toxoplasmosis, hydrocephalus or microcephaly is common.

HYPERPIGMENTATION. Hyperpigmentation of the skin over the cheeks, temples and around the mouth is seen in Kala azar. In onchocercosis, allergic dermatitis may result in hyperpigmentation of the area on the face, neck or ears.

JAUNDICE. In severe liver fluke infection, obstructive jaundice may be observed. In falciparum malaria, there is marked enlargement and tenderness of the liver, with jaundice appearing on second day.

LEUCOCYTOSIS. It is very common only in amebic abscess. Leucocytosis, followed by leucopenia, is common in many protozoan and helminthic infections.

LEUCOPENIA. It is generally seen in Kala-azar.

LYMPHADENITIS. It is common in filariasis. Axillary and inguinal lymph nodes are enlarged, painful and tender. In acute stage of Chagas' disease, there is a generalised lymphadenopathy.

LYMPHANGITIS. Acute lymphangitis is an early symptom of filariasis. It is followed by fever. When it occurs on a limb, it progresses distally.

LYMPHOCYTOSIS. It is generally seen in Chagas' disease.

LYMPH VARICES. Due to lymphatic blockage in filariasis, the lymphatic vessels of the inguinal and femoral areas are dilated. The soft lobulated swellings may rupture and drain.

MENINGOENCEPHALITIS. In African sleeping sickness, the symptoms of meningoencephalitis may result due to the invasion of the central nervous system by trypanosomes. There may be confusion, headache, drowsiness and, finally, coma. In Chagas' disease, the symptoms are similar but milder. Meningoencephalitis is also observed in falciparum malaria.

MICROCEHPHALUS. See HYDROCEPHALUS.

MONOCYTOSIS. In both protozoal and helminthic infection, monocytosis is a frequent finding.

MONOCARDIT. It is characteristic of Chagas' disease and trichinosis. In trichinosis, the migration of the larvae through the myocardium causes myocarditis. It is also seen in toxoplasmosis, as a result of invasion of toxoplasma in the myocardium.

MYOSITIS. Migration of *Trichinella spiralis* larva in the muscles causes myositis.

NEUROLOGICAL SYMPTOMS. See under MENINGOENCEPHALITIS.

NODULES, SUBCUTANEOUS. Onchocercomas, cysticercus larva of *Taenia solium* and *Echinococcus* cysts may be found in the subcutaneous tissues forming nodules of 0.5 to 3.0 centimetre in diameter.

OBSTRUCTION, INTESTINAL. Ascaris may cause complete intestinal obstruction in children with abdominal pain, vomiting, distension and hyperperistalsis.

OCULAR SYMPTOMS. See CONJUNCTIVITIS.

EDEMA. Migrating larvae of *Trichinella spiralis* may cause vasculitis leading to edema. The migration of adult *Loa loa* across the eyeball or lid may cause unilateral edema with local pruritis and intense pain. Calabar swellings are also seen in loiasis; while in onchocerciasis, there will be edema of face, neck, ears followed by an intense pruritus and erythema. The most common type is unilateral edema of eyelids (Romana's sign). Edema of the face and legs is seen in severe hookworm infection, fasciolopsis and diphyllobothriasis.

ONCHOCERCOMA. Adult worms of *Onchocerca volvulus* remain coiled underneath the skin, enclosed in a fibrous tissue capsule.

ORCHITIS. Recurrent attacks of hydrocele may cause orchitis in filariasis.

PAIN. Abdominal pain is said to accompany many of the intestinal parasitic infections. Severe pain may indicate intestinal obstruction, perforation and peritonitis or bile duct blockage in ascariasis.

PERITONITIS. Penetration of Ascaris through the wall of the intestine leads to peritonitis, with pain, abdominal distension and tenderness. Ulcers in severe amoebic dysentery may erode through the wall of the intestine to initiate peritonitis.

PNEUMONITIS. When the larvae of *Ascaris lumbricoides* breakout of the capillaries into the alveoli cause pneumonitis. In the neonatal period, acute toxoplasmosis causes pneumonitis.

PROTEINURIA. Proteinuria with hyaline and granular casts in the urine is common in falciparum malaria.

PRURITUS ANI. It accompanies pinworm infection. Sometimes, it may also be associated with migration of gravid proglottids of *Taenia saginata* out of anus.

PULMONARY SYMPTOMS, CHRONIC. Pseudotubercle formation in lungs around ova, of Schistosoma, which are carried to lungs. Chronic cough is characteristic of Paragonimiasis. Cough is the primary symptom in pulmonary echinococcosis.

RASH. In early stage of schistosome infection and in ascariasis, an allergic urticarial rash may appear. In the course of trichina infection, a macular or maculopapular eruption may be seen.

ROMANA'S SIGN. In early stage of *Trypanosoma cruzi* infection (Chagas' disease), unilateral edema involving both the eyelids may appear.

SPLENOMEGALY. In both African and American sleeping sickness, splenomegaly may be noticed. The spleen is said to enlarge downwards about an inch per month in Kala-azar. The spleen enlarges and becomes tender during an acute attack of malaria. Hepatic fibrosis caused by the egg deposited by *Schistosoma mansoni* and *S. japonicum* in the liver may result into splenomegaly.

TACHYCARDIA. It could be observed in African and American sleeping sickness, which is characterised by a fast pulse.

ULCERS, CUTANEOUS. Oriental sore or Delhi boil, caused by *Leishmania tropica*, is characterised by a shallow ulcer. *L. braziliensis* also produces cutaneous ulcerations which involve the nasal mucosa, the soft and hard palate, nasal septum, pharynx and larynx. *Dracunculus medinensis* initially produces blister which transforms into ulcer. Adult worm can be seen in the centre of the ulcer.

URETHRITIS. *Trichomonas vaginalis* causes 'non specific urethritis'.

VAGINITIS. In *Trichomonas vaginalis* infection, vagina is congested and there will be yellowish discharge.

WINTERBOTTOM'S SIGN. See LYMPHADENITIS.

CHAPTER 58A

IMMUNOPARASITOLOGY

Immunoparasitology is the study of the host response to parasites and of the evasion of parasites to the host's immune response. It has been demonstrated that numerous parasites species were capable of eliciting immune response by stimulating B Lymphoblasts in the lamina propria of the intestine to produce secretory Ig A (s Ig A). This immunoglobulin is believed to act non-specifically by preventing parasites from attaching to the mucosal cells. Furthermore, intestinal parasites can cause T cells to migrate to the lamina propria via the mesenteric lymph nodes and thoracic duct.

Parasitic infections rarely confer life long or complete immunity after primary infection. The primary infection with cutaneous leishmaniasis is possibly an exception.

During most parasitic infections, the host is protected against hyperinfection by the same parasite species. However, subsequent infection can occur after the disappearance or expulsion of the parasite from the host. In malaria and toxoplasmosis, continuous low level infection confers partial protection against the respective parasite species. This later phenomenon is known as *premunition*.

The immune responses may sometimes have the detrimental effects to the host. For example, prolonged exposure to *A. lumbricoides* may cause delayed hypersensitivity reaction. Schistosome-soluble egg antigen produces extensive granuloma formation, an anaphylactic shock may ensue due to hydatid cyst rupture and its fluid discharged into the visceral cavity of a sensitised patient. The crux of the problem is the antigenic complexity of parasite themselves. When the host responds to multiple antigens, it is difficult to isolate pure antigens and to determine which antigens and to determine which antigens trigger either humoral or cell mediated immunity.

Antibodies produced in response to protozoan parasites ordinarily belong to Ig G and Ig M classes. In most cases, it is non-specific and therefore does not confer protection. Exceptions are antibodies produced against *Toxoplasma gondii* possibly plasmodia. It has been well-established that cell mediated immunity determined by delayed hypersensitivity reaction is important in affording protection against many species of parasitic protozoa.

IMMUNITY TO PROTOZOA

Amebic dysentery. Though the immunity to *E. histolytica* infection has not yet been clearly defined, the immunity to this infection may exist. The indigenous residents of highly endemic areas may possibly become immune to local strains. Symptomless carriers may develop considerable tolerance to the parasite. Complement fixation test may become positive when the blood serum of infected individuals is brought into contact with the antigen extracted from the cultures of ameba. When this antigen is injected into the susceptible animals, it may protect these animals from *E. histolytica* infection; but it has been practically observed that the recovery from amebic dysentery does not confer an immunity against reinfection.

E. histolytica regularly invades human tissues and does cause immune responses. Antibodies of Ig G and Ig M classes can be demonstrated by passive hemagglutination, precipitation, fluorescent antibody techniques. These antibodies can be used for the diagnosis of amebic dysentery. However, the presence of specific antibody does not necessarily indicate active infection but rather an exposure to the organisms at some time. Skin tests give immediate responses in many patients indicating Ig E production and Arthus phenomenon can also be demonstrated. Skin tests for immediate and delayed hypersensitivity indicate past or present infection. Delayed hypersensitivity is depressed with liver abscess. To date, there is little direct evidence that immunoglobulin is protective.

Cell mediated immunity to *E. histolytica* can be demonstrated by delayed hypersensitivity skin test in many patients who do not have clinically evident disease and patients with amebic abscess of the liver have depressed cell mediated immunity to amebic antigen while retaining their ability to respond to other skin test antigens.

Visceral leishmaniasis (Kala azar). A long lasting immunity appears after the recovery from Kala-azar as the second attack of the disease does not occur. In endemic areas, many exposed persons may develop a mild type of the disease and recover without appreciable symptoms. In visceral leishmaniasis, delayed hypersensitivity occurs only after spontaneous recovery or chemotherapy and there is increased non-specific immunoglobulin level. Massive polyclonal hypergammaglobulinemia with little or no evidence of cell mediated immunity is the rule in visceral leishmaniasis.

Cutaneous leishmaniasis due to *Leishmania tropic* results in immune response characterised by little or no specific antibody but by strong cell mediated immunity. In endemic area, vaccination with virulent strains of the parasites derived from culture is a common practice to make certain that disfiguring lesions do not occur.

In *American leishmaniasis* (Espundia) due to *L. braziliensis*, both delayed hypersensitivity and elevated immunoglobulins are detected.

In *Malaria* immunity, there is a combination of power and process. This combination (a) prevents plasmodial infection, reinfection or superinfection; (b) destroys plasmodium; (c) limits its multiplication; (d) modifies its effects on the body; and (e) aids specifically in repair of tissue. The immunity may be natural or acquired. Natural immunity is genetic or innate, independent of previous infection, e.g., man is immune to avian malaria. Acquired immunity is due to antigenic stimulation by the parasite or its products. It protects against superinfection rather than against reinfection and it does not seem to persist much beyond the time when the plasmodia are eliminated from the body. Acquired immunity may be active or passive. Actively acquired immunity is due to malarial infection. Active immunity may be concomitant, i.e., present while there is parasitemia, or it may be residual persisting after eradication of parasites. Passive immunity is conferred by the maternal transfer. Infants less than six months old are protected from antibodies received by their mother's milk (WHO, 1991).

Premunition is concomitant or infection immunity tolerance is the term applied to an infection immunity which reduces the effects of a given number of parasites on the human host and also allows the infection without acute illness. There is variation in infection due to different strains of the same plasmodium as well as in different species. Malaria immunity is specific for homologous strains or species. In cellular immunity of malaria, reticuloendothelial system (lymphoid, macrophages) undergoes hyperplasia. Monocytes and specially the wandering cells found in the spleen, liver, bone marrow and general circulation originating as lymphocytes enlarge and become motile and phagocytic. They engulf rapidly merozoites, pigment, cellular debris and even whole parasitised red blood cells. As the disease continues these macrophages also engulf apparently normal uninfected erythrocytes, thus further adding to the anaemia caused by Plasmodium.

Humoral malaria immunity with formation of protective antibodies is more important. Malaria antibodies are closely associated with 7 S fraction of serum gammaglobulin and are developed during the infection. These antibodies have shown increased levels in the inhabitants of area of highly endemic area. This immune gammaglobulin has been found to have therapeutic and preventive action in malaria of children. These malaria protective antibodies have a powerful effect in stimulating the lymphoid-macrophage system. Besides, they seem to include lysins, agglutinins, precipitins, opsonins, complement fixing and cytoplasm modifying antibodies. Fluorescin tagged antibodies can be used to differentiate strains of plasmodia.

The exoerythrocytic forms induce little or no immuno response because *P. vivax* and other relapsing forms exist for extended period in the exoerythrocytic phase. The parasites in the blood induce an array of humoral responses in the host as demonstrated by complement fixation, precipitation, agglutination and fluorescent antibody reaction. Specific protective Ig G antibody was produced against merozoites.

The immune response that leads to protection is generally thought to be produced by complement independent antibody which inhibits entry of the merozoites into host erythrocytes. It has been shown that the people residing in endemic areas become increasingly less parasitemic with age and that children born in these areas appear to be protected during their first year of life by Ig G which crosses the placenta from the immune mother during gestation. Although all immune classes are elevated in the serum of malaria patients, it is the serum Ig G levels appear to correlate well with protection. The irradiated sporozoite antigens elicited an immune response in human volunteers but did not cause disease in man. Protection by this vaccine was fairly species specific.

In malarial infection, the reticuloendothelial system is hyperactive resulting in the removal of effected red blood cells, parasitised cells and parasitic metabolic byproducts. An intact spleen may be needed in addition to antibody production, because increased reticuloendothelial system clearance appears to be non-specific, since enhanced clearance may augment the immune response.

In summary, it appears that non-complement dependent Ig G antibodies to merozoite antigens are the main source of protection in malarial infection in the adult human, although the diverse antigens produced during the infection result in other types of immunity not yet fully understood.

World's first vaccine (synthetic peptide) against malaria was developed to prevent the invasion of red blood cells by raising antibodies against the micromerozoites. It is cheap and given in three doses against malaria caused by *P. vivax* and *P. falciparum*. *In late 1991*, this technology of vaccine preparation has been transferred to India, free of cost.

Toxoplasmosis

Toxoplasma infection results in the production of Ig G and Ig M anitbodies which are readily demonstrated by hemagglutination, complement fixation, fluorescent antibody technique and Sabin-Feldman dye tests. The mere presence of antibody is not sufficient for the protection as shown by the ability of the parasite to persist in the presence of high antibody titers and by the fact the passive transfer of antibody is not protective.

Cell mediated immunity is also involved in protection against Toxoplasma because delayed hypersensitivity develops early in toxoplasmosis and protection results only from infection with living organisms. Interferon is also produced. Inhibition of the multiplication of organism would effectively reduce the parasite burden.

It now appears that the macrophages inhibit multiplication of Toxoplasma both specifically or non-specifically.

Vaccination of population with strains of low virulence would probably be effective in establishing protection against Toxoplasma, but most persons develop adequate protection after natural infection. In order to prevent the intrauterine transmission of Toxoplasma in uninfected women of child-bearing age, this protection can be worthwhile.

African Trypanosomiasis

Greatly increased levels of immunoglobulins especially of the Ig M class are regularly present in infected animals. Specific antibodies do arise in trypanosomal infection.

The specific antibody can either lyse the parasites or clump them. Clumping allows for more efficient removal of the parasites by the reticuloendothelial system. Effective reduction of parasites numbers would protect the host. In fact, there are healthy carriers of *Trypanosoma rhodesiense* which usually produce a fatal infection; it implies that some protective mechanism must exist. However, the precise immunologic nature of this protection is obscure.

The multiplicity of antigenic variants observed makes vaccination an unlikely solution to African trypanosomiasis, unless common antigen can be found. Antigenic variation produces specific antibody sequentially.

American Trypanosomiasis

Antibody that can be detected by complement fixation test is produced during the course of the disease. This can be a guide for diagnosis, although the antibody cross-reacts with other flageliates, i.e., Leishmania. Antibody may persist after infection and therefore does not indicate active disease. High titer antibody does not appear to limit the infection is man. Acquired resistance to variant strains is probably the result of previous inapparent infection with strains of low virulence.

Activated macrophages can be demonstrated in *Trypanosoma cruzi* infection, although their role in protection has yet to be fully explained. Attempts to vaccinate against this disease might do more harm than good if such sensitised lymphocytes against shared antigens should develop.

IMMUNITY TO HELMINTHS

Helminths (trematodes, cestodes and nematodes) are metazoic (multicellular) organisms. The antigenic mosaics of these organisms are complex, making the isolation of medically important antigens difficult. Moreover, many helminths undergo life cycles during which more than one stage develops in the host. Eosinophilia and increased levels of Ig E antibody are indicative of helminthic infection. Eosinophilia readily attach to the cuticle of intestinal nematodes in the presence of specific antibody. Because eosinophils are known to release substances such as enzymes and prostaglandins, it is hypothesised that they play a part in worm expulsion. Experimental studies using a rodent hookworm, *Nippastrongylus braziliensis*, showed that a soluble factor secreted by helper T cells stimulate B cells in the mesenteric lymph nodes to produce specific Ig E antibody. Ig E appears to be involved in the worm expulsion by interfering with the metabolism of the worm by rendering the worms susceptible to a population of T cells capable of triggering worm expulsion.

Besides B and T cell involvement, immune responses to parasites may include inflammatory responses, macrophages activation, complement mediated cell lysis and interferon production. Thus the parasites do indeed trigger immune response by their hosts.

The eggs of *Schistosoma mansoni* have been shown to secrete unique antigens that induce granuloma formation, the various stages of developing nematodes have stage specific antigens to which the host responds by various ways and the special cells localised in the "neck" of *Trichinella spiralis* elicit specific antibody.

Nematodes, cestodes and trematodes all share common antigens. The two most frequent responses to helminths — eosinophilia and reaginic antibody (Ig E) — are both T cell dependent. In addition, certain helminths have been shown to potentiate the immune response to other antigens, perhaps by common metabolic byproducts acting as non-specific adjuvants.

Nematodes

Trichinosis

Specific immuno-diagnostic tests may be of great importance. The bentonite flocculation test for human trichinosis is of great value, because of its high degree of specificity. In addition, there are many other immuno-diagnostic tests including complement fixation, hemagglutination, flocculation, skin tests. Skin test produces both immediate and delayed hypersensitivity responses.

In man, infection with *T. spiralis* initially elicits Ig M antibody followed by Ig G response. Ig A antibody is not yet been reported, which is surprising, because the female worms are in the intestinal mucosa, a major site of Ig A production. The immediate hypersensitivity response shows that Ig E is also produced. Man develops both immediate and delayed hypersensitivity to Trichinella antigens which suggests that Ig E alone or in combination with mononuclear cells may mediate the protection. Although, Trichinella is extensively immunogenic in its hosts, it can also exert an immunosuppressive action.

Ascariasis

In *Ascaris lumbricoides* infection, specific antibody is detectable and Ig E is elevated. During the infection with Ascaris, immune responses to other unrelated antigens are potentiated.

Toxocara Infection

Toxocara canis, the dog intestinal round worm, is known to infect small children who ingest eggs in dirt. *T. canis* eggs produce a population of migrating larvae that are immobilised in the tissue of man and consequently never produce worms in the intestinal tract. The symptoms caused by the immobilised larvae is called *Visceral larva migrans*. This visceral larva migrans is characterised by high eosinophilia and chronic granulomatous growth associated with the migrating larvae; such larvae in the eyes of the infected children have been confused with retinoblastoma, the diagnosis is only after enucleation the affected eyeball. The specific immunodiagnostic methods have been developed that should allow the prompt diagnosis.

Filariasis. The excretory - secretory antigen of *B. malayi* are effective in inducing resistance against filarial parasites and thus have potential in immunoprophylaxis.

Trematodes

It is generally agreed that the protective immune response to schistosoma is mediated by antibody. However, in this disease and other helminth infections, there is evidence indicating that humoral and cellular protective mechanisms are interrelated. It is known that people residing in endemic areas become resistant to reinfection with schistosoma. It may be due to continuous exposure to small number of cercariae of zoophilic species. Newly invading schistosomes are rapidly killed or immobilised by the action of antibody. This *concomitant immunity* has been established as an important way in which host protection to reinfection may be achieved while allowing the original parasite to persist.

Ig G antibody that killed immobilised schistosoma have been demonstrated *in vitro*, but these antibodies do not protect against reinfection after passive transfer. On the other hand, certain antisera have successfully produced protection. Ig E production may be of one of the mechanisms by which the protection is achieved.

Cell mediated immune response may produce many lesions. In *S. mansoni* and *S. japonicum*, fibrosis of the liver is the main cause of death. The fibrosis may result due to delayed hypersensitivity reaction to antigens produced by the secretions from the eggs.

In *S. hematobium* infection, a granulomatous reaction early in the diagnosis may spontaneously subside. This abatement results from desensitisation by blocking antibody or anitgen-antibody complex produced within the granuloma itself. It is generally agreed that antibodies formed to the developing worms produced the reaction.

Human Ig E, Ig G-4 are responsible for the resistance to the infection with *S. hematobium*. Immunity to reinfection is due to Ig E, Ig G-4 acts as blocking antibody.

Cestodes

It is now established that the larval forms of the parasites which are tissue penetrators evoke humoral responses that protect the hyperimmunised host against new infection. Infection with cestodes is usually life threatening to man only when he acts as an unnatural intermediate host. *T. solium* from swine can develop extra-intestinally in man and can be found in any organ of the body. When the encysted parasite dies in the brain, tissue reactions with resultant central nervous system disorders and even death can occur.

Echinococcosis

Echinococcus granulosus normally forms fluid filled cysts in the liver, but this can also occur in the lungs and other parts of the body. These hydatid cysts are highly immunogenic and result in the production of high titers of reaginic antibody (Ig E) and other immunoglobulins. Cystic fluid from ruptured cyst can cause anaphylactic reaction and death. Little or no protection seems to be elicited by this highly immunogenic cestode because the hydatid cysts remain alive for years.

Casoni's skin test indicates the past or present echinococcosis resulting in both immediate and delayed hypersensitivity. The specificity of this test is doubtful, because of cross-reaction with other helminths. Diagnosis can be made by hemagglutination, complement fixation and flocculation tests using serum of the patient.

The life cycle of protozoa and helminths are complicated and the immune response to be effective has to interrupt the cycle at a stage when the parasite is accessible to the immune process.

Malaria infection is initiated by sporozoites which transform into exoerythrocytic schizonts in the liver and there is no recognisable immunity. The liver cells rupture and discharge their merozoites into the peripheral circulation then they invade the erythrocytes. At this stage, it appears that there is alteration in the permeability of the red cell membrane, so that the immunoglobulin molecules can enter and attack the parasite, *Plasmodium*. Antibodies are readily detectable in the serum and increased until the crisis 7 to 10 days later and then slowly decline. Because these antibodies are able to get access to the parasite only during a relatively short period of its life cycle, then the immunity is incomplete and the host usually fails to eliminate the parasite completely. Plasmodium like trypanosome is subject to antigenic variation and antigenically distinct forms may appear after each relapse. Immunity probably depends on the gradual build-up of antibodies to a group antigen common to all variants. The state in which the organisms persist in small numbers in the tissue in the presence of an immune reaction is called "preimmunition".

The adaptive phenomenon of antigenic variation is seen in trypanosome means that the immune response has great difficulty in coping with these parasitic variations so that in African sleeping sickness the parasite does not induce an effective immunity and the infected individuals develop progressive infection with the invasion of central nervous system and leading to death. Trypanosomiasis is associated with high levels of Ig M immunoglobulin in both the blood and cerebrospinal fluid. It is not certain if this is due to repeated new antigenic stimuli resulting from the changes in the organisms or if the parasite in some way influences directly the cells of the immune system. Increased immunoglobulin production is a common finding in protozoal infection and often affects all classes of immunoglobulins. Because usually less than 5 per cent of the total immunoglobulin appears to react specifically with the inducing parasite, it is probable that protozoa stimulate the lymphoid cells in a non-specific way to over-produce immunoglobulins (called paraglobulins).

Helminths like protozoa go through a complex life cycle and protective immune mechanisms probably act only at an early stage in the cycle. The main stimulus seems to be due to the antigens derived from adult worms and the immune mechanisms act on new parasites entering the body. A noteworthy point of these infections is the appearance of Ig G (reaginic) antibody with pulmonary eosinophilia and it seems likely that the immediate hypersensitivity reaction of anaphylactic type (type 1) is involved in the pathogenesis of helminth infection.

UNIT E

CHAPTER 59

PATHOGENS FROM THE SOIL

Bacterial pathogens of the soil (spore forming bacilli).

Most of the spore-forming bacilli of human or animal intestine are excreted through their faeces and contaminate the soil and form the spores under adverse conditions. In the human or animal tissue, these spores germinate into infectious bacilli, and produce diseases.

Gram-Positive Spore Forming Bacilli

Anaerobic	Aerobic
↓	↓
Spore bulging (Clostridium) (e.g., *Cl. tetani, Cl. welchil; Cl. botulinum*)	Spore central within the bacillus (e.g., *Bacillus anthracis*)

TETANUS, caused by *Cl. tetani*, occurs in man and animals, when a wound is infected with *Cl. tetani* under conditions that allow the organism to multiply and produce the toxin. Absorption of the toxin leads to hyperexcitability of voluntary musculature. The disease is characterised by increased muscle tonus and exaggerated muscular response to simple stimuli. *Trismus* occurs as early sign of tetanus in man, when jaw muscles are affected and the disease is called "lock jaw".

Cl. tetani are Gram-positive rod-shaped bacilli. They are motile with numerous peritrichous flagella. Their spores are spherical, terminal, larger than the diameter of the bacillus producing a typical "drum stick" appearance.

Cl. tetani are obligate anaerobes, grow best at 37°C in cooked meat medium.

The spores may be highly resistant to adverse conditions. They resist dry heat at 150°C for 1 hour. 5% phenol, iodine in watery solution and hydrogen peroxide (10 volumes) kill them within a few hours.

Tetanus toxin. It is an exotoxin and has two components : (a) Neurotoxic constituent (tetanospasmin) is the essential pathogenic constituent and has been separated as a pure crystalline protein which can kill mouse in a dose of 0.0000001 mg. It is an extremely powerful toxin, second in potency only to the exotoxin of *Cl. botulinum*.

(b) *Tetanolysin* is another constituent which causes lysis of red blood cells. It is oxygen labile.

Tetanus antitoxin is often called antitoxin serum (ATS). It can be obtained by immunising horse with toxoid. This serum is of great value in the prophylaxis of tetanus, when given immediately after wounding. Its use as a curative agent after the development of tetanus is less effective. At the international conference of Tetanus, Mumbai, it was decided that an initial dose of 10,000 units of antitoxin should be adopted in the treatment of adult cases of Tetanus, when intravenous antitoxin is prescribed, it should be preceded by a subcutaneous test dose, followed by an intramuscular test dose at half hour interval. The antitoxin should be diluted, warmed at room temperature and injected slowly into the recumbent patient.

Precautions while injecting antitoxin. Routine precautions should be taken before an antitoxin is administrated to avoid the risk of anaphylactic reaction following injection of antitoxin. Informations regarding previous serum injections, any history of asthma, infantile eczema, urticaria and other allergic conditions should be obtained from the patient. In the absence of the contraindications, the full dose of antitoxin may be injected, but a sterile syringe and needle with adrenalin (1 ml. of 1 : 1,000) solution should be ready. The patient should be kept warm before and after treatment and he should be under observation for at least 30 minutes after the injection.

If the patient has had a previous injection of serum, but gives no history of allergy, a subcutaneous test dose of 0.2 ml. antitoxin shall be given and a full dose of antitoxin may be given if no general reactions have occurred after 30 minutes. If the patient gives a history of allergy, the initial test dose should be 0.2 ml. of a 1 : 10 dil of antitoxin subcutaneously. If no general symptoms develop within 30 minutes, this may be followed by 0.2 ml. of undiluted antitoxin subcutaneously. The full dose may be given if there are no general reactions after a further dose.

Tetanus Toxoid. The toxin can be detoxified by the chemical (formaldehyde). During the conversion period the toxic part is destroyed leaving antigenic part intact. Thus the toxoid is an excellent immunising agent.

A course of three 0.5 ml. doses of tetanus toxoid (formol toxoid) with intervals of 6 to 12 weeks between the first two doses and 6 to 12 months between the second and third injections is proved valuable in the prevention of tetanus. A reinforcing (booster) dose of 0.5 ml. toxoid should be given at intervals of 5 to 10 years to maintain immunity.

Pathogenesis. Tetanus is usually the result of contamination of a wound with *Cl. tetani* spores from the soil. Deep punctured wounds, wounds associated with devitalised, necrotic tissue and wounds contaminated with soil, ionised calcium salts and salicylic acid favour the germination of spores of *Cl. tetani* and multiplication of this organism and production of the toxin. This tetanus toxin is absorbed by the motor nerve endings and spread up the space between the nerve fibres. It seems to act as excitant to the motor cells in anterior horn of the spinal cord and may diffuse in the CNS. It may also interfere with normal inhibition of motor impulses, thus producing early increase in tonus and tonic spasms of muscles and also impair the release of acetylcholine.

Laboratory diagnosis. can be done by microscopic examination of Gram-stained films of wound exudate for typical 'drum-stick' appearance bacilli. They grow in Robertson cooked meat medium or anaerobically in blood agar medium.

Chemotheraphy. A course of systemic penicillin or tetracycline therapy should be given in cases of established tetanus and, at the same time, antibiotics should be applied in and around wound.

Application to Nursing

Nurse should invariably disinfect and dispose-off all dressings soiled with the wound exudate. She should take utmost precautions while administrating antiserum to avoid the anaphylactic shock. She should wear gloves while dressing wound and then should not delay in treating wound.

GAS GANGRENE, caused by *Cl. welchii*, is characterised by rapidly spreading edema, necrosis and gangrene of the tissue and gas production. The infection results from the contamination of a wound with soil from manured or cultivated land, dirty clothing, street dust, etc. or from skin contaminated with intestinal organisms. The predisposing factors already discussed in detail with regard to tetanus are equally applicable in the case of gas gangrene. In pueperal sepsis cases and especially in case of septic abortion, the organism may gain access via the perineum to necrotic or devitalised tissues and set up a dangerous infection.

Cl. welchii is Gram-positive bacillus, occurring singly or pairs, is non-motile and often capsulated when seen in the tissues. Spores are formed outside of the body and are typically oval subterminal and slightly bulging (Fig. 59.2). They grow best anaerobically at 37°C in blood agar medium and Robertson cooked meat medium. They are saccharolytic and proteolytic; hence in Litmus milk medium, acid clot and gas production result, the gas breaks up the clot and produces the "stormy clot" reaction.

Toxin. Cl. welchii produces 12 types of toxin of which 4 major lethal toxins and 8 minor lethal or non-lethal toxin; out of these four major lethal toxins(α, β, ε), alpha toxin is produced by all types of *Cl. welchii*, but, notably by type A strain of *Cl. welchii* as the most important of the lethal toxins of the organism and is considered to be the main cause of the profound toxemia associated with gas gangrene in man. The alpha toxin is lethal, necrotising on intradermal, inoculation. It is a relatively heat stable enzyme, lecithinase C. In presence of Ca and Mg ions, it can attack phospholipid constituents of red blood cells.

Laboratory Diagnosis

Specimens of exudate should be taken from the deeper parts of the wound surface. The sterile swabs rubbed over the wound surface and soaked in the exudate serve the purpose (one swab for film preparation and another for the culture). If there are necrotic tissues in the wound, small pieces should be placed in a sterile screw capped bottle and used for microscopic examination and culture.

Chemotherapy. The common antibiotics are used in the following order of the activity, in general, tetracycline, penicillin, chloramphemicol. Severe wounds considered to be the gas gangrene demand intravenous gas gangrene antiserum in addition to *meticulous* removal of death tissue plus broad and parenteral antibiotics.

Prophylaxis of gas gangrene. A polyvalent serum is available for prophylactic use. The prophylactic dose, given intramuscularly, is 10,000 international units (IU) *Cl. welchii* antitoxin, 5,000 units *Cl. septicum* antitoxin and 10,000 units of *Cl. edematiens* antitoxin. The therapeutic dose given intravenously should be at least three times the prophylactic dose and it can be repeated if necessary. Monovalent serum can be used if the causal organism is identified. Reactions to antitoxin administrated intravenously may be severe and precautions should be taken.

Application to Nursing

Nurse should be aware that only autoclaving or hot air oven sterilisation or treatment of infected objects by sporocidal gases are necessary to prevent the transmission by fomites. Dressings should be burnt completely. Nurse and surgeon should wear gloves while dressing the oozing wound. Washed and wrapped gloves can be sterilised again, if necessary.

BOTULISM is a fatal form of food poisoning caused by consumption of preformed toxin of *Cl. botulinum* and characterised by pronounced toxic effects — oculomotor paralysis, pharyngeal paralysis, aphonia. The causal agent is Gram-positive *Cl. botulinum*. It occurs singly or in pairs, it is motile, its spore is oval, subterminal and slightly bulging. Its growth characteristic is similar to that of *Cl. welchii*. Spores of some strains of *Cl. botulinum* withstand moist heat at 100°C for several days. They are destroyed at 120°C (autoclaving). Insufficient heating in the process of preserving foods is an important factor in the causation of food poisoning, a great care should be taken to ensure that sufficient heating is achieved in all parts of the can while manufacturing canned food in canning factories. Home canning of foodstuffs can be done until the spores are ensured to be destroyed by sufficient heat.

Toxin. Toxin of Type-A *Cl. botulinum* has been isolated as a pure crystalline protein and is the most potent toxic substance in nature. The estimated lethal dose for a mouse is 0.000000033 mg., i.e., 1 Kg. of this toxin can kill whole world population.

Laboratory Diagnosis

Suspected food can be examined bacteriologically. The toxin can be demonstrated in the extract of macerated food and in the patient serum.

Application to Nursing

Nurse should not allow the patient to eat the canned food if the lids of the tin are bulging at both sides as it indicates the food is contaminated with *Cl. botulinum.* Antitoxin (10 ml.) can be given intramuscularly for prophylactic purposes and the toxoid in three doses for active immunity.

ANTHRAX is a zoonotic disease. It is primarily an infectious disease of domestic animals and is transmitted to man when he comes in contact with them.

Bacillus anthracis is the causal agent of anthrax. It is Gram-positive bacillus arranged in chains or in pairs or singly. In blood and tissue, it exhibits a distinct capsule when stained by polychrome methylene blue. The capsule is stained purplish and bacillus blue. It is called as methylene blue reaction of MC Fadyean which is very useful to recognise anthrax bacillus in blood films. Its spore, central, oval within the bacillus, can be stained by ordinary staining method.

B. anthracis grows best aerobically at 37°C. Its colonies appear under low power of microscope as lock of hair — "medusa head appearance".

Toxin. Anthrax bacillus produces a toxin - "anthrax toxin complex" which increases the permeability of blood vessels leading to the gelatinous edema and hemorrhage particularly in animals.

In man, the infection is acquired from animal source, usually through damaged skin or mucus membrane. The resulting lesion is usually described as a "malignant pustule". This starts as papule and becomes a blister within 48 hours and then a pustule with an increasing area of inflammation depending upon the resistance of the host.

Infection may also result from inhalation of spores carried in dust or filaments of wool from infected sheep as in wool factories — "Woolsorter's disease". The organisms settle in the lower part of the trachea or in large bronchus and an intense inflammatory lesion results with haemorrhage, edema, involvement of lungs, spread to the thoracic glands and diffusion into the pericardial and pleural cavities; considerable number of organisms are present in the lesion; a septicaemic condition or haemorrhagic meningitis may supervene. Infection of intestinal route is very uncommon.

Laboratory Diagnosis

Smears made from the exudate of malignant pustule or sputum of Woolsorter's disease patient are stained with Gram-stain. The finding of bacillus morphologically similar to *B. anthracis* is suggestive but not conclusive.

Chemotherapy. B. anthracis is sensitive to most antibiotics, hence treatment of malignant pustule and Woolsorter's disease is successful.

Application to Nursing

When taking care of a patient with anthrax, the nurse should wear rubber gloves and a rubber apron. Dressings contaminated with purulent exudates or, in fatal cases, fluids exudating from eyes, nose and mouth should be burnt promptly. Autoclaving or exposure to hot air oven at sterilising temperature or exposure to sporicidal gases for sufficient time is effective in destroying the spores. Pulmonary anthrax requires the same precautions of respiratory infections. In addition to these, the disinfectant-resistant spores of the exudates should be completely destroyed. Besides, the public health nurse should educate in explicit language the community that since the infected animal and dead carcases are potent source of infection to man, the farmers should avoid the contact of infected animals which should be buried very deep with lime. All fomites should *completely burnt.*

CHAPTER 60

MYCOSES

The diseases caused by Fungi are called mycotic diseases or mycoses.

They consist of two groups :

(a) Cutaneous mycoses (Skin, hair, nails affected);

(b) Systemic mycoses (internal organs affected).

(a) Cutaneous mycoses

Fungi penetrate the skin, hair and nails and grow as branching filaments or hyphae. Only the dead outer layer of these tissues is invaded; whereas the deeper or living layers cannot support the growth of hyphae.

In skin infection, the metabolites of the fungi diffuse into deeper living skin cells. People infected with these fungi become sensitive to these substances as a result there is skin response with a reddened erythematous area and itching. In the erythematous area, a little blister soon appears. The centre of the lesion becomes scaly and heal, it is then surrounded by an enlarging, red, outer ring covered with blister. These conditions are known as "ring worm".

In hair infection, the shaft of the hair — which is just formed above the living cells in the hair follicles — is attacked by superficial fungi (dermatophytes).

As the living cells continue to form the hair shaft, the infected portion of the shaft is brought upward. The penetration of hyphae of some fungi in the internal structure of the hair shaft may result in easy breakage of the hair within the hair follicle. In this condition, the infected area of the scalp appears *bald.*

In cases where the surface of the hair shaft is only infected by the hyphae of the fungi the hair breaks often and, thereby, the scalp appears as moth-eaten. The fungal infection of the hair of children is very common, compared to adults. Infective nails become yellow, black and brittle.

Tinea (Ringworm)

The medical term "tinea" implies the superficial fungal infection (ringworm) of the skin, hair and nails. *Tinea capitis* is the fungal infection of the hair of the scalp. When the foot is infected the condition is called "athlete's foot" or tinea pedis. Fungal infections of the nail and groin are named respectively as *Tinea unguium* and *Tinea cruris.*

Dermatophytes (*derm,* skin; *phyte,* plant) are fungi which are infectious. They are groups of related fungi which embraces three genera and 20 species. Species of fungi occurring in the skin, hair and nails of man and animals are fully responsible for the direct infection from one individual to another and their hyphae in the tissues may directly develop into chains of spores after a long time. Other types of the dermatophytes may live in soil; when they are rubbed on to the skin, they may cause the infection.

The infections caused by dermatophytes are collectively called dermatophytoses or dermatomycosis.

Dermatophytes and their location of the infections

1. Hair, skin, rarely nails.

   Microsporum canis (ringworm, tinea capitis in children)

   M. audouini (epidemic tinea capitis in children).

   M. gypseum (ringworm, tinea capitis).

2. Skin, hair and nails.

   Trichophyton mentagrophytes (athlete's foot, infection of nails and skin).

   T. rubrum (athlete's foot, tinea cruris, nail infection, sycosis*).

   T. tonsurans (tinea capitis), *T. schoenleini* (favus +)

3. Skin, nails, *not hair.*

   Epidermophyton floccosum (athlete's foot, tinea cruris, nail infection).

   *sycosis - pustular inflammation of the hair follicle of the face due to dermatophytes (barber's hitch).

   +favus - dermatomycosis of the scalp characterised by honeycomb-like, itching yellow crusts over the hair follicles.

Application to Nursing

The nurse should have the knowledge that the hyphae and spores of fungi can initiate the infection, if they are lodged on the skin or scalp of another susceptible individual. Therefore she should take precautions to dispose-off scale and stub of infected hair. She should also remember that the infected child can transmit his infection to his schoolmates and even to his pet animal. Dogs and animals should be carefully examined for scaly patches with loss of hair as they may become the source of infection to other human beings. Thus the owners of these animals should be advised to get these animals treated; if not responding to the treatment, they should be discarded.

Systemic Mycoses

The systemic mycoses are caused by fungi which occur in soil as saprophytes. The dust containing spores and hyphae inhaled by man may get lodged in the lung, they grow; if they overcome the host defense mechanism, they multiply and produce lesions in the lung and from these lesions they may be carried through the blood stream to various parts of the body where they set up the infection and lesions are produced. The lesion is limited to a small area of the lung in some people and may heal soon. Wounds of hands and feet are the portal of entry for soil fungi. Only few pathogenic fungi develop the infection.

Coccidioidomycosis

The causative agent, *Coccidioidoides immitis*, of the disease is commonly encountered in the soil of United States and grows as mould in soil. It is a *diphasic* fungus because it forms *spherule* in the tissue. Most of the people are infected by inhalation of dust laden with the fungus; they show only a mild influenza-like syndrome with fever.

Erythema nodosum. Painful red lumps appear on the legs of few patients. Pulmonary symptoms are very severe in some cases, resembling pneumonia, and in others they may be suggestive of tuberculosis. If localised, giant cavities are formed in the lungs. If the fungus is disseminated to various parts of the body, skin and bone marrow lesions may develop; meningitis is common and the patient will become seriously ill. In addition to the cultivation of the fungus, Skin test, *Coccidioidin* test, similar to tuberculin test is an useful test for diagnosis.

Histoplasmosis

Histoplasma capsulatum (diphasic fungus) causes histoplasmosis and grow commonly in the soil of United States. The human infection occurs through inhalation of its spore.

Some infected people experience symptoms like influenza or pneumonia or tuberculosis. The prognosis is grave if the pulmonary disease is severe. If the liver or spleen is affected through dissemination the patients are seriously ill.

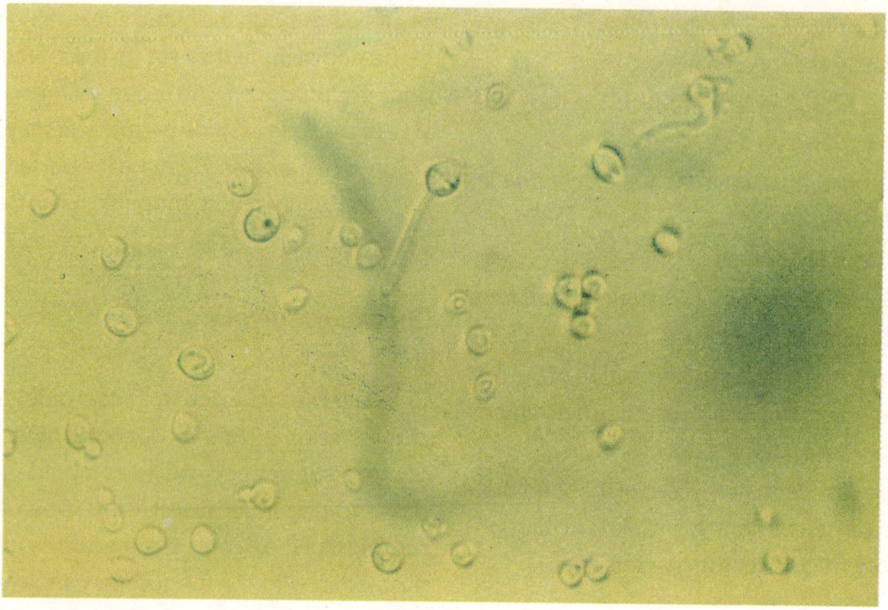

Fig. 60.1 : C. albicans with germ tube × 400

Skin test with histoplasmin and X-rays can be used for the diagnosis.

Blastomycosis, reported in United States of America and Canada, is caused by *Blastomyces dermatitis*, diphasic fungus. Lung infections begin with the inhalation of spore or hyphae. Dissemination may be to all parts of the body. Lesions on the skin and in the bones are especially common. Skin test with Blastomycin can be carried out.

Opportunistic mycoses. They are caused by a large number of soil fungi that are capable of producing infection in man under unusual conditions.

Candidiasis. It is caused by *Candida albicans* which is yeast-like organism commonly found in the mouth and the genital tract of healthy people, but under favourable conditions they multiply heavily (Fig. 60.1), invade the tissues (Fig. 60.2), and grow into long filaments (Fig. 60.3) and in the form of budding yeast-like cells and produce germ tube. New aniline blue dye method accurately identifies *C. albicans*.

Diabetes, debility, steroid therapy and the prolonged administration of antibiotics are the factors which promote the growth of *C. albicans*.

Candida vaginitis may occur in pregnant women. If the hands are wet for longer period, some people may develop skin lesions of the interdigital webs or of the finger nail.

Thrush

Though *C. albicans* is normal flora of the mouth of the genital tract, it may invade tissues, may set up the inflammation and produce pseudomembrane on the lip and the mouth. This condition is called "Thrush". It is also common in neonates who acquire this infection from the infected mothers while passing through the birth canal. Ordinarily, the bacteria of the genital tract suppress the growth of *C. albicans*; but if the patients are under antibiotic therapy for a longer period, the antibiotics may inhibit the growth of bacteria. As a result, *C. albicans* is free from the bacteria. Itching or perianal rash may also occur. Besides, if the

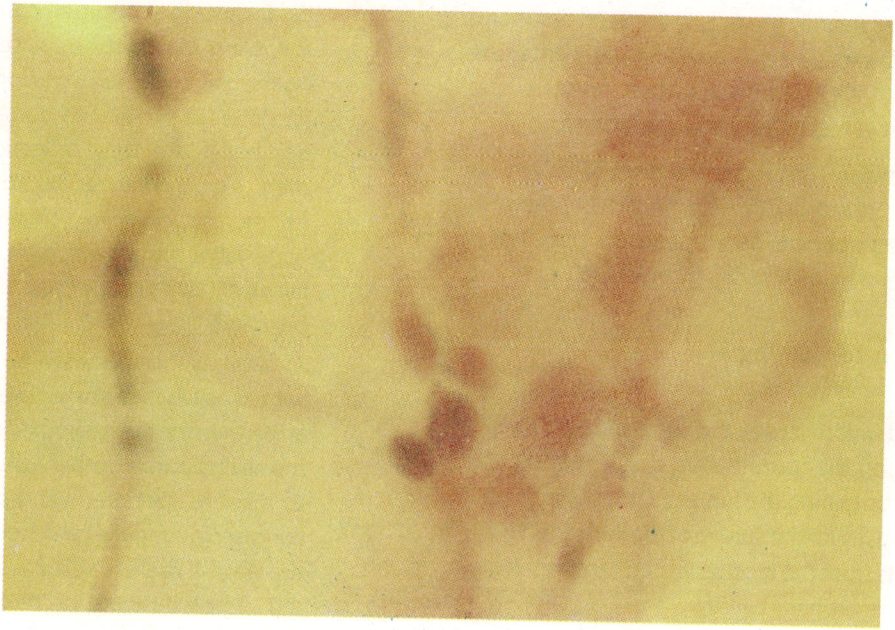

Fig. 60.2 : Candida albicans in tissue × 400

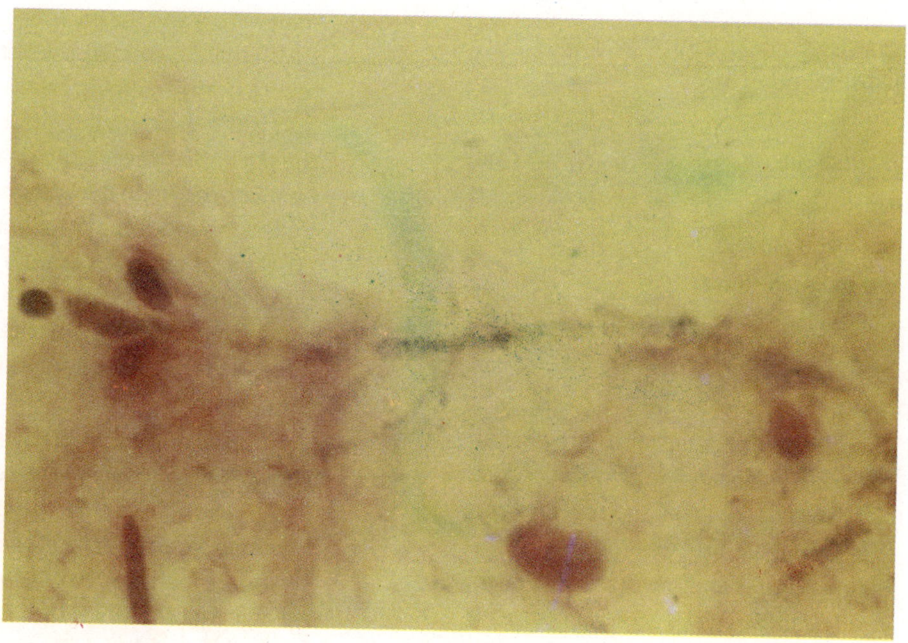

Fig. 60.3 : Candida albicans with long filaments × 400

lung tissue is damaged by tuberculosis or other diseases. *C. albicans* may multiply in the dead tissue and aggravate the infection. *C. albicans* rarely enter the blood stream; if it at all invades, it may cause vegetation of heart valves or lesions in the kidney.

Treatment. Nystatin is the drug of choice for candidiasis. Griseofulvin (oral administration). Betrafen cream and zole powder (local application) for 21 days are very effective for superficial mycoses.

Application to Nursing

In systemic mycoses, the nurse should take care to dispose-off the sputum, pus, dressing and other materials containing the fungus. Otherwise there is every possibility for the spread of the infection. Newly born infants from the mother with *C. albicans* vaginitis should be properly cared.

UNIT F

CHAPTER 61

RESPONSIBILITIES OF NURSES IN THE TRANSMISSIBLE DISEASES

The responsibilities of professional nurses are to assist the physician in :

1. the diagnosis;
2. the treatment; and
3. the prevention of the disease.

1. In the *diagnosis of the disease* a nurse can assist the physician for —

(i) The *collection of specimen.* If she has an excellent understanding of the procedure, she can collect herself the specimen for the diagnostic purpose, otherwise she may make preparation for the collection. Poorly and carelessly taken specimen is of no use for correct diagnosis of the disease.

(ii) *Labelling.* The nurse should be responsible to label the specimen containers the following information (a) the patients name; (b) case Registration number; (c) date; (d) physician's name; (e) ward number; (f) the site of collection of specimen (e.g., throat, cervix, abscess etc.). Adhesive tape is always preferable to the paper label, pasted with gum, which may fall off if it is not properly secured by rubber band.

As soon as the specimen is collected, it should be labelled immediately and kept aside; then the nurse should proceed with the next specimen, otherwise she is liable to mix the specimens and she may be confused during the peak hour of work in the ward. If there is a slightest suspicion, the samples should be discarded and, again, the new samples should be collected. Petri plate containing solid culture medium should be labelled on its *bottom* because its lid may be transposed. Specimen should be transmitted *immediately* to the laboratory, if there is delay, the specimen will dry and the microorganisms will perish, thereby there is possibility of wrong report. The microbiological diagnostic report is the deciding factor for the life of the patient, so, the life and death of a patient depend upon the laboratory report. Hence, the specimen collection, immediate transfer to the laboratory and quick processing in the laboratory are very important considerations for the correct diagnosis of the disease and for the life of the patient.

(iii) *Swabs.* The nurse should have the sound knowledge to collect the material for the bacteriological examination with the help of sterile swabs. Test tubes containing swabs are readily available in the bacteriological laboratory. It should be always borne in mind that while taking a swab for culture it is necessary to touch the lesion or spot from which the specimen is required with the help of sterile swab. The swab containing the specimen should be inserted quickly into the sterile test tube and sent immediately to the laboratory and used for the inoculation of the media in the microbiological laboratory.

(iv) *Throat culture.* During the collection of the specimens with the help of throat swab from the tonsils or from the pseudomembranes of the faucial region of the throat, it is necessary to have clear vision of the throat with good light by using tongue depressor or tea-spoon. The same procedure is applicable to septic sore throat and other throat infections.

Specimens for meningococci (causative organism of meningitis) should be collected from the nasopharynx with the help of the post-nasal swab by passing it back gently through the nostril. The specimen should be cultured and incubated *immediately*, because meningococci are very *fragile* and die rapidly.

In whooping cough, the specimen can be collected by exposing, in front of the mouth of the patient, petri plates containing media suitable for the growth of desired bacteria when the patient coughs. The spray of the sputum produced by cough inoculates the medium. The plate should be covered immediately with the lid and placed in the incubator in an inverted position.

(v) *Sputum.* The nurse should guide the patient to collect very carefully the sputum in the sterile wide mouthed cup of 2 oz capacity. The specimen must not consist of material from the mouth and throat (i.e., mucus, saliva, food particles). The sputum should be certainly collected direct after expectoration or after cough that brings *secretions up from the lungs* **(not from the throat)** and sent immediately to the microbiological laboratory. In case of infants, the sputum should be obtained by throat swab, since they swallow the sputum.

(vi) *Urine.* The nurse should invariably instruct the female patients to collect with extreme care the midstream urine (MSU) into a sterile test tube after separating the vulva so to avoid the contamination of urine by bacteria present on the skin and mucus membrane of the genitalia and the test tube should be closed quickly with sterile cotton plug and sent immediately to the laboratory. The first stream of urine should be allowed to run off to wash out any bacteria present in the urethra. The collection of urine by catheterisation can be done only by the physician with the assistance of the nurse.

(vii) *Faeces.* The nurse should collect *fresh* stool in a sterile container and send it to the laboratory for the isolation of dysentery, typhoid, paratyphoid bacilli and for the demonstration of eggs or cysts of the parasites (hookworm, tapeworms, protozoa). Mucus should be preferred particularly for the culture of dysentery bacilli and be sent to the laboratory by Stuart's transport medium or glycerol saline, as these bacilli are delicate. The collection of "rice water stool" in case of cholera should be carried out on a clean paper or leaf, but never from a bedpan, because the left-over disinfectant in the bedpan may destroy *Vibrio cholerae*. This method of collection of stool in sterile container should be strictly followed by the nurse to obtain the correct laboratory diagnosis.

(viii) *Blood for culture.* Blood should be collected in a sterile container for blood culture to diagnose septicemia or bacteriemia. In the early stage of bacteriemia (first week) in typhoid, *Salmonella typhi* (typhoid bacilli) can be isolated. The nurse should collect aseptically about ten ml of blood with a sterile syringe with extreme care and full responsibility. Before puncturing the skin over the vein, she should sterilise the skin with alcoholic solution of iodine (1 per cent) and remove the excess of iodine within 1-2 minutes with a sterile gauze soaked in 70 per cent ethyl alcohol. This is a valuable procedure to avoid the contamination of blood with staphylococci or other organisms from the skin.

The nurse should know very well that Trypticase soy broth can support early and rapid growth of all organisms responsible for blood infections and it can be used at bedside for the quick inoculation before the blood is clotted. In case the blood is to be sent to the laboratory, it should be mixed with an anticoagulant (sterile solution of sodium citrate), particularly for microbiological investigations, but, for chemical examination, sodium oxalate is mostly used to prevent clotting.

(ix) *Blood for serological tests.* The blood can be drawn at one puncture for culture, serology and microscopic examination. The blood for serology should be put into a clean, dry test tube without anticoagulant and this test tube should be kept in a slanting position on the working table till the blood is clotted. For blood grouping, it is convenient to have only a few drops of blood by puncturing the finger or ear lobe with the help of the sterile needle after sterilising the site with ethyl alcohol. A thin uniform blood film can be also prepared from a drop of blood on a clean slide.

(x) *Peritoneal and pleural fluids.* These specimens can be collected very carefully only by the physician, but the nurse should prepare the sterile needles, test tubes and other accessories and she is responsible for proper labelling and despatching the specimen promptly to the laboratory.

(xi) *Cerebrospinal fluid* (CSF). The site for lumbar puncture should be disinfected with extreme care beforehand and covered with sterile gauze after the needle is withdrawn. This is the responsibility of the nurse. The lumbar puncture is always made by the physician. The nurse should know that CSF is used for the diagnosis of meningitis (caused by meningococci, pneumococci, streptococci or other organisms) and it is turbid. White blood cells or leucocytes can be counted if the fluid is clear or cloudy and the differential counts of cells is also possible from the smear of the sediment. Albumin or globulin content can also be determined chemically. Both number of cells and the protein content may be much increased although the fluid remains clear. This can differentiate paresis from other form of neurosyphilis. In suspected cases of syphilis, CSF can be used for serological tests.

Reporting of the Results of Laboratory Tests

The nurse should read *at first* the results of the laboratory report, if the patient is in hospital and there is any abnormality in the report it should be brought *at once* to the notice of the physician, because he visits once or twice a day and he depends on the information provided by the nurse during his absence. Abnormal findings in the laboratory report may provide some indications for better diagnosis and treatment of the patient. If this information is delayed, the physician may delay necessary treatment required for the speedy recovery of the patient. Therefore, the nursing student should acquire a sound knowledge during her training period to read the laboratory report, since she will become a fully responsible professional nurse in the hospital.

2. *Assisting the physician in the treatment.* The nurse is fully responsible to carry out very carefully

the orders given by the physician regarding the treatments and medicines. Particularly, while administrating the antibiotics or chemotherapeutic agents, she should observe very strictly the time interval indicated by the physician. If she does not stick to the time interval, there is possibility of low concentration of antibiotics or chemotherapeutic agents in the blood which may result, ultimately, in the development of drug resistant microorganisms. Multiple drug resistant strains of *Staph. aureus* are very common in the hospital, because of the insufficient use of the antibiotics in the infection. In addition to the duties carrying out the orders of the physician, nursing care of the patient (e.g., bath, care of the skin and general cleanliness) should be taken by the nurse, which is one of the most important supportive treatments for the speedy recovery. Hygienic measures can prevent fecal contamination of food which may enter the mouth; thus, the transmissible intestinal infection can be ultimately prevented. The nurse should report immediately to the physician the untoward symptoms noticed during the treatment.

3. *Assisting in the prevention of transmissible diseases.*

(a) Inhibition, destruction and removal of microorganisms; and

(b) Assisting in the immunisation programme in the community are two most important nursing responsibilities to prevent the transmissible diseases, knowledge gained during the nursing training will aid these nursing responsibilities. For example, the knowledge of the transmissibility of the infection will help to protect the population from the known cases of the infectious diseases. The nurse administrates the antigens (vaccines) and antibodies during the outbreak of the infectious diseases in the community. Besides, she educates the community in clear explicit language about the danger of the spread of the infections amongst the population, their prevention and other hygienic measures to combat the transmissible diseases in the community population, e.g., destruction of the microorganisms excreted through body fluids and discharges. The carriers of the disease can be detected and treated by assisting the physician. In case of the outbreak of intestinal infections like cholera, the feces should be disinfected or destroyed or disposed-off away from the human dwelling. The vectors (flies) should also be destroyed by the use of insecticides. Thus, it can be concluded that the nursing responsibilities in transmissible diseases are the application of the nursing microbiology knowledge.

COLLECTION OF SPECIMENS AND DIAGNOSIS OF DISEASE

Diagnosis is the determination of the exact nature of the disease. The laboratory contributes to this diagnosis by finding and identifying the specific pathogens. The laboratory diagnosis is reached by three general methods — microscopic examination of material, cultivation of material, and serological tests. All laboratory diagnosis depends upon the specimens collected and care and intelligence used in collecting them. Since the nurse is responsible for collecting many of the specimens and for sending them to the laboratory, she should learn how and why this is an important factor in diagnosis.

The purpose of this exercise is to acquaint the student with the collection of specimens and to set the stage for the rest of the work in the microbiology laboratory.

There are a few general rules that can be followed for all specimens; however, each hospital and laboratory will have its own rules and regulations.

The following are general rules :

1. Secure an uncontaminated specimen.
2. Label it fully and accurately.
3. Handle it with care to avoid infection.
4. See that the specimens reaches the laboratory promptly.

The types of specimens collected for laboratory diagnosis are :

(1) Pus, (2) Sputum,(3) Feces, (4) Urine, (5) Spinal fluid, (6) Peritoneal and pleural fluids, (7) Blood, (8) Cultures from nose, throat, etc.

MATERIALS NEEDED

1. Sterile applicator or swab in test tube
2. Tongue depressors
3. Blood agar plates
4. Laboratory sheets used to record finding in the microbiology laboratory.

PROCEDURE OR INSTRUCTIONS

1. The students should work in pairs. The bottom of a blood agar plate should be divided into 2 parts. Each student will take a throat culture of the other and streak a half of the plate for each student. The throat culture is done as follows : hold the tongue with the tongue depressor with a sterile applicator touch the back of the throat, being careful not to touch the teeth or tongue. Labelled, incubated and examined after 24 hours or next day.
2. The laboratory record sheets should be filled up.
3. Serology tests from the laboratory should be understood as to how these blood tests are done for diagnosis.

QUESTIONS

1. What is the role of nurses in collecting specimens?
2. How a specimen of sputum is collected?
3. Into what part of the vertebral column is the needle inserted to obtain cerebrospinal fluid?
4. For what diseases is this fluid examined?
5. What is a paracentesis?
6. What is obtained?
7. Why it is necessary to do this procedure?

SECTION 8

CHAPTER 62

LABORATORY TECHNIQUES

Introduction

The intelligent use of laboratory services is necessary for the practice of good clinical medicine. The help of the microbiological investigations is quite essential for the correct diagnosis of many diseases and the selection of a suitable antibiotic for the treatment of the patient; without the knowledge of *in vitro* antibiotic sensitivity of the causative microorganisms, it may not be possible to treat accurately. Before undertaking *in vitro* antibiotic sensitivity test of the causal agents of the diseases, it is of great necessity to isolate these agents in pure culture for their identification by the various morphological characteristics after staining them with the appropriate stains and by their biochemical properties.

Parts of Microscope. Simple magnifying glasses were in use in ancient times, but, later, the combinations of two or more lenses arranged in a tube — so that one lens magnifies the image produced by another — is used, as in the compound microscope. This kind of microscope was originally developed in 1602-1680 by a Jesuit scholar, Athanasuis Kircher.

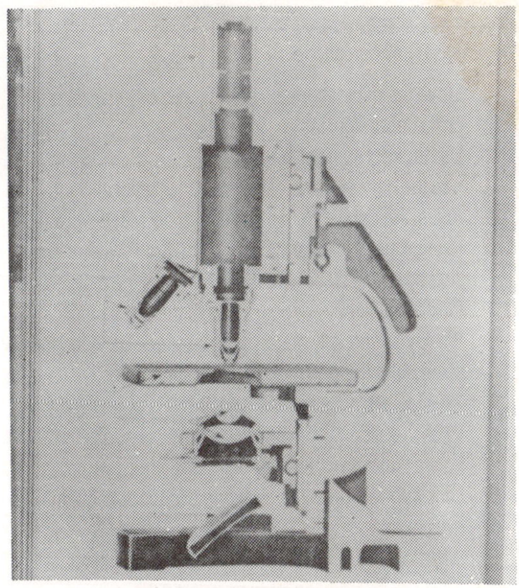

Fig. 62.1 : Microscope

The lens nearest to the object is known as the *objective.* The powerful microscope used in the microbiological laboratory has a very small objective lens with a very short focal distance. This lens should be very close to the object. The second lens, magnifying the image made by the objective, is some inches (cms.) above to the first lens. The eye is applied to the second lens which is called as *eyepiece* or *ocular.* Modern microscope has added accessory lenses — both objective and ocular — to make the image very clear and free from distortion, but the basic principles remain the same. The highest magnification given by an ordinary objective is about 90 x. This image is magnified by a 10 x ocular, giving a total enlargement of the image of 900 x. A good microscope with several combinations of object and ocular, giving total magnification of varying from 50 - 2,000 x are now available. A strong source of light is provided by a mirror by reflecting the light upwards through the object. A sub-stage condenser has a system of lenses, between the mirror and the object, which collects the light rays and brings them to focus on the objects so that the object is well-illuminated. An iris diaphragm is also included with the condensor to adjust the light.

The object mounted on a glass slide is placed on the flat metal plate/stage, which is between the condenser and the object. To correct the focal distance, the wheels are raised or lowered so that the object is focused. Large wheel for *coarse adjustment* and small wheel for fine adjustments are used. A *mechanical stage* can hold the slide in position and move the slide to various directions.

Oil immersion lens. The object lens commonly used in the microbiology laboratory to study the bacteria, is an *oil-immersion objective* (100 x) Fig. 62.1.

KEY STEPS	IMPORTANT POINTS
(A) *Focusing a Microscope:*	
1. Move the microscope so that it is directly in front of you on the laboratory table.	1. In-order to finish the assigned exercises, it is desirable that students learn how to focus an object with a microscope.
2. Use indirect sunlight or light.	2. Students who are beginning to use a microscope may have serious accidents with spilling of moist materials on a microscope if they tilt the body tube.
3. Use the concave side of the mirror for artificial light.	3. The body tube of a microscope is never tilted when using the oil immersion objectives. Experienced workers may tilt the body tube when examining dry preparations.
4. Adjust the condenser so that it is close with the stage.	4. The instructor will be able to determine if major or minor adjustments need to be made.
5. Using clips or the mechanical stage hold the slide to be studied on the stage so that the centre of the material on the slide is directly over the lens of the condenser.	5. Liquids or dirt on the stage may be transferred to the lenses. This might result in serious power damage to the microscope.
6. While you carefully observe the distance between the tip of the objective and the slide, lower the objective toward the slide. Do not allow the tip of the any objective to touch the slide.	6. Lens paper is a very fine paper which will not scratch or damage sensitive lenses. If dry lens paper may be moistened with a xylol to facilitate cleaning.
7. Focus first with low power objective whenever possible.	7. The oil immersion lens on the longest objective gives the highest magnification. The high magnification of the oil immersion objective is made possible because the oil used has almost the same power of refraction as the glass of the lens.
8. Look through the ocular with one eye while keeping both eyes open.	8. Tough while the microscope appears to be a sturdy instrument, it is a delicate, precise piece of equipment which has been assembled with extreme care.
9. While looking through the ocular, move the objective slowly away from the slide by turning the coarse adjustment screw *counterclockwise.*	9. The high dry and oil immersion objectives do not have a stop and may be damaged by accidental contact with the substage condenser.
10. When the object is focused as well as possible with the coarse adjustment screw, adjust and sharpen the focus further with the fine adjustment screw.	10. Covering a microscope protects it from unnecessary dust and dirt.
11. After you have focused the object.	11. The two arms of the base should be pointing away from you at right angles with the edge of the table.
12. Clearly with low power objective, turn the high power objective into position by moving it into place over the slide.	12. Indirect sunlight reflected from the clouds is the most acceptable source of light for microscope work.
13. To use the oil immersion lens for focusing raise the objective from the slide. Place a drop of immersion oil on the slide swing the oil immersion objective into place and by turning the coarse objective screw lower the tip of this objective into the drop of oil.	13. The concave mirror reflects the greatest number of light rays through the condenser. The light is optimum when a clear uniform circle of light is visible when you are looking through the ocular. Experience is needed in judging the optimum light requirements for microscopic work.
14. While looking into the ocular focus away from the slide slowly by turning the fine adjustment screw.	
15. Observe your slides with careful thought for detail.	
16. After you have completed your observation with the oil immersion lens screw the coarse adjustment to raise the objective from the stage and wipe the excess oil from the lens of the objective with dry lens paper.	
17. Put your microscope away in clean and good condition.	

KEY STEPS	IMPORTANT POINTS
(B) *Care of the Microscope* 1. Learn the essential points about the use of a microscope. 2. Keep the body of the microscope in a perpendicular position. 3. If your microscope is not functioning properly, report it to your instructor. 4. Keep the stage clean and dry. 5. Clean lenses with lens paper only. 6. Use special immersion oil with the oil immersion lens. 7. Carry each microscope with two hands. 8. Place the microscope on the desk gently. 9. When you leave a microscope, clean all lenses that you have used. 10. When you leave a microscope, place the low objective in position over the opening in the stage. 11. When you finish using the microscope, return to its case or cover it with a plastic protector.	14. When condenser is in this position the maximum amount of light is focused through microscope. 15. By placing the slide in this position you will be most likely to have the material you want to study in the correct position for focusing. 16. The lenses of objectives may be badly scratched if they contact a glass slide. While this precaution is not as essential when using the low power objective or when using important to develop habits so that you will observe the distance between the objective and the slide. After you have developed these habits you will never look in the ocular while the objective is moving toward the slide. 17. The low power objective gives you the smallest magnification (usually by using the smallest magnification first you can most easily adjust your thinking from a picture of gross to microscopic structure). When using the low power objective the object comes into focus when the lens of the objective is about 16 mm from the slide. 18. Closing one eye while working with a microscope may result in eye strain. 19. If you turn the coarse adjustment screw too rapidly, you will be likely to pass the focus of the object without seeing it. If you pass the point where the object comes into focus, you will have to lower the objective by looking at the relationship between tip of the objective as described in above No. 17. 20. This movement with the fine adjustment screw is not visible with naked eye but must be remembered when the objective is close to the slide. 21. You will need to remember that changing from a low magnification to a high magnification decreases the diameter of the material that you will see. Therefore, it is important that the particular material that you want to see with a higher magnification is in the center of the field as you see it with a lower magnification. 22. You should always observe the distance between the tip of the oil immersion objective downward. 23. If you miss the object by going beyond the focal distance and the objective is above the drop of oil, you must lower the objective again into the oil as explained in 13 and 14 above key steps of care of microscope. 24. After making careful observation draw what you have seen. 25. If non hardening oil is used cleaning with dry lens paper is usually sufficient. 26. See 9, 10 and 11 under Care of Microscope.

THE USE AND CARE OF THE MICROSCOPE

Objectives :

1. To introduce the student to the effectiveness of the microscope as a laboratory tool.
2. To demonstrate the correct ways of using a microscope.
3. To help the student to understand the precautions that must be taken to protect the microscope from damage.

Electron microscopy can be used to study the extremely minute objects and the inner, minute structure of bacteria and viruses. It makes possible magnification up to 300,000 diameters. Visible light consists of spectrum of electromagnetic waves with wave lengths ranging from about 4000 Angstrom units (Violet) to about 77,000 A° (Red), — A° = 1,000,000 mm. or 0.001 μ. Angstrom was a famous Swedish physicist.

Objects smaller than bacteria do not reflect such long waves to the eye in a clear pattern (i.e., are not resolved) and are, therefore, not clearly visible. Electrons create electromagnetic waves of very much shorter length (about 0.05 A°) and when focused magnetically as in electron microscope are capable of *resolving* objects much smaller than even the smallest bacteria of rickettsiae, particularly viruses and their internal structures. Electron waves are not visible to the human eye just as ultraviolet rays. The magnified image produced by electron beam in an electron microscope must, therefore, be viewed on a fluorescent screen similar to that used in clinical X-ray fluoroscopy, photographs of the images can be enlarged and are called as *electronographs*. There are other types of microscopes.

COMMON LABORATORY MEDIA

For rapid multiplication of bacteria in the laboratory, following growth requirements must be provided :

(a) Food — Most pathogenic bacteria require food as source of organic carbon and nitrogen;,

(b) Moisture—Since bacterial cell consists of water, moisture is essential for its growth;

(c) Temperature — For each species, there is a maximum and minimum temperature at which the growth is possible. The optimum temperature for most pathogenic bacteria is 37°C;

(d) Reaction — Like temperature, there is an optimum pH for each species. Usually most pathogens grow well at neutral or slightly alkaline pH (7.2);

(e) Oxygen — Certain bacteria grow in presence of molecular oxygen and are called as 'aerobes'; others, called as "anaerobes", will grow only in absence of oxygen.

Preparation of culture media. In the laboratory, bacteria can grow on "culture media" which are mixtures of suitable food materials required for bacterial growth. After preparation the pH of the media is adjusted by pH meter or comparator (Fig. 62.2) to 7.2 to 7.4. Prepared media are sterilised by autoclave and poured in Petri dish (plate), test tubes, flasks etc. They are incubated to check the sterility and finally they are stored in the refrigerator. For general application, the media are prepared from the base — peptone water (containing peptone, sodium chloride, water) — to which meat extract, blood, serum has been added. For solidifying the media, the agar or gelatin is added.

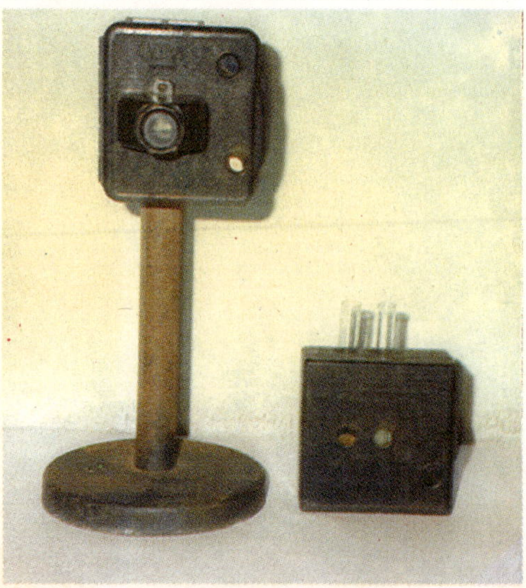

Fig. 62.2 : pH Comparator

COMMON LABORATORY MEDIA	
A. Liquid (broth)	B. Solid (agar)
(i) Peptone water.	1. Nutrient agar.
(ii) Nutrient broth.	2. Blood agar.
(iii) Glucose broth.	3. Chocolate agar.
(iv) Sugar medium.	4. Tellurite chocolate agar.
(v) Urea medium.	5. Loeffler serum.
(vi) Glycerolsaline.	6. Dorset's egg medium.
(vii) Cary Blair medium.	7. Lowensten Jensen medium
(viii) Stuart medium.	8. MacConkey agar medium.
(ix) V. R. medium.	9. Wilson and Blair medium.
	10. Robertson's cooked meat medium.
	11. Litmus milk medium.
	12. TSI medium.
	13. Simmon's citrate medium.

1. *Peptone Water.* Contains 1% peptone and 0.5% sodium chloride dissolved in water. It does not contain meat extract. The medium is colourless. Peptone water is used to study proteolytic activity of bacteria, viz; formation of indole and hydrogen sulphide (H_2S.) Motility of bacteria is best studied from peptone water culture; peptone water is used as a base for sugar media.

2. *Nutrient Broth.* It is a pale yellow coloured liquid. The first step is to prepare the meat extract. This is done by extracting meat in cold with water. It is then heated to coagulate the dissolved proteins and filtered. The filtrate is the required meat extract. Peptone and sodium chloride are added to the above for preparation of nutrient broth. It is sterilised by autoclaving. It is a common fluid medium for non-fastidious organisms and serves as a base for preparation of solid media.

3. *Glucose Broth* is a pale yellow liquid which contains basically nutrient broth to which one per cent glucose is added. It is mainly used to grow anaerobic streptococci.

4. *Sugar Media.* Various carbohydrates, alcohols etc. (designated as 'SUGAR') are fermented by bacteria with the formation of acid or acid and gas. Sugar media are used to study these fermentation reactions. Appropriate sugars are added to peptone water in the proportion of one per cent. A suitable indicator is also incorporated to detect the formation of acid. Usually Andrade's indicator is used, which is colourless in alkaline and neutral pH and turns pink in presence of acid. To detect the production of gas, a small tube (Durham tube) is placed in an inverted position in the medium. The air is replaced by fluid during sterilisation by heat.

Gas, if produced, is seen as a bubble at the top of the Durham tube. The sugar media are sterilised in a steam steriliser at 100°C for 20 minutes on THREE SUCCESSIVE DAYS. The common sugar media are Glucose, Sucrose, Lactose, Mannite, and Dulcitol. Note the coloured plugs to differentiate them (Glucose; Blue; Sucrose White. Mannite, Pink; Lactose, red; Du citol, Yellow).

5. *Urea medium.* It contains peptone, sodium chloride, glucose, buffer, 20% urea, phenol red, pH 6.8 - 6.9. After inoculation heavily with cultures and incubation at 37°C for 4 hrs, and then overnight, urease positive cultures produce purple pink colour due to a change in the colour of the indicator. Thus, urease producing organisms are identified.

6. *Glycerol saline Transport medium.* This medium contains glycerol, sodium chloride, buffer, phenol red, water. It is used to transport enteric bacilli to the laboratory. This fluid should not be used if it becomes acid, indicated by a change in colour to yellow.

7. *Cary Blair medium.* This is a buffered solution of sodium chloride, sodium thioglycollate, disodium phosphate and calcium chloride at 8.4. It is a suitable transport medium for *Vibrio cholerae.* At pH 7.4, it can be used to transport Salmonella, Shigella and Campylobacter.

8. *Stuart's transport medium* is composed of anaerobic salt solution, methylene blue, agar 0.6% pH 7.3 - 7.4. This is soft agar medium used to maintain the viability of gonococci on swabs during transport to the laboratory.

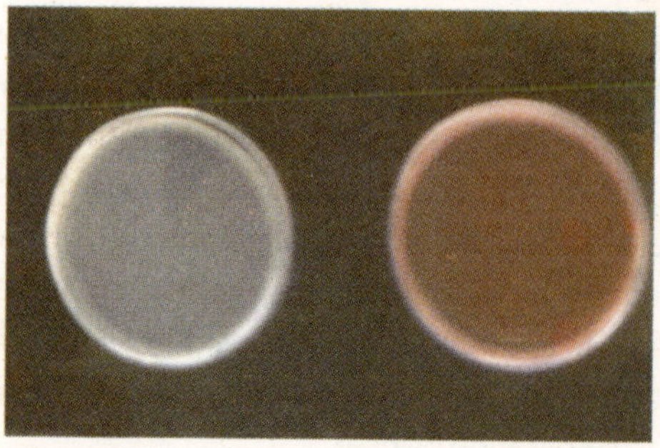

↬ **Fig. 62.3 :** (Left) Nutrient Agar
↬ **Fig. 62.4 :** (Right) Mac Conkey Agar

9. *Venkatraman-Ramakrishnan* (VR) medium. A simple modified form of this medium is prepared by dissolving 20 g. Crude sea salt and 5 g. peptone in one liter of distilled water and adjusting the pH to 8.6 - 8.8. It is dispensed in screw-capped bottles in 10 - 15 ml amount.

About 1 - 3 ml stool is to be added to each bottle. In this medium *Vibrio Cholerae* do not multiply, but remain viable for several weeks.

1. *Nutrient Agar* is prepared by adding agar to nutrient broth in proportion of 2 to 3 percent. The broth is put in the steamer to dissolve the agar. The agar broth fluid is filtered hot if necessary and autoclaved. It becomes solid when cooled. The medium is almost transparent. It is a common — purpose solid medium for growth of non-fastidious organisms, further it serves as a base for the 'Enriched media' (Fig. 62.3).

2. *Blood Agar* is prepared by adding defibrinated or citrated blood to nutrient agar in the proportion of 5 to 10 per cent. Blood is collected aseptically and added to the already sterilised nutrient agar which has been melted and cooled to about 55°C. The medium is used for the cultivation of fastidious organisms which fail to grow on nutrient agar.

3. *Chocolate Agar* is prepared by adding, the defibrinated blood, heated to 55°C, in the proportion of 5 to 10 per cent, to sterilised nutrient agar which has been melted and cooled to 55°C. It is opaque brown in appearance.

This medium is used for the cultivation of gonococci and meningococci which form greyish colonies.

4. *Tellurite Chocolate Agar.* It is heated blood agar to which potassium tellurite (0.04%) has been added. It inhibits the growth of many commensel organisms likely to be present in the throat but not the diphtheria bacilli and related organisms. Moreover these latter organisms form grey or black colonies on the medium as they reduce potassium tellurite. The medium is opaque brown in appearance.

5. *Loeffler's Serum.* Consists of human or animal serum added to Glucose broth. The collection of blood and separation of serum are carried out with aseptic precautions. The medium is solidified by inspissation. The medium is opaque white in appearance. It is mostly used for cultivation of the diphtheria bacillus. It can be employed to study proteolytic activity of bacteria (liquefaction of serum).

6. *Dorset's Egg Medium* is prepared by inspissating a mixture of whole egg fluid 3 part and saline 1 part. The medium is yellow and opaque. When glycerinated, the medium is used for cultivation of tubercle bacilli; without glycerine it is useful for the preservation of stock cultures of enteric bacilli.

7. *Lowenstein Jensen Medium :* It contains a number of mineral salt, glycerine, starch, egg proteins and malachite green. The last is a bactericidal agent. This medium is used for the cultivation of tubercle bacilli.

8. *MacConkey Medium.* (Bile salt lactose Neutral red agar). It is used for the isolation of intestinal pathogens. Bile salt inhibits the growth of Gram-positive cocci. Pathogenic Gram-negative enteric bacilli (Salmonella, Shigella) do not ferment lactose and form pale colonies. *Escherichia coli* (which are mostly commensels), on the other hand, ferment lactose producing acid and, therefore, their colonies are pink. The medium is thus both an inhibitory and differentiating one. A number of media are described which work on the same principles, viz., D.E.C. medium of Punja and Ghosh and Leifson's desoxycholate citrate medium etc. They differ from the basic medium described above in containing inhibitory substances other than bile salt. All appear reddish brown and transparent (Fig. 62.4).

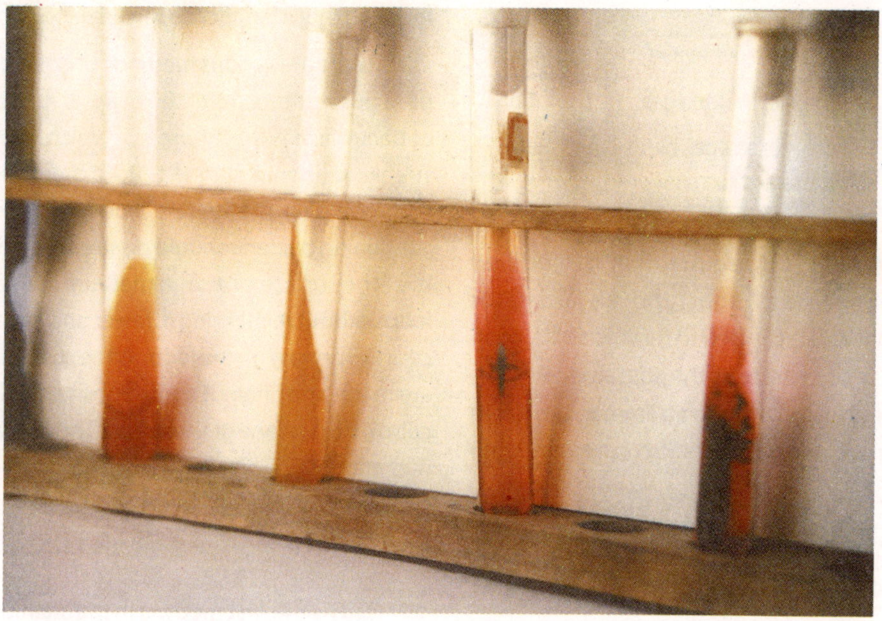

Fig. 62.5 : Triple Sugar Iron medium

9. *Wilson and Blair Medium.* This medium is utilised for isolation of typhoid and paratyphoid organisms from heavily contaminated material like sewage. It contains sodium sulphate, Bismuth ammonium citrate and brilliant green. The last even inhibits *Escherichia coli*. Typhoid and paratyphoid organisms form black colonies as they reduce to sulphate to sulphide in presence of glucose precipitating insoluble bismuth sulphide (which is black). It is also a differentiating and inhibitory medium.

10. *Robertson's Cooked Meat Medium.* Minced meat is boiled in alkaline water. Softened meat is then partially dried between folds of filter paper and added to nutrient broth. The medium is autoclaved for sterilisation. The medium is used for cultivation of anaerobic organisms.

11. *Litmus Milk Medium* is prepared by adding litmus solution to skimmed milk. The medium is autoclaved or boiled for sterilisation. It is used for studying proteolytic and saccharolytic activity *of Clostridium welchii.*

12. *Thiosulphate Citrate Bile Salt Sucrose (TCBS) Medium.* This medium containing thiosulphate, citrate, bile salt, bromothymol blue and sucrose is available commercially and is very widely used at present. *Vibrio Cholerae* produce large yellow convex colonies which may become green on continued incubation.

13. *Triple Sugar Iron (TSI).* This medium contains glucose, lactose and sucrose, phenol red indicator (to indicate fermentation), ferrous sulphate (to demonstrate H_2S, indicated by blackening of the butt). It is orange red when uninoculated. It is used to identify the enterobacteriacae. The glucose concentration is 1/10th of concentration of lactose and sucrose so to detect the fermentation of glucose alone. The small amount of acid produced by fermentation of glucose is oxidised rapidly in the slant which reverts to alkaline (red); in contrast, under lower O_2 tension in the butt, the acid reaction (yellow) is maintained. Free exchange of air may be permitted in the slant through the use of loose cotton plug to promote oxidation of acid produced by glucose fermentation in the slant. This reaction should be read after 24 hrs. incubation (Fig. 62.5).

Interpretation of Reaction

Reaction	Carbohydrate fermented	Organism
Acid butt.	Glucose with acid and gas.	*Esch. Coli.*
Alkaline slant.	Glucose with acid gas but not lactose and sucrose.	Proteus.

14. *Simmons' Citrate medium* is modified Koser's medium with agar and an indicator (bromothymol blue). It is used to test the ability of an organism to utilise citrate as the sole source of carbon and energy for growth and an ammonium salt as the sole source of nitrogen. It is also called as citrate utilisation test.

Result :

Positive = Blue colour and growth of bacteria.

Negative = Original green colour and no growth.

Both Wilson Blair and Lowenstein Jensen media are green. Wilson Blair, however, is usually poured in Petri dishes whereas Lowenstein Jensen medium has to be kept in screw capped bottles or tubes with paraffinised plugs.

Agar Agar. It is a polysaccharide prepared from a sea-weed grown on the Japanese and Chinese sea coasts. It is available in dry strands or in powder forms. It has no nutrient property and is used for solidifying the media. It does not set till it is cooled to 42°C. Therefore, blood, serum etc. can be added to nutrient agar at 55°C at which temperature the medium is still fluid and there is no risk of denaturation of the serum proteins added.

Inoculation of Culture Media

In clinical specimens (feces, sputum etc.), mixtures of microorganisms are very common. It is a *mixed culture*. In the microbiological laboratory, to study a causative agent of the particular disease, it is necessary to inoculate the specimens into the media and fish out a single bacterium from the *pure culture* for its further identification in the laboratory.

There are various methods of isolation of bacteria in pure culture (refer the chapter no 8 of isolation of bacteria in pure culture). Of which, the plating or streaking (inoculation of culture media) is the most common easy method — "Specimens or materials containing bacteria should be streaked several times over the surface of a solid medium with a platinum loop without recharging it; fewer and fewer bacterial cells will remain on the loop, as the successive streaks are made and finally it may deposit a single bacterial cell on the surface of the media. Thus separate colonies are obtained."

PREPARATION OF A SMEAR FOR STAINING

This is the first method in the staining of bacteria. Smears are made on a clean, grease-free, dry slide. For examining a culture on a solid medium, the required colony is touched with the tip of a platinum loop or wire and a small loopful of the material thus removed is mixed with a drop of water or normal saline to give a faint turbidity. Then the drop is spread into a thin film and allowed to dry in air or by gently warming over the flame. If the culture for examination be in a fluid medium, a drop of the medium is removed with the platinum loop and a film is prepared from it directly. Similarly, smears are prepared out of any fluid material like sputum, pus etc., collected from a patient.

At last, the smears are "fixed" by passing them through a flame four to five times. The fixation kills the bacteria and — by coagulating any protein contained in the preparations, makes the bacteria to adhere firmly to the slide (Fig. 62.6).

GRAM'S STAIN

1. The fixed smear is covered with Oxalated gentian violet; allow the stain to act for one minute.

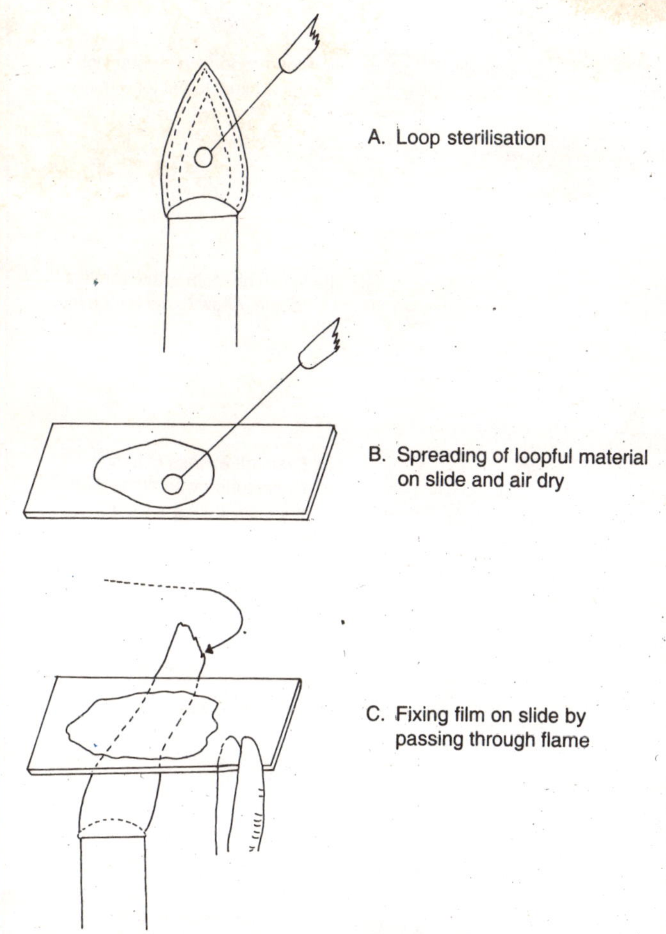

Fig. 62.6: Preparation of smear for staining

2. Pour off excess of the stain, holding the slide at an angle downwards, wash away the remain of the stain with water and add Gram's Iodine. Allow Gram's Iodine to act for *THREE* minutes.
3. Wash off Iodine with Ethyl alcohol, and continue with fresh alcohol drop by drop, until no more violet colour is removed from the film. This step is called *decolourisation.*
4. Wash with tap water.
5. Counterstain with safranin for *ONE* minute. Safranin stains only those bacteria which have completely decolourised by alcohol.
6. Wash with tap water and dry the smear between blotting paper. See that the smear is completely dry.
7. Examine under oil immersion lens (Fig. 62.7).

RESULT. With Gram's bacteria can be divided into two large groups:

1. Gram-positive; and
2. Gram-negative.

Gram positive bacteria retain gentian violet stain despite decolourisation and stained *violet.* Gram-*negative* bacteria loose completely the violet stain after decolourisation with alcohol and stain *red* by the counterstain, Safranin.

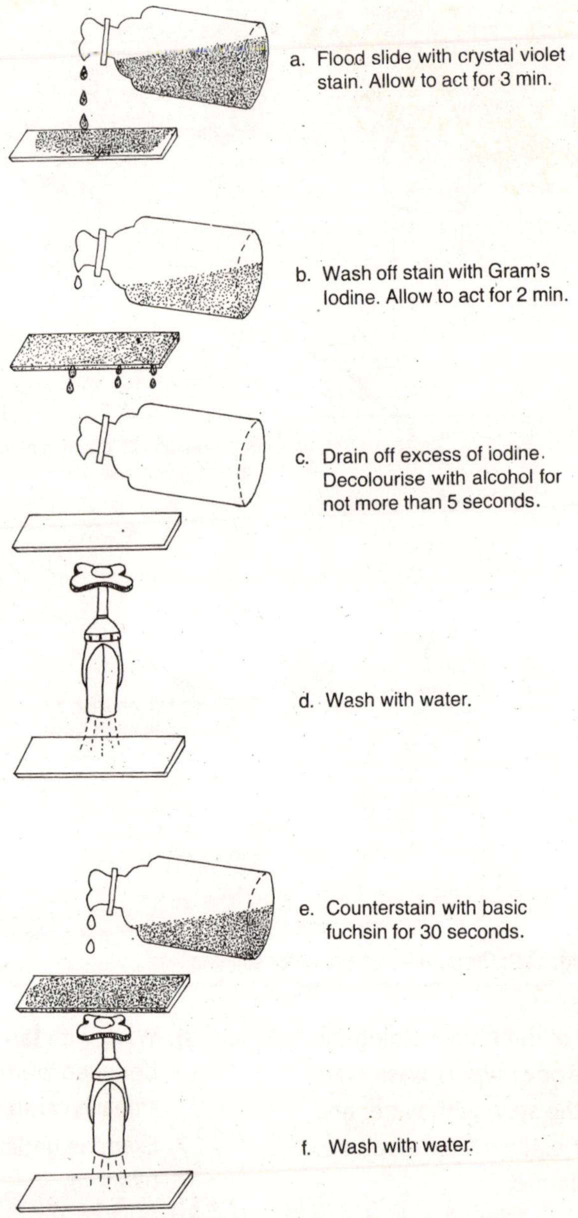

Fig. 62.7 : Gram Staining

Table : Classification of common bacteria according to their reaction to Gram stain

Gram-positive	***Gram-negative***
Bacillus subtilis	Pseudomonas
Bacillus anthracis	Salmonella
Clostridium tetani	Proteus
Clostridium welchii	Shigella **Contd.**
Staphylococci	*Escherchia coli*
Streptococci	*Vibrio cholerae*
Pneumococci	*Brucella abortus*
Mycobacterium tuberculosis	*Neisseria meningitidis*
Corynebacterium diphtheriale and diphtheroids.	*Neissera gonorrhoae*

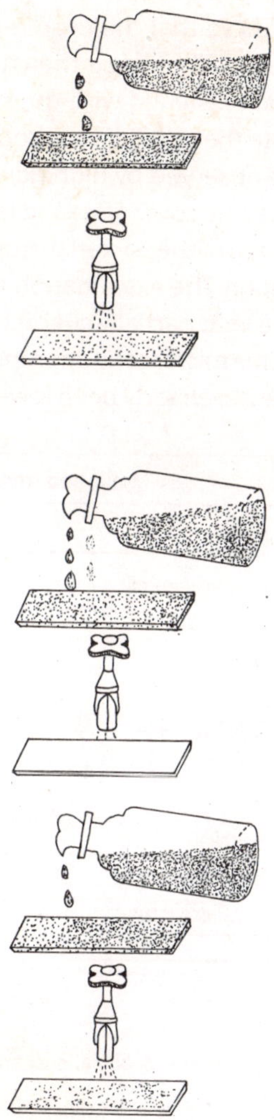

Fig. 62.8 : Ziehl Neelsen method

ZIEHL-NEELSEN (ZN) STAIN

Cell wall of certain bacteria (i.e., *Mycobacterium tuberculosis*) contains wax like substance known as "mycolic acid". Hence, these bacteria cannot be easily stained by Gram's stain. Heat or prolonged contact is required to drive the stain into the bacterial cells; once stained, they are not decolourised by mineral acids. They are called "acid fast bacilli" (AFB). So Ziehl-Neelsen stain has been devised to study their morphology microscopically :

1. Cover the fixed smear with carbol fuchsin. Now heat the smear gently from below till steam rises.
2. Allow the stain to act for *FIVE* minutes and, during this time, steam twice again. The stain must not be allowed to evaporate and dry on the smear.
3. Wash the smear well with tap water for *TWO* minutes.
4. Pour on the slide 20% H_2SO_4 from drop bottle. The red colour of the smear be-

comes yellowish brown. After ONE minute wash with tap water. If the red colour returns, pour acid again. The decoloursation is continued till, after washing, the film is only faint pink.

5. Wash well with tap water TWO minutes.
6. Counterstain with Methylene blue for 30 seconds.
7. Wash with tap water ONE minute and blot and dry.
8. Examine with oil immersion lens (Fig. 62.8).

Thus with Ziehl-Neelsen stain, acid fast bacilli (tubercle bacilli) are stained pink. Non-acid fast bacilli lose the pink colour by treatment with mineral acid and take the counterstain. They are stained blue.

Hanging Drop Method (for the study of motillty of bacteria)

Method. Take a "hollow ground glass slide" and cover the surface around the hallow with a thin layer of vaseline. By means of platinum loop which has already been sterilised by flaming, place a drop of bacterial suspension in the centre of a clean cover glass. The slide is then gently lowered on the cover glass so that the drop remains undisturbed in the hollow. The slide is then turned over and the drop is first examined with the low power objective to locate the edge of the drop. Then the motility should be observed by high power objective. The vaseline fixes the cover glass and tends to prevent the evaporation of the bacterial drop during prolonged observation. The examination should be performed with the light partially cut off, i.e., with the iris diaphragm of the microscope appropriately closed, after the condenser already been lowered down (Fig. 62.9).

Motile and Non-motile Bacteria

Motile	*Non-motile*
Escherichia coli	Shigella
Salmonella	*Mycobacterium tuberculosis*
Vibrio	*Corynebacterium diphtheriae*
Pseudomonas	and diphtheroids.
Spirillum	All cocci (Staphylococci,
Treponema	Streptococci, Meningococci,
Leptospira	Gonococci, Pneumococci)
Borrelia	*Clostridium welchii*
Clostridium tetani	*Bacillus anthracis*
Bacillus subtilis	

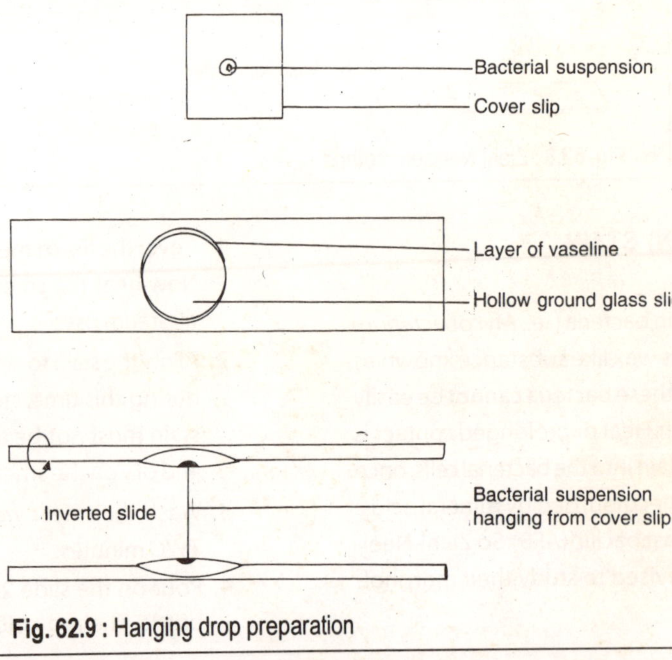

Fig. 62.9 : Hanging drop preparation

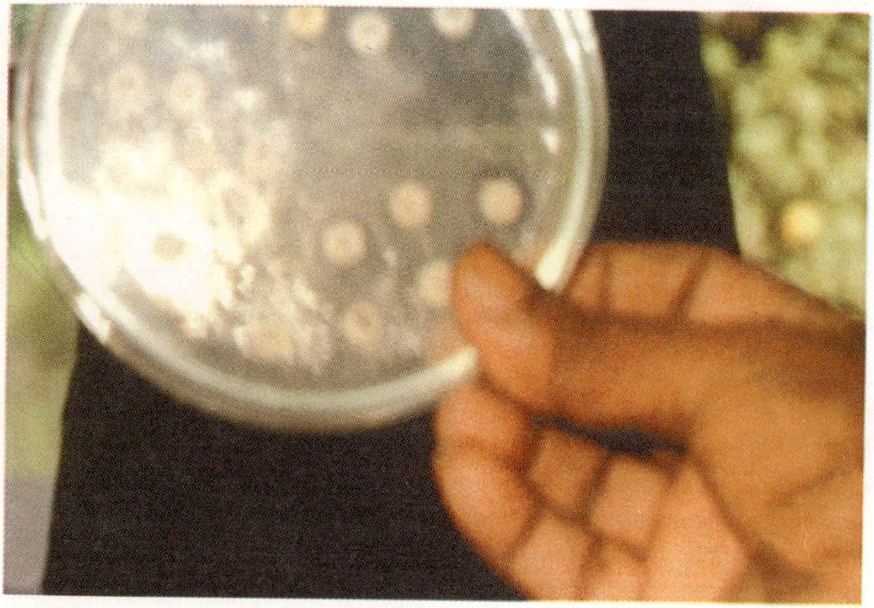

Fig.62.10: Antibiotic sensitivity test

Antibiotic Sensitivity Test

Subcultures of the test organisms are made in broth and incubated for 6 - 18 hours. Any density of inoculum may be used but, in most cases, the surfaces of cultures plates may be sown with broth containing approximately 100 million cells per ml. After drying the surface, the previously prepared disks of filter paper saturated with various concentrations of antibiotics are applied, the plates are incubated and the zone of inhibition is measured. A zone of inhibition of growth around the disk may indicate that the antimicrobial agent is either bactericidal. (S = bacteria are sensitive) or merely bacteriostatic (R R = bacteria are relatively resistant) or bacteria are resistant (R = resistant). If the test organism is not resistant to the antibiotic, zones of complete inhibition of the growing organism are found around the disks containing the effective antibiotic (Fig.62.10).

Culture and sensitivity test report of diagnostic microbiological laboratory.

Culture-organism isolated. *Staphylococcus aureus*

Sensitivity. Penicillin — R
Tetracycline — S
Gentamycin — S
Streptomycin — R R

(R = resistant; S = sensitive; RR = relatively resistant).

SEROLOGY

Serology is the study of reaction between antigen and antibody and is grouped broadly as follows:

1. Agglutination (in which particulate antigen is involved); and

2. Precipitation (in which soluble antigen is involved).

1. *Agglutination*	2. *Precipitation*
(a) Widal test	(a) VDRL test
(b) Weil-Felix test	(b) Kahn test
(c) Brucellosis test	(c) Wassermann test (complement fixation)
(d) Cold agglutination test	(d) Agar gel precipitation test (counter immunoelectro-phoresis)
(e) Paul-Bunnel test	(e) Fluorescent antibody test
(f) Rose Waaler test or test for Rheumatoid arthritis	

(g) Latex agglutination test for Rheumatoid arthritis
(h) Coombs' test

(f) Antinuclear factor test
(g) Antitoxin toxin neutralisation test (Skin tests)
(h) Antistreptolysin-O titre.
(i) Reverse passive hemagglutination (RPHA) test
(j) Enzyme Linked Immunosorbent Assay (ELISA) test
(k) Western Blot test (ELISA and Western Blot are used respectively, to screen and confirm AIDS)

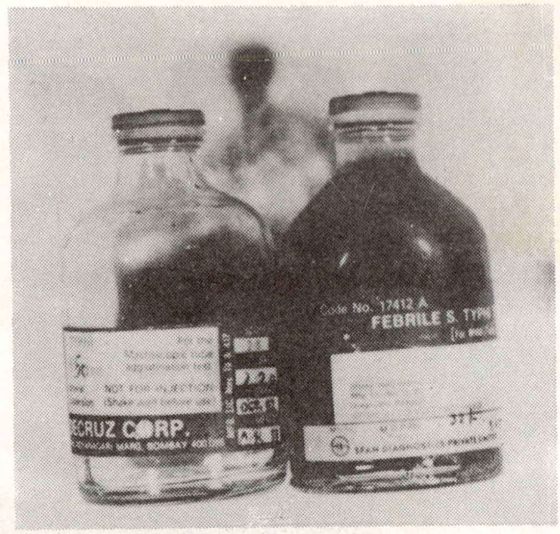

Fig. 62.11: Widal antigen in bottle

1. Agglutination

Serological techniques are of considerable importance in identifying unknown antigens and detecting the presence of antibody in the serum of infected or immunised subjects.

Agglutination tests are performed by mixing a serial dilution of antiserum with a suspension of bacterial cells or particles. These methods are used to examine sera for antibodies against Salmonella and Brucella and, using standard antisera to identify the unknown organisms.

The basic principle of the techniques of agglutination tests in enteric fever (typhoid or paratyphoid) is to examine the serum *quantitatively* for agglutinin towards a particular organism. For this purpose, the method usually adopted is to mix varying dilutions of serum (made up in saline solution) in narrow tubes with a fixed quantity of a uniform and stable suspension of the organism or its antigen. These mixtures are kept at 37°C or 50 - 55°C in a water bath for a certain length of time and then examined for *visible* agglutination of the suspension. The agglutinated antigens tend to sediment and the reaction can also be evaluated by the amount of deposit in the tubes and the clarity of the supernatant fluid. The strength can be stated in terms of the highest dilutions (titers) that produce the agglutination.

The measuring titer. The titer of an antiserum is the number of antibody units per unit volume of the original serum; thus if the last tube, showing a reaction, e.g., agglutination, contains 1 ml volume and is a dilution of 1 : 128 of the original serum, the titer of the serum is 128 units of antibody per ml of the serum.

At least, 5 ml of blood should be obtained by vein puncture and the blood is immediately transferred from the syringe to a dry well-stoppered sterile bottle or tube and allowed to clot; when the serum has separated, it is pipetted off into a sterile tube.

(a) Widal test

In the routine laboratory diagnostic Widal reaction, the patient's serum is tested simultaneously with the antigen of each organism likely to be responsible for enteric fever in the particular region, e.g., *Salmonella typhi* or *S. paratyphi* A or B or C. Additional information can be obtained by testing separately for H and O agglutinins. Thus, Widal test generally involves parallel tests with different Salmonella group of organisms and also different forms of the same organism.

In addition to the test with typhoid-paratyphoid organisms, it is the practice of many laboratories to test also for *Brucella melitensis* agglutinins and, if considered necessary, with non-motile strains of proteus ox19, ox2 and oxk for typhus fever, thus increas-

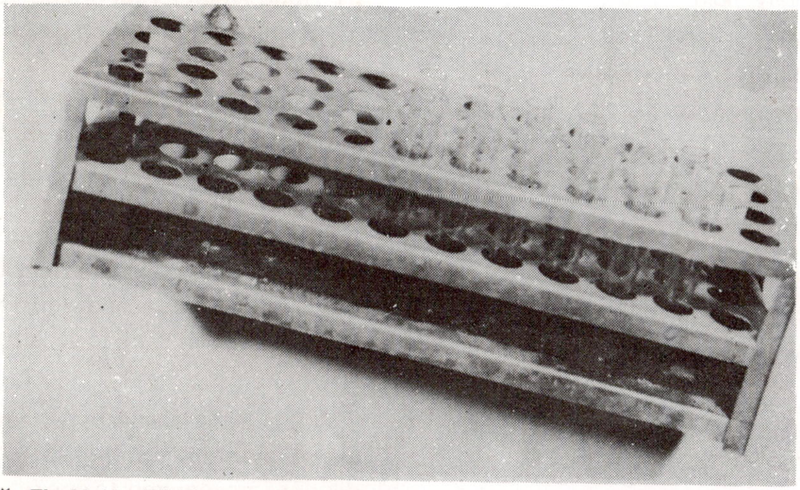

Fig.62.11a: Widal tube agglutination test

ing the number of parallel tests. This is called as "Triple Widal".

Master (1 : 15) dilution of the patient's serum is first prepared, thereafter a series of doubling dilutions are made in narrow tubes. Then, 0.4 ml of the bacterial antigen is added in each tube.

To observe H type (loose cotton wool) agglutination, it is usually sufficient to incubate at 37°C for 2 hours and leave for half an hour at room temperature. "Large flake" clumping or agglutination can easily be detected with naked eye. The flocculi can also sediment rapidly and the deposit is quite perceptible in the narrow tube (Dreyer's tube).

Compact agglutination of O type settles down in round bottom tubes (Felix tubes) kept in the first row of test tube rack and its readings should be made after 4 and 24 hours of incubation as these forms of reactions develop slowly. The control tube contains saline only. The clumps are small, granular, and visible with the help of hand lens.

O agglutination is always positive as O antigen is common to all Salmonella. If O and H agglutinations are positive, then it is diagnosed as Typhoid since the causative agent, *S. typhi* contains both O and H antigens.

If AH agglutination is positive, then it is considered as paratyphoid caused by *S. paratyphi* A.

Widal test report of diagnostic laboratory.

I. For *Typhoid*

	Titer	
S. *typhi* O	— 1 : 60	Typhoid (Positive)
S. *typhi* H	— 1 : 240	

S. paratyphi A— Negative

S. paratyphi B — Negative

S. paratyphi C — Negative

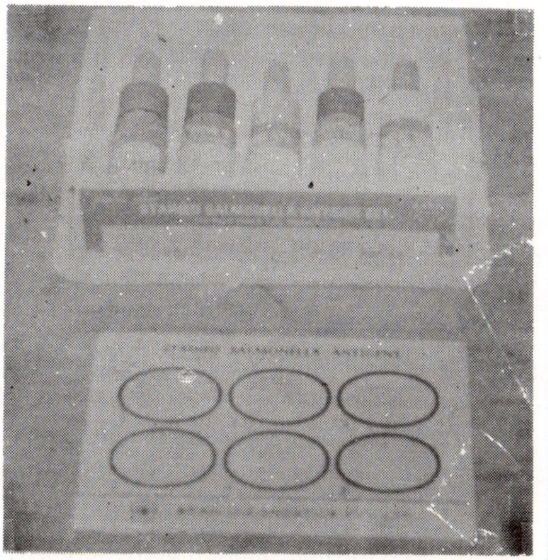

Fig.62.11b: Widal plate agglutination test

II. For *Paratyphoid*

S. *typhi* O	—	1 : 60
S. *typhi* H	—	Negative
S. paratyphi A	—	1 : 120 Paratyphoid by S. paratyphi A - positive
S. paratyphi B	—	Negative
S. paratyphi C	—	Negative (Fig. 62.11a, b)

The same agglutination techniques of Widal test are also applicable to diagnose brucellosis, typhus fever in man. A titer of 1 : 40 or 80 International Units (IU) per ml. is considered positive for Brucellosis (c) and a titer of 200 or a peak titer of 1,000 - 5,000 is positive for Typhus fever (b).

(d) Cold Agglutination Test

In cases of primary atypical pneumonia caused by *Mycoplasma hominis,* the serum may agglutinate at low temperature group O human red blood cells. To a series of doubling dilutions of patient's serum (1 : 8 to 1 : 2,048) an equal volume of 0.2 per cent of suspension of washed group O human erythrocytes is added. The mixtures are kept in the refrigerator at 0° - 4°C overnight. Agglutinations are observed with naked eye. A titer of 1 : 32 to 1 : 64 is considered significant.

(e) Paul-Bunnel Test

An agglutinin for sheep red blood cells is present in the serum and is of diagnostic significance during and after the attack of infectious mononucleosis.

Test. The patient's serum is heated at 55°C for 20 minutes and series of doubling dilutions of this serum is made from 1 : 16 to 1 : 1,024. The control tube contains saline only. 0.5 ml. of a 1 per cent suspension of saline washed sheep red blood cells is added to each tube containing diluted serum. The tubes were thoroughly shaken and incubated at 37°C for four hours. Tube showing agglutination of red blood cells is the final dilution of the serum. A suggestive titre is 1 : 128; a significant titre is 1 : 256.

(f) Rose Waaler Test or Test for Rheumatoid Arthritis or Serum Factor

Sheep red blood cells sensitised with rabbit anti-sheep erythrocytes serum are agglutinated by the sera of 70 - 80 per cent patients with rheumatoid arthritis and positive reaction occurs in some 2 - 5 per cent of normal subjects. Serum factor is macroglobulin which is an index of inherited metabolic disturbances which predisposes an individual to rheumatoid arthritis and is an antibody to denatured gamma globulin.

Previously inactivated patient serum is diluted in two fold steps from 1 : 2 to 1 : 1,024. Two sets of dilutions are required; to one set is added an equal volume of sensitised red blood cells and the second set receives the same volume of unsensitised red blood cells of sheep and acts as control. The tubes are incubated at 37°C and then placed in the refrigerator until the cells have completely settled. The last tube or last wall of perspex plastic plate, if used, shows a definite hemagglutination at the end titre. Serum titre of 16 or more is taken as positive in rheumatoid arthritis.

(g) Latex Agglutination Test for Rheumatoid Arthritis

To one drop of diluted patient's serum on the latex plate, one drop of latex antigen is added and mixed thoroughly with the plastic stick. Latex agglutination indicates that the test is positive.

(h) Coombs' Test

Mechanism. In Coomb's antiglobulin test, the red blood cells (RBCs) anti-D antibody (IgG) cannot link two red cells for aggluination. Addition of Coombs' serum (antiglobulin, AHG) has brought about agglutination by linking two attached immunoglobulins to one another. It may be direct or indirect Coombs' test. Both these tests can detect incomplete antibodies.

(A) *Direct Coombs' test* detects autoimmune hemolytic anemia, erythroblastosis fetalis.

Method. To remove serum proteins except globulin, RBCs are washed three times in saline by centrifugation. When washed RBCs are mixed with AHG in presence of bovine albumin, there will be agglutination of RBCs in positive cases.

(B) *Indirect Coombs' test* can detect anti Rh antibody in serum of Rh negative pregnant women of Rh positive huband.

Method. Saline washed Rh positive group O red cells are mixed with patient's serum and incubated at 37°C for 30 minutes. Red cells are washed three times in saline. These washed cells are mixed with Coombs' serum. Clumpling of RBCs occurs, if positive.

Precipitation

(a) Venereal Disease Research Laboratory (VDRL) flocculation test is simple, rapid, sensitive screening test used to diagnose syphilis.

One drop (0.05 ml) of inactivated patient's serum is placed on a VDRL glass plate and one drop of diluted VDRL antigen Cardiolipin, 0.03 per cent; Lecithin, 0.24 per cent and cholesterol, 0.9 per cent), is added on the serum and the whole plate is rotated on VDRL rotator for 3 to 4 minutes, visible aggregation or precipitation indicates a positive reaction.

(b) *Kahn flocculation Test* to diagnose syphilis. The test for each serum is set up as follows;

Tube	1	2	3
Add diluted antigen	0.05 ml	0.025 ml	0.0125 ml
Add serum	0.15 ml	0.15 ml	0.15 ml

The tubes are shaken in Kahn shaker machine for 3 minutes and incubated at 37°C for 20 minutes.

Then add saline 1.0 ml. 0.5 ml. 0.5 ml.

Readings are now made after the appearance of precipitates.

The control is set up as follows:

Tube	1	2	3
Add diluted antigen	0.05 ml	0.025 ml	0.0125 ml
Add saline	0.15 ml	0.15 ml	0.15 ml
Shake tubes and incubate as above			
Then add saline	1.0 ml	0.5 ml	0.5 ml

Reading: ++++ = large floccules at the bottom of the Kahn tube; – = minute floccules just visible throughout the tube.

(c) *Complement fixation test* (CFT) is frequently employed with soluble antigen for the detection of antibody, even 0.08 μg of antibody nitrogen can be detected. It is very sensitive and specific. Both bacterial and viral infections can be diagnosed with this test.

When antigen and antibody reaction is specific, the complement is fixed. This reaction cannot be seen with the naked eye; but it can be observed with the help of hemolytic system (Sheep RBCs + Hemolysin); if the complement is fixed, there is no hemolysis (*Positive*); if the complement is free, there is hemolysis (test is negative).

Antigen + Antibody	+ Complement	+ Hemolytic
(Specific)	(fixed)	system (sheep RBCs + Hemolysin)

Result = No hemolysis (Positive)

Antigen + Antibody	+ Complement	+ Hemolytic system
(not specific)	(free)	

Result = Hemolysis = (Negative)

When CFT is employed for the diagnosis of syphilis, it is called Wassermann test:

(d) *Agar gel precipitation technique.* In this test, the antigen and antibody diffuse is the gel and form a line of precipitation when they meet. When this basic principle is adopted in electrophoresis apparatus, it is known as *Counter immunoelectrophoresis* (CIEP).

(e) *Fluorescent antibody technique.* There are two main methods used in immunofluorescent work : the direct and indirect methods. The direct method consists of bringing fluorescein tagged antibodies in contact with antigens fixed on a slide, allowing them to react, washing off the excess of antibody and examining under the fluorescence microscope. The site of union of the labelled antibody with the antigen can be determined by the apple green or orange yellow fluorescent area on the slide.

The indirect method is used to detect both specific antibody in sera and also, as a direct method, for identifying antigens. For the detection of antibody, a slide on which a preparation of the antigen on the slide is flooded with the specific serum, and, after an interval, the excess serum, is washed off. The localisation of the antibody on the antigen preparation is then visualised under fluorescent microscope by layering the slide with the fluorescein labelled antibody specific for the serum proteins of the serum under test. The most suitable type of labelled antibody is that directed primarily against the globulin fractions of the test serum, i.e., fluorescein labelled anti-globulin serum.

(f) Antinuclear Factor Test

Sera that are able to induce the formation of Lupus erythematosus (LE) cells contain the antinuclear antibody (ANP) which react with the nuclei of tissue cells. This factor present in the connective tissue disease (Serum Lupus Erythematosus, SLE) can be detected by the application of indirect fluorescent antibody technique.

(g) Antitoxin

Toxin neutralisation test is very useful to detect the toxigenicity of certain strains of bacteria, e.g., *Clostridium tetani* in mice. The control mouse, which has already been protected passively by Antitetanus serum (ATS) against tetanus, will survive, as the toxin is neutralised by antitetanus serum; the mouse which receives the toxin of toxigenic strain of *Cl. tetani*, will show the symptoms and die of tetanus. The same principle is applicable in skin tests — Schick skin test to diagnose diphtheria and Dick test to diagnose scarlet fever.

(h) Anti-streptolysin-O (ASO) titer

Anti-streptolysin-O *(ASO) titer* is useful for the detection of clinically significant levels of Antistreptolysin-O antibodies found in the serum of persons following infection with a streptolysin-O producing strain of streptococci.

The ASO titer, expressed in Todd units, is the reciprocal of the serum dilution which completely neutralises the streptolysin-O. A serum with a titer of 166 Todd units should show no hemolysis.

(i) Reverse Passive Hemagglutination (RPHA) test

This test is a useful sensitive test to detect HB_sAg in serum hepatitis patient. Besides, it is simple and specific.

A simple and convenient testing procedure to detect HB_sAg :

25 μl diluent should be added into U or V cavity plates; then 7 μl test specimen (patient serum) should be added into the same cavity and mixed; 25 μl of sensitised sheep erythrocytes should be added and mixed again. The test should be kept at room temperature for 2 hours.

Interpretation. Reactive screening test result - The cell settling pattern will appear as a large diffused pattern; non-reactive test result - a distinct compact bottom of cells.

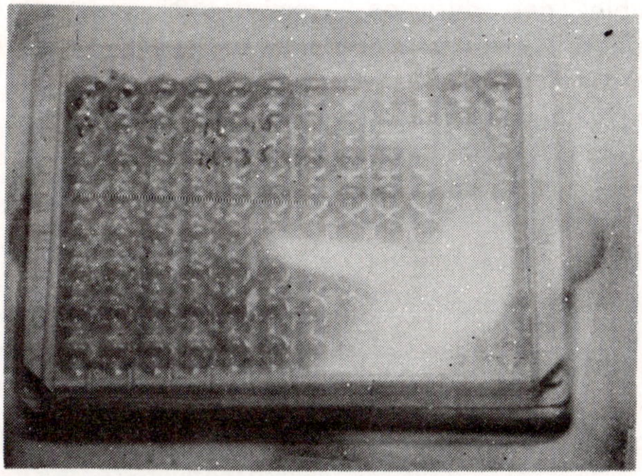

Fig. 62.12: ELISA test in perspex plastic plate

(j) Enzyme Linked Immunosorbent Assay (ELISA) Technique

In the micro-ELISA for detection of antibody, the antigen is coated onto the surface of wells in microtitration plate. The patient serum is then added and time is allowed for an antigen-antibody reaction to occur. An *enzyme labelled specific* antiglobulin is then added, which attaches to the antigen-antibody complexes. Any untreated antiglobulin is washed away. An *enzyme substrate* is then added which is acted upon by the attached enzyme producing a colour which can be measured colorimetrically or interpreted visually. Incubation with enzyme substrate produces a yellow orange colour in the test well, if anti-HIV is present in the sample. Commonly used enzymes are Horse Radish peroxidase (HRP) or phosphatase. Penicillinase prepared in India is also useful and cheaper than other enzymes.

ELISA test is widely used to diagnose viral (AIDS, Hepatitis bacterial and parasitic diseases (Fig. 62.12).

Principle of the Test

Soild phase antigen — **HIV** —
- anti-HIV (Positive sample)
- (anti HIV) HRP labelled antibody

+ substrate

(k) Western Blot test

Western Blot test is used to confirm HIV in patient sera screened positive for AIDS. This test is carried out only in AIDS Reference Laboratory (National Institute of Virology, Pune; All India Institute of Medical Sciences, New Delhi; India).

RECENT PARASITIC SEROLOGY

Serological tests are most helpful when the diagnostic forms cannot be readily demonstrated as in tissue infection such as amebic liver abscess (ALA), trichinosis, visceral larval migrans, toxoplasmosis.

Immunodiagnostic tests to detect parasitic antigens have been described for a number of infections and could eventually replace morphological diagnosis of many parasites. Monoclonal antibodies may be particularly helpful in developing sensitive and specific antigen detection tests.

Antigenic structure of parasite is complex and cross-reactions in serological tests are common. Newer tests using different or more purified antigens have given better results. Various types of tests have been described. Agglutination tests use whole organisms or antigen coated particles such as in bentonite flocculation (BF), indirect hemagglutination (IHA) and latex agglutination (LA). Complement fixation (CF) test has been widely used but is being superseded by newer tests. Precipitin tests include capillary precipitin, double gel diffusion, counterimmunoelectrophoresis (CIE) and circumlarval precipitin. Indirect immunofluorescence (IIF) has been widely used in parasitic serology and is readily adapted to detect Ig M antibody. Recent test development has emphasised Enzyme linked immunosorbent assay (ELISA) and soluble antigen fluorescent antibody (SAFA) such as Automated fluoroimmunoassay (FIAX) system, although some improved tests are based on modification of older methods (e.g., IIF, CIE). Thus improvements in serological methods and antigens are causing rapid changes in parasitic serology.

Cross-reactions are common and sensitivity and/or specificity of some tests may be poor. In addition, serology may not distinguish between previous and active infection. Thus, for some infection, serology may be useful in screening person who have visited an endemic area, whereas they are of little value in diagnosing infection in residents of the endemic area. The presence of antibody does not necessarily indicate immunity.

Immunodiagnostic procedures for detecting antigen or antibody in parasitic diseases are numerous and are changing rapidly.

ELISA Technique

In the micro-ELISA for detection of antibody, the antigen is coated on to the surface of wells in microtitration plate. The patient serum is then added and time is allowed for an antigen-antibody reaction to occur. An enzyme labelled specific antiglobulin is then added, which attaches to the antigen-antibody complexes. Any unattached antiglobulin is washed away. An enzyme substrate is then added which is acted upon by the attached enzyme producing a colour which can be measured colorimetrically or interpreted visually. Commonly used enzymes are peroxidase of phosphatase. Penicillinase is found useful, cheaper and can be prepared in India.

In recent years, ELISA is used to assist in the diagnosis of malaria, amebiasis, schistosomiasis, onchocerciasis, leishmaniasis, echinococcosis, trypanosomiasis, trichinellosis and toxoplasmosis. ELISA is sensitive and specific than other serological tests.

Amoebiasis. Serodiagnostic procedure depends on the type of infection present, a very low degree of sensitivity is found with sera from asymptomatic carriers, increased sensitivity from patients with amebic dysentery and the greatest sensitivity with sera from those patients with extraintestinal disease. The CF has been generally replaced by IHA, CIF and indirect fluorescent antibody (IFA) procedures, these three tests have more or less the same degree of sensitivity.

A new fluorescence (FIAX) technique — in which the fluorescence is measured in a fluorometer — is a new test that has been adapted to routine diagnosis of amebiasis. The technique has been developed for detection of antigen in feces. The sensitivity of this test is quite good, although the only parasite detected is *E. histolytica*.

Invasive amebiasis by *E. histolytica* can be detected by a very recent technique — cellulose acetate precipitin (CAP) test.

Dot immunobinding assay (DIB) and sandwich ELISA can be used in the diagnosis of invasive amebiasis. Both tests are equally specific and sensitive. DIB, easier to perform is less expensive and recommended for detection of antibody in patients with invasive amebiasis (amebic liver abscess — ALA) in India (1992).

Giardiasis. ELISA is compared with microscopy for detection of Giardia fecal antigens. ELISA was highly sensitive and specific either visually (95 and 97 per cent, respectively) or by optical density determination (99 and 96 per cent, respectively). ELISA is extremely effective for epidemiology study.

Toxoplasmosis. The methylene blue dye (MBD) test — Sabin-Feldman dye test — has been used for many years for the serological diagnosis of toxoplasmosis. This procedure has been replaced by the IHA and IFA procedures, both of them are technically simple to perform and utilise a killed antigen rather than live organisms (used in MBD test). All these procedures are equally sensitive and specific procedure can be performed using specific conjugates of Ig M

— although the interpretations of the results are difficult. Congenital infections are generally indicated when sera from newborns are positive with Ig M conjugates.

Ig M antibody methods may give both false positive and false negative results, because of rheumatoid factor, blocking antibody and the induction of factor Ig M antibody against maternal globulin. The double sandwich ELISA test has eliminated many of these problems. The combination of IFA and IHA procedures allows more accurate interpretation, because a different type of antigen is used for each test.

Tests for Ig M antibody (Ig M fluorescent antibody or double sandwich ELISA technique) are particularly useful for establishing recent toxoplasma infection, because titers appear early (as early as five days after infection) and disappear within several months. Ig M antibodies are elevated in acute disease. CFT using soluble toxoplasma antigen becomes positive three to six weeks after infection, rises for two to eight months, and falls to a very low level after one to two years.

Very recently, the direct agglutination test with 2 mercaptoethanol (Ad-2ME) and immunofluorescent antibody test (IFAT) are used in the diagnosis of toxoplasmosis. The former is little superior to the latter.

Pneumocystosis. The tests of choice for pneumocystis are the CF and IFA tests and can detect 85 per cent infected patients. A direct fluorescent antibody test has been developed for the detection of organisms in mucus and sputum smears and tissue biopsies.

During the last few years, CIE and ELISA were evaluated. They are not still easily available. They lack specificity and sensitivity; so they are not used successfully in routine clinical diagnosis. The development of culture technique for this organism may lead to more specific antigen production.

Leishmaniasis. The serological procedures (IHA, IFA and CF) are available for visceral leishmaniasis and are quite helpful in making diagnosis and IFA is being used routinely with excellent results using amastigote antigen for cutaneous leishmaniasis. The IFA test is more specific than ELISA for diagnosis of cutaneous leishmaniasis, but neither is satisfactory as microscopic examination. Both methods were acceptable for the diagnosis of visceral leishmaniasis when promastigote forms of *L. donovani* were used as antigen. ELISA test, using promastigotes as antigen, is probably the most practical for testing number of sera. The IFA technique employing either amastigotes or promastigotes as antigen has been used as direct agglutination test (DAT) of fixed promastigotes. There may be cross-reaction with serum of patient infected with *T. cruzi*. The leishmanin skin (delayed hypersensitivity) test is negative in cases of active visceral leishmaniasis (AVL).

In 1995, an immunodot assay was developed for serodiagnosis of AVL which utilises protein. A colloidal gold as the visualising agent. The test is simple requires few reagents and can be completed in 2 hours. It is sensitive and specific for AVL and generally corelates with ELISA. Either whole blood or sera in minute quantities may be used as test antibody.

Besides indirect ELISA tests for *L. donovani* antibody was carried out with enzyme labelled protein A or protein G instead of anti-immunoglobulin. It was found that this modification improved the positive/negative discrimination. In addition, antibody could be measured in human sera (e.g., dogs).

In 1995, monoclonal antibody L_{12} F_7 against the antigen of *L. donovani* promastigotes was labelled with peroxidase and used in dot-ELISA test for detecting circulating antigen in sera of cases with visceral leishmaniasis. The results showed that monoclonal antibody can be used in dot-ELISA for diagnosis of visceral leishmaniasis. It is of special significance that this method can be used as simple and reliable tool for filed evaluation of therapeutic effectiveness for visceral leishmaniasis.

A technique that may permit direct and rapid diagnosis of cutaneous leishmaniasis as well as differentiation of leishmania is blotting with radiolabelled DNA probes.

A positive leishmanin skin test and serum antibody can be demonstrated in patients by the time a cutaneous lesion has ulcerated. These tests remain positive in mucocutaneous disease. Serological tests are not useful in the diagnosis, because antibody levels are low. Positive skin test and serological test can reflect a previous rather than a current leishmanial infection. A direct agglutination test (DAT) is useful and sensitive in the diagnosis of cutaneous leishmaniasis.

Chagas disease. Serological testing is generally not needed for diagnosis of acute disease. Parasite-specific Ig M antibody detected by immunofluorescence or direct agglutination does not become positive until twenty to forty days after the onset of symptoms. The diagnosis of *Chronic* Chagas disease requires demonstration of antibody to *T. Cruzi* in the presence of characteristic cardiac abnormalities. In 1995, in Brazil, American trypanosomiasis (*T. Cruzi*) can be diagnosed by testing blood donor for infection by G-agglutination test (WHO). HIA and IIF tests are also used.

African sleeping sickness. Several immunodiagnostic tests have been developed for African trypanosomiasis IFA, ELISA, Capillary hemagglutination (HA) test that are useful for epidemiological surveys. However, no serological test provides sufficient definite information for treatment of a patient without demonstration of the organism. A card agglutination test (CATT) has been produced in late1996. It is simple, specific, sensitive. It is yet to be fully evaluated.

Malaria. A variety of serological tests have been developed for malaria, but are not usually used for the diagnosis of clinical infection. They are particularly useful for epidemiological survey and detection of infected blood donors. Those most commonly used are indirect immunofluorescent (IIF) and IHA tests. IIF titres equal to or greater than 1 : 64 are suggestive of recent infection with plasmodium. These serological tests showed a false positive rate of 1 per cent or less and have a sensitivity of over 95 per cent. Development of natural immunity in *P. falciparum* malaria can be detected by Western blot. The rather inovative title "ABC - ELISA" is merely a novel abbreviation for avidin-biotin complex ELISA. It is useful method for malaria serology in the field and is most recent. A conventional ELISA is carried out but instead of enzyme labelled antiglobulin, biotin labelled antiglobulin followed by avidin labelled enzyme (1 additional step). The results of this new test correlated well with those of obtained by immunofluorescence and was better than those of the conventional ELISA.

The IFA test and micro-ELISA test for detection of antimalarial antibodies have little value in endemic areas. Recently, monoclonal antibody has been introduced for the detection of plasmodial antigen in human blood for the diagnosis of malaria by IFA technique.

In India, IIF test is used for the diagnosis of malaria by using *P. falciparum* antigen. The diagnostic titre is 1 : 80. Besides, 80 per cent seropositivity was observed by mean ELISA — optical density values to both *P. falciparum* and *P. vivax.*

Plasmodial antigen can be detected by monoclonal antibody as a screening procedure for blood donors in transfusion medicine in epidemic countries like India.

Cryptosporidiosis. A serological test has been described (J. Clin. Microbiol. 18 : 165, 1983).

Trichinellosis. Diagnosis is often established indirectly by serological tests, some are commercially available. The most commonly used are bentonite flocculation (BF), fluorescent antibody (IIF) and Complement fixation (CF). The bentonite flocculation (BF) is very sensitive and usually becomes negative two to three years after an infection; thus, a positive test usually indicates active infection. The test becomes positive after the third week of infection and is most helpful when a fourfold rise in paired sera can be demonstrated. The CF test detects antibodies slightly earlier than the BF test. IIF is considered to be as good as the BF test and most sensitive.

Filariasis. Serological tests using extracts of *Dirofilaria immitis* as antigen include IHA and BF, but they allow only a diagnosis of filarial group rather than the species. Moreover, there is cross-reactivity with other parasite (false positive) as well as many false negative.

Western blot technique and ELISA can be used to detect *B. malayi* in filarial sera of different groups of patients.

Schistosomiasis

Several serological tests (Cholestrol-lecithin flocculation, BF, CF and IFA) are used for the diagnosis of schistosomiasis, all share problems of specificity and sensitivity. There has been increased use of IFA procedure which uses section of adult worm for the antigen and proved to be most sensitive technique (less cross reactivity with other sera).

The circumoral precipitin test is used extensively for diagnosis of *S. japonicum* infection. ELISA technique is sensitive as the IFA and CF titers with adult worm using as antigen, but indicates that ELISA was more specific.

Cysticercosis. IHA was 85 per cent reactive with sera from proved cases of human infection. The double diffusion was sensitive using both animal and human sera. Cross-reaction with sera from patients infected with Echinococcus species, *T. saginata* and Coenurus species have been reported.

Echinococcosis. The IHA, IFA and immunoelectrophoresis (IE) procedures are considered to be the test of choice for the diagnosis of echinococcosis, IHA and BF are routinely used at Centre for Disease Control (CDC), USA, the IHA is most sensitive. Much IHA titers usually indicate the presence of hydatid disease. IE test has been evaluated in many countries, a double diffusion band 5 (DD^5) test has been reported to be more sensitive and more specific than IE test. CIE test has also been reported to be specific and sensitive and ELISA has also been evaluated. IHA titer of 1 : 256 is considered significant and is positive in 88 per cent of people with non-calcified hepatic cyst. Low titer with any of these tests do not necessarily mean infection, since sera from patients with other conditions, such as liver cirrhosis and collagen diseases, cross-react. Cross reaction with the cestode larvae such as cysticercus are also common. In addition, patients with calcified hepatic cysts or cysts of lung frequently have negative serology.

Visceral larva migrans. Serological tests may aid in establishing the diagnosis. Different methods vary in sensitivity and specificity. The ELISA using embryonated egg extract as antigen offers much better sensitivity and specificity and cross-reacting with Ascaris antibody can be removed by preadsorption. In visceral larva migrans, a significant titre is 1 : 321 whereas if ocular toxocariasis is suspected a titer of 1 : 8 is significant.

Strongyloidiasis. The results of the indirect agglutination test with newly developed gelatin particles were found to be quite comparable to those of IHA and ELISA. The test is simple and rapid to perform for mass screening for human strongyloidiasis very recently, the sensitivity, specificity, positive and negative predicted values of ELISA test using F_2, protein fraction from *S. stercoralis* were 95, 96.4, 95 and 96.4 per cent, respectively, as the latest observation. Immunoblot can be useful in the diagnosis of human strongyloidiasis.

Filariasis. In India, very recently, Dot-ELISA in detection of *W. bancrofti* filarial antibody was compared with standard ELISA, the dot-ELISA was found more sensitive. Besides, ELISA developed using soluble antigen of adult *B. malayi* gave positive responses in 95 per cent cases in India.

Onchocercosis can be diagnosed by recent immunoblot test.

Dracunculosis : Most recently, the Falcon assay screening test — enzyme linked immunosorbent assay (FAST-ELISA) and enzyme linked immunoelectrotransfer blot (EITB) techniques are used to test human sera with *D. medinensis* adult worm antigen.

Following serological tests are performed at Centre for Disease Control (CDC), USA (1990).

Diseases	Tests	Diagnostic titers
Amebiasis	HIA	1 : 256
Ascariasis	ELISA	1 : 128
Babesiosis	IIF	1 : 16
Chagas' disease	CF	1 : 8
Cysticercosis	IHA	1 : 128
Echinococcosis	IHA	1 : 256
Filariasis	IHA	1 : 128
Leishmaniasis	DAT	1 : 64
Malaria	IIF	1 : 64
Paragomoniasis	CF	1 : 8
Pneumocystosis	IIF	1 : 16
Schistosomiasis	IIF	Positive
Strongyloidiasis	IHA	1 : 64
Toxocariasis	ELISA	1 : 32
Toxoplasmosis	IIF, IIF - Ig M+	1 : 256; 1 : 64
Trichinellosis	BFT	1 : 5

IHA — Indirect hemagglutination;
CF — Complement fixation;
DAT — Direct agglutination test;
IIF — Indirect immunofluorescence;
BFT — Bentonite flocculation test;
ELISA — Enzyme Linked Immunosorbent Assay; + Any IIF - Ig M titer to toxoplasmosis in an infant less than two years old is strongly suggestive of infection.

The diagnostic titres given are highly suggestive of clinical disease, but a fourfold rise in titer is stronger evidence.

Infections due to Toxoplasma Gondii and *Trypanosoma Cruzi*

The advent of Polymerase Chain Reaction (PCR) has opened up the possibility of isolating DNA sequence from ancient samples from museum specimens and archeological findings. As majority of these molecules in these ancient samples are degraded to such an extent as to preclude any other molecular technique, PCR with its remarkable sensitivity can be employed to amplify the existing few molecules to an appreciable extent which can then be further studied.

For example, for the diagnosis of infections caused by RNA viruses by PCR, RNA has to be first converted into the complementary DNA (C DNA). C DNA is obtained by a reverse transcriptase assay using RNA as the template. This step takes 2 hours. The C DNA thus obtained is next used as the template in the PCR assay.

Serological tests which have wider use are commonly carried out and most of these tests are well-standardised. Howerver, serological tests are essentially indirect tests except when antigens are detected. The more direct tests involve demonstration of the pathogen or pathogen specific nucleic acid (DNA or RNA) in the clinical diagnosis.

Therefore, the Polymerase Chain Reaction offers a rapid, sensitive and a very specific diagnostic approach for protozoal diseases caused by *Toxoplasma gondii* or *Trypanosoma cruzi*.

CULTIVATION OF ANIMAL VIRUSES

Viruses can be grown only within living host cells, as they gain access to the energy-producing systems and protein synthesising machinary which they lack :

(a) Experimental animals,
(b) Chick embryos, and
(c) Tissue cultures.

(a) *Animal inoculation* was only old method available at that time by which the recognisable disease and death can be demonstrated. The presence of inclusion bodies in the tissues is the evidence of virus infections. The poliomyelitis virus can cause paralysis.

(b) *Chick embryos* (Fig. 62.13) provide more satisfactory hosts, because they are clean and bacteriologically sterile and have no specific protective immune system to counteract the virus infections. Poxviruses, vaccina, herpes virus can grow on chorio-

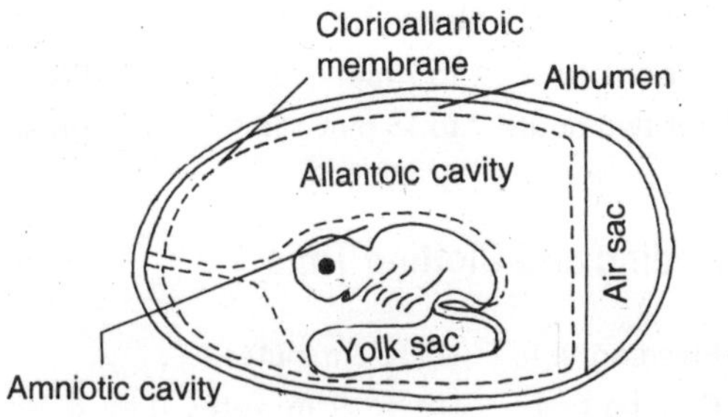

Fig. 62.13 : Chick embryo

allantoic membrane (CAM, Fig. 62.13) and produce characteristic visible lesions. Influenza viruses multiply in the lung cells of the embryo and the cells lining allantoic cavity. Rickettsiae and psittacosis lymphogranuloma group grow well in yolk sac and kill the embryo.

(c) *Tissue cultures* of human or simian cells are the most frequently used and are relatively simple to prepare in large quantities that are required by modern diagnostic virological methods. Suspensions of cells dispersed from tissue fragments or bulk cultures of cell lines (human amnion cell; monkey kidney cell; squamous cell carcinoma of the cervix uteri - He La cells; and HEP2 strain of from an epithelioma) are obtained by tryptin digestion. The cells adhere to the walls of the test tube and grow out to form a sheet — *monolayer*, which can be observed *in situ* under the low power objective of the microscope.

After inoculation into monolayer cell culture, a virus causes degeneration of the cell sheet. This progress of the infection (cytopathic effect CPE) can be studied under the low power objective of a light microscope and the cells may become rounded, shrivelled, ballooned or fused together to form a multinucleate syncytial masses, ultimately all cells are affected and get detached from the wall of the test tube.

CULTIVATION OF FUNGI

Cultivation of fungi can be done on Sabouraud's medium at room temperature. The growth characteristic of each fungus can be studied along with its morphology, after staining with Lactophenol blue, under low or high power objectives of light microscope.

STUDY OF BLOOD CELL (Hematology)

Human blood cells are of three types :

1. Erythrocytes (red blood cells);
2. Leucocytes (white blood cells);
3. Thrombocytes (blood platelets).

In man, red blood cells (RBC) are round, devoid of nucleus, smaller than white blood cells. The cytoplasm of red blood cells contains a respiratory pigment called hemoglobulin which imparts red colour. Due to hemoglobulin, red blood cells help in transportation of respiratory gases, i.e., O_2 and CO_2.

White blood cells (WBC) are nucleated, colourless, irregular in outline and devoid of respiratory pigment. The cytoplasm of most of the white blood cells contains some granules and accordingly they are classified into two main groups : granular and agranular leucocytes.

According to the nature of these granules, granular leucocytes are further classified into three types : (a) Neutrophils; (b) Acidophils (Eosinophils) and (c) Basophils.

(a) *Neutrophils :* Granules of neutrophils as the name suggests, show neutral property. Their nuclei consist of three to five lobes. Sixty to seventy per cent of total leucocytes are of this type. They act as phagocytes and are also known as polymorphs.

(b) *Acidophils :* Granules of acidophils are alkaline in nature and are stained by acidic stains. Their nuclei are bilobed. Their percentage is very little, i.e., about 1 to 4 per cent of total leucocytes. They are also called as eosinophils.

(c) *Basophils* are acidic in nature and stained by alkaline or basic stains. Their nuclei consist of three to five lobes. Their percentage is the least, i.e., 0 to 1.0 per cent of total leucocytes.

Agranular leucocytes are of two types :

(I) Monocytes, and (II) Lymphocytes. Monocytes are largest leucocytes, while lymphocytes are smallest. The nucleus of monocyte is crescentic, while that of lymphocytes is round. The number of monocytes is about 2 to 6 per cent, while that of lymphocytes is about 25 per cent of total leucocytes. Lymphocytes, being smallest in size, can pass through the very thin wall of blood capillaries and, therefore, they are found in lymph. Hence, they are called as lymphocytes.

Thrombocytes are small, oval or spindle shaped fragments of special large cells found in the bone marrow. Therefore they are devoid of nucleus and short lived. They distintegrate easily when they come out of the bleeding wound and help in clotting.

Hemoglobin (Hb) Report

Blood counts : Peripheral venous blood.

Hb. gms % *normal* (for adults)

(Male, 13.5 to 18 g%; Female, 12 to 16 g%)

Total RBC /cmm (M, 4.6 to 6.2 millions/cmm;
F, 4.2 to 5.4 millions/cmm.)

Total WBC /cmm (4000 to 10,000/cmm).

Differential Leucocyte Count (DLC) :

Polymorphs	60 to 70%
Lymphocytes	20 to 30%
Eosinophils	1 to 4%
Monocytes	2 to 6%
Basophils	0 to 1%

Erythrocytes Sedimentation Rate

	Males	Females	
After one hour	1 to 7 mm	3 to 12 mm	Wester-
After two hours	7 to 15 mm	10 to 18 mm	green
			method.

Bleeding and Clotting Time

Bleeding time	Up to 5 minutes.
Clotting time	Up to 9 minutes (Lee & White method).

Blood indices

PCV %	(42 to 60%)
MCV	cmm (82 to 90 cmm).

Blood Examination for Parasites

The blood provides the most common medium for recovery of human parasites at various stages. From this source, routine diagnosis is made of malaria, African trypanosomiasis, most types of filariasis, less frequently Chagas' disease and rarely Kala azar and toxoplasmosis.

Preparation of Films

Thin film on one slide. A drop of blood is taken at the end of the slide. A spreader is held at an angle of 45°C and pushed in the opposite direction to make a smear.

Thick film on one slide. Four drops of blood are placed at the corners of a half inch square slide and joined to form a thick film. A glass slide with corners cut at one end or the coverslip of a hemocytometer can be used as spreader.

Examination of Blood for Malarial Parasites

Time for taking blood. The blood specimen should be obtained several hours after the paroxysm has reached its peak, because the parasites are more easily detected in the film.

The schizogony of *Plasmodium vivax, P. malariae* and *P. ovale* can readily be demonstrated in the peripheral blood during both the febrile and afebrile periods. The best time for demonstrating *P. falciparum* is few hours after the febrile paroxysm reaches its peak, because *P. falciparum* disappears from the peripheral blood during the afebrile period. Generally, the blood film should be taken when the patient is seen first and therefore.

It will be useful to have both thin and thick films, either on one slide or on two different slides and to examine them after staining. The thin film is examined to identify the parasites.

Stains

1. *Leishman's Stain.* Leishman's stain should be poured on the smear and diluted twice its volume with neutral distilled water. The diluted stain is allowed to remain on the slide for 10-15 minutes, and then the slide should be washed with running tap water, dried and examined under an oil immersion lens.

2. *Giemsa Stain.* The diluted Giemsa stain is poured over the film and kept for 30 to 45 minutes. The film is washed with running water and dried. The stain is examined under an oil immersion lens.

Examination of Blood for Microfilariae

Blood should be collected between 10 p.m. an 2 a.m. for microfilariae are of nocturnal periodicity. A thick film of blood is prepared and kept covered. The next morning, it is dehemoglobinised by the slide being put in water, dried and fixed in methyl alcohol and then stained with Leishman's stain or Giemsa stain. Microfilaria may be detected occasionally even in a thin film.

STOOL EXAMINATION FOR PARASITES

The entire stool specimen should be examined macroscopically for its consistency and component elements (feces, mucus, blood tissue elements and undigested food) and for parasitic segments of *Taenia saginata, T. solium,* whole adult worm of *Ascaris lumbricoides, Ankylostoma duodenale, Trichuris trichiura, Enterobius vermicularis* and various intestinal flukes.

During the identification of eggs, one should pay attention to shape, size, colour and marking on the surface of egg shell, the presence of granules, ovum or a differentiated embryo, the existence of an operculum and the three pairs of embryonic hooklets in cestodes. For detection of helminthic eggs, only an unstained preparation is necessary (Fig. 62.14a, b).

Methods of Examinations of Stool, and in detecting parasitic infection is as follows :

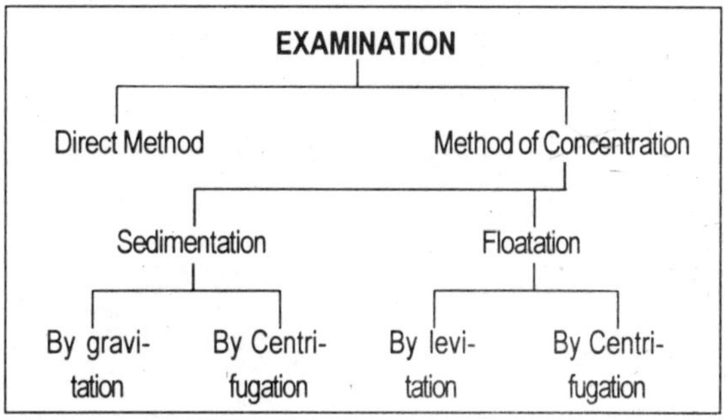

1. Direct method is commonly used. Two cover glass preparations are prepared on one microscopic slide for apart from each other.

   1. *Saline preparation.* 1-2 mg. of the fecal material should be mixed in a drop or two of physiological salt solution for the left hand preparation and
   2. *Iodine preparation.* 1-2 drops of iodine solution should be mixed with 1-2 mg. of the fecal material for right hand preparation. Cyst forms and living parasites can be detected in the saline preparation. Nucleus, glycogen mass of the protozoan cyst of *E. histolytica* and the flagella on the parasite can be studied in iodine preparation.

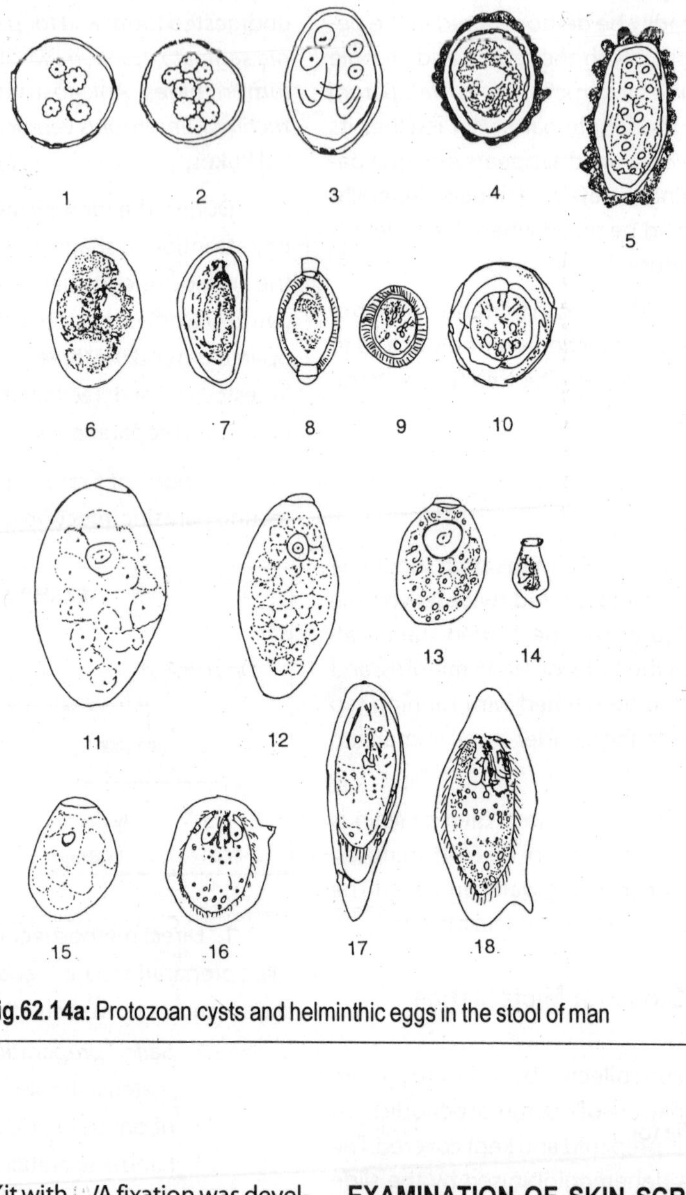

Fig.62.14a: Protozoan cysts and helminthic eggs in the stool of man

Trichrome stain Kit with PVA fixation was developed for the simplified staining of intestinal parasites. The cytoplasm of these organisms, cysts or trophozoites stain blue green with a purplish tint. The nuclear chromatin, chromatoid bodies, ingested RBCs and bacteria stain red or purple red.

A pseudo-parasite is an object which resembles a parasite or egg of a parasite. A wide variety of objects which resemble parasites may be found in stool specimens.

EXAMINATION OF SKIN SCRAPINGS FOR IDENTIFICATION OF MITES

A small quantity of skin scraping is taken in a test tube to which 10 per cent potassium hydroxide is added. The material is boiled for 10 minutes and kept in a stand to settle the sediment. A drop of sediment should be taken on a slide with the help of a pipette, covered with a cover slip and examined under low and high power objectives.

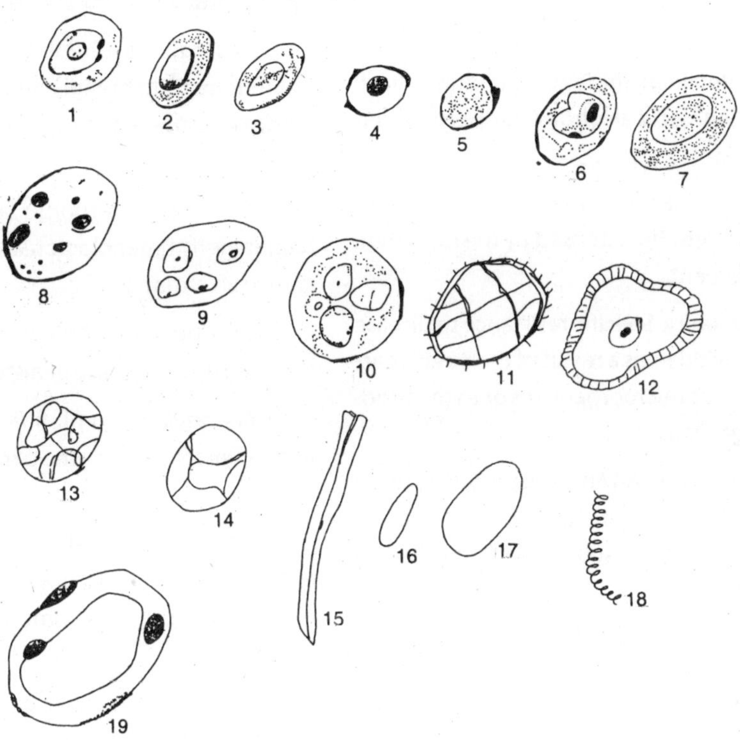

Fig. 62.14b : Pseudoparasites

EXAMINATION OF URINE

Urinary tract infection can be confirmed by routine microscopy by presence of pus cells and by culture of urine or preferrably centrifuged deposit on the laboratory media for the characteristic growth of organisms and the ultimate morphological identification of organisms.

APPLICATION TO NURSING

Though the nurse may not be well-acquainted with the handling of the microscope, staining and other laboratory techniques, she will be able to recognise the difficulties of the laboratory procedures and at the same time she will be able to differentiate Gram-negative and Gram-positive bacteria and the antibiotics effective on these broad groups of bacteria and the ultimate selection of an antibiotic for the treatment. If a knowledgeable and professional nurse can recognise the problems and difficulties faced in the laboratory, she will be able to collect and handle the specimens, so that these specimens can be processed easily in the laboratory for the correct results. The same methods of handling of sterile materials in the hospital wards and in public health nursing by the nurse should be followed in the microbiology laboratory to avoid the contamination.

If the nurse has a sound knowledge of interpretation of the report of serology, blood examination for parasites, stool and skin scraping examination, she will be of great assistance in reporting immediately to physicians for the diagnosis and the appropriate treatment.

TECHNICAL TERMS

Microbiology

Acid-fast. Retaining the initial stain and difficult to decolourise with acid alcohol. A property of certain bacteria.

Actinomycetes (ak-tin-o-*mye*-seets). Gram-positive bacteria that are characterised by the formation of branching filaments.

Active immunity. Specific resistance to disease acquired by individuals as a result of their own reactions to pathogenic microorganisms or to the products of such organisms.

Adaptive enzyme. An enzyme produced by an organism in response to the presence of the enzyme's substrate or related substance. Also called induced enzyme.

Adenovirus. A group of icosahedral double stranded DNA viruses.

Adjuvant. A substance that when injected together with antigen increases antibody production.

Aerobs (air-obe). An organism that requires oxygen for growth and can grow under an air atmosphere. Compare *Anaerobe.*

Aerosol. Atomised particles suspended in air.

Agar (ah gar). A dried polysaccharide extract of red algae used as a solidifying agent in microbiological media.

Agglutination (uh-gloo-tin-ay-shunt). The clumping of cells.

Alga pl. algae (*al*-guh-*al*-jee). Any member of a heterogeneous group of eukaryotic, photosynthetic and unicellular or multicellular organisms.

Allergy. A type of antigen-antibody reaction marked by an exaggerated physiological response to a substance in sensitive individuals.

Aminoglycoside antibiotics. A class of antibiotics which disrupt the normal synthetic sequence of protein synthesis.

Amophitrichous (am *fit*-rik-us). Having a single flagellum at each end of a cell.

Anaerobe (*an* uh-robe). An organism that does not require O_2 to obtain energy, cannot grow under an air atmosphere and for which O_2 is toxic. Compare *aerobe.*

Anamnestic response (an-am-*ness* tick). The heightened immunologic reaction to a second exposure to an antigen.

Anaphylatoxin. A complement derived peptide that causes the release of histamine mast cells.

Anaphylaxis (an-uh-fi-*lak*-sis). Hypersensitivity in an animal following the parenteral injection of an antigen.

Angstrom (A°) 1/10 of nanometre. Conventionally used for measuring wavelengths. Also used to express dimensions of some intracellular stricture of microbes.

Antibiosis (an-tee-bye-o-sis). An antagonistic association between two organisms in which one is adversely affected.

Antibiotic (an-tee-bye-ot-ik). A substance of microbial origin that has antimicrobial activity in very small amount.

Antibody (an-ti-bod-ee). Any of a class of substances (Proteins) produced by an animal in response to the introduction of an antigen.

Antigen (an-ti-jen). A substance that when introduced into an animal body stimulates the production of specific substances (antibodies) that react or unite with the substance introduced (antigen).

Antimicrobial agent. Any chemical or biological agent that either destroys or inhibits the growth of microorganisms.

Antiseptic. Acting against or opposing sepsis, putrefaction or decay by either preventing or arresting the growth of microorganisms.

Antiserum. Blood serum that contains antibodies.

Antitoxin. An antibody capable of uniting with and neutralising a specific toxin.

Arthropod. An invertebrate with jointed legs (insect).

Arthrospore. An asexual spore formed by the fragmentation of the mycelium.

Ascitic fluid. Serous fluid that accumulated abnormally in the peritoneal cavity.

Asepsis. A condition in which harmful microorganisms are absent.

Aseptic technique. Precautionary measures taken to prevent contamination.

Assay. The quantitative or qualitative estimation of the components of a drug.

Asymptomatic. Exhibiting no symptoms.

Autoclave. An apparatus using pressurised steam for sterilisation.

Autoimmune disease. A condition in which the body develops an immunological reaction against its own tissues.

Autolysis. The disintegration of cells by the action of their own enzymes.

Bacillus. Any rod-shaped bacterium.

Bacteriemia. A condition in which bacteria are present in the blood stream.

Bactericide. An agent that destroys bacteria.

Bacteriolysin. An agent or substance that causes the disintegration of bacteria.

Bacteriophage. A virus that infects bacteria and causes lysis of bacterial cells.

Bacteriostasis. The inhibition of the growth and reproduction of bacteria without killing them.

Bacteriostatic. Inhibiting the growth of bacteria without killing them.

Bacterium. Any of a group of diverse and ubiquitous prokaryotic single celled microorganisms.

BCG Vaccine. Bacillus Calmette-Guerin Vaccine, an attenuated strain of Mycobacterium tuberculosis bovis strain against tuberculosis.

Bergey's Manual. An international reference work which classifies and describes bacteria.

Beta haemolysis. A clear zone of haemolysis around certain bacteria growing on blood agar medium.

Binomial nomenclature. The scientific method of naming plants, animals and microorganisms, because species names consist of two terms.

Blood plasma. The fluid portion of fresh blood.

Blood serum. The fluid expressed from clotted blood.

BOD. Biochemical oxygen demand.

Botulism. Food poisoning due to the toxin of *Cl. botulinum.*

Bronchi. Branches of trachea.

Brownian motion. A peculiar dancing movement shown by fine particles or bacteria.

Bubo. Swollen infected lymph nodes.

Capsid :The protein of a virus.

Capsomere. A morphological subunit of a capsid seen under electron microscope.

Capsule. An envelope or slime layer surrounding the cell wall of certain bacteria.

Carrier. A person in apparently good health who harbours a pathogenic microorganism.

Catalase. An enzyme that converts hydrogen peroxide into water and oxygen.

Cell. The microscopic functionally and structurally basic unit of all living organisms.

Cell wall. A rigid external covering of the cytoplasmic membrane.

Chemotherapy. Treatment of the disease with the use of chemicals.

Chromatin body. Bacterial nuclear material.

Coagulass. An enzyme of staphylococci that causes the coagulation of blood plasma.

Colony. A microscopically visible growth of microorganisms on a solid culture medium.

Commensalism. A relationship between members of different species living in the same cultural environment in which one organism benefits from the association but the other is not affected.

Competitive inhibition. The inhibition of the action of an enzyme by a non-substrate molecule occupying the site on the enzyme that would otherwise be occupied by the substrate.

Complement. A normal thermolabile protein constituent of blood serum, that participates in antigen-antibody reactions.

Complement fixation. The binding of the complement to an antigen-antibody complex so that the complement is unavailable for a subsequent reaction.

Conjugation. A making process of temporary fusion of the mating partners and the transfer of genes and it occurs in unicellular organisms.

Contamination. The entry of undescribable organism into some material or object.

Culture. A population of microorganisms cultivated in a medium.

Cytoplasm. The living matter of a cell between the cell membrane and the nucleus.

Cytoplasmic membrane. A thin layer under the cell wall consisting of phospholipids and proteins and it is responsible for the selective permeability properties of the cell. Also called plasma membrane.

Diplococci. Cocci occurring in pairs.

Disinfection. An agent that frees from infection by killing the vegetative cells of microorganisms.

Ecology. The study of the interrelationships that exist between organisms and the environment.

Odema or *oedema.* The excessive accumulation of fluid in body tissue.

Electrophoresis. An electrochemical process in which suspended particles with an electric charge migrates in a solution under the influence of an electric current.

Endemic. With reference to a disease, one that has a low incidence but which is constantly present in a particular geographic region.

Endospore. A thick-walled spore formed in the bacterial cell. Very resistant to physiological and chemical agents.

Endotoxin. A heat stable toxin which consists of lipopolysaccharide it is located in the outer membrane of Gram-negative bacteria and is liberated only when the bacteria disintegrate.

Enteric. Pertaining to the intestine.

Enterotoxin. A toxin specific for cells of the intestine.

Epidemic. With reference for a disease, one that displays a sudden increase in incidences in a particular geographic region.

Epidemiology. The study of the occurrence and distribution of disease.

Etiology or *aetiology.* The study of the cause of a disease.

Exotoxin. A toxic protein excreted by a microorganism into the surrounding medium.

Facultative anaerobe. An organism which does not require O_2 for growth (but may use it if available) which grows well under both aerobic and anaerobic conditions and for which oxygen is not toxic.

Fastidious organisms. An organism that is difficult to isolate or cultivate on ordinary culture media because of its need for special nutritional factors.

Fermentation. The anaerobic oxidation of compounds by an enzyme action of microorganisms, neither gaseous oxygen nor a respiratory chain is involved in this energy-yielding process. An organic compound is the electron acceptor.

Fibrinolysin. A substance produced by haemolytic streptococci, that can liquefy clotted blood plasma or fibrin clots. Also called streptokinase.

Fimbriae. Surface appendages of certain Gram-negative bacteria composed of protein subunits. They are shorter and thinner than flagella. Also called *pili.*

Flagellum (pl. flagella). A thin filamentous appendage on cells responsible for swimming motility.

Fluorescence microscopy. Microscopy in which cells or their compounds are stained with a fluorescent dye and thus appear as glowing objects against a dark background.

Fomites. Inanimate objects that carry viable pathogenic microorganisms.

Food poisoning. Stomach or intestinal disturbances due to food contaminated with certain microbial toxins.

Frei test. A skin test to determine sensitivity to the agent that causes lymphogranuloma venereum.

Fungicide. An agent that kills or destroys fungi.

Fungus. A microorganism that lacks chlorophyll and is usually filamentous, a mould or yeast.

Gamma globulin. A fraction of serum globulin that is rich in antibodies.

Gastroenteritis. Inflammation of the mucosa of the stomach or intestine.

Genome. A complete set of genetic material, i.e., a complete set of genes.

Genus. A group of very closely related species.

Germ. A microbe, usually a pathogenic one.

Germicide. An agent that kills pathogenic microorganisms.

Giardiasis. Disease of human small intestine caused by *Giardia lamblia.*

Globulin. A protein soluble in dilute solution of neutral salts but insoluble in water. Antibodies are globulins.

Glucan. A polymer of glucose.

Gram-negative bacteria. Bacteria that does not retain crystal violet-iodine complex when subjected to the Gram technique and thus acquire the colour of the dye (usually red dye) that is used to counterstain the cells.

Gram-positive bacteria. Bacteria that retain the crystal violet-iodine complex when subjected to Gram technique and thus appears violet.

Gram stain. A differential stain by which bacteria are classed as Gram-negative or Gram-positive.

Granules metachromatic. Intracellular granules of polyphosphate found in certain microorganisms such granules stain deep violet colour when stained with methylene blue.

Growth curve : A graphic representation of the growth of bacteria in a culture medium.

Hanging drop technique : A technique in which microorganisms are observed suspended in a drop of fluid.

Hapten. A simple substance that reacts like an antigen *in vitro* by combining with antibody but cannot induce the formation of antibodies by itself.

H antigen. A type of heat-labile protein antigen found in the flagella of certain bacteria.

He La cells. A pureline of human cancer cells used for the cultivation of viruses.

Helix. A coiled spiral form.

Hemagglutination or *haemagglutination.* The agglutination (clumping) of red blood cells.

Hemoglobulin or *haemoglobulin.* The constituent of red blood cells that gives them their colour and carries oxygen.

Hemolysin or *haemolysin.* A substance produced by microorganisms that lyses red blood cells liberating hemoglobin. Also can refer to a type of antibody that acts in conjunction with complement to cause the lysis of red blood cells.

Hemolysis or *haemolysis.* The process of dissolving of red blood cells.

Hemorrhagic or *haemorrhagic.* Showing evidence of hemorrhage (bleeding).The tissue becomes reddened by the accumulation of blood that has escaped from capillaries into the tissue.

Heterophilic antibody. An antibody that reacts with microorganisms or cells that are unrelated to the antigen that stimulated production of the antibody.The agglutination of *Proteus sp.*cells by serum from typhus fever patients is an example.

Heterophile antigen. An antigen that reacts with antibodies stimulated by unrelated species.

Heterotroph. A microorganism that is unable to use the carbon dioxide as its sole source of carbon and requires one or more organic compounds.

Humoral immunity. Immunity arising from the formation of specific antibodies that circulate in the blood steam in response to the introduction of an antigen.

Hyalurinadase. An enzyme that catalyses the breakdown of hyaluronic acid. Also called spreading factor.

Hypersensitivity. Extreme sensitivity to foreign antigens, e.g., allergens.

Hypha. One filament or thread of a mycelium.

Icosahedron. A solid formed of 20 triangular faces and 12 corners, the geometrical shape of many virions.

I D U. An antiviral agent, 5-iodo-2-deoxyuridine.

Immune serum. Blood serum that contains one or more specific antibodies.

Immunity. A natural or acquired resistance to a specific disease.

Immunisation. Any process that develops resistance (immunity) to a specific disease.

Immunoelectrophoresis. A technique which employs a combination of immunodiffusion and electrophoresis to identify various antigens.

Immunogenicity. The capacity to stimulate the formation of specific antibodies.

Immunoglobulin. Any of the serum proteins such as gamma globulin that possess the antibody activity.

Imperfect fungi. Fungi that do not have a sexual cycle.

IMV_1C. A group of tests used to differentiate *Escherichia coli* from Enterobacter aerogenes.

Inactivate. To destroy the activity of a substance, e.g., to heat blood serum to 60°C for 30 min. to destroy complement.

Inclusion bodies. Discrete assemblies of virions and/or viral components that develop within virus-infected cells.

Incubation. In microbiology, the subjecting of cultures of microorganisms to conditions (especially temperatures) favourable to their growth.

Incubation period. The time between the exposure to an infection and the appearance of symptoms or the time period during which microorganisms inoculated into a medium are allowed to grow.

Indicator. A substance that changes colour as conditions change, e.g., pH indicators reflect changes in acidity or alkalinity.

Infection. A pathological condition due to the growth of microorganisms in a host.

Infectious. Capable of producing disease in a susceptible host.

Inflammation. A tissue reaction resulting from irritation by a foreign material and causing a migration of leucocytes and an increased flow of blood to the area producing swelling, reddening, heat, pain and tenderness.

Inhibition. In Microbiology, the prevention of the growth or multiplication of microorganisms.

Inoculation. The artificial introduction of microorganisms or other substances into the body or into a culture medium.

Inoculum. The substance containing microorganisms or other substances that are introduced into the body or into a culture medium.

In situ. In the original or natural location.

Interferon. An antiviral substance produced by animal tissue.

In vitro. Literally, 'in glass', pertaining to experiments carried out in test tubes.

In vivo. Within the living organisms. Pertaining to the laboratory testing of agents within living organisms.

Isoantibody. An antibody found only in some members of a species that acts upon cells or cell components of other members of the same species.

Isoantigen. A tissue-specific antigen present in one individual of a species but not in another. Also called allo-antigen.

Kahn test. A flocculation test for the diagnosis of syphilis.

Lag phase. A period of slow orderly growth when a medium is first inoculated with a culture.

Laminar airflow. The flow of air currents in which streams do not intermingle, the air moves along parallel flow lines.

Liquefaction. The transformation of a gel into a liquid.

Litmus. An indicator for pH and oxidation or reduction.

Lophotrichous. Having a polar tuft of flagella.

Lypholisation. The preservation of biological specimens by rapid freezing and rapid dehydration in high vacuum.

Lysin. An enzyme, antibody or other substance capable of disrupting or disintegrating cells (lysis).

Lysogenic bacteria. Bacteria that carry prophages.

Lysogeny. The state of a bacterium that is carrying a bacteriophage (often as a prophage) to which it is not itself susceptible.

Medium, pl. media. A substance used to provide nutrients for the growth and multiplication of microorganisms.

Mesophile. A bacterium growing best at the moderate temperature range 25 to 40°C.

Mesosomes. Membrane invaginations in the form of convoluted tubules and vesicles.

Metachromatic granules. See granules, metachromatic.

Microserophile. An organism that requires low levels of oxygen for growth but cannot tolerate the level of 21 per cent oxygen present in an air atmosphere.

Microbe. Any microscopic organism; a microorganism.

Microbiology. The study of organism of microscopic size (microogranisms) including their culture, economic importance, pathogenicity etc.

Microorganism. Any organism of microscopic dimensions.

Mould. A fungus characterised by a filamentous structure.

Monoclonal antibody. A specific antibody produced by hybridoma cells.

Mordant. A substance that fixes dyes.

Morphology. The branch of biological science that deals with the study of the structure and form of living microorganism.

Mycology. The study of fungi.

Mycoplasma. A member of a group of bacteria lacking cell wall.

Mycosis. A disease caused by fungi.

Mycotoxin. Any toxic substance produced by fungi.

Naked virion. A non-enveloped virus.

Nanometer. A unit of length equal to one billionth of a meter, or 10^{-9} m; 1 millimicrometer. Abbreviation; nm.

Negri bodies. Minute pathological structures (inclusion bodies) found in certain brain cells (hippocampus) of animals infected with rabies virus.

Nematode. Round worm.

Nomenclature. Any system of scientific names such as those employed in biological classification.

Nosocomial disease. Disease acquired in hospital.

O antigen. Polysaccharide antigen found in the body of bacterial cell. Also called as somatic antigen.

Ocular micrometer. Eyepiece of a microscope with a scale in divisions.

Oxidase. An enzyme that brings about oxidation.

Pandemic. A world-wide epidemic.

Passive immunity. Immunity produced by injecting serum containing antibodies.

Pasteurisation. The process of heating a liquid food or milk to a controlled temperature to destroy harmful or pathogenic microorganism.

Per os. Through the mouth.

pH. A symbol for the degree of acidity or alkalinity of a solution.

Phagocyte. A cell capable of digesting microorganisms or foreign particles.

Pilus pl. pili. Any filamentous appendage other than flagella on certain Gram-negative bacteria. Also called fimbria.

Pinocytosis. The uptake of fluid and soluble nutrients through small invaginations in the cell membrane that form intracellular vesicles.

Precipitin. An antibody causing precipitation of soluble antigen.

Psychrophile. A cold-loving microorganism growing at 6°C.

Ptomaine. Substances that are produced during the putrefaction of animal or plant protein and cause food poisoning.

Pure culture. A culture containing only one species of organism.

Pus. The fluid product of inflammation containing serum, protein, bacteria, dead cells and leucocytes.

Putreaction. The decomposition of proteins by microorganisms producing disagreeable odour.

Reagin. Antibodies against cardiolipin.

Reticulo endothelial system. A system of cells in various organs and tissues (spleen, liver, bone marrow) that are important in resistance and immunity.

Rickettsiae. Obligate parasitic bacteria of arthropods, many are pathogenic to human and other animals.

RPR test. Rapid plasma reagin test, a macroscopic precipitation screening test for detection of Wassermann antibodies in the serum of syphilitic patients.

Salmonellosis. An infection by Salmonella species that affects the gastrointestinal tract.

Shick test. A skin test used to determine the susceptibility of a person to diphtheria.

Schuitz-Charlton reaction. A skin test used to diagnose scarlet fever.

Sepsis. Poisoning by the products of putrefaction, a severe toxic state resulting from an infection with pyogenic microorganisms.

Septicaemia. A systemic disease caused by the invasion and multiplication of pathogenic microorganisms in the blood-stream.

Serology. Study of reaction between antigen and antibody in the laboratory.

Serotype. A subdivision of species based on its antigenic composition. Also called serovar.

Smear. A thin layer of material, e.g., a bacterial culture spread on a glass slide for microscopic examination. Also called film.

Species. The basic taxonomic group.

Spiriltum. A rigid helical bacterium.

Spirochaete. A helical bacterium which is flexible and has periplasmic flagellum.

Staphylococci. Spherical cocci occurring in grape like clusters.

Sterile. Free of living organisms.

Sterilisation. The process of making sterile; the killing of all forms of life.

Stock culture. Known species of microorganism maintained in the laboratory.

Stain. All descendants of a pure culture.

Streaked-plate method. A procedure for separating cells on a sterile agar surface so that individual cells will grow into distinct, separate colonies.

Streptobacilli. Rod-shaped bacteria in chain.

Streptococci. Spherical bacteria in chain.

Streptokinase. See fibrinolysin.

Subclinical. Pertaining to infection so minor that there are no detectable clinical signs or symptoms of the infection.

Subcutaneous. Beneath the skin.

Subtrate. The substance acted upon by an enzyme.

Suppuration. Formation of pus.

Susceptibility. A state of being exposed to infection.

Symbiosis. The living together of two or more organisms; microbial association.

Synergism. The ability of two or more organisms to bring about changes.

Syphilis. A venereal disease caused by *Treponema pallidum.*

Terminal disinfection. The disinfection of a room or building after it has been vacated by a patient who had a contagious disease.

Terminal infection. An infection with pathogenic microorganisms that terminate into the death of the host.

Tetanus. A disease caused by *Clostridium tetani.*

Thermolabile. Destroyed by heat at temperature below 100°C. Opposite thermostable.

Tinea. Ringworm which is caused by fungi.

Tissue. A collection of cells causing a structure.

Toxemia. The presence of toxins in the blood.

Toxigenicity. The ability to produce the toxin.

Toxin. A poisonous substance such as bacterial toxin elaborated by a bacterium.

Toxin-antitoxin. A mixture of toxin and antitoxin containing slightly more toxin than antitoxin.This was formerly used to produce active immunity.

Toxoid. A toxin that has been treated to destroy the toxic properties without affecting its antigenic properties.

Tyndallisation. A process of fractional sterilisation with flowing steam.

Urease. An enzyme that catalyses the hydrolysis of urea.

Vaccination. Inoculation with a biological preparation (in vaccine) to produce immunity.

Vaccine. A preparation of killed or attenuated microorganisms or their components that is used to induce active immunity against the disease.

VDRL test. Venereal Disease Research Laboratory test used to screen reagin antibodies in serum of syphilitic patients.

Vector. An agent (insect) which transforms a pathogen from one organism to another.

Venereal. Sexually transmitted.

Viable. Capable of living, growing and developing alive.

Vibriso. A curved or comma shaped bacterium.

Vincent angina. Ulcerative condition of gums caused by a spirochaete with a fusiform bacillus.

Viremia. The presence of virus in the blood.

Virion. Complete mature virus particle.

Viropexis. Phagocytosis of whole virion by phagocytic cells.

Virucide. An agent that kills the viruses.

Virulence. The degree of pathogenicity exhibited by a microorganism.

Virus. An obligate intracellular parasitic entity that is smaller than bacteria which can be seen only under electron microscope.

Voges-Proskauer test. A test for the presence of acetylmethyl carbinol to assist in distinguishing between species of coliform groups.

Volutin. See granule, metachromatic.

Wassermann antibodies. Antibodies against cardiolipin. Also called reagins.

Wassermann test. A complement fixation test for syphilis.

Weil-Felix test. An agglutination test for typhus using *Proteus sp.* as antigen.

White corpuscles. A leucocyte of the blood.

Widal test. An agglutination test for typhoid.

Yeast. A kind of fungus that is unicellular and lacks typical mycelium.

Yolk sac. The membrane of covering the yolk of an egg.

Zoonosis. An animal disease transmitted to human being.

PARASITOLOGY

Abscess. Latin : Abscedere to go away, to separate circumscribed collection of pus in tissue.

Accole'. French : *accolter* to embrace. Referring to the form of *Plasmodium falciparum* which adheres to the surface of red cells as a thin strip of cytoplasm.

Acetabulum. Latin : *acetabulum* a little cup to hold vinegar. The sucking cup of flukes.

Aedes. Greek : *aedes* = odious, annoying. A genus of mosquitoes.

Alae. Latin : *ala* = wing. Referring to the hyaline wings at the anterior end of Enterobius.

Amoeba (Ameba). Greek : *amoibe* = change. A genus of protozoa which changes shape by extending pseudopodia.

Ankylostoma. Greek : *agkylos* = curved, bent; *stoma* = mouth. Refererring to the head which is bent backward. A genus of hookworms.

Anopheles. Greek : *an* without, *opheles* help. The harmful one. A genus of mosquitoes.

Antenna. Latin : *antenna* sail yard. The feeder of insects.

Arthropoda. Greek : *arthron* = joint, *poda* pleural of *pous* foot. The phylum of animals having jointed limbs.

Ascaris lumbricoides. Greek : *askaris* intestinal worm; Latin : *lumbricus* = earthworm, Greek. *eidos* = form. The large intestinal round worm.

Axonema. Greek : *axon* = axis, *ne* = thread. The intracellular portion of the flagellum in flagellates.

Axostyle. Greek : *axon* = axis, *styles* = pillar. The axial supporting structure in flagellates.

Babesia. In honour of Victor Babes, Rumanian bacteriologist, 1854 - 1926. A genus of the Haemosporidia, which contains the species causing Texas cattle fever.

Balantidium. Greek : *balantidion* = little bag. A genus of ciliata.

Bilharziasis. After Theodor Bilharz, helminthologist, 1825-62. Infection with *Schistosoma hematobium.*

Binary. Latin : *Bini* = two, at a time. Referring to the equal parts into which protozoa divide.

Bursa. Latin : *bursa* = purse, sac. A posterior expansion of the cuticle of some nematodes which serves as a clasper.

Calabar. A district, river, and town in Southern Nigeria.

Casoni's test. After Tommaso Casoni, Italian physician. Skin test for hydatid disease.

Cerceria. Greek : *Kerkos* = tail. The tailed larval stage of flukes.

Ceateda. Greek : *Kestos* = girdle, *eidos* form resembling Tapeworm.

Chagas' disease. After Carlos Chagas, Institute Owsaldo Cruz, Rio de Janeiro, 1879-1934. Infection with *Trypanosoma cruzi.*

Charcot - Leyden crystals. After Jean Martin Charcot, French neurologist, 1825-93, and Ernst Victor Von Leyden, german physician, 1832-1910. Colourless, pointed crystals found in sputum in bronchial asthma and in faeces in amoebic dysentery and other ulcerative disease of the colon.

Chromatin. Greek : *Chroma* = colour. The deeply staining protoplasmic material within the nucleus of the cell.

Chromatoidal. Greek : *Chroma* = colour, eidos form. Resembling chromatin in affinity for stains.

Chrysops. Greek : *Chrysos* = gold, *ops* face. A genus of biting flies.

Ciliata. Latin : *Cilium* = eyelash. A class of protozoa.

Cirrus. Latin : *Cirrus* = Curl. Slender, flexible appendage, the male copulatory organ of flatworms.

Clonorchis sinensis. Greek : *Klon* = branch, *orchis* testicle; pertaining to Sinae, i.e., Latin name for oriental people or Chinese. The Chinese liver fluke.

Coccidiosis. Greek : diminutive of *kokkos* = berry, Infection with Coccidia, e.g., *Isospora hominis.*

Commensal. Latin : *Cum* = together, *mensa* = table. Companion at the table. An organism living in or on another, partaking of its food but not harming it.

Copopodas. Greek : *Kopa* = our, *pous* = foot, *poda* = feet. Small Crustacea.

Coracidium. Greek : diminutive of *Korex* = hooklet (originally crew) Larval stage of *Diphyllobothrium latum.*

Cosmopolitan. Greek : *Kosmos* = world, *polites* = citizen. At home in any country.

Crithidisa. Greek : diminutive of *Krithai* = barley. A stage in the life cycle of *Trypanosoma.*

Crustacea. Latin : *Crusta* = crust, the hard surface or shell of a body. Class of Arthropoda including lobster, crab, shrimp.

Cryptozoite. Greek : *Kryptos* = hidden, *zoion* = animal. A stage in the life cycle of plasmodium.

Culex. Latin. *Culex* = gnat. A genus of mosquitoes.

C. fatigans. Latin : *fatigare* = to hunt down.

C. pipiens. Latin : pipira to chirp.

C. quinquefasciatus. Latin. *quinque* = five, *fasciatus* — past participle of *fasciare* = to envelop with hands (*fascia* = band).

Culicoides. Latin : *Culex* gnat, Greek : *eidos* = form. Resembling Culex. The punkies or biting midges.

Cyclops. Greek : *Kylops* = round-eyed. A genus of small crustacea, the intermediate host of *Diphyllobothrium latum* and *Pracunculus medinensis.*

Cyst. Greek : *Kystis* = bladder. The immotile, resistant stage of protozoa. In pathology, a sac with a distinct wall containing fluid or other material.

Cysticercoid. Greek : *Kystis* = bladder, *kerkos* = tail, *eidos* = form. Resembling a cysticercus, but with a small bladder without fluid. A stage in the life cycle of *Hymenolepis nana.*

Cysticercosis. Infection with cysticercus, the larval stage of *Taenia.*

Cysticercus. Greek : *Kystis* = bladder, *kerkos* = tail. The larval stage of *Taenia.*

C. bovis. Latin : *bos* = cattle. The larval stage of *Taenia saginata.*

C. Cellulosae : Latin diminutive of *cella* = cell. The Cysticercus of "Cell tissue". The larval stage of *Taenia solium.*

Cytoplasm. Greek : *Kytos* = hollow vessel, hence cell, *plasma* = a thin molded, hence the viscous matter of a cell. The cytoplasm of a cell other than that of the nucleus and inclusions.

Cytopyge. Greek : *Kytos* = hollow vessel, cell, *pyge* = bullock. The excretory orifice of certain protozoa.

Diaptomus. Greek : *diaptoma* from *diapiptein* = to slip away. A genus of small Crustacea, the intermediate host of *Diphyllobothrium latum.*

Diphyllobothrium latum. Greek : *dis* = double, *phyllon* = leaf, *bothrion* = groove; Latin : *latus* = broad. The broad fish tapeworm.

Diptera. Greek : *dis* = double *pteron* = wing. The order of the Arthropoda which includes the mosquitoes and flies.

Dirofilaria immitis. Latin : *dirus* = terrible, *filum* = thread; *immitis* = merciless. The filaria of the dog, the dog heart worm.

Diurnal. Latin : *dies* = day. Relating to daytime.

Donovania. In honour of C. Donovan, born 1863, pathologist in Madras (Chennai), India. Bacteria causing granuloma inguinale.

Dracunculas medinensis. Greek : diminutive of *drakon* = dragon; probably from Medine, French Sudan, or Medina, Saudi Arabia. A tissue roundworm, the Guinea worm.

Echinococcus granulosus. Greek : *echinos* = hedgehog, *Kokkos* = berry; Latin : *granulum* = a little grain, a small particle. The hydatid worm.

Ectoplasm. Greek : *ektos* = outside, external, *plasma* = a thing molded, hence the viscous matter of a cell. The outer, more compact layer of the cytoplasm.

Endemic. Greek : *en* = in, *damos* = the people. Constantly present in the people of a certain area.

Endoplasm. Greek : *endon* = within *plasma* = a thing molded, hence the viscous matter of a cell. The inner portion of the cytoplasm of a cell.

Entamoeba histolytica. Greek : *entos* = within, *amoiba* = change, *histos* = web, hence the tissue, *lyein* = to dissolve. The causative organism of amoebiasis.

Enterobius vermicularis. Greek : *enteron* intestine, *bios* = life; Latin : *vermicularis* diminutive of *vermia* worm. The seat worm or pinworm.

Entomology. Greek : *entomon* = insect, past participle of *entamein* = to cut in, because insects appear cut in, or almost divided, *logos* = word, science. The study of insects or of arthropods in general.

Espundia. Spanish : Tumour, ulcer, Mucocutaneous leishmaniasis.

Estivoautumnal malaria. Latin : *aestivus* = belonging to the summer *autumnus* = fall. Falciparum malaria.

Fasciola. Latin : Diminutive of *fascis* = bundle, referring to the appearance of the reproductive organs. A genus of hermaphroditic flukes.

Fasciolopsis buski. Latin : diminutive of *fascis* bundle, Greek : *Opsis* = appearance, after George Bush, surgeon in London, 1807-86. The giant intestinal fluke.

Faeces. Latin : plural of *faex* = yeast, i.e., residue after fermentation. Faeces are the excrement.

Filaria. Latin : *filum* = thread. The tissue roundworms.

Fuadin. Antimony compound named in honour of Ahmed Fuad, Pasha, King of Egypt from 1922-36. Used in the treatment of a number of parasitic infections.

Gamete. Greek : Gamein to marry. The mature sexual cell in the life cycle of *plasmodium*.

Gametocyte. Greek : *gamein* = to marry. *Kytos* = hollow vessel, hence cell. The sexually differentiated but immature cell in the life cycle of *Plasmodium*.

Genal. Latin : *gena* = cheek. Pertaining to the cheek, the anterior part of the side of the head of an insect.

Giardia lamblia. In honour of Professor Alfred. Giard, biologist in Paris, France, 1846-1908 and Dr. Wilhelm Dusan Lambl, Bohemian physician, 1824-95. An intestinal flagellate.

Glossina. Greek : glossa = tongue. A genus of bitting flies. *G. palpalis*. Latin : from *palapare* = to touch.

Guinea worm. Guinea, a coast region of West Africa, *Dracunculus medinensis*.

Helminths. Greek : Plural of *helminth* = worms. The parasitic worms.

Haematuria. Greek : *haima* = blood, ouron urine. Discharge of bloody urine.

Hermaphrodite. Greek : *Hermaphroditos* the son of Hermes and Aphrodite. Organism with male and female reproductive organs.

Hexacanth. Greek : *hex* = six, *pous* = foot, poda = feet.

Hyaline. Greek *hydatis* = a watery vesicle. The larva of *Echinococcus granulosus*.

Hydrocephalus. Greek : *hydor* = water, *Kephale* = head. A condition in which the amount of cerebrospinal fluid is increased.

Hymenolepis nana. Greek : *hymen* = membrane, *lepsis* = shell; Latin : *nanus* = dwarf. The dwarf tapeworm, the eggs of which have a thin membrane.

Infect. Latin : *in* = and *facere* = to put into. The establishment of a pathogenic organism (except arthropods) upon or within a host.

Infest. Latin : *infestere* = to attack, to molest. The establishment of arthropods upon or within the host.

Kala-azar. Hindi : *Kala* = black, *azar* = febrile disease. Infection with *Leishmania donovani*.

Karyosome. Greek : *Karyon* = Kernel, hence nucleus like body. The nucleolus like body within the a nucleus of protozoa.

Kinetoplast. Greek : *Kinetos* = movable, *plastos* = formed. Kinetonucleus closely associated with the blepharoplast of haemoflagellates.

Leishmania donovani. After Sir William Boog Leishman, British army surgeon, 1865 - 1926, and C. Donovan - 1863, pathologist in Madras (Chennai), India. Species of haemoflagellates causing Kala-azar.

Leptomonas. Greek : *leptos* = delegate, *monas* = unit. The flagellate stage of Leishmania.

Loa. Congo dialect : worm. A genus of filarial worm.

Macrogametocyte. Greek : *makros* = large, *gamein* to marry, *kytos* = hollow vessel, hence cell. The female sexual stage in the life cycle of Sporozoa.

Malaria. Italian : *mala* = bad, *aria* = air. Infection with *Plasmodium sp.*

Mastigophora. Greek : *mastix* = whip, flagellum, *pherein* = to bear. A class of Protozoa.

Maurer's dots. After Georg Maurer, 1860-1919, German physician in Sumatra (1888-1905). Irregular, red-staining dots or lines in erythrocytes infected with *Plasmodium falciparum.* Maurer's dots were discovered and described by Schiffner in 1889. Maurer devised an important staining technique for them in 1902.

Merozoite. Greek : *meros* = part, *zoion* = animal. A stage in the life cycle of plasmodium.

Metacercaria. Greek : *meta* = after, *kerkos* = tail. The larval stage of flukes which follows the cercaria stage.

Metazoa (Singular metazoan). Greek : *meta* = after beyond, *zoion* = animal. Animals that came after the protozoa, characterised by segmentation of the ovum.

Microgametocyte. Greek : *mikros* = small, *gamein* = to marry, *kytos* hollow vessel cell. The male sexual stage in the life cycle of sporozoa.

Miracidium. Greek : *meirakidion* = little boy. The ciliated larva which hatches from the egg of flukes.

Mosquito. Spanish : diminutive of musca fly. A member of the family culicidae, order Diptera.

Necator. Latin : *necator* = killer, slayer. A genus of hookworm..

Nemathelminthes. Greek : *nema* = thread, *helmins* = worm. The roundworms.

Nematoda. Greek : *nema* = thread, *aidos* = form. Roundworms.

NMN Medium. Devised for the culture of hemoflagellates by Novy and mcNeal in 1904 and modified by Nicolle in 1908.

Onchocarca volvulus. Greek : *Onkos* = hook, tumour, *kerkos* = tail; Latin : *volvare* to twist. A filarial worm.

Onchosphere. Greek : *Onkos* = hook, tumour, *sphaira* = sphere. A stage in the life cycle of tapeworm.

Oocyst. Greek : *Oion* = egg, *kystis* = bladder. A stage in the life cycle of sporozoa.

Ookinete. Greek : *Oion* = egg, *kinesis* = motion. A stage in the life cycle of plasmodium.

Operculum. Latin : *Operculum* = cover, lid. Referring to the lid of eggs of certain flatworms.

Paragonimus. Greek : *para* = bed side, *gonimos* = generative. A genus of flukes.

Parasite. Greek : *parasitos* = he who eats at some one else's table. An animal or plant which lives upon or within another organism.

Parasitology. Greek : *para* = bedside, *sitos* = food, *logos* = word, science. The study of parasites.

Paroxysm. Greek : *Paroxynein* = to sharpen. A sudden severe attack in a disease.

Pathogenesis. Greek : *Pathos* = disease, *genesis* = origination. The origination and development of a disease.

Pathogenic of or pertaining to pathogenesis. Causing disease.

Pathognomonic. Greek : *pathos* = disease, *gnome* = a sign. Characteristic of a disease, distinguishing it from other diseases.

Phlebotomus argentipes. Greek : *phlebs* = vein, *tommein* = to out; Latin : *argentum* = silver, *podes* = feet. A genus of blood-sucking flies, the sand flies.

Planorbis. Latin : *planus* = flat, *orbis* = circle. A genus of snails, the intermediate host of *Schistosoma mansoni.*

Plasmodium. Greek : *plasma* = a thing molded, hence the viscous matter of a cell, *eidos* = form, resemblance. A genus of sporozoa which contains the parasites causing malaria.

Plasmodium falciparum. Latin : *falx* = sickle, *pario* to bring forth.

Plasmodium vivax. Latin : *vivax* = vigorous.

Platyhelminthes. Greek : *platys* = wide, flat, *helmins* = worm. Flatworms.

Proboscis. Greek : *proboskis* = trunk (of an elephant). The tubular process of the head, especially of insects and arachnids, made up of various mouth parts.

Procarcoid. Greek : *Pro* (occurring) before, *karkos* tail, *eidos* = form. A stage in the life cycle of some tapeworms.

Proglottid. Greek : *proglottis* = the tip of the tongue. A segment of Taenia.

Protozoa (Singular protozoon). Greek : *protos* first, *zoion* = animal. The phylum of uninuclear animals.

Pseudopodia. Greek : *pseudes* = false, *poda* = plural of *pous* = foot. Footlike. A temporary protrusion of the cytoplasm of amoeboid cells serving locomotion and feeding.

Pyrogenic. Greek : *pyr* = fire, hence fever, *gennan* to produce. Producing fever.

Redia. After Francesco Redi, Italian naturalist, 1626-97. Larval stage of flukes, found in snails.

Rhabditiform. Greek : *rhabdos* = rod, *eidos* = form. A stage in the life cycle of some roundworms.

Rhizopoda. Greek : *rhiza* = root, *poda* plural of *pous* = foot. The class of protozoa which move by means of pseudopodia : the amoeba.

Rostellum. Latin : *rostellum* = the little beak. A prolongation of the scolex.

Schistosome. Greek : *Schistos* = split, *soma* = body. A genus of flukes, the blood flukes.

Schistosoma hematobium. Greek : *haima* = blood, *bios* = life.

Schistosoma mansoni. After Sir Patrick Manson, 'the father of Tropical Medicine', 1844 - 1922.

Schizogony. Greek *Schizein* = to split, *gonos* = generation. Asexual multiplication by multiple fission. The nucleus divides into several, after which the cell divides into as many as they are nuclei.

Schizont. Greek : present participle of *schiseisn* to split. The stage in the life cycle of plasmodium, which precedes the merozoite stage.

Schuffner's dots or *granules.* After William Schuffner, German pathologist, 1867 - 1949, who discovered and described Acidophilic stippling of erythrocytes parasitised by *Plasmodium vivax* or *ovale.*

Scolex. Greek : *Skolex* = worm (Plural agolices). The anterior end of a tapeworm by which it attaches to the wall of the intestine, commonly referred to as head.

Simulium. Latin : *simulare* = to stimulate. This genus includes the black flies and buffaloe.

Sparganum. Greek : *Spargana* = diaper referring to early childhood. The larval stage of the fish tapeworm, which is infective to man.

Sporocyst. Greek : *Sporos* = seed, *kytos* = cell. The oocyst of plasmodia after sporczoites have developed within it the larval stage of flukes in snails from which eventually cercariae develop.

Sporogony. Greek : *Sporos* = seed, *gonos* = generation. Sexual reproduction by the formation of spores. The life cycle of plasmodium in the mosquito.

Sporozoa. Greek : *Sporos* = seed, *zoion* = animal. The class of plasmodium that form spores in their life cycle.

Sporozoite. Greek : *Sporos* = seed, *zoion* = animal. The end product of sporogony. The stage of Plasmodium transmitted to man by the mosquito.

Stoma. Greek : *Stoma* = mouth. A minute opening.

Strobila. Greek : *Strobile* = twisted. The complete tapeworm including scolex, neck and proglottides.

Stromas. stromas = bed. The supporting framework of an organ.

Strongyloides stercoralis. Greek : *Strongylos* = round, *eidos* = form; Latin : *stercus* = dung. An intestinal roundworm, the cause of strongyloidiasis.

Symbiosis. Greek : *Symbiosis.* = living together. The mutually advantageous association between organisms of different species.

Taenia. Greek : *taina* = ribbon. A genus of tapeworm.

Taenia saginata. Latin : *Saginare* = to fatten. The beef tapeworm.

Taenia solium. Arabic *sosi* = chain. The pork tapeworm.

Tenemnus. Greek : *teinein* = to strain. The painful straining to empty the bowels or bladder, without the evacuation of faeces or urine.

Toxoplasma gondii. Greek : *toxon* = bow, *plasma* = a thing molded, hence the viscous matter of a cell; the gondii in a small North African rodent : A protozoon.

Trematode. Greek : *trema* = hole, *eidos* = form, i.e., having holes. Referring to acetabula. The flukes.

Triatoma. Latin : *tria* = three; Greek : *tomos* = sectioned. A genus of Hemiptera (true bugs).

Trichinella. Greek : diminutive of *thrix* hair. The Trichina worm.

Trichocephalus trichiurus. Greek : *thrix* = hair, *kephale* = head; *thrix* = hair, *oura* = tail. Synonyms of *Trichuris trichiura*. The whipworm.

Trophozoite. Greek : *trophe* = nutrition, *zoion* = animal. The motile stage of protozoa.

Trypanosoma. Greek : *trypanon* = auger, borer, *soma* = body. A genus of haemoflagellates.

Tsetse. South African Dutch from Bantu. *Onomatoposic* (initative in origin) 'fly'. Species of genus Glossina.

Vacuole. Latin : *Vacuus* = empty. Cavity in the cytoplasm.

Wuchereria bancrofti. After Otto Wucherer 1820-73, who described the microfilaria, in 1866, in Bahia, Brazil; after J. Bancroft, English physician, 1836-94, who discovered the adult worm of this species, in 1876, in Australia. A species of the filarial worm.

Xenodiagnosis. Greek : *Xenos* = foreign, *diagnoskein* = to learn thoroughly. Diagnosis by finding the causative organism in an arthropod infected from the patient.

Xenopsylla cheopis. Greek : *Xenos* = foreign, guest, *psylla* = flea; *cheopis* = king of Egypt, 2900-2877 B.C. The tropical rat flea.

Zoonosis. Greek : *Zoon* = animal, *nosos* = disease. Disease of animals transmitted to man.

Zygote. Greek : *Zygon* = yoke. A stage in the sexual life cycle of sporozoa. The cell resulting from the union of microgamete and macrogamete.

NOTES

INDEX

A

B

C

F

G

H

I

O

P

Q

R

S

T

U

V

W

X

Y

Z